AF767987

# Cannulated Screw Fixation

## Principles and Operative Techniques

**Springer**
*New York*
*Berlin*
*Heidelberg*
*Barcelona*
*Budapest*
*Hong Kong*
*London*
*Milan*
*Paris*
*Santa Clara*
*Singapore*
*Tokyo*

Stanley E. Asnis, M.D. Richard F. Kyle, M.D.
Editors

# Cannulated Screw Fixation
## Principles and Operative Techniques

*With 190 Illustrations*

Springer

Stanley E. Asnis, M.D.
Department of Orthopaedics
Cornell University Medical College
Hospital for Special Surgery
New York, NY 10021; *and*
North Shore University Hospital
Manhasset, NY 11030, USA

Richard F. Kyle, M.D.
Department of Orthopaedic Surgery
University of Minnesota
Chairman
Department of Orthopaedic Surgery
Hennepin County Medical Center
Minneapolis, MN 55404, USA

Library of Congress Cataloging-in-Publication Data

Cannulated screw fixation: principles and operative techniques /
(edited by) Stanley E. Asnis, Richard F. Kyle.
p. cm.
Includes bibliographical references and index.
ISBN-13:978-1-4612-7503-9 e-ISBN-13:978-1-4612-2326-9
DOI: 10.1007/978-1-4612-2326-9

1. Bone screws (Orthopedics) 2. Internal fixation in fractures.
I. Kyle, Richard F. II. Asnis, Stanley E.
(DNLM: 1. Bone Screws. 2. Fracture Fixation, Internal—methods.
HE 185 T3553 1996)
RD103.I5T49 1996
B17.1'B—dc20
DNLM/DLC
for Library of Congress 96-10770
CIP

Printed on acid-free paper.

© 1996 Springer-Verlag New York, Inc.
Softcover reprint of the hardcover 1st edition 1996

All rights reserved. This work may not be translated or copied in whole or in part without the written permission of the publisher (Springer-Verlag New York, Inc., 175 Fifth Avenue, New York, NY 10010, USA), except for brief excerpts in connection with reviews or scholarly analysis. Use in connection with any form of information and retrieval, electronic adaptation, computer software, or by similar or dissimilar methodology now known or hereafter developed is forbidden.
The use of general descriptive names, trade names, trademarks, etc., in this publication, even if the former are not especially identified, is not to be taken as a sign that such names, as understood by the Trade Marks and Merchandise Marks Act, may accordingly be used freely by anyone.
While the advice and information in this book are believed to be true and accurate at the date of going to press, neither the authors nor the editors nor the publisher can accept any legal responsibility for any errors or omissions that may be made. The publisher makes no warranty, express or implied, with respect to the material contained herein.

Production coordinated by Chernow Editorial Services, Inc. and managed by Karen Phillips; manufacturing supervised by Joe Quatela.
Typeset by Asco Trade Typesetting Ltd., Hong Kong.

9 8 7 6 5 4 3 2 1

ISBN-13:978-1-4612-7503-9

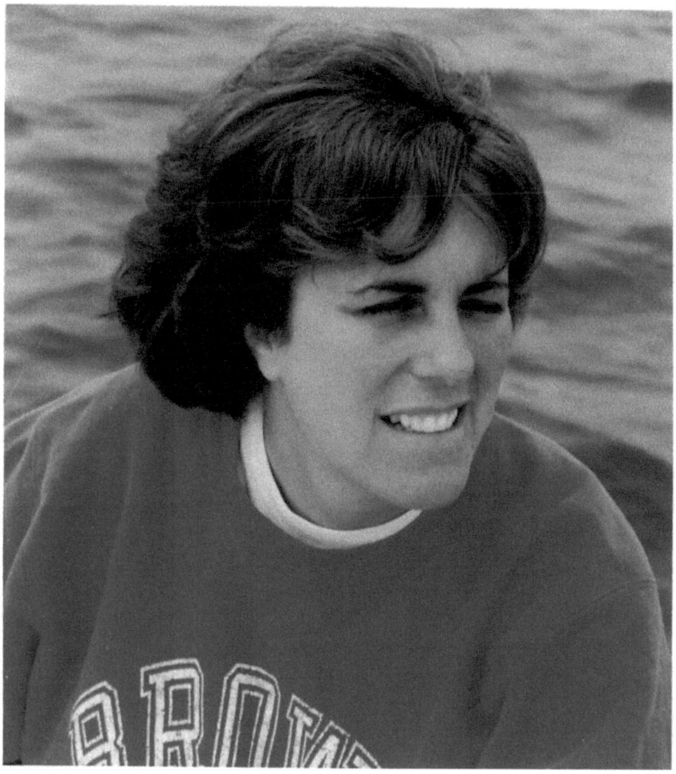

1944–1995

*To Elaine, the most talented individual whom I have ever known. A person with the amazing ability to bring out the best in anyone who was lucky enough to know her. You are the one to whom I owe everything. Elaine, you will always be my best friend, my most beautiful rose, my true companion.*

*With all my love, now and forever,*

*Stan*

# Preface

Bone screws are among the oldest means of internal fixation for fractures. Despite the continual use of these amazing machines, our understanding of the mechanical principles of the screw–bone complex in fracture care is still limited but rapidly growing. Chapters 1 and 2 reexamine the principles of screw biomechanics as well as the characteristics of the materials and techniques used to manufacture screws.

With the advent of improved radiographic techniques, image intensified fluoroscopy, and computed tomography, the surgeon can better understand the fracture that he is presented with and plan appropriately. With a cannulated screw system and intraoperative fluoroscopy, the surgeon can frequently limit his exposure and still obtain very accurate screw placement. Chapter 3 deals with the radiation to the patient and physician and methods to minimize exposure.

The remainder of this book gathers the clinical experience and techniques of experts of fixation in the different anatomical areas. The knowledge of internal fixation is rapidly growing. It is our goal to give the reader an update on the understanding of cannulated screw fixation principles as well as specific clinical techniques. The clinical chapter authors give their preferred screw systems and procedures; however, they realize that there are many variations that can be successfully employed. The orthopaedic surgeon is encouraged to apply those basic principles of cannulated screw fixation that apply to each specific case and use his initiative to best fix the fracture. This will help to improve our skills and increase our knowledge of this old but most-challenging field of medicine—fracture care.

Stanley E. Asnis, M.D.
Richard F. Kyle, M.D.

# Foreword

For the last decade, cannulated screws have crept quietly into a place of prominence and utility in contemporary orthopaedic surgery. Despite their pivotal role as an adjunct to the new minimally invasive surgery, they have not been formally recognized as have their cousins —the plate, intramedullary nail, and external fixator. Dr. Stanley E. Asnis pioneered the development of cannulated screws for the fixation of femoral neck fractures in the early 1980s and has worked steadily to expand the indications and perfect the technique for their use. The thoroughness and detail of this reveal his high level of scholarship book and focused expertise. The text begins with a group of chapters on materials, manufacturing, biomechanics, and radiation safety. The remainder of the chapters cover individual anatomic areas and pathologic entities, where cannulated screws can be employed to great advantage. Comprehensive scientific discussions and extensive technical information contained in the text are complimented by numerous excellent illustrations. Dr Asnis and an experienced group of contributors provide formal recognition for the now well-established technique of cannulated screw fixation by bringing together its many technical nuances under a single cover.

Along with the arthroscope and image intensifier, the cannulated screw has been a major facilitator of minimally invasive surgery. In the past, screw fixation of fractures usually required extensive surgical exposure of bone fragments and substantial soft tissue stripping. This resulted in increased postoperative pain and a greater risk of infection and nonunion. The success of operative arthroscopy has opened a new era of minimally invasive surgery. In comparison to open arthrotomies, the use of multiple small incisions for arthroscopy portals has led to rapid patient recovery and lower complication rates. Continued improvement in image intensification and development by manufacturers of a wide array of cannulated screws has permitted many fractures that previously required open surgery to be fixed percutaneously. Reduction of fractures can be achieved with radiographic control and provisionally fixed with the cannulated screw guide wire. Because the cannulated screw is inserted over the guide wire, the surface area of bone that must be stripped of soft tissue need only be slightly larger than the diameter of the screw.

Manufacturing steps necessary to produce the cannulated screw make them ten times more expensive than an equivalent screw without cannulation. Use of this more expensive implant is more than justified if it allows a patient to be treated with minimally invasive surgery. As cost reduction of medical care is now a national priority, it is incumbent on surgeons to avoid gratuitous expenses in implant selection. The use of cannulated screws during open reduction, which affords broad exposure of bone fragments, is not warranted. Fixation can usually be accomplished by traditional methods that employ provisional Kirschner wire fixation and standard lag screws. Read carefully, the information in this book can steer orthopaedic surgeons to the proper indications and correct use of this new technology.

Bruce D. Browner, M.D.
Gray-Gossling Professor,
Chairman
Department of Orthopaedics
University of Connecticut Health Center
*and*
Director of Orthopaedics
Hartford Hospital

# Contents

# Contributors

*Neel Anand, M.D.*
Senior Clinical Associate, Department of Orthopedic Surgery, Cornell University Medical College, Hospital for Special Surgery, New York, NY 10021, USA

*Stanley E. Asnis, M.D.*
Clinical Associate Professor, Department of Orthopaedic Surgery, Cornell University Medical College, Hospital for Special Surgery, New York, NY 10021; and North Shore University Hospital, Manhasset, NY 11030, USA

*Mathias P.G. Bostrom, M.D.*
Senior Clinical Associate, Department of Orthopedic Surgery, Cornell University Medical College, Hospital for Special Surgery, New York, NY 10021, USA

*Jens R. Chapman, M.D.*
Assistant Professor, Department of Orthopaedic Surgery, University of Washington, Harborview Medical Center, Seattle, WA 98104-2499, USA

*Charles N. Cornell, M.D.*
Associate Professor of Surgery, Cornell University Medical College, Hospital for Special Surgery, New York, NY 10021, USA

*David M. Dines, M.D.*
Clinical Assistant Professor, Department of Orthopaedic Surgery, Cornell University Medical College, Director, Division of Orthopaedic Surgery, North Shore University Hospital, Manhasset, NY 11030, and Hospital for Special Surgery, New York, NY 11021, USA

*Paul J. Duwelius, M.D.*
Assistant Professor, Division of Orthopaedics and Rehabilitation, Oregon Health Sciences University, Portland, OR 97201-3098, USA

*Jens J. Ernberg, M.S.*
Design Engineer, Department of Biomedical Engineering, Hospital for Special Surgery, New York, NY 10021, USA

*Richard M. Harrington, M.S.*
Research Engineer, Department of Orthopaedics and Biomechanics, University of Washington, Harborview Medical Center, Seattle WA 98104-2499, USA

*David L. Helfet, M.D.*
Associate Professor, Department of Orthopaedic Surgery, Cornell University Medical College, Director, Orthopaedic Trauma, Hospital for Special Surgery, New York, NY 10021, USA

*Jesse B. Jupiter, M.D.*
Associate Professor, Department of Orthopaedic Surgery, Harvard Medical School, Director, Orthopaedic Hand Service, Massachusetts General Hospital, Boston, MA 02114, USA

*Richard F. Kyle, M.D.*
Associate Professor, Department of Orthopaedic Surgery, University of Minnesota, Chairman, Department of Orthopaedic Surgery, Hennepin County Medical Center Minneapolis, MN 55404, USA

*Robert A. McGuire, Jr., M.D.*
Professor of Orthopaedic Surgery, University of Mississippi Medical Center, Jackson, MS 39216, USA

*Dana C. Mears, M.D., Ph.D.*
Clinical Associate Professor, Department of Orthopaedic Surgery, University of West Virginia, Shadyside Hospital, Pittsburgh, PA 15232, USA

*Eric C. Mirsky, M.D.*
Senior Orthopaedic Resident, Department of Orthopaedic Surgery, Mount Sinai School of Medicine, New York, NY 10021, USA

*W. Gordon Monahan, Ph.D.*
Director of Medical Physics, Department of Radiology, North Shore University Hospital, Manhasset, NY, 11030, USA

*Brian J. Padrta, M.D.*
Foot and Ankle Fellow, Tampa Orthopaedic Program, Tampa, FL 33617; and Northwest Orthopaedic and Fracture Clinic, Sacred Heart Doctors Building, Spokane, WA 99204, USA

*Alexandra Page, M.D.*
Clinical Associate, Department of Orthopaedic Surgery, Cornell University Medical College, Hospital for Special Surgery, New York, NY 10021, USA

*Robert E. Schwartz, M.D.*
Clinical Instructor, Department of Orthopaedic Surgery, Cornell University Medical College, North Shore University Hospital, Manhasset, NY 11030, USA

*Bruce A. Seideman, M.D.*
Clinical Instructor, Department of Orthopaedic Surgery, Cornell University Medical College, North Shore University Hospital, Manhasset, NY 11030, USA

*Nicholas A. Sgaglione, M.D.*
Clinical Assistant Professor, Department of Orthopaedic Surgery, Cornell University Medical College, North Shore University Hospital, Manhasset, NY 11030, USA

*David C. Templeman, M.D.*
Associate Professor, Department of Orthopaedic Surgery, University of Minnesota, Hennepin County Medical Center, Minneapolis, MN 55415, USA

*Allen F. Tencer, Ph.D.*
Research Engineer, Department of Orthopaedics and Biomechanics, Harborview Medical Center, University of Washington, Seattle, WA 98104-2499, USA

*Arthur K. Walling, M.D.*
Director, Tampa Orthopaedic Program, and Head, Section of Foot and Ankle Surgery, Florida Orthopaedic Institute, Tampa, FL 33617, USA

*Lon S. Weiner, M.D.*
Chief of Trauma, Department of Orthopaedics, Lenox Hill Hospital, New York, NY 10021, USA

# 1

# Materials and Manufacturing of Orthopaedic Bone Screws

Jens J. Ernberg and Stanley E. Asnis

## Brief History of Metallic Materials Used in Orthopaedic Applications

Reports of the use of metal implants in the reduction and fixation of human bone fractures date as far back as the late eighteenth century. Procedures were performed in a nonsterile operating environment, consequently putting the patient at an extremely high risk of postoperative infection. The implants consisted primarily of wires and pins used to assist bone fracture healing. Metallurgical techniques such as alloying (the introduction of impurities to metal substrates to enhance their properties) had not been discovered at that time. Instead, materials including iron, silver, gold, and platinum were used in their "pure" states. Unfortunately, these metals proved to be inadequate both in terms of mechanical strength and chemical stability when introduced into the highly corrosive in vivo environment.

With the rapid evolution of chemical analysis a great number of newly identified metals were soon introduced. Impurities of different concenrations and chemical configuration were discovered in ores of the same metal originating from alternate sources. Chemists and metallurgists alike began to understand that the constituents of these metal mixtures determined their chemical, physical, and mechanical characteristics.

In 1786 a number of investigators independently confirmed that steel consisted of an alloy of iron containing carbon. Due to the abundance of natural iron ore deposits, steel and iron became increasingly popular for a variety of applications. As a result, metallurgical studies performed during the better part of the nineteenth century concentrated on iron and chemically engineered iron alloys.

Early microscopic studies revealed that iron existed in a number of chemical phases depending primarily upon temperature conditions. Similarly, steel was observed to undergo a complete change in phase when hardened. During these early studies, metallurgists invested considerable time tabulating the properties of a great number of the alloys with respect to phase, microstructure, and chemical composition. In association with alloy categorization, Josiah Gibbs developed a graphical method depicting the dependency of the microstructural phase on temperature and chemical constitution.

X-ray diffraction was introduced as a method for crystal analysis by Lawrence Bragg in 1912. Subsequently, metal structures that had previously been described on a microscopic level could be studied at an atomic level. Crystal organization and grain boundary interfaces were extensively researched. Simultaneously, mathematical models that described properties such as strength, ductility, and elasticity emerged. Laboratory mechanical testing methods to validate these models were established and standardized. As a result, metallurgists were able to correlate material properties and failure mechanisms with crystal orientation and imperfections in the crystal structure.

In the period between 1920 and 1950, research in orthopaedic materials concentrated primarily on developing and manipulating alloys to conform with the stringent requirements set by the in vivo environment. Stainless steel alloys remained the material of choice for most orthopaedic applications largely due to strength considerations. Corrosion, however, was a significant concern particularly when steel was implanted with other metallic materials. Stainless steel plates were shown to disintegrate when fixed to the bone with nickel alloy screws. In the early 1900s, a number of orthopaedic surgeons experimented with a variety of materials, analyzing tissue reactions and material dissolution. Stainless steel alloys containing nickel and chrome were observed to perform favorably over other stainless steel mixtures.

Despite few research efforts toward developing new alloys, Vitallium, a cobalt based alloy, was introduced to the orthopaedic community in 1929. Vitallium demonstrated excellent mechanical strength and remained surprisingly inert when implanted into the body. Titanium, which proved to be remarkably resistant to corrosion when used in underwater installations, was also labeled as a promising contender for implantation. Titanium was first tested in vivo in 1947 and showed encouraging results. Unfortunately, pure titanium was not strong enough, and further alloying was required before it could be used successfully in high-load applications.

In recent years metallurgical research in orthopaedics has focused on the development of new materials rather than trying to modify existing metals. Unfortunately, materials research is expensive and it is difficult to economically justify the development of new materials for relatively small markets such as orthopaedic implants. Therefore, many of the materials currently used have come from developments made in other, more cash-intensive, industries. Titanium alloys, for example, were first used by the aerospace industry because of their high strength-to-weight ratio. Nevertheless, great advances have been made in orthopaedic materials research; surgeons and design engineers are presently faced with an enormous variety of implantable materials to choose from. Many materials have been manipulated chemically and mechanically to perform appropriately depending on the environment in which they are implanted and on the function that they are expected to perform. The most commonly used metal alloys in orthopaedic implants today are iron alloys (stainless steels), cobalt alloys, and titanium alloys.

## Definitions

**Alloys:** Alloys are materials composed of two or more elements, one of which is a metal. Alloys of the same metal containing different quantities and types of elements will have different physical, mechanical, and chemical properties.

**Bar stock:** The material from which a product is to be fabricated is termed stock material. To reduce the number of material removal operations that need to be performed on the part, the geometry of the stock material should as closely as possible approximate the final product shape. Stock material is generally provided in bars of simple geometry: rectangular bars, cylindrical bars, rectangular blocks, etc. Bar stock is the consolidated term for raw materials provided in bar configurations.

**Boring:** Boring can be described as internal turning. It is a machining operation that is used to produce internal cylindrical or conical surfaces. Tools used in boring are called boring bars.

**Brittle:** Materials that allow little or no plastic deformation before rupture are termed brittle.

**Broaching:** Broaching is a machining process that is comparable to sawing except the cut is performed in a single pass of the broach. The broach is the consolidated term for the tools used in broaching. Generally broaches are used in the machining of noncircular holes, slots, and other recesses of geometry that may be difficult to produce with other machining processes. The geometry of the broach is the inverse geometry of the surface that is to be machined and consists of cutting teeth that run the full length of the tool. Each row of teeth, which spans the full periphery of the tool, is set slightly higher than the row that precedes it; the amount of material removed by each row of teeth equals the difference in tooth height between two succeeding rows. The broach is translated relative to the work, or in a single stroke to produce the final surface.

**Casting:** Products that are produced by pouring a chosen material in its liquid state (usually molten metals) into a cavity are said to be cast; the process is commonly termed casting or molding. The tools used in casting are the inverse geometry of the final product and are known as casting dies. One advantage of the casting process is that a number of time-consuming and costly machining operations can be avoided. Similarly, materials that may be difficult to machine due to material hardness, for example, can be produced through casting.

**Cold working and hot working:** The mechanical strength or resistance to plastic flow of most metals can be enhanced by first deforming the metal plastically by a certain amount. If this deformation, otherwise known as working of the material, occurs at a temperature higher than the material's recrystallization temperature, the operation is known as hot working. If the deformation is performed below the recrystallization temperature, the operation is known as cold working.

**Cutting tool:** Cutting tools perform the actual material removal. The cutting tools are mounted in the machine tools that control the movement of the former with respect to the workpiece.

**Deflection rate:** Deflection rate is the speed at which deformation of a material is taking place.

**Die:** Die is the consolidated term used to describe a tool that represents the inverse geometry of the final product. In casting, for example, the cavity in which the molten metal alloy is poured is the inverse geometry of the final product and is known as a casting die. In screw thread manufacturing a die cutter is a tool that resembles a nut, where the internal threads are the inverse geometry of the threads that are to be produced. The threads in the die consist of sharp cutting edges that get progressively deeper along the length of the nut to facilitate material removal. The final threads in the die are the exact inverse geometry of the desired thread configuration.

**Drilling:** Drilling is a cutting operation used to produce round holes in a material. The tools employed in drilling are known as drills or drill bits and consist of cylindrical shafts with helical flutes spanning the length of the tool body. The flutes act as a channel for the removal of chips produced at the cutting site. The drill nose generally consists of two sharp cutting flutes that are the sites for chip removal.

**Ductile:** A material that is able to resist extensive plastic deformation or elongation without fracture is known as a ductile material (antonym: brittle).

**Elastic behavior of a material:** Materials that return to their original shape once applied external forces are removed from them are said to behave elastically.

**Elastic modulus (Young's modulus):** When loads that do not exceed the yield strength of an elastic material are applied to a structure, the strain seen in the material is directly proportional to the stress (Hooke's law). The proportionality constant is known as the elastic modulus or Young's modulus of elasticity. The slope of a curve plotting the stress in the material against material strain (in the elastic region of the material) is equivalent to the modulus of elasticity.

**Endurance:** The ability of a material to resist cyclic loading without failure is known as endurance or resistance to fatigue. The endurance limit or fatigue strength of a material may lie well below the materials yield strength.

**Fatigue:** Fatigue is the term used to describe the degradation of the mechanical properties of a material as a result of repeated loading and unloading. Fatigue limit is the load at which a material, when subjected to repetitive loading, will fail after a specified number of loading cycles (fatigue limit is usually determined in a laboratory test where the fatigue strength is the stress at which the material will resist ten million loading cycles without failure). Fatigue failure is material rupture as a result of repetitive loading.

**Feed:** The feed is the amount of material that is removed with every passage of the cutting tool over a workpiece.

**Forging:** Forging is a process whereby a metal is worked in the plastic region of the stress-strain curve for the material via locally applied compressive forces. Loading is performed by manual or power hammers, presses, or other specially designed machines. The structure is essentially deformed into the desired configuration. Generally forging applies to hot-working processes where the deformations are performed at temperatures higher than the recrystallization temperature of the material.

**Grinding:** Grinding is abrasive machining. Material removal is performed by small cutting edges on abrasive particles embedded in the surface of the tool. Another example of abrasive machining or grinding is sandpapering. Grinding is often used to machine hard materials that are difficult to cut with conventional tools.

**Hardness:** Hardness is the resistance to permanent indentation of a material when a static or dynamic load is applied to it. Material hardness is difficult to determine, and there are a number of experimental tests that try to explore material hardness. Other definitions that may appear in the literature are resistance to wear, energy absorption during impact loading, resistance to scratching, and resistance to cutting or drilling.

**Machining:** Machining is the general term used to describe material removal from a core stock to produce a final product of specified geometry and surface finish.

**Milling:** Milling is a basic machining process in which material is removed by feeding the workpiece into a rotating cutter or by having the rotating cutter advance into a stationary workpiece. The cutter generally consists of multiple cutting teeth and material can thereby be removed at high rates. Milling provides good surface finish characteristics.

**Passivation:** Passivation is the formation of carefully controlled oxides on the surfaces of metals to prevent electrochemical degradation or corrosion of the material in vivo. The oxide surfaces are generally produced by submerging the metal in an acidic solution. Passivation is routinely performed on all metal orthopaedic implants.

**Plastic deformation:** When an elastic material is loaded beyond its yield strength, plastic deformation occurs. The material retains permanent deformation upon removal of the load.

**Powder metallurgy techniques (P/M):** Powder metallurgy is a process where finely powdered materials of desired concentration are blended, pressed into the product shape under the application of considerable pressure, and finally sintered or heated. The heating temperature is generally lower than the melting point of the more important constituents of the powder blend. The mixture is heated until the surfaces of the particles bond and the desired material properties are achieved. The product is less likely to contain the defects consistent with casting or cold/hot working techniques. The composition of the powder determines the mechanical and chemical properties of the final product.

**Strain:** When external loads are applied to a structure the material is deformed. This deformation is termed strain. Strain is a measure of the change in length of an object as a result of an applied load divided by the object's original length (strain is a dimensionless number and is frequently expressed as a percentage).

**Stress:** To resist external loads applied to a structure, internal forces are produced. Stress is the force or load being transmitted divided by the cross-sectional area transmitting the load [units are pounds per square inch (English) and megapascals or newtons per square millimeter (SI)].

**Tap:** Cutting an internal thread by means of a multiple-point cutting tool is known as tapping. The tool used to produce the threaded hole is called a tap. The tap is essentially the inverse geometry of the internal thread to be machined where the threads consist of sharp cutting edges. To ease machining, the threads on the tap increase gradually in height up to the desired thread depth. The amount of material removed with every revolution of the tap is the difference in heights between two successive rows' thread cutters.

**Toughness:** Toughness is used to describe the work per unit volume that is required to fracture a material. If one performs a tensile test (tensile loading of a specimen of known geometry to establish mechanical properties of the material) and plots the load versus deformation of the material, the area under the graph up to the fracture of the material will be equivalent to the fracture toughness.

**Turning:** Turning is a machining operation used to produce external and internal cylindrical or conical surfaces. The workpiece is rotated about the central axis of the cylinder to be machined and the cutting tool is advanced into and fed longitudinally along the workpiece. A conical surface will be produced if the cutting tool is fed at an angle to the axis of rotation as the work is advanced longitudinally.

**Ultimate tensile strength:** When a structure of elastic material is subjected to tensile loads (forces that cause tension in the material), the material will behave elastically to the yield point of the material. Beyond this point plastic deformation will occur. The ultimate tensile strength of a material is the stress at which the material ultimately ruptures.

**Work-holding device:** The device that is used to hold the workpiece in the machine tool while a machining operation is being performed is known as the work-holding device. An example of a work-holding device is a vise.

**Workpiece (also known as the work):** The core material from which a part of specified geometry and surface finish is to be fabricated is termed the workpiece or the work.

**Yield strength:** In an elastic material there is a stress limit at which the material ceases to deform elastically. The stress in the material at the elastic limit is known as the yield stress (yield strength). If loads that exceed the yield strength of the material are applied to the structure, the stress will no longer be proportional to the strain.

## Metals Used in Orthopaedic Bone Screws

Orthopaedic bone screws are now most commonly manufactured in alloys of two metals: titanium and stainless steel. Of the stainless steels, 316L and 22-13-5 are the most frequently used alloys. Ti-6Al-4V is the titanium alloy of choice and is currently used in multiple orthopaedic applications. Cobalt alloys are generally tough to machine due to their hardness. Their high cost also makes it difficult to support their use economically, despite the potential benefits that the material may provide (Table 1.1).

### Stainless Steel

Stainless steels have been used in orthopaedics since they were first discovered in the 1700s. Unfortunately the early alloys demonstrated poor resistance to corrosion, and rusting of the implants was not uncommon. When alloyed with chromium, however, a corrosion-resistant oxide film develops naturally on the implant surface. The film is impervious to aggression by body fluids, thus protecting the implant from dissolution. Chromium is generally added in moderation due to high cost and its tendency to harden the material.

**TABLE 1.1.** Specifications of metals used in bone screws.

| Material | Young's modulus (GPa) | Yield strength (MPa) | Ultimate tensile strength (MPa) | Fatigue strength (MPa) 10 million cycles |
|---|---|---|---|---|
| ASTM 316L Stainless steel | 195 | 250 (hf)<br>310 (cw) | 550 (hf)<br>655 (cw) | 379–414 (cf)<br>414–448 (cw) |
| ASTM 22-13-5 Stainless steel | 193 | 827 (hf)<br>993 (cw) | 1,069 (hf)<br>1,262 (cw) | 414 (hf)<br>483 (cw) |
| Titanium alloy Ti-6Al-4V | 110 | 795 | 985 | 520 |

cf, cold forged; cw, cold worked; hf, hot forged.

Passivation is a process whereby the implant is submerged in acid for cleaning purposes following machining. This procedure enhances the formation of the protective oxide film. Passivation is performed routinely with all implanted metals.

American Standard for Testing and Materials (ASTM) F138 and F55, known as 316L stainless steel, are ductile steels commonly used in orthopaedics including bone screws. The 316 steels are generally casting alloys (produced by mixing the elements included in the alloy in their molten state followed by casting into bars) composed of approximately 18% Cr, 15% Ni, and 3% Mo; the remaining fraction consists of iron.

The ASTM 22-13-5 stainless steel is an iron alloy containing approximately 22% Cr, 13% Ni, and 5% Mo. It is stronger than 316 and is frequently used in forging where ductility combined with high ultimate tensile strength is desired. Nickel and molybdenum are the principal components that provide additional strength to this alloy. Chromium is added for corrosion-resistance purposes.

Stiffness of stainless steel remains relatively unchanged for almost all alloys. Yield strength, ultimate strength, and endurance (resistance to fatigue), on the other hand, are largely determined by chemical composition. Small changes in the concentration of one component of the alloy may lead to significant alteration in mechanical strength. Material strength can be further adjusted through mechanical manipulation of the material at room temperature (cold working), or at slightly elevated temperatures (hot working). Hence, steel alloys have a particularly wide range in strength. When compared with other alloys used in orthopaedic implants, stainless steels have moderate yield strengths, yet demonstrate high ductility even after considerable cold working. Their low cost also makes them popular.

### Titanium Alloys

Titanium alloys were introduced relatively recently to the orthopaedic community. Therefore, only a few alloys are available on the market. ASTM F136, commonly known as Ti-6Al-4V, is currently the most widely used titanium alloy. Pure titanium is fairly weak. Ductility and yield strength can be controlled over a considerable range by varying the oxygen content of the metal. Titanium is relatively inert and effectively resists the corrosive in vivo environment.

Titanium has an elastic modulus that is roughly half of that of cobalt chrome and stainless steel. It has low ductility and can fail by brittle fracture. Nevertheless, the vanadium adds strength to the titanium, and its high strength-to-weight ratio make it an attractive option for many orthopaedic applications.

## Screw Manufacturing

To fully understand the steps involved in the manufacturing of orthopaedic bone screws, a review of the fundamentals of machining is necessary. The general machining terminology and the various material removal operations that may be employed during screw production will be described.

*Machining* is the general term used to describe the removal of material from a core stock to produce a final product of specified geometry and surface finish. The orthopaedic industry is regarded as being particularly machining intensive. Essentially all metallic orthopaedic implants are subjected to some form of machining during their production life. The machining operations may involve simple low-precision cosmetic cleanup of castings or forgings, but could also include material removal operations such as drilling, turning, or milling requiring tight tolerances.

Although machining in its broadest sense has existed since early man, it was not until the dawn of the industrial era that considerable research was invested toward a better understanding of the mechanics of material removal. These efforts were rewarded with staggering progress in production efficiency, yet the process of material removal at the level of the metal chip remains poorly understood. Models used to describe the chip removal process are often simplified and are based on major assumptions. Essentially, metal cutting can be described as a localized shearing process of considerable strain (deformation) carried out at a very high deflection or strain rate. This relatively unconstrained process is unique and lacks parallels in other areas of materials engineering, making it difficult to model accurately. The process is further complicated by the number of variables that are introduced with the choice of work piece material, tool material and geometry, temperature fluctuations, and ambient operating conditions. Thus the science of chip formation and surface generation is one of high complexity that extends beyond the scope of this chapter.

The *workpiece*, popularly termed the work, is the core material from which the final product is to be machined. The workpiece is mounted on a machine tool, which is the consolidated term for machines used in cutting and material removal processes. *Work-holding devices* are used to hold the work in the machine tool during the machining operation. These work-holding devices are often custom produced to accommodate the particular part that is being manufactured, and the specific operation that is being performed. The actual machining of the material is performed by the *cutting tool*. Standard cutting tools of different geometry and material configurations are available on the market. As with the work-holding devices, tools can be custom manufactured when unusual geometry is specified. The cutting tools are mounted on the machine tool. Material removal is performed by translating the work relative to the cutting tool, moving the cutting tool with respect to the material, or a combination of the two.

The important parameters set by the machine tool operator during manufacturing include *speed, feed rate,* and *cut depth*. The speed refers to the relative velocity of the cutting tool with respect to the workpiece. The feed rate, which is the increment the tool is advanced with every pass over the material, determines, together with the cut depth, the volume of material that is removed during each tool pass. These variables are largely dependent upon the material being machined, the ambient conditions, and the machining operation being carried out. Generally the cutting speed is deduced from a standard chart that lists suggested tool speeds with respect to the cutting tool material, the work material, and the specific process being performed. Similarly, suggested feed rates and cutting depths for common operations have been charted by the large cutting tool and machine tool manufacturers.

The material properties of the workpiece are an important consideration when determining the setup parameters for the machining operation. Materials of higher strength, for example, require greater work input for material removal. These materials also cause greater tool and workpiece deflection, resulting in increased heat generation from frictional forces. The heat, in turn, can affect surface finish, machining precision, and tool life expectancy. Similarly, if the material contains abrasive or harder constituents, such as the carbides in steels, accelerated tool wear may result. Also, ductile materials that allow extensive plastic deformation before rupturing require an increased work input for material removal and generate considerable frictional heat. Ductile materials produce long chips that remain in contact with the tool for an extended time. Consequently, additional friction and temperature elevation can occur, which may be detrimental to the life expectancy of the cutting tool.

The cutting tool is one of the most important components in the machining process. With increased computer and robot control of material removal operations, requirements on tool precision and reliability have escalated. Some of the largest advances in the machining industry over the last decades have been in the development of new cutting tools. A wide variety of tools with different material properties, performance capabilities, and cost are currently available on the market. Cutting tool choice depends on a number of parameters, including the material properties of the workpiece, the characteristics of the product being machined (geometry, specified surface finish, etc.), machine tool capabilities (structural rigidity, horsepower, etc.), and the available support systems (sensors, skilled machine tool operator, etc.). The tool is frequently the limiting factor in the machining operation. Cutting speed, feed rate, and cutting depth are often determined by the material properties of the cutting tool. Rates of material removal must be maintained at a low-enough level to allow for an extended tool life expectancy. Currently, the most commonly used cutting tool materials are high-speed steels (HSS) and cemented carbides.

Cutting tools are subjected to severe operating conditions where temperatures may exceed 1000° Celsius. Therefore, some of the desirable characteristics for cutting tools include high hardness; favorable resistance to abrasion, cutting edge chipping, and wear; high toughness; high hot hardness; strength to resist bulk deformation, inertness, or low affinity with work material; adequate thermal properties; and high stiffness. There are a large variety of tool materials that meet the requirements set by the machining process. The tool materials vary considerably in composition and cost depending on the properties of the workpiece to be machined and the operation being performed. Harder materials with high wear resistance are more difficult to machine and require tougher, more expensive tools. Tool material hardness and resistance to wear can be controlled by adding different concentrations of elements to the bulk material of the tool. Molybdenum, vanadium, cobalt, tungsten, and chrome can be added to iron to improve strength and resistance to wear, for example. Fabrication of tools made from these materials is challenging and they are generally cast, wrought (hot or cold worked), or sintered using powder metallurgy techniques. The sharp cutting edges can then be perfected with multiple grinding operations. Aside from HSS, cast cobalt, carbides, ceramics, diamond, and cubic boron nitrides are commonly used materials in tooling. In some cases the cutting portion of the tool is coated locally with harder, more abrasion-resistant, and more chemically inert materials.

In addition to improving the strength and resistance to wear of the tool material, tool geometry plays an important role in machining. The shape of the tool determines the mechanical advantage that it has over the work and the ability of the tool to shear off material. The geometry of the tool is a science requiring a good understanding of material shear planes, tool forces, deflections, and chip formation, which is beyond the scope of this chapter.

An important method for extending tool life expectancy was first described by Frederick Taylor in the early 1900s. The process involves the administration of copious amounts of fluid to the material removal surfaces. The fluid is commonly termed cutting fluid and serves multiple purposes. Taylor demonstrated that cutting rates could be more than doubled, while maintaining the same tool life expectancy, when water was pumped to the cutting site. The cutting fluid acts as a coolant for both the workpiece and the cutting tool, thus contributing to maintenance of tool hardness and dimensional control. The fluid also reduces friction at the cutting surface, again preventing excessive temperature escalation. Similarly, the fluid acts as a method of transportation, to guide the metal chips away from the cutting site. A considerable amount of energy used in the cutting process is converted to heat. The majority of the heat generated is transferred to the chip. Therefore, the chip removal function performed by the cutting fluid further assists in cooling the area immediately surrounding the cutting site.

In summary, there are a number of variables that the designer and manufacturer must be aware of when developing a product. The object geometry, specified surface finish, and required tolerances will determine the appropriate sequence of machining operations that must be performed to create the product from a bar of stock material. Once the operation order has been defined, the parameters for each machining step need to be established. These parameters include tool speed, feed rate, and cutting depth, which together govern the rate of material removal. Material removal rate is, in turn, largely dependent on the properties of the cutting tool, the design and model of the machine tool, and the tolerance requirements for the cut being made. If the cut is a preliminary roughing cut, the precision level is minimal and large material removal is limited only by the quality of the tool and the material properties of the workpiece. In high-precision cuts material is removed in smaller increments, making certain tool accuracy is maintained and the surface produced is within the specified tolerances. A profuse amount of cutting fluid is usually delivered to the cutting site. This can be done either manually or by an automated pumping mechanism. The purpose of the fluid is to reduce friction, maintain temperature levels at a reasonable level for extended tool life expectancy, and transport the severed metal chips away from the cutting area.

## Machining Operations in Screw Manufacturing

There are seven commonly used methods of material cutting: shaping, turning, milling, drilling, sawing, broaching, and grinding (abrasive machining). Of these, turning, drilling, broaching, milling, and grinding are applied in the manufacturing of orthopaedic bone screws. The following sections discuss the steps involved in screw production in chronological order. The method of material removal is described briefly and different methods of performing each operation are explored.

*Bar stock* is the initial material from which the screw is manufactured. Almost all machined metals are alloys of one form or another and are cast, rolled, or drawn into rods, bars, sheets, or other geometric configurations. Manufacturers try to ensure that the stock material closely approximates the final geometry of the product, since removed material automatically goes to waste. Similarly, if the stock geometry is close to the final product shape, fewer material removal operations are required to finish the piece. Lead times, material costs, tooling costs, and costs associated with the setup of machining operations including tool changes can be reduced through a wise choice of initial stock geometry.

For screw manufacturing, the stock material is generally purchased in cylindrical rod form. The rod diameter coincides with or closely approximates the largest diametric dimension of the screw being produced. Therefore, the stock geometry generally corresponds to the screw head diameter. It is advisable to inspect stock material for quality assurance as it is brought into the shop from outside vendors.

### Turning

*Turning* is the first operation performed on the cylindrical rods. It is one of the most commonly used processes when machining external cylindrical or conical surfaces. The operation consists of rotating the workpiece, while the cutting edge of a tool is advanced into the material, perpendicular to its axis of rotation. As the tool contacts the workpiece, the process of material removal is initiated. At the same time the tool is displaced longitudinally, parallel to the axis of rotation of the piece, removing a layer of material along the length of the work. When taper geometry is turned, the tool is translated at an angle to the axis of rotation of the work. Turning is a single-point cutting operation, meaning that the material is being removed at a single site (at the tool's cutting edge). The machine tool used to perform turning operations is known as a lathe.

The cylindrical bar stock is turned to the profile geometry of the screw. The screw head is machined to the appropriate dimensions and the shank behind the thread is turned to design specification (length and diameter). The segment of the screw body that will ultimately be threaded is machined to the outer diameter of the screw threads. The turning operation also cuts the bar stock to the appropriate screw length. The resulting cylinder of varying diameter is popularly called a *blank* (a screw without threads).

### Broaching

Once the screw blank has been machined, the geometry for accepting the driving element is produced. Hexagonal or other multiple edge driving elements are generally used for the insertion of orthopaedic bone screws. These allow controlled insertion with high surgical precision.

For odd-shape geometry holes and counterbores, such as hexagonal driving element recesses, *broaches* are commonly used. Broaches are not unlike the trial rasps used to clear out the proximal geometry of the femur in noncemented total hip replacement procedures. The broach tool is the inverse geometry of the profile that is to be machined and is composed of a series of cutting teeth evenly distributed along its length. Each level of teeth is set slightly higher than the previous one and material is removed at an increment equal to the height difference between two successive rows of cutting teeth. For shallow counterbored holes such as those produced to accept driving elements, cutting teeth are unnecessary and the tool functions as a punch. The tool represents the exact geometry of the hexagonal screwdriver where the edges have been sharpened. The recess is produced by a combination of shearing and plastic deformation. The problem encountered during this process is the removal of chips generated during the cutting process. These can be compressed into the bottom of the counterbored hole and they interfere with the proper machining and shaping of the recess for the screwdriver.

A counterbore hole or drill hole of diameter approximately equal to the distance between opposite flats in the hexagonal recess is bored or drilled into the screw head prior to performing the broaching operation. (*Boring* is a turning operation used to machine internal cylindrical and conical surfaces.) The depth of the hole is the specified depth of the driving element recess. The entrance of the drill hole is chamfered to facilitate centralizing of the broach in the hole. The chamfer also helps the surgeon engage the driving element into the screw during surgery. The counterbore hole reduces the removal work that needs to be carried out by the broach and provides a void where chips generated during broaching can migrate to. The hexagonal broach cuts six vertices concentric with the circular hole, converting the hole to a hexagonal recess.

## Gun Drilling

Many orthopaedic screws used today are cannulated. The cannulation allows the surgeon to pass the screw over guide pins that predetermine the screw's path. Some companies use hollow stock to manufacture cannulated bone screws and are subsequently able to avoid the machining step involved in producing central cannulation. It is difficult, however, to appreciate hole concentricity and straightness when buying hollow stock from vendors; most companies prefer to handle this sensitive step in the machining of bone screws themselves.

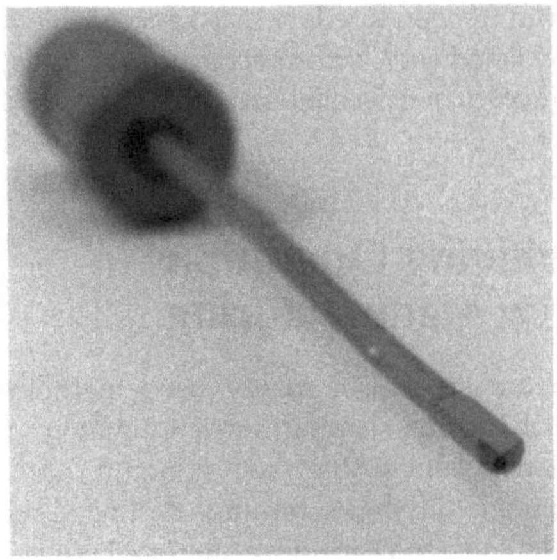

FIGURE 1.1. The gun drill is used to cut the cannulation into the screw blank. It has cutting edges and itself is cannulated to allow for cooling fluids to be transported to the cutting surface.

Cannulations are produced by a special type of drilling operation known as *gun drilling*. Most drilling operations performed in a machining setting are carried out using a long, relatively flexible tool with two cutting edges (flutes) (Figure 1.1). Cutting occurs within the workpiece and the chips generated are transported from the cutting surface though helical flutes that extend along the length of the drill bit body. Drilling is a high-friction operation generating substantial heat. This is supplemented by the hot, newly removed chips that are transported from the site at a relatively slow rate. Feeding cooling fluids to the cutting surfaces is difficult, as it must be done against the flow of chip expulsion. Drilling deep holes becomes particularly arduous as the high temperatures tend to dull the drill and reduce precision. In addition to heat generation, drift of the drill bit is not uncommon during the machining of deep holes. The result is loss of concentricity and hole straightness.

*Gun drills* or *deep hole drills* were developed especially for the creation of deep holes with a high level of precision. The drills are designed with a central channel through which cooling fluid can be administered to the cutting site. The fluid helps to maintain temperatures at a reasonable level and accelerate the exportation of the chips along the external flute on the drill bit. The drills are also produced in stiffer materials that discourage drifting of the drill and subsequent loss of concentricity. Gun drilling also produces holes of finer finish than traditional drilling. It is, however, a relatively time-consuming process.

For screws produced with a central cannulation, the cannulation is machined immediately after the broaching of the driving element recess.

## Machining of Screw Cutting Flutes in Self-Tapping Bone Screws

The next step in screw production involves orthopaedic screws designed for self-tapping. Self-tapping screws are produced with sharp *cutting flutes* at the leading end of the threaded portion of the screw. The flutes are *milled* into the thread blank. The intent of the flutes is to cut through the bone and facilitate screw insertion. *Tapping* is the process of cutting internal threads into a material. Pretapping of the bone is performed when bone screws are used to prepare the bone to accept the screw threads. This is advantageous in cortical bone, but may not be necessary in cancellous bone. Tapping may reduce the torque needed to place the threads through dense cortical bone, but in cancellous bone it may decrease the ultimate holding and compressive power of the screw. Flutes are also milled into the opposite end of the thread blank. These are called *reverse cutting flutes,* which allow the thread to cut its way out of the bone after fracture healing.

## Thread Machining

There are a number of methods that are used to produce external threads on screws. These include cutting, rolling, and casting. Rolling is by far the most common method of mass production of screw threads for machine applications. Rolling involves forming the threads by forcing the material through die wheels. The die wheels replicate the desired thread geometry. As the material is pushed through the dies, the thread geometry is created mechanically from the screw blank. One advantage of rolling is that the material is cold or hot worked during the process, thereby increasing the material's yield strength. Similarly, the probability of producing local stress risers through material undercuts or scratching is greatly reduced. Rolling does require very ductile materials, however, and the process is rarely used in the production of orthopaedic bone screws.

Casting is used very rarely in the production of threaded components. It may be an attractive solution for the production of bio-resorbable or plastic screws.

Cutting is by far the most common method of material removal in the manufacturing of threaded components in the orthopaedic industry. Thread cutting can be divided into a number of different categories and manufacturing methods may vary considerably. Threads can be cut through turning, milling, or grinding operations, or by using cutting dies.

### *Thread Turning*

There are some basic requirements when thread geometry is machined on a lathe. First, the tool must be accurately shaped and properly mounted in the machine tool, as thread cutting is a *form-cutting* operation (Figure 1.2). Form

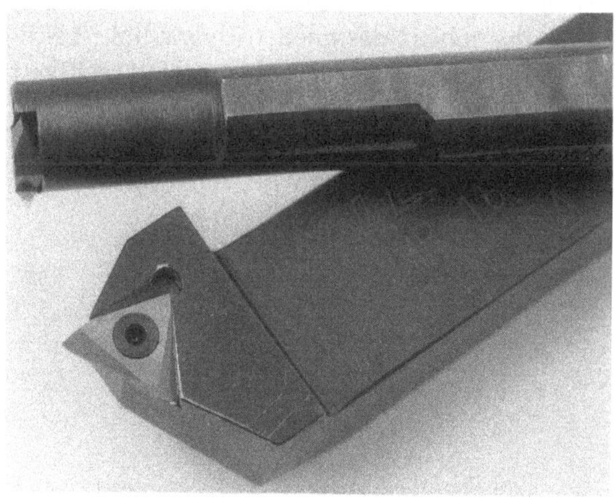

**FIGURE 1.2.** Two separate lathe tools are demonstrated. The one on top is a cutting edge mounted on a boring bar. It is used on a lathe to cut internal threads. The bottom instrument is a cutting tool used on the lathe to cut external screw threads.

cutting means that the cut produced is entirely determined by the geometry of the tool used and its position in the machine tool relative to the workpiece. Second, the tool must be able to advance longitudinally, parallel to the axis of rotation of the workpiece. The machine operator will specify the increment that the tool travels for every revolution of the workpiece. This translation determines the lead of the screw (the amount the screw will advance with every revolution). The initial step in thread turning, therefore, is to choose a tool that reproduces the geometry of the thread. The tool is then brought to the surface of the workpiece, and a first pass of the tool over the material is carried out. A scratch depicting the path of the tool is thereby etched on the surface of the workpiece; the machine tool operator is able to check whether the machine is set up correctly. Gradual increments of material can then be removed with each passage of the cutting tool until the desired geometry is achieved. The final passes are performed with very little material removal for fine surface finish with a high level of precision.

## Thread Milling

High-precision threads can be produced by *milling* operations. Milling is a material-removal operation similar to turning or drilling, except that the tool is designed with multiple cutting edges (Figure 1.3). The tool is rotated relative to the workpiece and multiple cutting teeth contact the workpiece surface. The workpiece is simultaneously translated relative to the tool. Hence, two feed rates may be specified: one feed rate specific to each cutting edge of the tool and one overall feed rate of the tool relative to the workpiece. In thread manufacturing, the milling tool consists of cutting edges mounted on an annulus concentric to the workpiece. The cutting edges are mounted at an angle to the transverse plane of the cylinder; this allows the lead to be cut. The tool is first moved in to the specified thread depth. The workpiece is then rotated through the full thread length of the screw. As with thread turning, milling is a form-cutting operation that requires the tool to be correctly mounted with respect to the workpiece. The tool geometry must also accurately replicate the thread geometry.

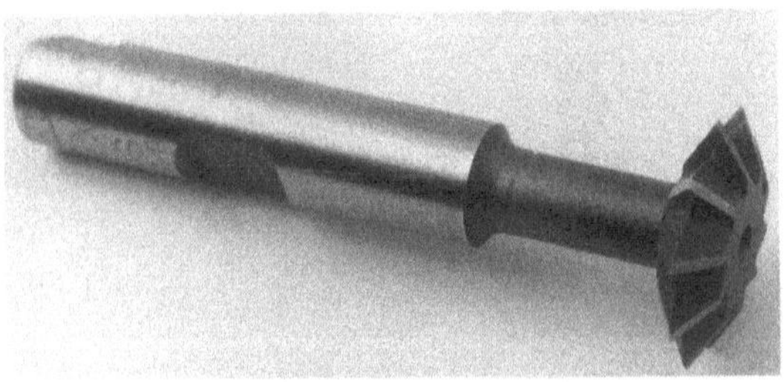

**FIGURE 1.3.** Milling is a machining process in which material is removed by feeding the workpiece into a rotating cutter or by having the rotating cutter advance into a stationary workpiece. The cutter generally consists of multiple cutting teeth and material can thereby be removed at high rates.

Thread milling can also be performed with a tool that replicates the exact geometry of one thread. The tool has several cutting edges of the same geometry. During the milling operation the tool is translated along a helical path, which equals the thread lead, about the cylindrical shaft to be machined. At the same time, the tool is rotated about its own axis.

## Thread Grinding

*Grinding* is another method of cutting screw threads. Grinding is an abrasive material-removal operation. Sharp edges of abrasive particles, such as ceramics or glass, perform the actual cutting. They are mounted on belts, propelled freely against the machined surface, or are closely packed into grinding wheels or stones. Grinding wheels are most frequently used in thread-cutting procedures. The grinding wheels accurately reproduce the thread geometry that is to be cut. Material is removed with great accuracy at small increments. Grinding makes machining of hardened materials possible, and is commonly used in orthopaedic screw thread machining. The finish achieved with abrasive techniques is particularly good. The grinding wheel rotates on an axis parallel to the axis of the screw. At the same time the screw is rotated counter to the wheel and translated longitudinally along its axis. Again, the longitudinal translation of the work for every revolution is equal to the thread lead.

### *Thread Cutting Using Dies*

Thread cutting using *dies* is a quick way of producing external threads. The dies are essentially nuts with hardened internal cutting threads. The internal threads in the die are the inverse geometry of the threads being produced (Figure 1.4). The thread cutters start small and successively increase to the final geometry of the thread. The gradual buildup in thread height facilitates the cutting process. One of the problems with die cutting is that once the threads have been cut, the removal of the die can only be done by unthreading it from the workpiece. This increases lead times and production costs. There are self-opening dies currently available that can be released from the thread once the latter has been cut. Dies, however, are rarely used in orthopaedic bone screw production.

Thread cutting is the final machining operation performed on the screw before it is subjected to final cleaning and passivation. The threads are inspected for defects, and sharp edges are deburred manually. The screw is subjected to rigorous quality control inspections at all levels in the production line.

Final electropolishing and passivation is performed on the screw to clean the material after machining. In addition to removing cutting fluid and other impurities from the material, passivation increases the material's resistance to the corrosive in vivo environment.

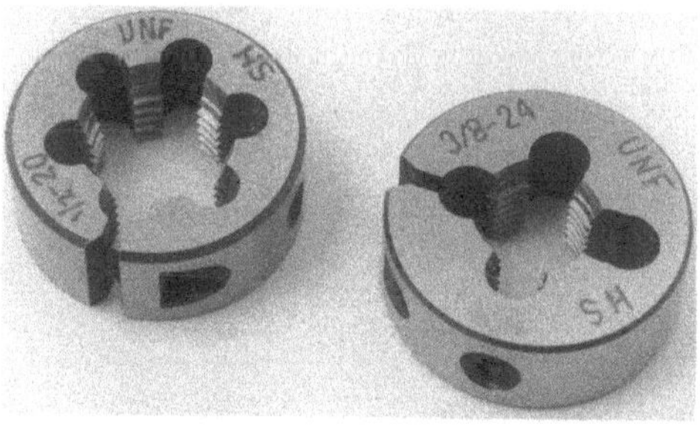


**FIGURE 1.4.** A die cutter is a tool that resembles a nut in which the internal threads are the inverse geometry of the threads that are to be produced. The threads in the die consist of sharp cutting edges that get progressively deeper along the length of the nut to facilitate material removal. The final threads in the die are the exact inverse geometry of the desired thread configuration.

## Practical Significance

The manufacturing of a bone screw is a series of very precise procedures. The material is first selected for the desired characteristics of the screw in light of the workability of the metal. Alloys of titanium or stainless steel have been used more widely. The material is then cut into bar stock of dimensions close to that of the largest dimensions of the screw. For screw manufacturing, the stock material is generally purchased in cylindrical rod form approximating the largest diametric dimension of the screw being produced. The screw is then machined from this workpiece. The alloy is then *turned* on a lathe to the profile geometry of the screw. The screw head is machined to the appropriate dimensions, and the shank behind the thread is turned to design specification (length and diameter). The segment of the screw body that will ultimately be threaded is machined to the outer diameter of the screw threads. The resulting cylinder of varying diameter is popularly called a *blank* (a screw without threads).

The recess for accepting the screwdriver is produced. Hexagonal or other multiple edge driving elements are generally used for the insertion of orthopaedic bone screws. A counterbore hole or drill hole of diameter approximately equal to the distance between opposite flats in the hexagonal recess is bored or drilled into the screw head. To produce the hexagonal recess, broaches are commonly used.

The cannulation is then added to the blank by gun drilling. Gun drilling must be exact with tight tolerances. For example, to place a 2-mm cannulation in a 100-mm 22-13-5 stainless steel screw, a slightly less than 2-mm-diameter drill must itself drill through a piece of steel 100 mm thick without deviation. The drill must have a central channel through which cooling fluid can be delivered and metallic debris can be washed away. This is a rather elaborate process that can be performed today with high-precision instrumentation.

The next step in screw production involves machining of the threads. The cutting flutes are first milled into the thread cylinder. The final bone thread can be machined by a number of processes, e.g., turning, milling, or grinding operations, or by using cutting dies. Grinding is among the most frequent techniques used for cutting threads in orthopaedic screws.

Electropolishing and passivation are performed on the screw to clean the material after machining and increase the material's resistance to the corrosion.

## Bibliography

Avallone EA, Baumeister T III. *Mark's Standard Handbook for Mechanical Engineers,* 9th ed. New York: McGraw-Hill, 1987.

Bechtol CO, Ferguson AB Jr, Laing PG. *Metals and Engineering in Bone and Joint Surgery.* Baltimore: Williams & Wilkins, 1959.

Black J. *Orthopaedic Biomaterials in Research and Practice.* New York: Churchill Livingstone, 1988.

DeGarmo PE, Black JT, Kohser RA. *Materials and Processes in Manufacturing,* 7th ed. New York: Macmillan, 1988.

Mears DC. *Materials and Orthopaedic Surgery.* Baltimore: Williams & Wilkins, 1979.

Oberg E, Jones FD, Horton HL. *Machinery's Handbook,* 22nd ed. New York: Industrial Press, 1987.

Rostoker W, Galante JO. Material for human implantation. *J. Biomechanical Engineering* 1979; 101(2):2–14.

# 2

# Biomechanics of Cannulated and Noncannulated Screws

Allen F. Tencer, Stanley E. Asnis, Richard M. Harrington, and Jens R. Chapman

The bone screw is a mechanical device that converts the torque applied during its insertion into a compressive force between the two components that it is placed through, as shown in Figure 2.1. The basic nomenclature used in discussing screws is given in Figure 2.2.[1] The root diameter is the diameter of the inner core of the screw, that is at the base of its threads. The pitch defines the distance between threads, and the lead is the linear distance that the screw advances with each complete turn. The pitch is usually equal to the lead in a classic single-helix screw. The major diameter is the dimension to the outside edges of the threads.

In the design of the geometry of a bone screw there is a trade-off between the inherent strength of the screw itself and its ability to gain purchase in bone. Essentially, for a given size of screw, deeper threads (to a point) increase purchase strength but decrease screw strength. Parameters that control the holding strength of screws in bone are the geometry of the screw, namely its outside and root diameters, thread pitch, length of purchase in bone, and thread profile,[2] as will be discussed in detail below. In addition, a most important factor is the strength of the bone into which the screw is placed. The factors that govern the strength of the screw itself are the geometry of its cross-sectional area, the material from which it is made, and the type of finish of its surface, especially around the junction between the thread and the root, which can create stress concentrations. These stress concentrations give rise to local areas of higher stress than in the rest of the body of the screw and can be the source of cracks that may cause fatigue of the screw. In the following sections we consider the specifics of both holding power and the strength of bone screws, and the particular effects of cannulation (creating a hole down the center) on strength and holding power. We then present biomechanical considerations related to cannulated screws.

## The Torsional Strength of Screws

There are at least two different mechanisms by which a screw can break, as shown in Figure 2.3. One is due to the application of excessive torque to overcome resistance of the screw to insertion, caused possibly by having too small a pilot hole, or an untapped hole in hard bone. High stresses may develop in the screw if there is significant resistance to insertion, causing the screw to shear at a cross section, and leave a part lodged in bone. This may also happen during removal if bone grows intimately to the threads of the screw.[3] A second mechanism of breakage results from bending of the screw as a cantilever, with the shaft end lodged in bone and a load applied transversely to the long axis of the screw. This may occur, for example, with a plate that loads the screw transverse to its head if it is not tightened sufficiently against the bone surface.

Failure of the screw by shearing may occur when the screw is inserted without correct sizing of the pilot hole, without tapping (in hard bone) or due to a lack of lubrication. The coefficient of friction between metal and bone is approximately 0.4.[4,5] When axial force is produced in tightening a screw, friction results from the screw threads sliding against bone. Approx-

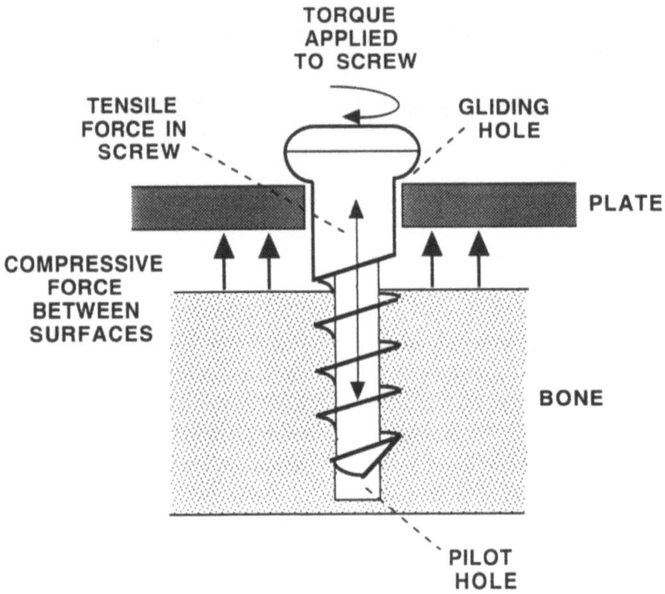


**FIGURE 2.1.** The function of a screw. The shaft passes through a gliding hole, and the thread is captured in a pilot hole, so that applying a torque to the screw draws the two components (plate and bone in this example) together. As they compress together, an opposing tensile force is produced in the screw.

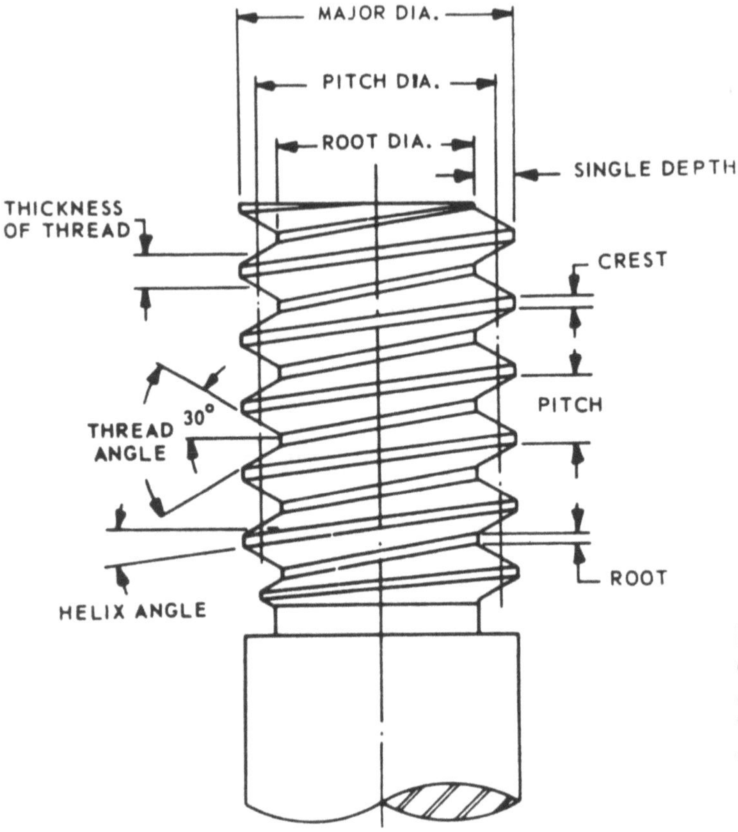


**FIGURE 2.2.** Basic nomenclature of a screw. Of particular note are the *pitch* (distance between threads), the *root diameter* (diameter at the base of the threads), and the *major diameter* (outside diameter of the screw).

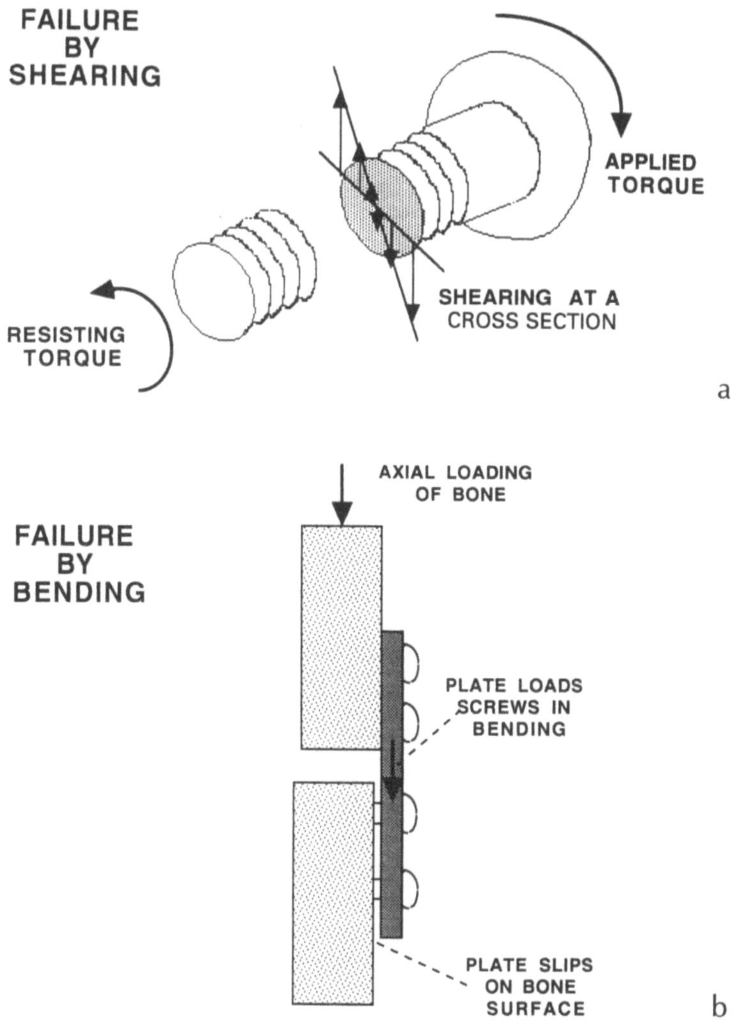


**FIGURE 2.3.** Mechanisms of failure of a screw: (a) Shear failure due to excessive torque. (b) Bending failure due to loading of the plate against the screw.

imately 42% of the torque applied is lost in overcoming friction.[4] The resistance of the screw to insertion for one of these reasons causes the surgeon to increase the torque applied, therefore increasing the shear stress in the screw. The shear stress developed in a screw, shown in Figure 2.3a, is due to twisting of one cross section against another. The stress magnitude depends directly on the torque applied and inversely on the cube of the diameter of its cross section, given by the simple formula[6]

$$\tau = 16T/(\pi d^3)$$

where

$\tau$ = shear stress

$T$ = applied torque

$d$ = root (minor) diameter of the thread

The load exerted on the screw is governed by the maximum torque that the surgeon can apply and the resistance of the screw to insertion, while the stress generated is a result of the torque applied and its root diameter. The cross section is dependent on the size and type of screw selected by the surgeon. For a given size,

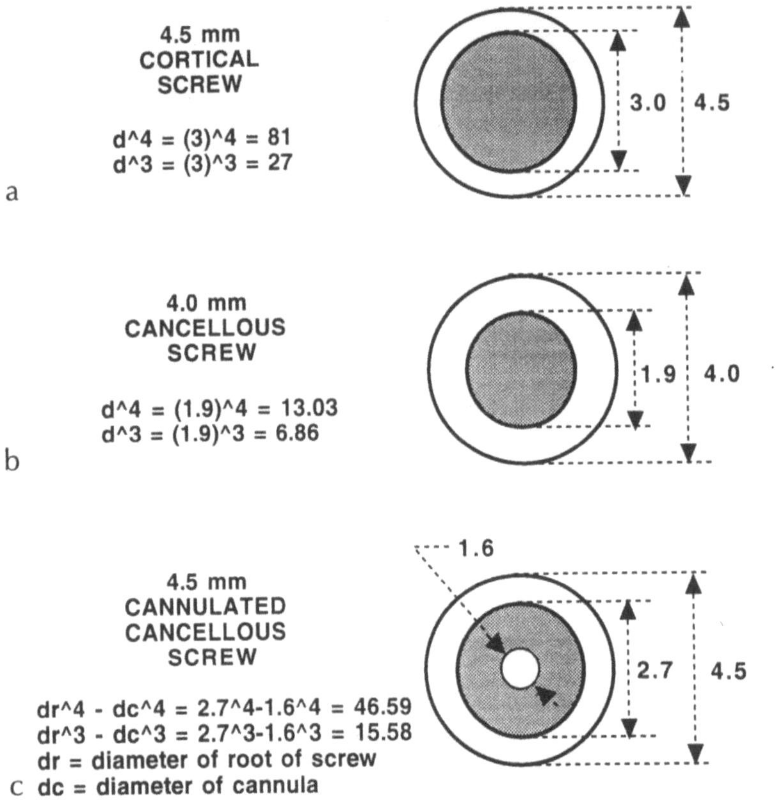


**FIGURE 2.4.** A comparison of the cross-sectional dimensions of three typical bone screws: (a) cortical screw, (b) solid cancellous screw, (c) cannulated cancellous screw. (*Note*: Screws are of similar dimensions, but this does not imply that they are similar in function.) (Data taken from catalog of Synthes Ltd., Paoli, PA.)

fine-threaded or small-pitch (cortical) screws have threads that are shallower; therefore, they have a larger root diameter than do coarse-threaded or large-pitch (cancellous) screws (Figure 2.4). A second parameter that affects the torsional strength is cannulation. A cannulated screw, due to the presence of a bore for the guide wire, has less material in the cross section of the body. Shown in Figure 2.4 are the cross-sectional dimensions of some typical cortical, cancellous, and cancellous cannulated screws of nearly equal size (from Synthes Ltd., Paoli, PA). In these examples, a solid cancellous screw of size nearly equal to a cortical screw can support about 25% of the peak shear stress that the cortical screw can sustain. In comparison, the cannulated screw, which has a larger minor diameter to compensate for the central bore, can sustain 227% of the shear stress of the solid cancellous screw and 58% of that of the cortical screw.

The relationship between the ultimate torsional strength of screws and their cross-sectional dimensions was demonstrated by Hughes and Jordan[6] (Figure 2.5) as well as by Ansell and Scales.[7] If an orthopaedic surgeon can typically apply a torque from 26 to 53 inch-pounds,[8] then it is possible, considering Figure 2.5, to shear a screw with a minor diameter as large as 0.115 inch (2.92 mm) during insertion if it jams.

An important question in determining the actual torsional strength of screws is the effect of variations in dimensions of the screw due to manufacturing tolerances. Standards govern the allowable tolerances in screw dimensions.[9] For cortical screws of 4.5-mm outer diameter, the allowable dimensional tolerance, shown in Fig-

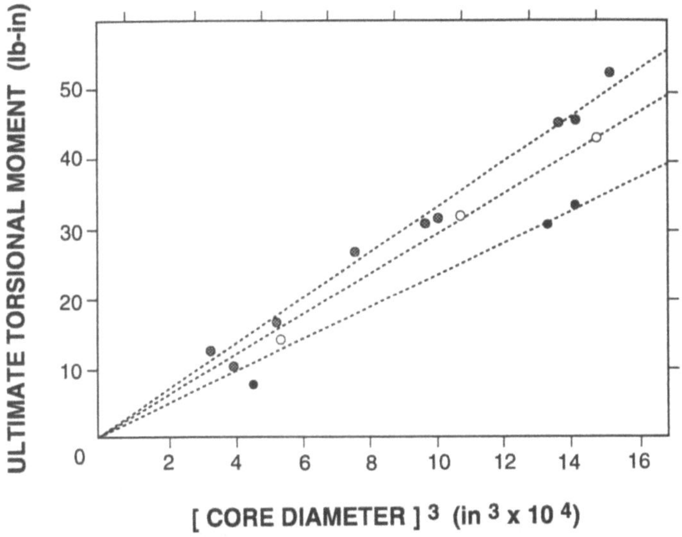


FIGURE 2.5. An experimentally derived relationship between the torsional strength of bone screws and the cube of their root diameters. (Reprinted with permission from Hughes and Jordan.[6])

ure 2.6, results in a variation of +10%, −14% in the cube of the cross-sectional area, and ultimate torsional strength. For a cannulated screw, using the same dimensional tolerances (±0.10 mm) for the root diameter and the bore of the cannula of the screw shown in Figure 2.4 results in an estimated variability in the torsional strength of ±24%. These larger variations are the result of the tolerances on both the root diameter and the cannula itself. However, the larger root diameter of a cannulated screw accommodates this larger potential variability since for equivalent sizes it is considerably stronger than a solid cancellous screw, as discussed above.

The specific potential for screw breakage by shearing depends upon the torque applied, which is governed by the factors that resist insertion of the screw. Perren et al.[4] quote the loss of torque toward screw-plate friction as 43% and toward screw thread-bone friction as 42%, leaving 15% of the applied torque for transformation into axial force. Hughes and Jordan[6] estimate that for an untapped screw in cortical bone, 35% of the applied torque goes into cutting threads, 50% is lost as friction between the undersurface of the screw and the object (i.e., bone or plate) that it seats against, and 10% is used to overcome friction between the screw threads and bone, leaving 5% as useful work (i.e., for compressing surfaces together). In contrast, with a lubricated tapped hole (in cortical bone), friction decreases to half, no work is lost in cutting threads, and the useful work due to applying torque to the screw increases to about

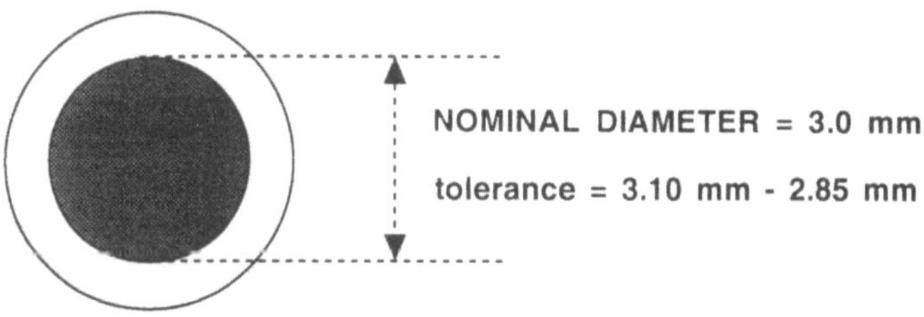


FIGURE 2.6. The variability in root diameter of a 4.5-mm cortical bone screw (per ASTM F 543) due to allowable manufacturing tolerances.

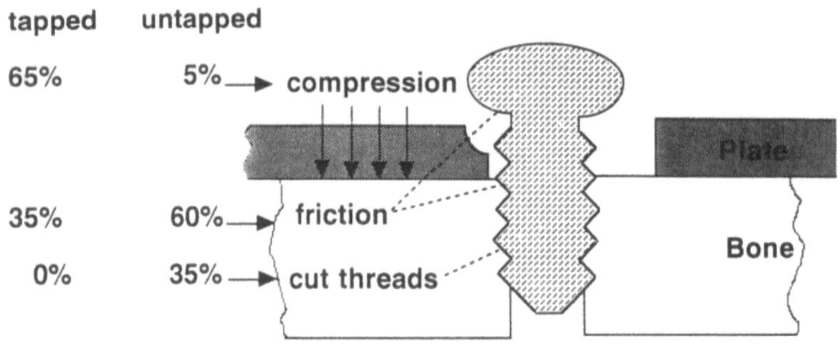


**FIGURE 2.7.** The factors causing resistance, and requiring higher insertion torque, during insertion of a screw (adapted from Perren et al.[4]).

65%, as shown in Figure 2.7. Therefore, the potential for screw failure by shearing is lessened by tapping and application of lubrication. To emphasize this last point, the torque applied to a screw in a tapped hole in cortical bone goes to overcome mainly the friction between the underside of the screw and whatever it seats against (i.e., a plate or bone) and to compressing the two components being fixed together.

In summary, one mechanism of screw failure occurs by shearing or twisting of the screw due to excessive applied torque. The stress that the screw is exposed to depends upon the resistance to insertion, typically caused by the need for self-tapping and friction between the screw threads and bone. Stress magnitude within the screw depends on the cube of the diameter of the cross section at the root of its threads. For similar sizes, a cortical screw can withstand about four times the stress of a solid cancellous screw and 1.7 times the stress of a cannulated cancellous screw; therefore, care should be taken during insertion and tightening of cannulated screws in dense cancellous bone or if they are placed through cortex. In addition, dimensional variations during manufacturing can potentially further change (increase or decrease) the failure stress of a cannulated screw by up to 25%.

## The Bending Strength of Screws

The prime function of a screw is to generate a compressive force between the two components that it is inserted into. In addition, increasing the compressive force that the screw generates relieves the bending loading on it, as shown in Figure 2.3, and significantly increases its fatigue resistance (Figure 2.8).[10] The shaft of the screw glides through the first component, as the screw thread advances into the second (Figure 2.1). The actual compressive force produced between components depends upon three factors. One is the pitch of the screw, which converts the rotational motion into a linear advance. A fine-pitched screw moves a smaller amount linearly for a given angular rotation (Figure 2.9), and therefore has a greater mechanical advantage and produces greater compression. In effect, the screw has more leverage. A second factor is the frictional resistance against the screw threads and underside of the head (Figure 2.7), which absorbs some of the work put into turning the screw. Third, if the material that the screw is placed into is relatively weak in shear (for example osteoporotic bone), the screw may strip the threads with loss of compression. The relationship between torque applied to typical bone screws (Synthes, Paoli, PA) and the compressive force generated from experimental measurements is shown in Figure 2.10.[11]

The compressive force generated between a plate and a bone surface has an important effect on the strength of the screw itself (Figure 2.8). Taking the example shown in Figure 2.3, where a plate is placed to transfer load across a fracture gap in which there is minimal bone-to-bone contact, the screws compress the plate against the bone and the frictional force generated prevents slippage of the plate. Functional load applied to the plate via bone is transmitted

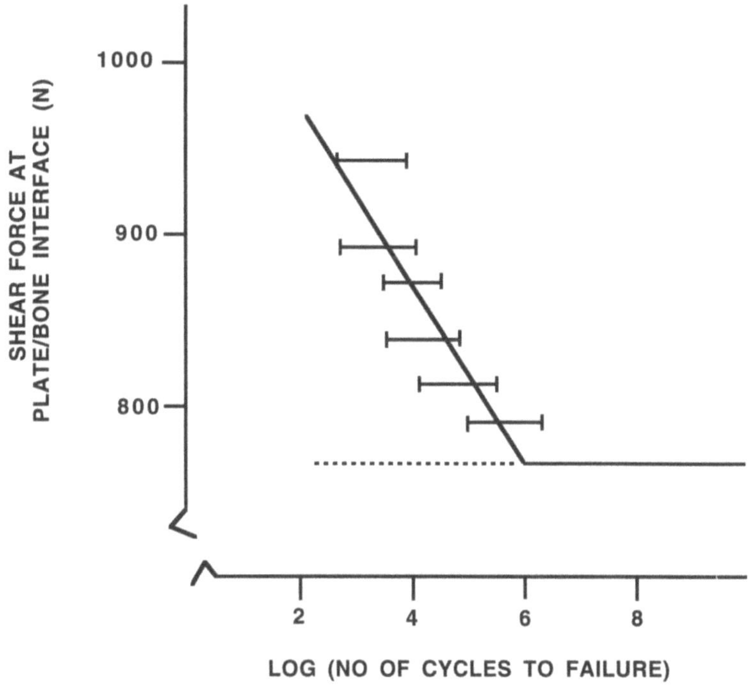


**FIGURE 2.8.** Relationship between the sheer force acting at the plate/bone interface (with the compressive force between plate and screw constant) and the number of cycles to failure of the screw by bending fatigue (adapted from Zand et al.[10]).

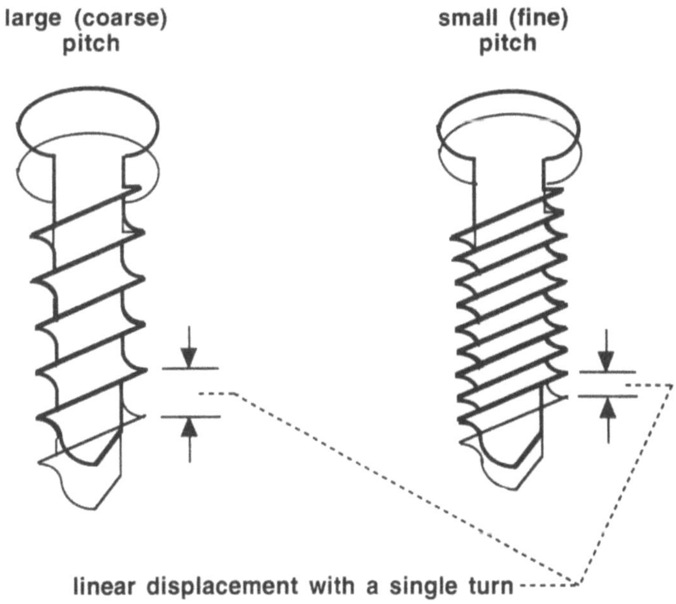


**FIGURE 2.9.** The effect of thread pitch on the linear advance of a screw for a single turn.

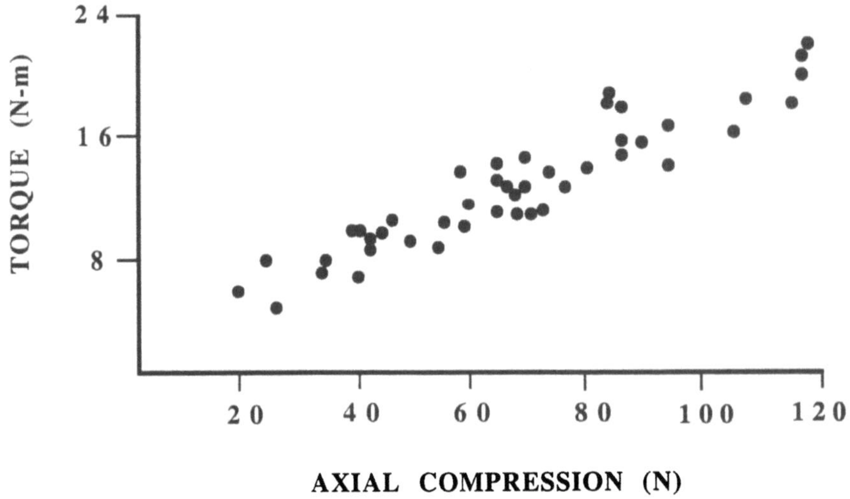


**FIGURE 2.10.** Experimentally measured relationship between the torque applied to a screw and the resulting compressive force between the two surfaces (adapted from Nunamaker and Perren[11]).

down the plate, and due to the frictional force between plate and bone, it is transmitted back into bone on the other side of the fracture gap. If the plate slips, load is applied directly to the screws in a direction transverse to their long axes, producing cantilever bending in the screws. The fatigue life of a screw is significantly reduced if it is loaded transversely by the plate (Figure 2.8).[11] The tensile stress at the surface of the root of the screw is inversely proportional to the moment of inertia of the cross section (i.e., to the diameter to the power of 4).[12] Relative to the 4.5-mm-diameter cortical screws in which theses cyclic loading tests were performed, and based only on cross-sectional dimensions (i.e., without consideration of materials) (Figure 2.4), a solid cortical screw can support 6.2 times the maximum bending stress of a solid cancellous screw of equivalent diameter and 1.7 times the stress of a cannulated cancellous screw. Estimating the actual fatigue lives of the different screws is more complicated, depending on materials and surface finish; however, it is clear that the fatigue life of a cannulated screw will be greater than that of a solid cancellous screw.

In summary, it is important to apply as much torque as possible to a screw to generate the frictional force that holds, for example, a plate against bone, and prevents slipping of the plate so that the screws become loaded in bending. Cyclic bending loading significantly decreases the fatigue life of the screw. On the other hand, if over-torqued in poor bone, the screw thread may strip (shear) and lose all purchase. Cannulated cancellous screws can support 358% of the bending stress of solid cancellous screws of similar diameter, if made of equivalent materials.

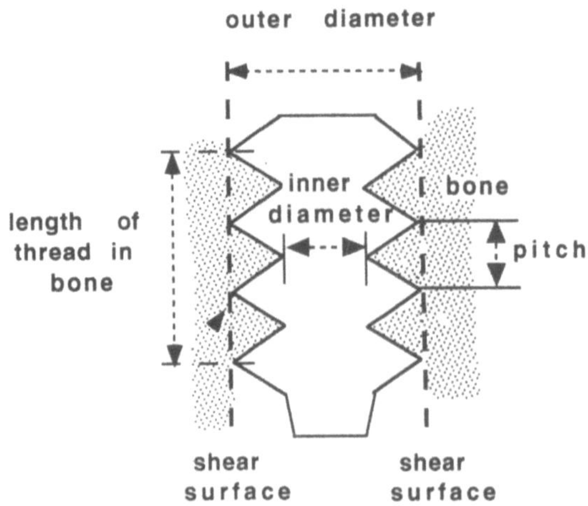


**FIGURE 2.11.** Schematic representation of the relationship between screw geometry, bone shear strength, and the pullout force of the screw in bone.

## Screw Holding Power

The resistance to pullout, or holding power of a screw in a porous material such as cancellous bone, is dependent on six factors. Three are related to the geometry of the screw: its outer diameter,[13] its length of engagement in bone including the degree to which it passes through cortex,[14] and the geometry of its threads including depth and pitch[15–17] but not tooth profile.[15,18] The other three factors relate to preparation of the hole into which it is placed: the shear strength of the bone that the threads engage,[17,19–25] pilot hole size,[4,19,26] and tapping.[17,27,28] For fixed-hole preparation techniques including pilot hole size and not tapping (in porous material) the other four factors described above can be related to holding strength, shown schematically in Figure 2.11, and given quantitatively by the following relationship, which has been shown experimentally to explain 97% of the variability in pullout strength of nontapped screws placed in porous foam (shown to be equivalent to cancellous bone but less variable) (Figure 2.12)[17]:

$$F_s = S \times A_s = S \times (L \times \pi \times D_{\text{major}}) \times TSF$$

where

$F_s$ = predicted shear failure force (N)

$S$ = material ultimate shear stress (MPa)

$A_s$ = thread shear area (mm$^2$)

$L$ = length (mm)

$D_{\text{major}}$ = major diameter (mm)

$(L \times \pi \times D_{\text{major}})$ = area of a cylinder of diameter $D_{\text{major}}$ and length $L$

$TSF$ = thread shape factor (dimensionless) $= (0.5 + 0.57735d/p)$

$d$ = thread depth (mm) $= (D_{\text{major}} - D_{\text{minor}})/2$

$D_{\text{minor}}$ = minor (root) diameter (mm)

$p$ = thread pitch (mm)

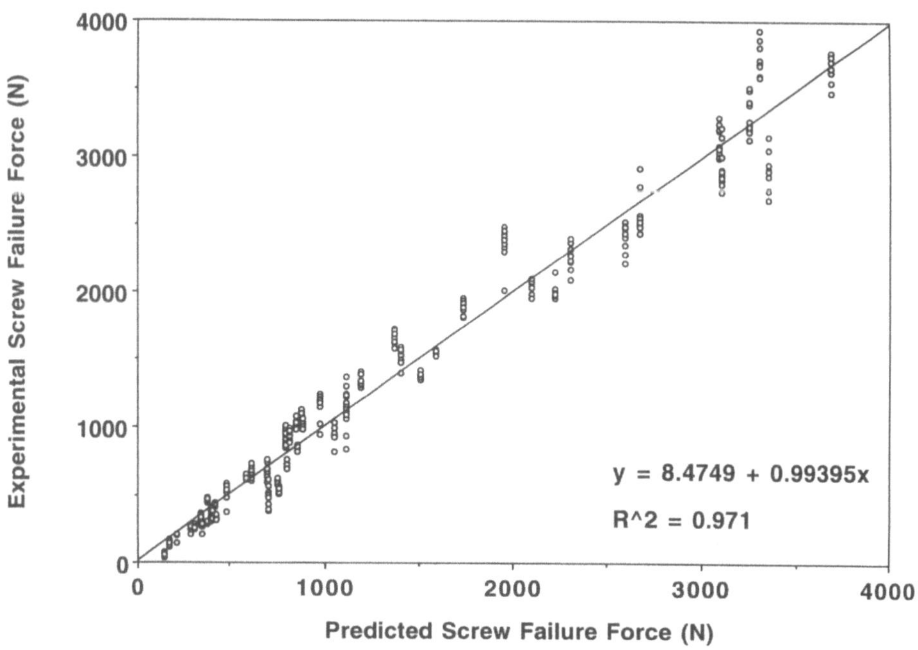


**FIGURE 2.12.** Relationship between experimentally derived pullout force and that predicted by the equation relating pullout strength to shear strength, and screw geometry (adapted from Chapman et al.[17]).

## Major Diameter and Length of Engagement

In pullout, a screw may fail in one of two ways, as illustrated in Figure 2.13. A wedge of bone may pull out with the screw, indicating failure of bone, or the screw may shear bone, carrying material between the threads as it fails.[29] The relationship given above applies to this latter mode of failure, which always happens for screws placed into cancellous bone and usually occurs in cortical bone. In simple terms, this relationship says that if pullout failure occurs along an interface between the screw and bone, the strength of the interface can be determined from its area and the maximum shear stress that it can support. Multiplying the two should give the resisting shear force, which is equal to the pullout force of the screw. The area of the interface along which the screw shears is the area of a cylinder of diameter equal to the screw major diameter and length equal to the length of thread engagement in bone. The thread shape factor (TSF) accounts for the effect of screw thread geometry and will be discussed later.

## Bone Shear Strength

The relationship between bone shear strength and screw holding power is extremely important (Figure 2.14).[23,24] The shear strength of bovine bone has been found to relate to the apparent density by the following power law relationship[30]:

$$S = 21.6\ \rho^{1.65}$$

where

$S$ = shear strength (MPa)

$\rho$ = apparent density of trabecular bone (g/cm$^3$)

a

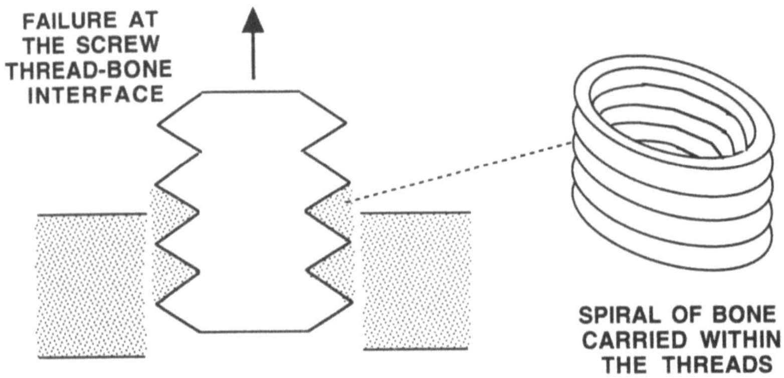


b

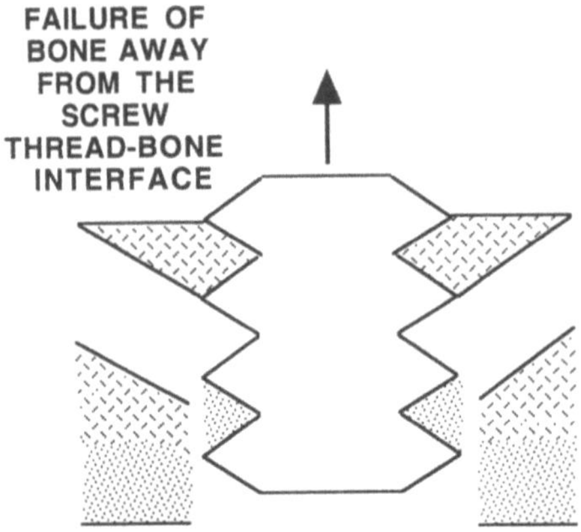


**FIGURE 2.13.** Two different mechanisms of failure in screw pullout. (a) Failure at the bone/screw thread interface with shearing of bone. A cylinder of bone is carried within the threads. (b) Failure of bone, typically in cortex.

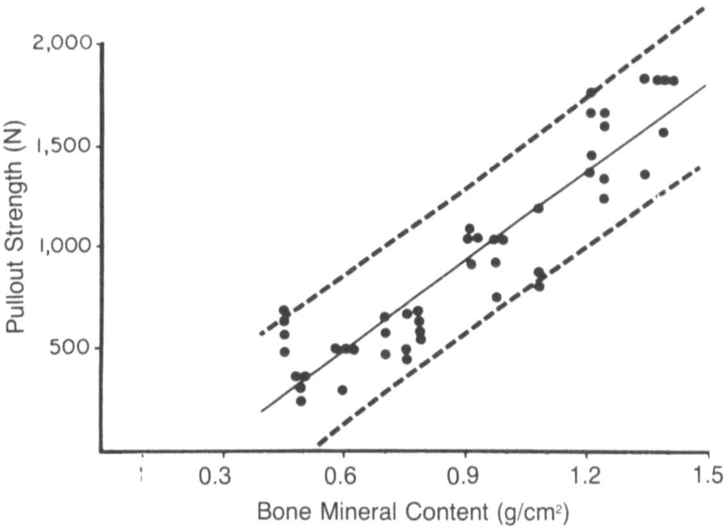


**FIGURE 2.14.** Relationship of screw pullout strength to bone density in vertebral bodies. (Reprinted with permission from Trader et al.[24])

Therefore, doubling the density of trabecular bone increases its shear strength and its screw holding power by 3.14 (i.e., $2^{1.65}$).

## Thread Shape

The thread shape factor (TSF) is defined as 0.5 plus a constant times the ratio of thread depth to pitch.[31,32] Conceptually, this means that the TSF (and screw holding strength) increases as *thread depth becomes larger* (i.e., increased difference between screw major and minor diameters) and *pitch becomes smaller*. Figure 2.15 shows that if the thread angle is kept constant, increasing thread depth also increases pitch, and decreasing pitch decreases thread depth. This demonstrates the practical limits on increasing TSF. For a given thread shape, increasing the TSF would require making the angle of the thread smaller, in effect making it thinner and weaker. For commercial cannulated and noncannulated cancellous bone screws, actual thread dimensions and corresponding TSFs are given in Table 2.1.

These concepts relating to the TSF have recently been confirmed experimentally. DeCoster et al.[16] show that the pullout strength of screws increases with a larger ratio of major to minor diameters (i.e., smaller minor diameter and larger thread depth). Similarly, using a smaller pitch increases pullout strength. Asnis et al.[33] also confirm the effects of thread pitch, maintaining constant depth, in custom-fabricated screws tested in porous foam. By decreasing the angle of the thread tooth, they were able to develop TSF values that varied from 0.74 to 1.55 in different diameter screws. When TSF values increased above 1.0, relatively little increase was found in pullout strength (Figure 2.16), which demonstrates the practical upper limit of altering screw thread geometry. The thread shape may become too long and narrow so that the material (bone or foam) within the threads now fails by bending instead of by shear.

It is interesting to note that the measured TSF for small noncannulated screws is 0.85, while that for cannulated screws ranges from 0.70 to 0.73 (Table 2.1). To allow space for the cannula, the minor diameter of these screws have been increased. If the screws have equivalent major diameters, cannulation decreases the thread depth, and thus the TSF (Figure 2.17). The holding power of currently available cannulated cancellous screws should therefore be lower than similarly designed solid cancellous screws. We have indeed found this to be the case. Figure 2.18 shows results of both experimentally derived and predicted measures of the pullout strength of 4.0-mm cancellous screws. The difference in TSF between cannulated and solid cancellous screws was 16% and the mean

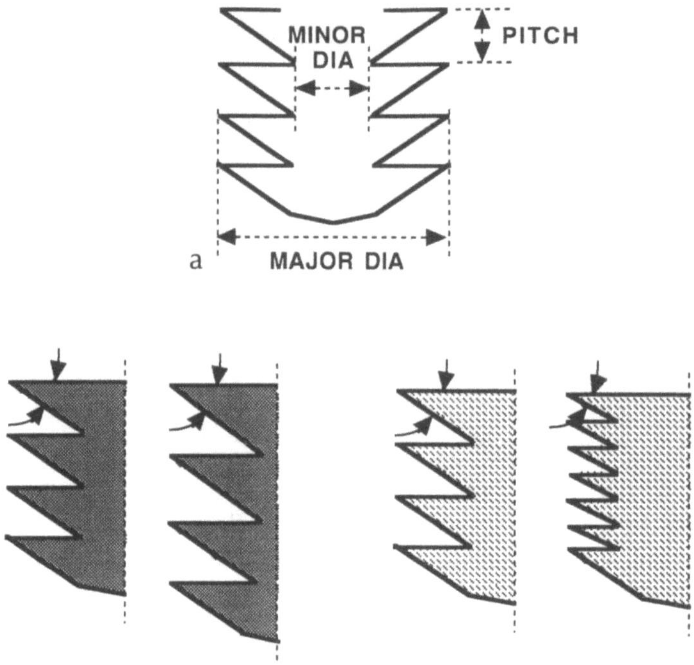


**FIGURE 2.15.** The effect of changing thread shape factor. (a) The geometric factors of the screw that can be altered. (b) If the thread angle is kept constant, increasing thread depth while maintaining the same thread angle results in increased pitch. (c) In contrast, decreasing thread pitch while maintaining the same thread angle results in decreased thread depth.

**TABLE 2.1.** Dimensions of commercial cancellous bone screws.

| Manufacturer | Item number | Thread type | Major diameter | Minor diameter | Thread depth ($d$) | Pitch ($p$) | TSF |
|---|---|---|---|---|---|---|---|
| | | | *Small* | | | | |
| Synthes | 207.40 | NonCan | 4.0 | 1.9 | 1.05 | 1.75 | *0.85* |
| Synthes | 205.40 | Cannul | 3.5 | 2.5 | 0.50 | 1.25 | *0.73* |
| Richards | 121840 | Cannul | 4.0 | 2.75 | 0.63 | 1.75 | *0.71* |
| Ace Med | 14225-40 | Cannul | 5.0 | 3.75 | 0.63 | 1.80 | *0.70* |
| | | | *Large* | | | | |
| Synthes | 216.60 | NonCan | 6.5 | 3.0 | 1.75 | 2.75 | *0.87* |
| Synthes | 208.60 | Cannul | 7.0 | 4.5 | 1.25 | 2.75 | *0.76* |
| Zimmer | 1146-60 | Cannul | 7.0 | 5.0 | 1.00 | 2.75 | *0.71* |
| Ace Med | 14088-60 | Cannul | 6.5 | 5.25 | 0.63 | 1.85 | *0.70* |
| Richards | 121632 | Cannul | 6.5 | 4.7 | 0.90 | 2.12 | *0.75* |

Thread type: Cann = cannulated; NonCan = noncannulated. All dimensions are in mm. Thread shape factor (TSF) $= 0.5 + 0.57735\ d/p$. Manufacturers: Ace Med: Ace Medical Co., Los Angeles, CA 90061; Richards: Richards Medical Co., Memphis, TN 38116; Synthes: Synthes (U.S.A.), Paoli, PA 19301; Zimmer: Zimmer, Warsaw, IN 46580.

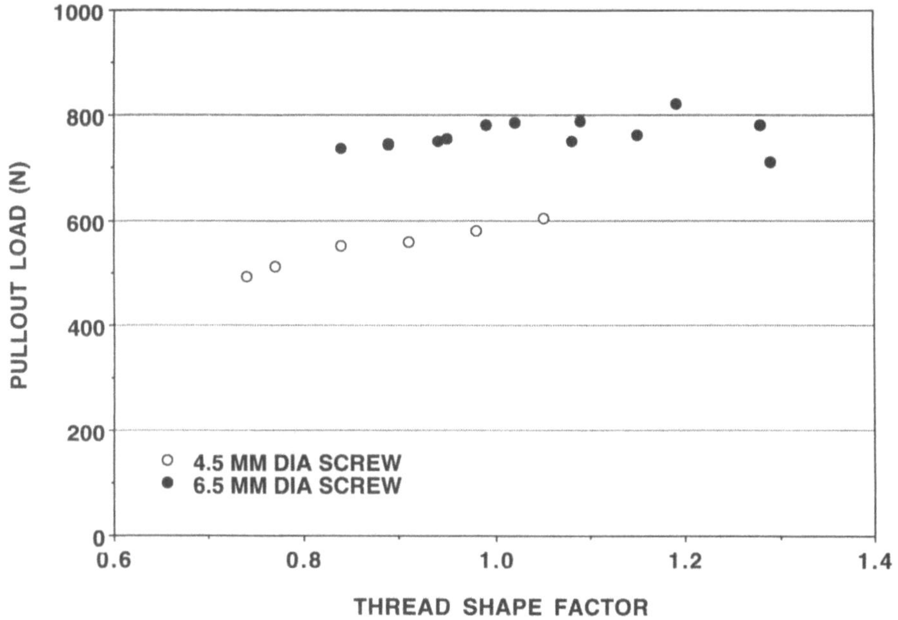


**FIGURE 2.16.** The effect of thread shape factor on screw pullout strength (adapted from Asnis et al.[33]).

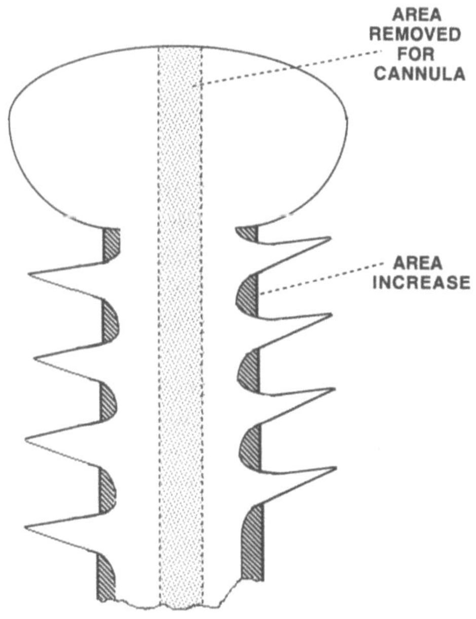


**FIGURE 2.17.** In order to allow for the cannula, the minor (root) diameter of the screw is increased. In some cases the major (outer) diameter may also be increased (see Table 2.1).

experimentally measured difference in pullout strength was 20%. Hearn et al.[34] found no statistical differences in the pullout strength between solid 6.5-mm cancellous screws (TSF = 0.87) and 7.0-mm cannulated cancellous screws (TSF = 0.76, Table 2.1). For the screws of this comparison the TSF was 12.6% lower with cannulation; however, the major diameter was increased from 6.5 to 7.0 mm (7.7%), thereby offsetting the effect of decreased TSF. Therefore, to obtain equivalent purchase in bone, the cannulated screws selected should be slightly larger than solid screws. This conclusion is further supported by the work of Leggon et al.,[35] who compared both small and large cannulated and noncannulated screws. The small screws had equivalent major diameters (3.5 mm) and cannulated screws were found to have 20% less holding power in cortex, similar to our findings. The large screws, similar to the ones tested by Hearn et al., showed no differences in pullout strength.

In designing a screw, the size of the cannulation and outer thread diameter are determined, then the root diameter can be specified. Theoretically if the outer diameter and the root diam-

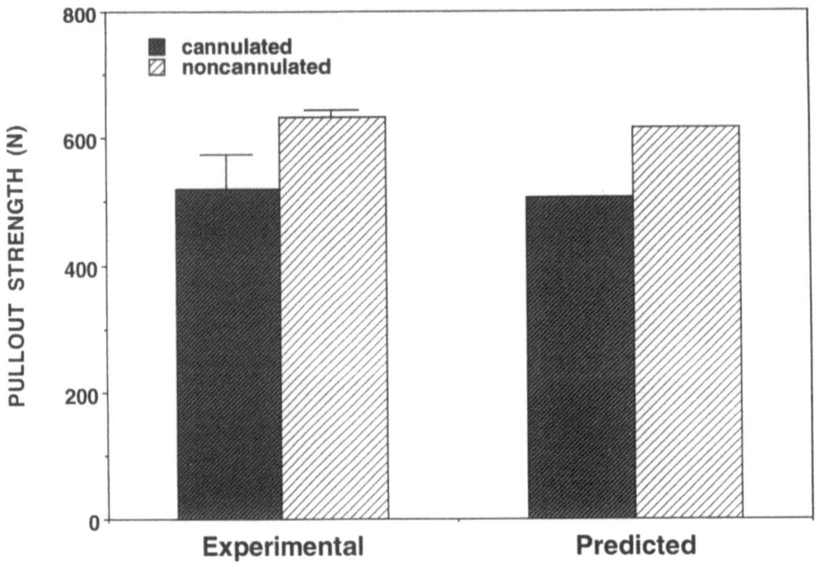


**FIGURE 2.18.** A comparison of the experimentally measured and predicted pullout strengths of cannulated and solid cancellous screws in porous foam (adapted from Chapman et al.[17]).

eter are known, the ideal pitch can be calculated. If we assume a target TSF = 1, then

$$TSF = (0.5 + 0.57735\, d/p) = 1$$

$$0.57735\, d/p = 0.5$$

$$p = 1.1547\, d,$$

or the ideal pitch should be approximately 1.15 times the thread depth $[(D_{\text{major}} - D_{\text{minor}})/2]$. For a 6.5-mm cannulated screw with a 6.5-mm major diameter and a 4.8-mm minor diameter,

$$p = 1.1547 \times [(6.5 - 4.8)/2]$$

$$p = 0.98 \text{ mm}$$

(most commercial 6.5-mm cannulated screws have a pitch of approximately 2.5 to 2.75 mm).

## Pilot Hole

Preparation of a screw hole requires drilling a pilot hole and possibly tapping. Hughes and Jordan[6] show that there is a critical pilot hole size (in relation to the screw diameter) in rigid materials (e.g., cortical bone) beyond which the pullout strength of the screw drops dramatically, but below which there is no effect. In their studies, this pilot hole size was approximately 90% of the screw major diameter. In materials simulating hard cancellous bone, the critical pilot hole size was 68% to 74% of the screw diameter, while for soft cancellous bone these values decreased to between 49% and 63% (Figure 2.19).[19] Currently, standards define the appropriate pilot drill sizes that are supplied by manufacturers.[36]

## Tapping

Tapping is necessary to allow the penetration of screws into hard materials such as cortical bone. For screws inserted into nontapped holes in cortical bone, a considerable fraction of the torque applied to the screw head is used to tap the threads, which reduces the percent applied torque that can be used to create compression between surfaces clamped by the screw, and increases the shear stress in the screw. The pullout strength of tapped screws is also significantly greater.[28] In lower-density materials (such as cancellous bone) the resistance to penetration of a screw into a nontapped hole is lower and shear failure of the screw becomes less of a concern. In this case, tapping has been found to significantly decrease pullout strength, with the greatest decreases occurring in the softest materials (Figure 2.20). In cancellous bone, the mean decrease was 30% (SD = 34%).

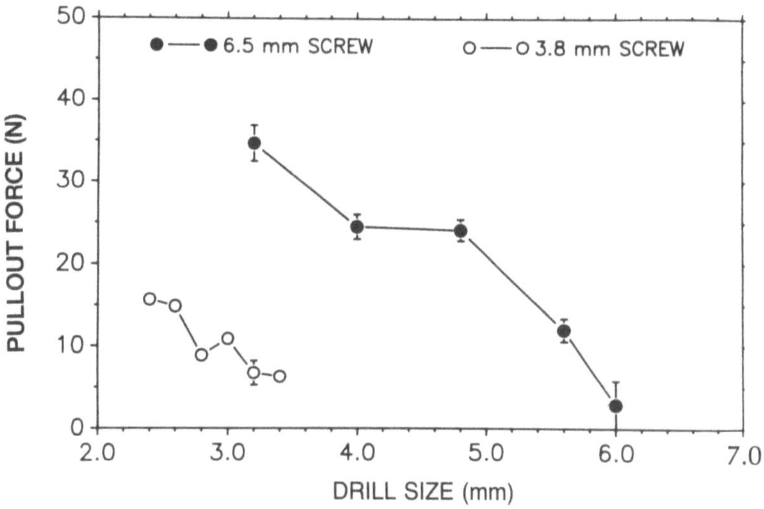


**FIGURE 2.19.** Measured pullout force of 6.5- and 3.8-mm cancellous screws in low-density material for different pilot drill sizes. (Reprinted with permission from Finlay et al.[19])

Tapping, apart from cutting threads, removes additional material from the hole, which enlarges it. Since the pilot hole size was shown above to have different effects on screw pullout strength depending on material density, it is not surprising that tapping would have little effect in hard materials and a progressively larger effect in softer, porous materials. Shown in Figure 2.21

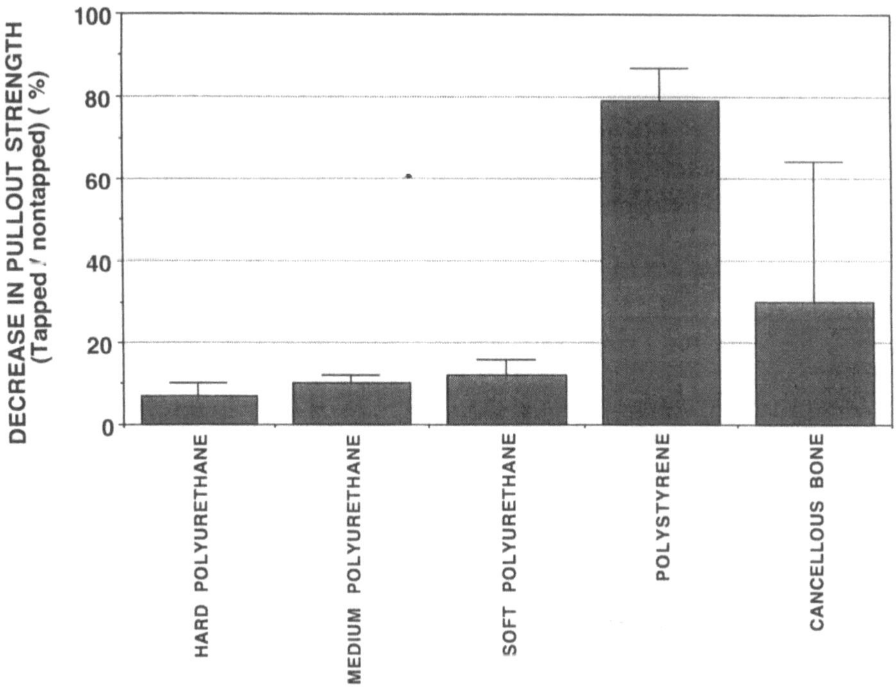


**FIGURE 2.20.** Mean percent decreases in screw pullout strength in porous materials as well as cancellous bone due to tapping holes before insertion of screws compared with not tapping (adapted from Chapman et al.[17]).

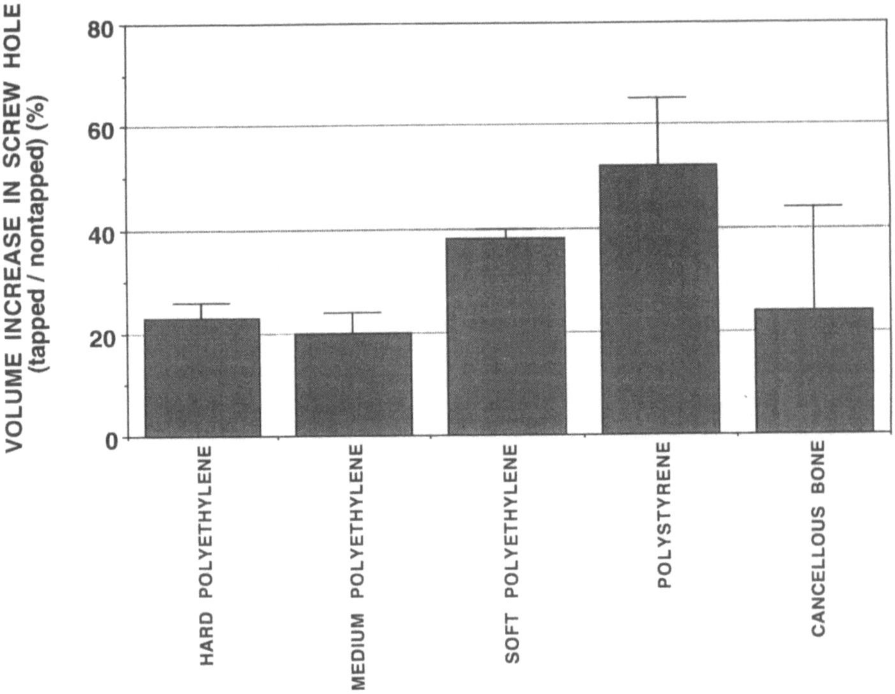


**FIGURE 2.21.** The percent increase in volume within a screw hole due to drilling and tapping before screw insertion as opposed to just drilling a pilot hole (adapted from Chapman et al.[17]).

are measurements of the change in volume in screw holes that had been only drilled compared with those that had been drilled and tapped.[17] These findings have been confirmed also by Hearn et al.[27]

## Self-Tapping

A screw can be made self-tapping by machining cutting channels, or flutes, into its tip. As the screw is turned, these sharp flutes cut the bone in preparation for the threads further along the screw shaft. This increases the torque of screw placement by 35–40%.[4] Using saline as an insertion lubricant, however, significantly reduces the insertion torque of the self-tapping screw. It has been found that the holding power of the first few fluted threads of the self-tapping screw tip are 17–30% less than the normal threads further up the shaft. The amount of decrease depends on the thread diameter. In the cortical screw this might significantly decrease the holding power in bone with a thin cortex. In this case, there could be a significant loss of thread surface area holding the far cortex. This can be corrected in cortical bone by driving the tip of the screw with the cutting flutes beyond the far cortical surface (beyond the bone). In cancellous bone the cutting flutes may be much less of a factor. The decrease in holding power may be small and a function of the small decrease in total thread area. Schatzker et al.[37] found no significant difference in vivo in holding power between non–self-tapping and self-tapping screws.

## In Vivo Effects

The holding power of screws in cortical bone increases significantly with time in vivo, as shown by Schatzker et al.[37] Increases ranged from 24% to 59% depending on screw type (Figure 2.22), due to bone consolidation and densification around the screw threads.[3,37]

## Summary

The holding power of a screw in bone is dependent on several factors, some of which

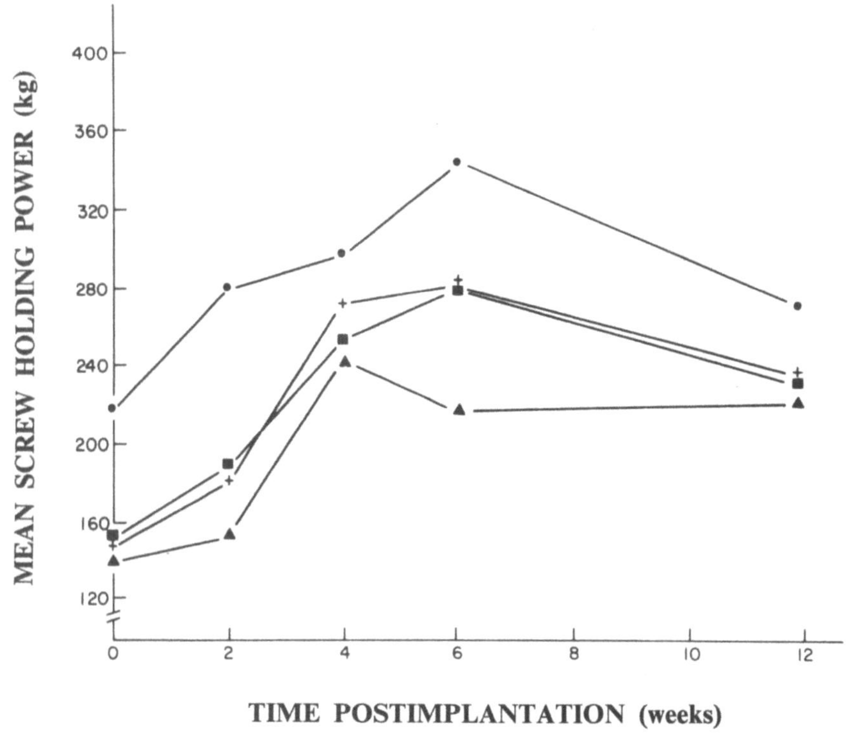


**FIGURE 2.22.** Mean holding power of screws in vivo as a function of time postimplantation. (Reprinted with permission from Schatzker et al.[37])

involve the size and design of the screw and some of which depend upon the density of the bone and its type and thickness at the site of use. Holding power increases with increased screw diameter and length of engagement, decreased pitch, and smaller minor diameter. The pitch on currently used cannulated screws could be decreased to improve holding strength. Not tapping is advantageous, especially in softer cancellous bone where there is little concern about screw breakage and more concern that using a tap removes material from the hole and therefore decreases holding power.

## Aspects of Design of Bone Screws

Perren et al.[4] provide an excellent discussion of the design features of bone screws. Different drives are found in the heads of screws from different sources. As shown in Figure 2.23, a simple slot is not effective for the transmission of torque and may strip easily. In addition, it is difficult to align the screwdriver without visualization of the slot. Cruciate or crossed slot drives are more effective for torque transmission but are sensitive to misalignment of the screwdriver. The hexagonal head driver makes a strong and alignment-insensitive connection with the screw but is somewhat difficult to manufacture, especially considering the necessity for the close tolerance fit to the head of the screw.

The undersurface of the screw head is normally spherical, which allows for transmission of force to a plate even if the screw is not aligned perpendicular to it, a frequent occurrence in surgery. The shaft of the screw may be equal in diameter to the major diameter of the threads (Figure 2.23). This type of screw provides greater strength and the gliding shaft maintains alignment of the threaded end in the hole. It is typically used in inclined holes to prevent the screw from becoming misaligned. The screw hole must be overdrilled to allow the smooth

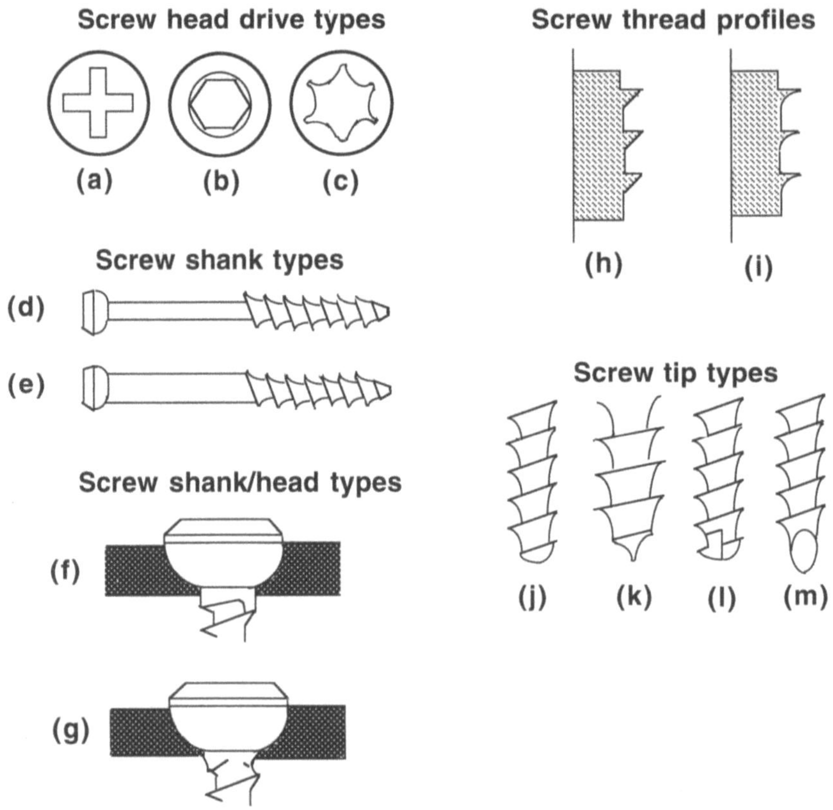


**FIGURE 2.23.** Some features of bone screw design. Head drive connections: (a) cruciate, (b) hexagonal, (c), star, (d) cancellous lag screw with smooth shaft diameter equal to that of thread root, (e) lag screw with shaft equal in diameter to major diameter of screw thread, (f) screw with thread/head shaft connection diameter equal to thread major diameter causes stresses in bone hole, (g) undercut shaft fits into bone hole. Bone screw thread profiles: (h) asymmetric thread with sharp connections to the screw shaft, (i) asymmetric AO thread with rounded corners. The upper surface of the thread contacts bone and resists pullout in an upward direction. Screw tips: (j) blunt, (k) corkscrew, (l) self-tapping with flutes, (m) self-cutting with trochar.

shaft to glide, adding an extra step to the surgery. To avoid this extra step, which may add considerable time to the procedure if many screws are used, some lag screws have smooth shafts that are of diameter equal to that of the root of the threads. These screws have obviously weaker shafts, a fact that should be appreciated. Fully threaded screws have been improved by undercutting or decreasing the diameter of the cross section of the small transition region between the end of the thread and the head (Figure 2.23). Previously, this oversize region (in relation to the hole in bone) caused significant bone expansion stresses by being forced into a hole of smaller diameter.

## Threads

Threads for use in bone are mainly asymmetrical (Figure 2.23). The surface of the thread, which transfers load to bone-resisting pullout, is nearly perpendicular to the direction of pullout force to provide maximum load transmission. The thread widens at its base to form a buttress that resists bending of the thread under load. The rounded corners at the junction of the base of the thread and the screw shaft reduce the stress concentrators, which are associated with sharp corners. The Herbert screw[38] is a unique device that has threads of different pitch on its two ends, and no head. The intention is for the screw to be buried beneath a bony surface. The coarser pitch moves the screw a greater distance through bone with each turn than does the finer pitch end. However, the screw is a single unit; therefore, as the screw is turned, the bone surfaces must come together, creating compression. Tips of screws may vary in shape, typically having a trochar point to allow self-drilling and -tapping, self-cutting flutes for self-tapping, or a blunt tip that requires separate drilling and tapping (Figure 2.23).

## Cannulated Screws

Cannulated screws have major advantages. Placing the guide wire first allows for accurate visualization of the path of the screw, which can be critical in certain circumstances. If the guide wire position must be changed, it can be done without enlarging the hole and sacrificing purchase strength. Also, the guide wire may aid in reduction of the fragment. Placing the screw requires first positioning the guide wire, then using a cannulated drill, a cannulated tap (if necessary), and finally inserting the screw. In many systems, these steps can be reduced by placing a self-cutting, self-tapping cannulated screw directly over the guide wire.

## Cutting Flutes

The cutting flutes of self-tapping screws can differ greatly. For bone screws the rake of the cutting flute becomes important (Figure 2.24). The cutting flutes can have negative, neutral, or positive rakes. Although a positive rake may be slightly weaker mechanically, it is a sharper flute, which requires less cutting force and generates lower rises in temperature.[39] The positive-rake cutting tip appears very effective when used in bone. It cuts like a chisel, and is only sharp when being turned in the clockwise direction.

# Biomechanics and the Design of Cannulated Screw Systems

The specific design and biomechanical considerations of a cannulated screw system are an expansion of many of the principles already discussed. The design of the jigs, guide pins, and measuring devices, and the interrelationship between these components and the screw are as important as the cannulated screw itself. The advantages of using guide pins and cannulated screws over primary screw placement are many:

- The cannulated system provides the ability to more accurately place the screw and predetermine its optimal position and length by the use of guide pins.
- A smaller initial defect is made in the bone, minimizing injury to the bone structure.
- Changes in position of the guide pin will usually have little or no deleterious effect on the final function of the bone screw and its ability to compress and hold bone.
- Guide pins can be used readily with power drills and placement jigs.
- They can be placed accurately in bone under fluoroscopic control where direct visualization is limited or impossible.
- They can readily be placed in patterns through jigs allowing controlled positioning with relation to other guide pins.
- They can be placed relatively atraumatically and maintain the proper position of the bone fragments as the screw is being inserted.
- Guide pins can also aid in the reduction of fractures. A free fragment can have a guide pin placed into it to be used as a handle in reduction. Once proper alignment is achieved it is driven through the distal fragment, holding reduction and establishing the final fixation screw position.

## The Guide Pin

There are several considerations in design of the guide pin. The strength and stiffness of the shaft of the guide pin is determined by its dimensions, just as for screws. Its torsional stiffness increases as the fourth power of its radius [polar moment

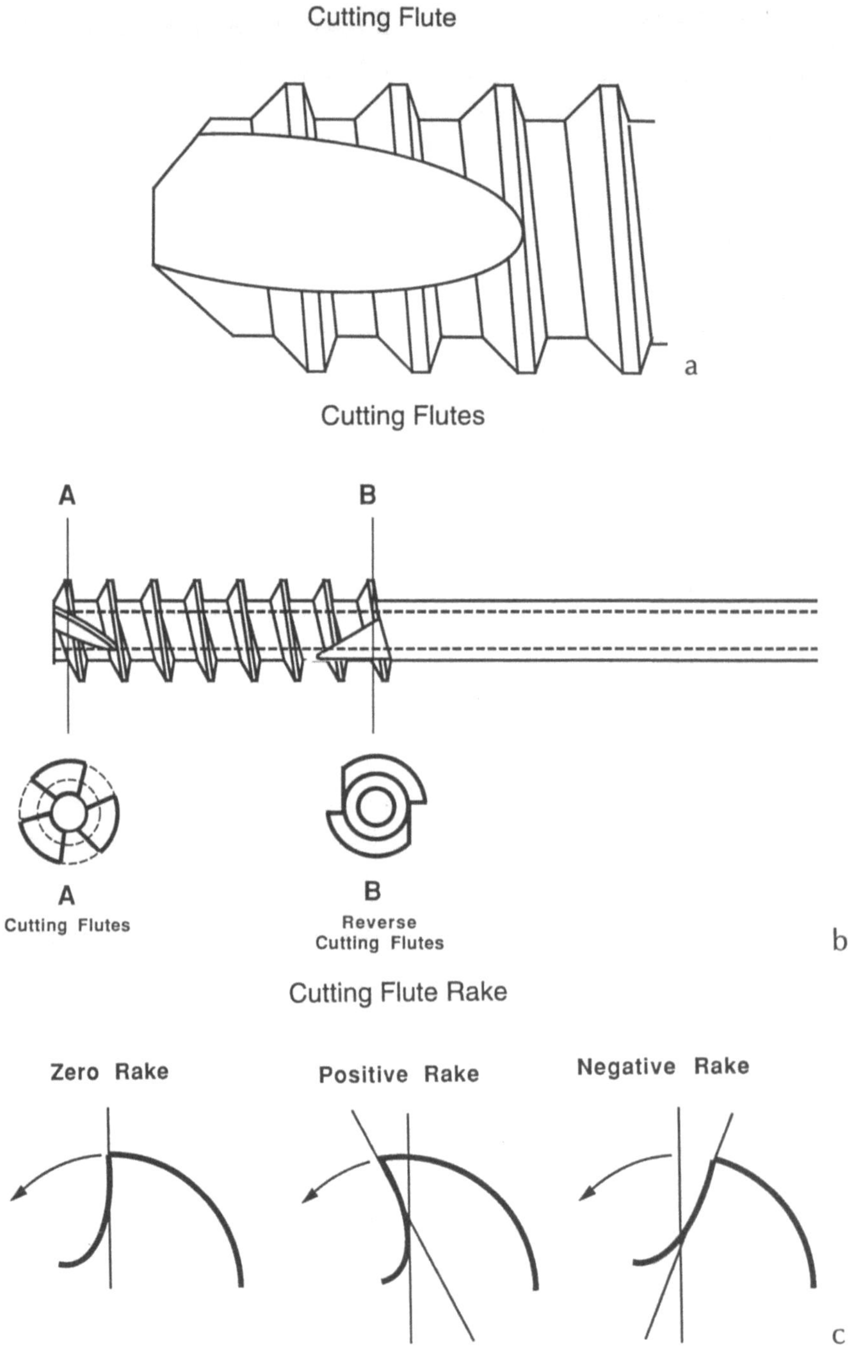


**FIGURE 2.24.** (a) A common cutting flute used on solid cortical bone screws. This allows the screw to be used without tapping and cuts the way for the thread. (b) The thread and shaft of a 6.5-mm cannulated cancellous bone screw. The tip of the cannulated screw may have cutting flutes to allow self-cutting and self-tapping. The end of the thread, just past the junction with the shaft, may have a reverse cutting flute to aid in removal. (c) The rake of the cutting flute may be negative, zero, or positive. The positive raked flute is sharpest and generates the least heat with installation. (Rake is the angle between the vertical line and edge of the screw.)

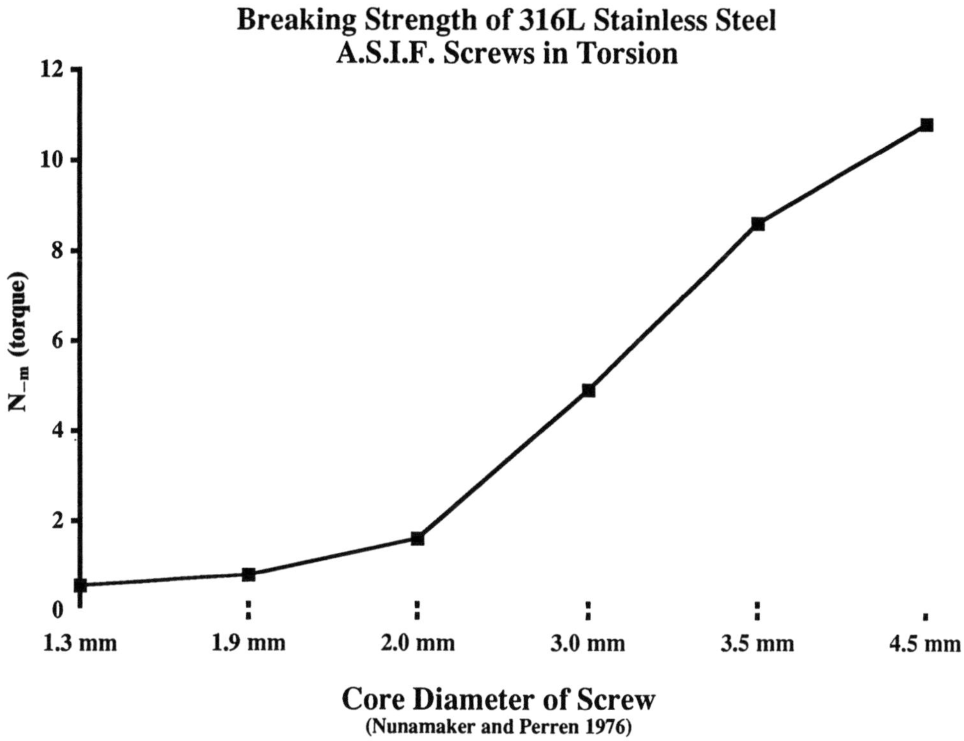


**FIGURE 2.25.** The breaking strength of a screw increases dramatically once the core diameter exceeds 2.0 mm (adapted from Uhl[40] and Nunamaker and Perren[11]). This is the same for guide pins.

of inertia $= (\pi R^4)/2$] and bending stiffness as the third power of its radius [area moment of inertia $= (\pi R^3)/2$]. The strength of a pin increases rapidly as its size increases beyond a 2-mm diameter[11,40] (Figure 2.25). Although a stronger and stiffer pin may be advantageous, this must be weighed against loss of strength of the screw caused by increasing the diameter of its cannulation. On the other hand, small pins can bend and jam in the screw or drill.

## Guide Pin Tip

The guide pin tip is usually threaded. This is done primarily to help temporarily fix the pin in bone. As the cannulated screw passes over the pin, its tip will prevent forward motion. It also helps fix the pin when overdrilling or tapping is required. If a screw is to be changed for one of longer length, the threads help keep the guide pin in place. Placing threads on the end of the guide pin does weaken its tip. The strength and stiffness of the threaded area is determined by the core or root diameter of the thread, which is less than that of the smooth part of the pin.

The junction of the thread and the smooth shaft is a potential weak point. A thread with a uniform root diameter results in a weaker junction with the smooth shaft than a tapered root that starts with the same diameter as the smooth shaft and decreases toward the tip (Figure 2.26). If too weak, bending or breakage at this junction can be a problem when the screw is being placed. If the guide pin is bent, the stiffer screw that takes a straight path will cause increased stress at the bend as it tries to straighten the pin. (If there is any difficulty in withdrawing the guide pin after screw placement, back the screw out part way, remove the pin, and advance the screw again without the guide wire.)

On occasion a drill may be used as a guide pin. If its length and diameter are the same as that of the guide pin it may be used directly and

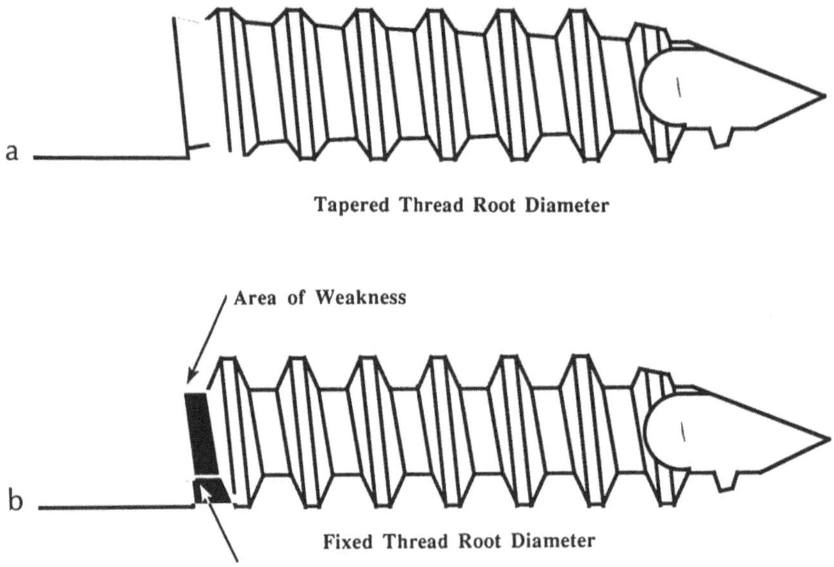


**FIGURE 2.26.** The root diameter of the threaded part of the guide pin can be (a) tapered toward the diameter of the smooth shaft, or (b) fixed in diameter, which causes a stress riser at the junction with the smooth shaft where there is a sharp change in diameter.

depth measurements may be taken from it. One example of this is its use in a slipped femoral capital epiphysis where the bone is very dense. Caution is necessary as the screw is driven over the drill. Since bone chips are trapped between the screw and the drill, jamming of the screw can occur. The sharp-tipped drill is then more likely to turn and advance forward than a guide pin with a threaded tip. If a drill is to be used as a guide pin, the position of its tip must be monitored with fluoroscopy. It should be removed after the screw has advanced only part way.

The guide pin essentially takes the place of the pilot hole used for placing solid screws. The pilot hole should be kept under a critical size to maintain maximum pullout strength of the screw thread. As we have previously discussed, for soft cancellous bone this critical pilot hole size is between 49% and 63%, whereas for hard cancellous it is 68% to 74% of the outer diameter of the screw threads. Since the guide wire diameter is always smaller than the root diameter of the screw, there is less chance of overenlarging the pilot hole with a cannulated screw.

## Guide Pin Depth Measurement

The larger guide pins are often marked for direct reading. This may be done with etched numerals or with rings or other markings. Direct reading depth gauges placed along the exposed portion of the guide pin are simple to apply and very easy to read.

## Jigs

A major advantage of the cannulated screw system is the ability to place the guide pins, and ultimately the screws, in a specified geometric relationship with each other. This is accomplished with the use of jigs. A common example of this is when multiple parallel screws are used for the fixation of intracapsular hip fractures. The simplest jig is a metallic block with a pattern of parallel holes. Assuming that the pins do not bend after leaving the jig guide hole, their positional accuracy is great. As an example, the Howmedica fixed jig, 25 mm in width, used to place parallel 3.2-mm pins in the hip, allows a deviation of only 0.3 mm for every 25 mm of advancement of the pin. This accuracy is based on the allowable tolerances of the jig guide holes and pin diameters.

## Cannulated Screw Head

The screw head has two basic functions: (a) to allow insertion of the driver, and (b) to serve as a buttress for the bone fragment and produce compression. The fit of the screwdriver bit is more critical for the cannulated than for the solid screw. The screw head has either an internal hexagonal recess to work with a cannulated screwdriver, or an external hexagonal or square head and a cannulated wrench (Figure 2.27). The internal recess design allows use of a less-bulky screwdriver and permits a spherical outer shape to the screw head. This can be important in screw removal. Bone growing around a screw head with an external hexagonal head makes removal difficult, since bone must be removed to allow engagement of the wrench. If two external hexagonal screw heads touch, they will lock. The advantage of using the external hexagonal head is the strength provided to the coupling with the driving wrench. The round head with an internal recess puts more demand on the screwdriver tip. The screwdriver hexagonal tip must be small enough to fit within the recess in the screw head, yet itself must be cannulated, leaving little material in it. In addition, the screw head–shaft junction strength is important. The internal hexagonal recess removes material from the head. If this recess is too deep, strength may be lost at the head–shaft junction.

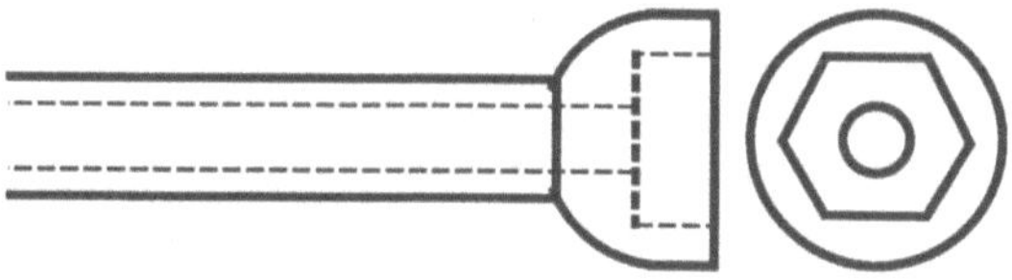


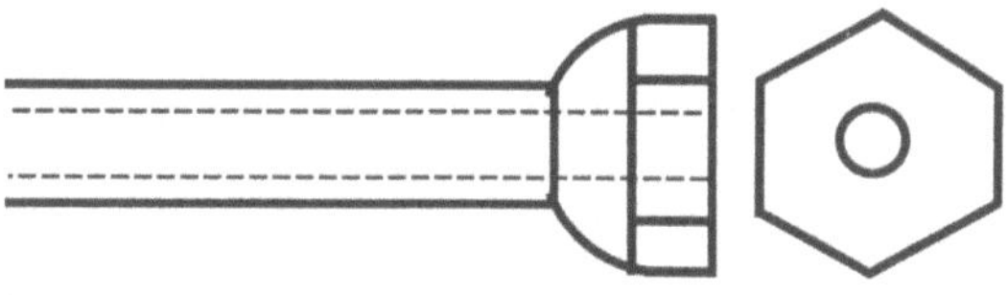


**FIGURE 2.27.** The cannulated screw head may have (a) an internal hexagonal recess, or (b) an external hexagonal shape.

## Cannulated Screw Shaft

The shaft of the cancellous lag screw has two basic functions: (a) to connect the head of the screw that is located in one bone fragment to the thread in the other fragment, and (b) to generate compression of the bone components through internal tension in the shaft. To maintain strength the shaft of the cannulated screw is often designed slightly larger than that of a solid screw of comparable size. Since the stiffness of a cylinder in bending is a function of the third power of its radius, a small increase in the outer radius of the shaft will compensate for the cannula. Figure 2.4 shows an example of this for medium-sized screws of comparable dimensions. This does not appear to be a problem in the larger screws, but in smaller screws leaving a cannulation large enough for a stiff guide wire may require the shaft diameter to be significantly increased or the screw will be considerably weaker.

There may be a misconception that a solid screw is always stronger than a cannulated screw of equivalent outer thread diameter. The 6.5-mm cannulated screws usually have a slightly larger shaft (root) diameter than their solid 6.5-mm counterparts. A solid 6.5-mm screw may have a 3.0-mm thread root diameter, while the Howmedica 6.5-mm cannulated screw has a root diameter of 4.8 mm. If the cannula is 2 mm in diameter, the area and polar moments of inertia of the cannulated screw would be 102.6 $mm^3$ and 514.8 $mm^4$, compared with 27 $mm^3$ and 81 $mm^4$, or 3.8 and 6.4 times greater, respectively, than those of the solid screw.

## Cannulated Screw Thread

The threads of the screw have three basic functions: (a) to transform torque applied to the screw into axial force, (b) to act as an inclined plane and gain mechanical advantage in the conversion of torque to compression, and (c) to resist pullout in the host material. As previously discussed, the ability of a screw thread to hold in bone without stripping is related to the geometry of the screw thread: its outer diameter, its length of engagement in bone, particularly cortex, and the geometry of its threads including depth and pitch, as well as the shear strength of the bone it is placed into. This is given by the relationship described previously:

$$F_s = S \times (L \times \pi \times D_{\text{major}}) \times TSF$$

When comparing cannulated screws with solid screws of nearly equivalent dimensions, in similar bone stock, the thread shape factor (TSF) becomes important. The TSF relationship given above states that screw holding power is directly proportional to thread depth and inversely proportional to pitch. Deeper threads with a greater difference between the outer and root diameters and thread forms with a smaller pitch, or more threads per inch, should have greater purchase strength. The problem in verifying these relationships is that in using commercially available screws, several variables always change together. We have manufactured custom screws in which these variables were varied individually.[33] The holding power of these custom screws were then tested using synthetic polyurethane materials to simulate cancellous bone of different densities. One material simulated moderate (0.15 g/cc), and one dense (0.22 g/cc) cancellous bone. The results of these studies indicate that the most important factor in screw holding power is the density of the host material followed by the outer diameter of the thread. With decreased pitch compared with those of commercially available screws (more threads per inch), there is an increase in pullout strength. This progresses to the point where the TSF is slightly greater than 1.0. Similarly, thread depth has an effect. A screw of 6.5-mm outer diameter and root diameter of 3.5 mm has significantly greater holding power in the lower density material than one with a root diameter of 4.2 mm, although there is no significant difference in the higher density material.

## Clinical Significance of Screw Thread Form

The cannulated screw must have a larger root diameter than the solid screw to allow room for the cannula. This does decrease its holding power, because the thread depth is smaller. The decrease in holding strength may be theoretically compensated for by decreasing the thread pitch (increasing the number of threads per inch). This can be determined by the given formulae. Clinically, cannulated screws appear to function well and in a practical sense may have more than adequate holding power. When comparing the holding power of different cannulated screws, the surgeon may apply the principles given in making his choice of the appropriate device.

## Cutting Tip

The tip of the cannulated screw is most important in screw function. In solid screws, tips may have a trochar to allow self-drilling and -tapping, self-cutting flutes for self-tapping, or a blunt tip that requires predrilling and tapping (Figure 2.23). The screw tip design may significantly decrease the screw's holding power in bone. In cancellous bone pretapping can decrease pullout strength approximately 30% (Figure 2.20). Tapping as a separate procedure removes additional material from the hole, enlarging it (Figure 2.21).

It appears that a cannulated screw designed for cancellous bone should be self-cutting and -tapping. The cutting flutes should direct bone chips away from the cannula and place them in a position to be packed by the oncoming threads. As previously discussed, one way to accomplish this is to place cutting flutes that have a positive rake into the first couple of threads. This removes minimal metal and causes very little change to the overall thread surface area. As the screw advances, it chisels into the bone and directs the chips to be packed against the screw threads. The tip of the screw only cuts when rotated clockwise. The tip is blunt when turned counterclockwise (removal direction). Another advantage of this type of tip is in percutaneous procedures. After the guide pin is placed, the screw is advanced through the soft tissue while turning it in a counterclockwise direction. The tip doesn't cut or wind the soft tissues. When cortex is reached the rotation is reversed to clockwise, allowing it to cut into bone.

## Summary

Cannulated screw systems can help the surgeon to position, determine length, and accurately place the final screw and have major advantages in maintaining the reduction and control of fracture fragments during the procedure. The principles that govern screw strength and holding power should be appreciated by the surgeon. There are also major differences between different cannulated screw systems in relation to sizing and tip design. The surgeon should appreciate the differences, since this will allow accurate selection according to specific clinical needs.

## Summary

A number of factors interact to control the performance of a screw placed in bone. These include the density of the bone into which it is placed, the geometry of the screw itself, and the technique of preparation of the hole. A screw functions to transfer the torque applied to it into a compressive force between the two objects that it is placed into. The compressive force that can be produced is directly dependent on the purchase of the screw in bone, as well as the torque that can be applied and the strength of the screw. Both the outside diameter of the screw and its purchase length in bone govern the pullout (purchase) strength. For screws of equal length and size, decreasing the minor (root) diameter decreases the strength of the screw but increases its purchase strength. Decreasing pitch (increasing the number of threads per inch) also increases purchase strength. There are practical limits to the geometrical modifications that can be made to improve purchase strength, in order to preserve sufficient strength of the threads in bending (i.e., in resisting pullout) and the root of the screw in shear (i.e., resisting torsional failure).

Tapping plays an important part as well. In dense (cortical) bone, tapping is occasionally necessary so that sufficient torque transmitted by the screw is used to create compressive force instead of being absorbed by cutting threads. On the other hand, for low-density (cancellous) bone, tapping is detrimental since it enlarges the hole and reduces purchase strength. In these circumstances, the bone is usually weak enough so that resistance to insertion is not an important issue.

Cannulated screws provide significant advantages over solid screws when the screw must be carefully positioned, and they aid in gaining control and temporary reduction of fracture components. On the other hand, especially with small screws, the existence of a cannula in the center of the screw reduces torsional strength significantly. For cannulated and solid screws of equal major diameter, the minor diameter of the cannulated screw is designed to be larger to increase torsional strength. This reduces the thread depth and the holding power of the screw. Some manufacturers, recognizing this, provide cannulated screws of larger diameter than equivalently sized solid screws. Another method for increasing cannulated screw purchase strength may be to make these screws with a finer pitch than is currently used.

## References

1. Albright JA, Johnson TR, Saha S. Principles of internal fixation. In: Ghista DN, Roaf R, eds. *Orthopedic Mechanics: Procedures and Devices*. New York: Academic Press, 1978.
2. Chapman JR, Harrington RM, Lee K, Tencer AF. Factors affecting the holding power of cancellous bone screws. *J Biomech Eng* 1995; in press.
3. Uhthoff HK. Mechanical factors influencing the holding power of screws in compact bone. *J Bone Joint Surg* 1973;55B:633–639.
4. Perren SM, Cordey J, Baumgart, F, Rahn BA, Schatzker J. Technical and biomechanical aspects of screws used for bone surgery. *Int J Orthop Trauma* 1992;2:31–48.
5. Hayes WC, Perren SM. Plate bone friction in the compression fixation of fractures. *Clin Orthop* 1974;89:236–240.
6. Hughes AN, Jordan BA. The mechanical properties of surgical bone screws and some aspects of insertion practice. *Injury* 1972;4:25–38.
7. Ansell RH, Scales JT. A study of some factors which affect the strength of screws and their insertion and holding power in bone. *J Biomech* 1968;1:279–302.
8. von Arx C. Schububertragung durch reibung bei der plattenosteosynthese. *Med Diss Basel* 1973.
9. *Standard specification for cortical bone screws*, Designation F 543-82. Philadelphia: American Society for Testing and Materials, 1989;13.01:106–108.

10. Zand MS, Goldstein SA, Matthews LS. Fatigue failure of cortical bone screws. *J Biomech* 1983; 16:305–311.
11. Nunamaker DM, Perren SM. Force measurements in screw fixation. *J Biomech* 1976;9:669-675.
12. Young WC. *Roark's Formulas for Stress and Strain*, 6th ed. New York: McGraw-Hill, 1989.
13. Benterud JG, Husby T, Graadahl O, Alho A. Implant holding power of the femoral head: a cadaver study of fracture screws. *Acta Orthop Scand* 1992;63:47–49.
14. Daum WJ, Tencer AF, Cartwright TJ, Simmons DJ, Woodard PL, Koulisis CW. Pullout strengths of bone screws at various sites about the pelvis—a preliminary study. *J Orthop Trauma* 1988; 2:229–233.
15. Krag MH, Beynnon BD, Pope MH, Frymoyer JW, Haugh LD. Weaver DL. An internal fixator for posterior application to short segments of the thoracic, lumbar, or lumbosacral spine. *Clin Orthop* 1986;203:75–98.
16. DeCoster TA, Heetderks DB, Downey DJ, Ferries JS, Jones W. Optimizing bone screw pullout force. *J Orthop Trauma* 1990;4:169–174.
17. Chapman JR, Harrington RM, Lee KM, Anderson PA, Tencer AF. Factors affecting the pullout strength of cancellous bone screws. *J Biomech Eng* 1994; submitted.
18. Koranyi E, Bowman CE, Knecht CD, Janssen M. Holding power of orthopedic screws in bone. *Clin Orthop* 1970;72:283–286.
19. Finlay JB, Jarada I, Boune RB, Rorabeck CH, Hardie R, Scott MA. Analysis of the pull-out strength of screws and pegs used to secure tibial components following total knee arthroplasty. *Clin Orthop* 1989;247:220–231.
20. Brantley HEV, Mayfield JK, Koeneman JB, Clark K. The effects of screw size and bone density on pedicle screw fixation and stiffness. *Orthop Res Soc* 1994;19:718.
21. Wilkinson TL, Laatsch TR. Lateral and withdrawl resistance of tapping screws in three densities of wood. *Forest Products* 1970;20:34–41.
22. Zdeblick TA, Kunz DN, Cooke ME, McCabe R. The relationship between insertional torque, bone mineral density, and pedicle screw fatigue pullout strength. *Trans 39th Orthop Res Soc* 1993;18:235.
23. Wittenberg RH, Shea M, Swartz DE, Lee KS, White AA III, Hayes WC. Importance of bone mineral density in instrumented spinal fusions. *Spine* 1991;16:648–652.
24. Trader JE, Johnson RP, Kalbfleisch JH. Bone mineral content, surface hardness, and mechanical fixation in the human radius. *J Bone Joint Surg* 1979;61A:1217–1220.
25. Zindrick MR, Wiltse LL, Widell EH, Thomas JC, Holland RW, Field BT, Spencer CW. A biomechanical study of intrapeduncular fixation in the lumbar spine. *Clin Orthop* 1986;203:99–112.
26. Evans M, Spencer M, Wang Q, White SH, Cunningham JL. Design and testing of external fixator bone screws. *J Biomed Eng* 1990;12:457–462.
27. Hearn TC, Surowiak JF, Schatzker J. Effects of tapping on the holding strength of cancellous bone screws, *Vet Compar Orthop Traumatol* 1992; 5:10–12.
28. Yovich JV, Turner AS, Smith FW, Davis DM. Holding power of orthopedic screws: comparison of self-tapped and pretapped screws in foal bone. *Vet Surg* 1986;15:55–59.
29. Lyon WF, Cochran JR, Smith L. Actual holding power of various screws in bone. *Ann Surg* 1941;114:376–384.
30. Stone JL, Beaupre GS, Hayes WC. Multiaxial strength characteristics of trabecular bone. *J Biomech* 1983;16:743–752.
31. Appendix A5—Design of special threads. In: *Screw-Thread Standards for Federal Services*, FED-STD-H28. Washington, DC: Interdepartmental Screw-Thread Committee, National Bureau of Standards, General Services Administration, 1978; 46–52.
32. Oberg E, Jones FD, Horton HL. Working strength of bolts. In: Ryffel HH, ed. *Machinery's Handbook*. New York: Industrial Press, 1987; 1068–1069.
33. Asnis S, Ernberg JJ, Bostrom MPG, Harrington RM, Tencer AF. Cancellous bone screw design and holding power. Scientific exhibit, 62nd Meeting of the American Academy of Orthopaedic Surgeons, Orlando, FL, February 16–20, 1995.
34. Hearn TC, Schatzker J, Wolfson N. Extraction strength of cannulated cancellous bone screws. *J Orthop Trauma* 1993;7:138–141.
35. Leggon R, Lindsey RW, Doherty BJ, Alexander J, Noble P. The holding strength of cannulated screws compared with solid core screws in cortical and cancellous bone. *J Orthop Trauma* 1993; 7:450–457.
36. *Standard reference chart for pictorial cortical bone screw classification*, designation F544-77. Philadelphia: *American Society for Testing and Materials*, 1989;13.01:109–112.
37. Schatzker J, Sanderson R, Murnaghan JP. The holding power of orthopedic screws in vivo. *Clin Orthop* 1975;108:115–126.
38. Lange RH, Engber WD, Glad RW, Purnell ML. Biomechanical and histological evaluation of the Herbert screw. *J Orthop Trauma* 1990;4:275–282.
39. Oberg E, Jones FD, Horton HL. In: Schubert PB, ed. *Machinery's Handbook*, 20th ed. New York: Illustrated Press, 1976;1800–1804.
40. Uhl RL. The biomechanics of screws. *Orthop Rev* 1989;18:1303.

# 3

# Fluoroscopic Procedures in Orthopaedics: Radiation Exposure of Patients and Personnel

W. Gordon Monahan

One of the major advantages to cannulated screw techniques is the ability to accurately place screws in an area without direct anatomic exposure and visualization. Guide pins, usually inserted under fluoroscopic observation, are used for trial positioning. However, this necessitates some radiation exposure to the patients and surgical team. Using modern fluoroscopic techniques, how significant is this exposure and what methods can be used to minimize this potential hazard?

As with any exposure to ionizing radiation, there is a risk of radiation-induced conditions being produced. The serious radiation-induced effects of concern are categorized as deterministic or stochastic. A deterministic effect is one that increases in severity with increasing absorbed dose (e.g., lens opacification, skin erythema, and decreased sperm production). In a stochastic effect, the probability of occurrence increases with increasing exposure; however, the severity is independent of the magnitude of the absorbed dose (e.g., cancers and genetic effects). Deterministic effects occur only after relatively high exposures to radiation,[1] whereas the induction of stochastic effects is considered to be the principal hazard of exposures to low doses of ionizing radiation. The objective of a radiation protection program is to prevent the occurrence of deterministic effects and to limit the risk of stochastic effects to a reasonable level. This objective can be accomplished by ensuring that all radiation exposure is As Low As Reasonably Achievable (ALARA). This is the general philosophy of a radiation protection program along with the inclusion of economic and social factors.

## Radiation Units

Figure 3.1 shows schematically an x-ray beam passing through air. In the path of the beam are situated two parallel metal plates that are connected to a battery and a sensitive current meter. As the x-rays interact with the air in the volume defined by the parallel plates, electrons and ionized air molecules are produced that experience the attractive force of the charged metal plates. The amount of current conducted is proportional to the radiation exposure rate. The formal definition of the unit of radiation exposure (the roentgen) was adopted by the International Commission on Radiological Units and Measurements in 1928, some 33 years after Wilhelm Roentgen discovered x-rays. The original definition was that one roentgen (R) of radiation produces one electrostatic unit (esu) of charge per cubic centimeter of air at standard temperature and pressure (STP). The modern equivalent in SI units is $2.58 \times 10^{-4}$ coulombs/kg of air. In more familiar terms, the entrance skin exposure to a patient in a typical fluoroscopic procedure is 3 to 5 R/min.

While radiation exposure is a measure of the number of incident x-rays, radiation dose is the amount of energy deposited per unit mass of air or a particular tissue. The x-ray–absorbing ability of various tissues depends on their atomic composition and density in addition to the energy of the incident beam. Because bone has a much higher effective atomic number than muscle or water, the dose to bone will be about 3.5 times greater for the same exposure of low-energy x-rays. The dose in tissue will also vary with depth. Imagine a series of parallel plate

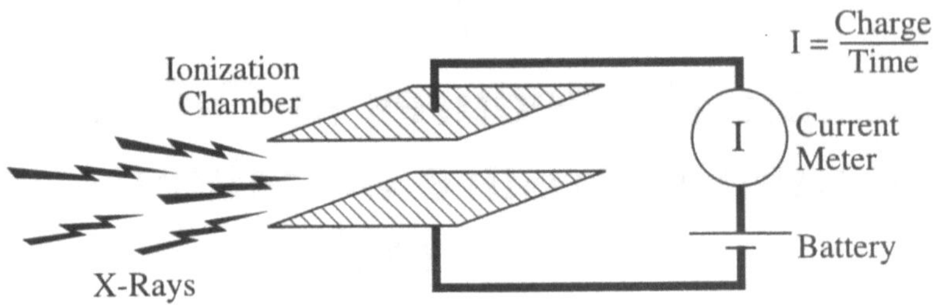


**FIGURE 3.1.** The ionization chamber is used to measure radiation exposure. X-rays cause ionization in the air between the chamber plates and the measured charge (Q) is proportional to the radiation intensity. The current, which is defined as the charge per unit time, is therefore proportional to the radiation exposure rate.

chambers placed in the path of an x-ray beam. The air in the first chamber will remove some of the x-rays from the beam so that the next chamber in line will receive a lower exposure and therefore a smaller dose. This reduction in exposure and dose would be maintained along the series of chambers. In an actual patient exposure, about one percent of the incident x-ray beam will exit the surface of the patient farthest from the x-ray source.

The unit of absorbed dose in SI units is the gray (Gy), which is equal to the radiation necessary to deposit one joule of energy in one kilogram of irradiated material. In the older centimeter-gram-second (cgs) units, the unit of absorbed dose is the rad, which is equal to 100 ergs per gram (1 Gy = 100 rad). Since different kinds of radiation (i.e., x-rays versus high-energy neutrons) cause varying degrees of biologic damage for the same absorbed dose, the absorbed dose equivalent has been defined for radiation protection purposes. The absorbed dose equivalent in sieverts (Sv) is equal to the absorbed dose in grays times a quality factor that is dependent on the biologic effectiveness of the radiation. The older unit is the rem (1 Sv = 100 rem). For x-rays, the quality factor is 1; therefore, the absorbed dose in grays is identical to the absorbed dose equivalent in sieverts. In addition, for soft tissue the exposure in roentgens is approximately equal to the absorbed dose in rads or the absorbed dose equivalent in rems. The entrance dose to a patient's soft tissue during fluoroscopy will therefore be 3 to 5 rem/min. For a more detailed description of radiation units the reader is referred to one of the standard textbooks on the physics of radiology.[2]

## Imaging Equipment

The imaging chain used in fluoroscopic procedures consists of an x-ray tube source in coaxial alignment with an image intensifier that is optically coupled to a television camera. The output image is viewed by the physician on a TV monitor. The principal advantage of this x-ray imaging system is the tremendous image brightness gain that is achieved by the image intensifier tube. This enables viewing of the fluorescent images in reasonable ambient lighting. The two factors that contribute to the gain of the image intensifier are (1) the energy increase of the electrons accelerated from the photocathode to the output screen and (2) the minification of the input image from an image receptor diameter of 15 to 30 cm to the output of 2.5 cm. The combination of these two factors yields a brightness gain of several thousand compared with a fluorescent screen alone, which is used in most static, x-ray imaging procedures. The only disadvantage of the image intensifier–TV tube imaging combination is the slightly reduced spatial resolution compared to a film-screen system.

### Resolution

Spatial resolution in an image intensifier–video camera fluoroscopy system is limited by the x-ray tube focal spot size, the input screen thickness of the image intensifier, and the number of lines used in the video camera. The choice of each of these elements in the various system components represents a design trade-off with other important characteristics. The focal spot size must be large enough to produce sufficient x-ray tube output while not degrading image resolution. Typical x-ray tube focal spot sizes that accomplish these design objectives are 0.5 to 0.9 mm. The image intensifier input screen must be thick enough to stop a good percentage of the incident photons, so that patient exposure can be kept as low as reasonably achievable while not reducing spatial resolution due to light diffusion in the screen. The cesium iodide (CsI) input screens have detection efficiencies of 50–60%[3] and, in addition, the CsI crystals can be aligned with the direction of the incident x-ray beam to reduce the lateral spread of light photons, which degrades spatial resolution. The number of TV lines in the video image is interdependent with the frame rate, which must be fast enough to capture motion without appearing jerky. Standard TV uses a frame rate of 30 frames/second and 525 lines/frame. Some current fluoroscopy C-arms offer 1023-line TV components and a proportionately reduced frame rate.

A good way to represent image resolution is to look at the contribution from each of the components as a function of object magnification. Following the example given by Sprawls,[4] Figure 3.2 shows the blur (reciprocal of resolution) for a typical image intensifier–video system. Ideally, each structure in the object should project onto the image plane with its correct geometric magnification. In actual practice, each structure in the object is enlarged beyond this size due to the extended focal spot size and the spreading of light in the screen. The specific situation illustrated is a 23-cm image intensifier, 1000-line TV, and an x-ray tube with a 0.6-mm focal spot. Since most applications will involve geometric magnification less than 1.5, the maximum blur of the system will be approximately 0.3 mm. While this degradation in image quality

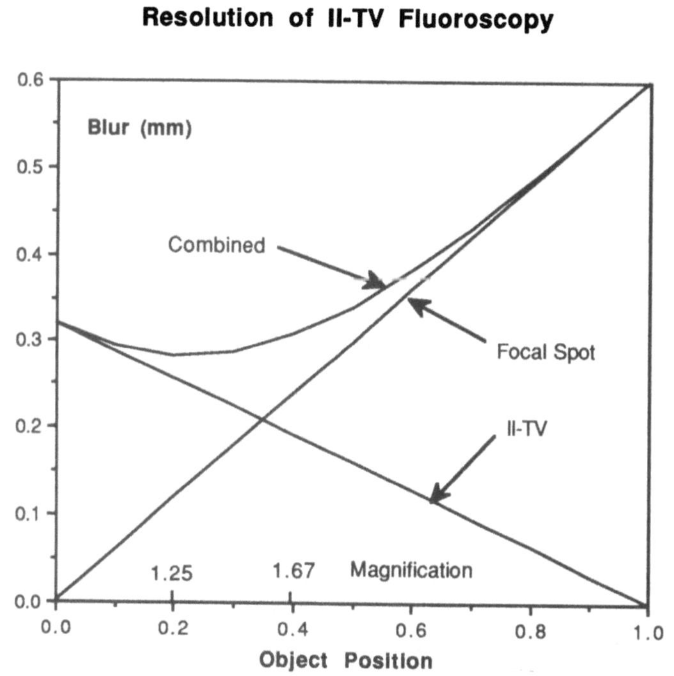


**FIGURE 3.2.** Estimated blur (reciprocal of resolution) for a 23-cm image intensifier optically coupled to a 1,000-line video camera using an x-ray tube with a 0.6-mm focal spot. The theoretical maximum resolution of this system is 3 line pairs/mm.

is acceptable in practice, a twofold improvement could be obtained, if needed, by using the electronic magnification capability of the image intensifier. However, the use of 2× electronic magnification will result in a 2 to 4× increase in patient exposure depending on the automatic brightness control setting.

## Automatic Brightness Control

As a patient is dynamically fluoroscoped, the changing field of view produces different x-ray absorption, which results in the image intensifier being exposed to different intensities of radiation. Without a compensating mechanism in place, the video screen intensity would be constantly changing during the movement of the image intensifier. In fluoroscopy, an electronic control system is used to keep the video image at a constant brightness level. This system works by either placing a photodetector in front of the video camera or using an internal camera signal to monitor the light level. This information is used in a feedback circuit to alter either the kilovoltage of the x-ray generator or the anode current of the x-ray tube, which controls radiation output. If the light signal is too low, the kilovoltage is increased to enhance the penetration of the x-ray beam. To avoid degrading the image contrast, the x-ray tube current will also be controlled to change the input exposure to the patient. By controlling these tube parameters, the automatic brightness system can maintain a constant intensity at the video camera and therefore keep constant illumination at the video monitor.

## Primary and Scattered Radiation

X-rays originate at the focal spot of the x-ray tube and the beam is confined by the collimator to irradiate the image receptor surface area. This cone of radiation, which passes through the patient and produces the two-dimensional image on the TV monitor, is called the primary beam. There are three processes that occur when x-rays at diagnostic energies interact with matter: coherent scattering, photoelectric effect, and Compton scattering. In a photoelectric interaction the x-ray is completely absorbed by giving its energy to an atomic electron. Coherent scattering constitutes about 5% of the possible events and results in a deflection of the incident photon in another direction without a loss of energy. Compton scattering is responsible for most of the scattered radiation in soft tissue. In a Compton interaction the photon divides its energy between an outer-shell electron and a secondary photon. The incident photon transfers only about 10–20% of its original energy to the orbital electron, so the scattered photon will penetrate tissue nearly as well as the primary beam. These scattered photons produce the radiation hazard for personnel.

The angular distribution of secondary photons is nearly isotropic at the energies used in fluoroscopy. Some convenient tables[5] have been compiled from experimental measurements of scattered radiation and are used in calculating personnel exposures. The amount of scattered radiation at 90° to the primary beam axis depends on the incident field size and the subject thickness. A good rule of thumb is that scattered radiation is 0.1% of the entrance exposure to the patient. At one meter from the beam axis.

## Regulations

There are two primary Federal regulations[6] that apply to C-arm fluoroscopy systems. One addresses the beam collimation and image receptor alignment and the other the maximum entrance skin exposure to the patient. The primary radiation beam must be contained within the image receptor input area. This requirement ensures that the patient receives only radiation that will contribute to the procedure and that personnel will be exposed only to scattered radiation, which is approximately 0.1% the intensity of the primary beam. In addition, for machines with automatic exposure control the maximum entrance exposure rate to the patient is limited to 10 R/min. Some machines have a high-level control mode of operation that must be accompanied by an audible signal when in use and the exposure rate is limited to 20 R/min.

**TABLE 3.1.** Summary of NCRP recommendations for annual radiation dose limits.*

| Class exposed | Rems | mSv |
|---|---|---|
| Occupational | | |
| Stochastic | 5 | 50 |
| Nonstochastic | | |
| Lens of eye | 15 | 150 |
| All other areas | 50 | 500 |
| Lifetime cumulative | 1 × (age in years) | 10 × (age in years) |
| Public | | |
| Effective dose equiv. | 0.1 | 1 |
| Embryo-fetus | | |
| Total dose equiv. | 0.5 | 5 |
| Dose equiv. (1 mo.) | 0.05 | 0.05 |

* Excluding background and medical exposures.

The high-level mode should always be used for short periods of time and never for routine operation.

## Radiation Hazards

Occupational and public radiation dose limits have been recommended by the National Council on Radiation Protection and Measurements.[7] These limits do not include exposure from natural background radiation and exposures received as a patient for medical purposes. A condensed version of these guidelines is given in Table 3.1.

The values given in Table 3.1 should be treated as upper limits of dose rather than design limits for radiation shielding. Even though the NCRP recommends a maximum annual permissible dose of 5 rem, the average annual dose equivalent of monitored hospital workers in 1989 was 140 mrem. The greatest radiation risk to the orthopaedic surgeon is to the head, neck, and hands. Average annual radiation doses to these areas have been reported in the 200 to 800 mrem range.[8]

The lifetime effective dose equivalent of 1 rem times the worker's age in years is consistent with the acceptable risk being comparable to or less than those in other safe industries. The average fatal accident rate in safe industries is about 1/10,000/yr.[1] The risk of developing a radiation-induced fatal malignancy during a worker's lifetime is 4/10,000/rem. Assuming a 30-year working career and multiplying by the maximum permissible annual whole-body dose of 1 rem/yr yields (30 yr × 1.0 rem/yr × 4/10,000/rem) 1.2/100, which is similar to the safe industry lifetime risk of 0.5% for a 50-year working life. The lifetime risk to the average radiation worker is about one-fourth of the maximum risk.

## Patient Exposure and Risk

Patients receive primary plus scattered radiation. The primary radiation is confined to a small fraction of the total body surface area. The scattered radiation is similar in intensity to that experienced by the surgical staff; however, since the patient is only involved in a single procedure, the scattered radiation exposure is insignificant in comparison to the primary. Keep in mind that dose is energy deposited per unit mass of tissue. To account for the difference in radiating a small volume of tissue and using risk factors based on whole-body irradiation, a set of weighting factors[1] has been derived from experimental data. These are given in Table 3.2.

Since the average fluoroscopic exposure time in most orthopaedic procedures is less than 5 minutes,[8] the average patient entrance exposure to the area of interest would be about 15 R. A weighting factor of 0.05 could be used to compare this limited area irradiation with an equivalent whole-body irradiation. The effective dose equivalent to the whole body would be about

**TABLE 3.2.** Tissue-weighting factors.

| 0.01 | 0.05 | 0.12 | 0.20 |
|---|---|---|---|
| Bone surface | Bladder | Bone marrow | Gonads |
| Skin | Breast | Colon | |
| | Liver | Lung | |
| | Esophagus | Stomach | |
| | Thyroid | | |
| | Remainder | | |

750 mrem. The radiation detriment to an individual patient who undergoes an orthopaedic procedure would therefore be at the same level as the detriment experienced by the orthopaedic surgeon on a yearly basis (3/10,000 risk of developing a fatal malignancy per procedure). While this risk to the patient is justified by the benefit received from the procedure, special shielding considerations must be made for pregnant patients and when the gonads are in the primary beam.

## Radiation Protection

There are three ways to limit the amount of radiation exposure to both patients and personnel: time, distance, and shielding. Fluoroscopy time is monitored and an audible alarm is sounded after 5 minutes of exposure. This timer is then reset by the technical staff. It is good practice to note the total fluoroscopy time in the patient log book, so that retrospective dose calculations can be made and used to streamline procedures. The total fluoroscopy time should be kept to a minimum to keep patient and personnel exposures as low as possible.

The second factor to use in controlling radiation exposure is distance. The patient should be positioned as close as possible to the image receptor and as far as possible from the x-ray source in order to minimize patient exposure. Since the intensity of any radiation from a point source decreases inversely with the distance from the source squared, personnel can be strategically positioned about the patient to minimize this component of exposure. If it is not necessary for assisting physicians or technical staff to be in close proximity to the central axis of the x-ray beam, then considerable dose reduction can be achieved by positioning the staff at larger distances from the beam axis. If a person moves from 1 m to 2 m distance from the x-ray field of view at the patient, the exposure is reduced by a factor of four.

The third factor in exposure reduction, shielding, is accomplished by personnel wearing lead aprons, thyroid shields, and protective eyeware and the use of transparent leaded plastic barriers. The recommended apron for fluoroscopic procedures is one with 0.5 mm lead equivalence. This thickness of material will remove more than 95% of the incident radiation. These are supplied in either single- or double-piece construction for reducing the physical strain of wearing this protection.

## Example

A physician is standing 50 cm perpendicular to the x-ray beam axis and performing 5 minutes of fluoroscopy time during a procedure. Assume that the patient's entrance exposure is 3 R/min (typical for an average-size patient) and that 0.1% of the radiation is scattered at 90°, 1 m from the beam axis. The total exposure to the surface of the physician's lead apron would be

$$(3\,\text{R/min}) \times 0.001 \times 5\,\text{min} \times 4 = 60\ \text{mR}.$$

The factor of 4 is due to the ratio of 1 m to 0.5 $m^2$ to account for the geometry. Since the apron will absorb at least 95% of the incident radiation, the exposure to the physician's trunk would be

$$60\,\text{mR} \times 0.05 = 3\,\text{mR}.$$

Thus, with this exposure for a single procedure the physician could perform 33 procedures per week and not exceed the recommended maximum permissible body dose. However, if the eyes were unprotected, the maximum dose to the lens would limit the number of procedures to just five (300 mrem/week divided by 60 mR/procedure). This illustrates the importance of wearing thyroid and eye shields. Figure 3.3 shows the amount of x-radiation that is transmitted by a lead apron (or thyroid shield) and protective eyeware. As can be seen in the plot, less than 3% of the incident radiation is trans-

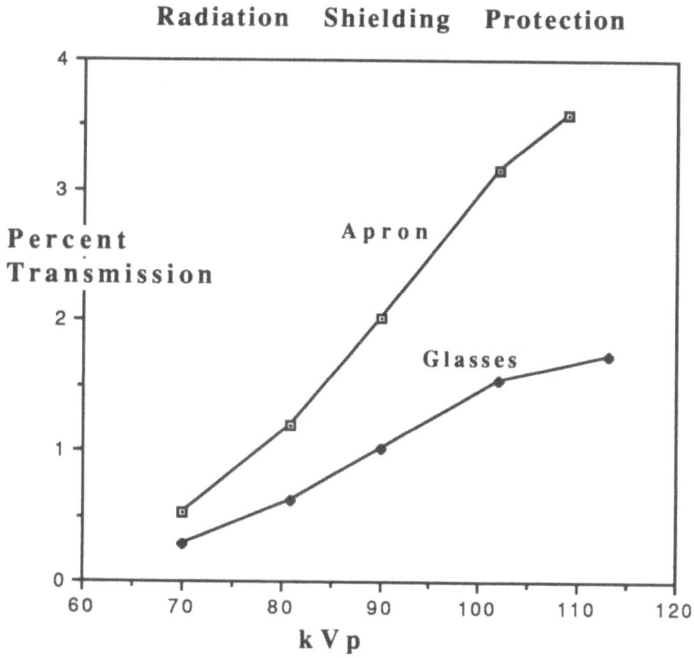


FIGURE 3.3. The plot shows the measured transmission of x-rays at different kilovoltages for a lead apron and protective glasses. The recommended lead aprons that should be worn for radiation protection are 0.5 mm lead equivalent. The protective eyeware that was tested is 0.75 mm lead equivalent.

mitted through these protective shields. In the previous example, a physician wearing protective eyeware and a thyroid shield would be limited only by the body exposure.

## Radiation Field Distribution

The main source of exposure to personnel during fluoroscopy examinations is scattered radiation from the patient and structures in the field of view of the x-ray beam. The volume of material in the primary beam consists of a cone with its apex at the focal spot of the x-ray tube and its base at the image receptor, the entrance window of the image intensifier tube. From this cone, x-rays are scattered nearly uniformly in all directions. Since the probability of Compton scattering is fairly constant along the axis of the cone, the intensity of scattered radiation will be proportional to the primary beam intensity with depth in the patient. The highest intensity of scattered radiation will occur on the side of the patient nearest to the x-ray tube and be about 10% of that value on the exit side of the patient. For this reason, the x-ray tube should be positioned under the table or on the opposite side of the patient from the personnel in order to reduce their exposure.

Two factors must be remembered when considering the scattered radiation spatial distribution: (1) the intensity decreases as the distance from the beam axis squared, and (2) at 1 m from the beam axis the magnitude of scattered radiation is about 0.1% of the patient's entrance exposure. The 0.1% is a conservative estimate of the actual amount of scatter, which depends on field size and patient thickness; it therefore contains a safety factor of 2 to 5 times. An example of the radial falloff of radiation exposure in the horizontal plane is given in Figure 3.4. The data in this demonstration were taken with a survey meter placed at certain radial distances from the source-to-receptor axis. The phantom was a 20 × 20 × 20 cm block of polystyrene and the technique factor used simulated a typical fluoros-

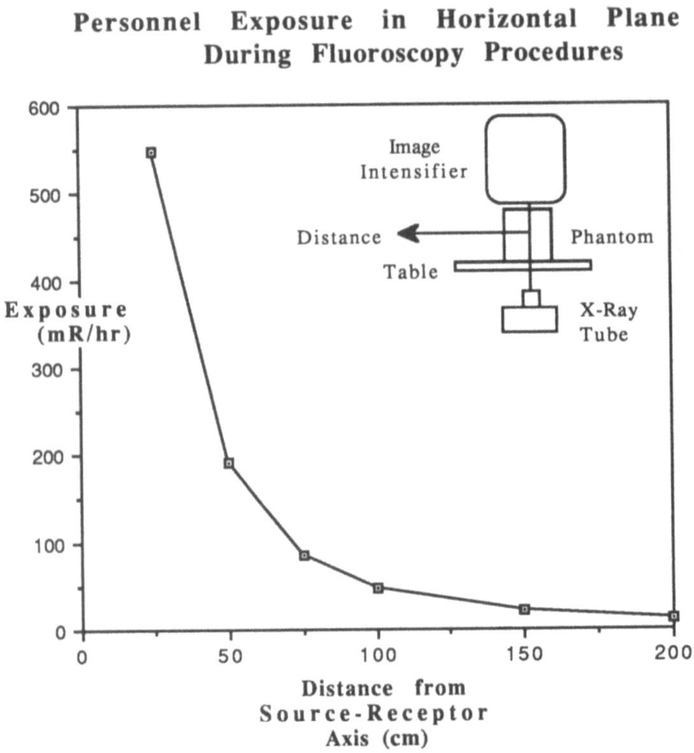


**FIGURE 3.4.** The measured exposure varies as the reciprocal of the distance from the source–image receptor axis squared. The x-ray technique factors used in this demonstration were 80 kVp and 2 mA. The phantom consisted of a cube, 20 cm on a side, of polystyrene.

copy application—80 kVp and 2 mA. As can be seen in the plot, the intensity decreases by a factor of four as the distance goes from 50 cm to 100 cm. Working backward from the exposure at 1 m (50 mR/hr), we can estimate the phantom's entrance exposure:

$$(50 \text{ mR/hr}) * (1000)/(60 \text{ min/hr}) = 5/6 \text{ R/min}.$$

In an actual measurement it was 2.2 R/min. Using the rule of thumb factor of 0.1% of the entrance exposure for the calculation of scattered radiation at 1 m results in a safety margin of 1.8 times. The rule of thumb factor will always be an overestimate of the actual exposure to scattered radiation.

Figure 3.5 shows the exposure distribution in the vertical plane. The isoexposure lines clearly illustrate the greater intensity of radiation on the beam entrance side of the phantom. To use the information in these two figures for different technique factors, simply multiply the exposure rate in the figure by

$$(\text{new mA}/2) * (\text{new kVp}/80)^2.$$

## Recommendations to Reduce Radiation Exposure

In keeping with the principle of radiation protection against ionizing radiation exposure "as low as reasonably achievable" (ALARA), the following techniques as recommended in the literature[9] are suggested for routine use.

1. Always obey the rules of radiation protection—time, distance, and shielding. These three parameters are under the control of the system operator. You can minimize the fluoroscopy time and position your personnel

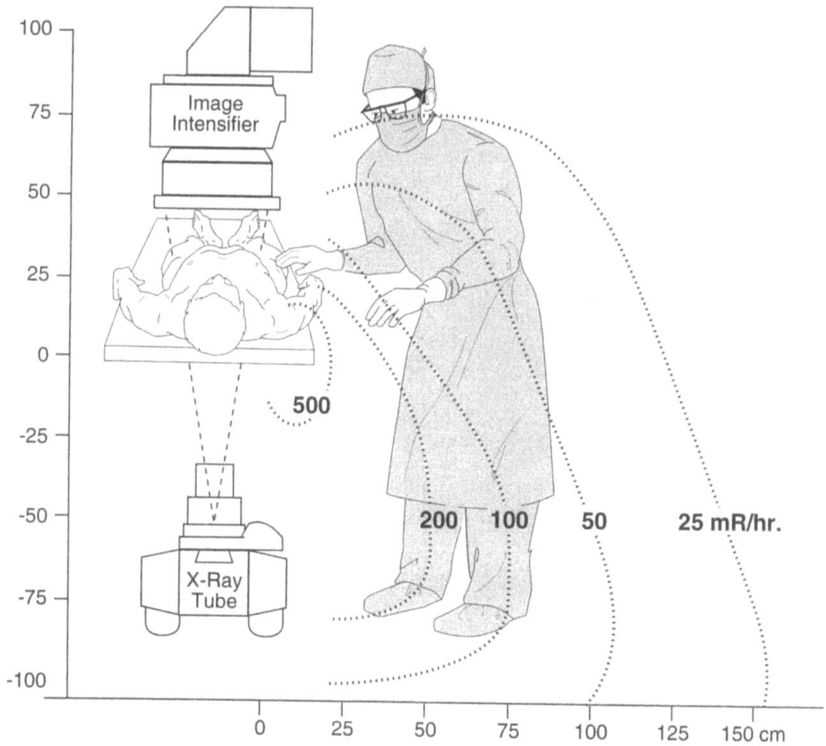


**FIGURE 3.5.** The scattered radiation is more intense on the entrance side of the x-ray beam. To minimize radiation exposure, personnel should work on the image intensifier side of the patient.

either behind appropriate barriers or at a safer distance from the radiation source.

2. Most modern C-arms are equipped with a pulsed fluoroscopy mode, where the x-ray tube is pulsed in synchronization with the television frame rate. This results in an exposure reduction of 3 to 10 times. A last image hold feature will also reduce fluoroscopy time.
3. Some automatic exposure systems give the operator three choices for input exposure to the image intensifier—low, medium, and high. If sufficient image quality can be obtained with the use of the low setting, then a reduction in radiation exposure of possibly 50% can be achieved.
4. To keep the scattered radiation intensity as low as possible, set the minimum useful field size with the collimator and keep the image intensifier in close proximity to the patient.

In summary, these techniques can easily be used to reduce or keep to a minimum the radiation exposure of both patients and personnel. Always be sure to properly wear your film badges, so that an accurate record of your radiation exposure is recorded. If you have any questions regarding radiation protection or wish to obtain another opinion concerning existing exposure levels for the procedures that you perform, consult your radiation safety officer.

## References


1. *Limitation of Exposure to Ionizing Radiation.* NCRP Report No. 116. Bethesda, MD. National Council on Radiation Protection and Measurements, 1993.
2. Curry TS, Dowdey JE, Murry RC. *Christensen's Physics of Diagnostic Radiology.* Malverne, PA: Lea & Febiger, 1990.
3. Mistretta CA. X-ray image intensifiers. In: Haus AG, ed. *The Physics of Medical Imaging: Recording*

*System Measurements and Techniques*. New York: American Institute of Physics, 1979;182–205.
4. Sprawls P. *Physical Principles of Medical Imaging*. Rockville, MD: Aspen, 1987.
5. *Structural Shielding Design and Evaluation for Medical Use of X-rays and Gamma Rays of Energies up to 10 MeV*. NCRP Report No. 49. Bethesda, MD: National Council on Radiation Protection and Measurements, 1976.
6. *Federal Performance Standard for Diagnostic X-Ray Systems and Their Major Components*. Federal Register Vol. 59, No. 96. Washington, DC: U.S. Government Printing Office, 1994.
7. *Radiation Protection for Medical and Allied Health Personnel*. NCRP Report No. 105. Bethesda, MD: National Council on Radiation Protection and Measurements, 1989.
8. Sanders R, Koval KJ, et al. Exposure of the orthopaedic surgeon to radiation. *J Bone Joint Surg* 1993;75-A:326–330.
9. Goldstone KE, Wright IH, et al. Radiation exposure to the hands of orthopaedic surgeons under fluoroscopic x-ray control. *Br J Radiol* 1993;66: 899–901.

# 4
# Intracapsular Hip Fractures

Stanley E. Asnis and Richard F. Kyle

Hip fractures represent a major component of health care in the United States. Current estimates of hip fractures are at approximately 250,000 per year.[1] The fractured hip represents a significant contributor to morbidity and disability of the elderly and is associated with increased mortality in the first year after fracture of approximately 12–20% higher than in persons of similar age and gender who have not suffered a fracture.[2] The average age of fracture is 78 years for women and 72 years for men. Women sustain approximately 80% of these fractures and the fracture rate doubles for each decade after the age of 50. In those patients who survive fracture, almost half spend time in a long-term care institution[1] and 15–25% for at least one year.[2] Because of its frequency among the fastest growing portion of our population, hip fractures represent a major health concern with costs to society that exceed $7 billion annually.[3]

## Structural Anatomy

In the adult hip the neck-shaft angle is approximately $130° \pm 7°$ and the femoral neck anteversion is $10° \pm 7°$ and does not vary by sex.[4,5] The femoral head is slightly oblong with an average size of 40 to 60 mm.[6] The hip capsule is attached anteriorly at the intertrochanteric line, whereas posteriorly the lateral half of the femoral neck is extracapsular.[7] The portion of the neck that is intracapsular has no periostium, and fractures must heal by endosteal union. The femoral head and neck are supported by a trabecular network as initially described in 1838 by Ward.[8] The primary compression trabeculae concentrate at the medical femoral neck, then fan out under the superior dome of the femoral head (Figure 4.1). The primary tensile trabeculae make an arch from the fovea medially to the lateral femoral cortex just distal to the greater trochanter laterally. Secondary compressive and tensile trabeculare orient themselves according to Wolf's law to increase the structural strength. Singh et al.[9] have found that with aging and osteopenia there is a progressive sequential loss of these trabeculae, thus decreasing structural strength. The trochanteric and secondary compression and tensile trabeculae are lost first, especially in Ward's triangle. As osteopenia continues the primary tension trabeculae become interrupted and lost, followed lastly by the loss of primary compression trabeculae. In that the average age of patients with intracapsular hip fracture is in the seventh decade and those patients with an intracapsular hip fracture may represent a more osteopenic population, femoral head and neck bone density are most important in fixation. The trabecular bone within the femoral neck is often of very low density and is unable to support the fixation device alone, necessitating the utilization of the femoral neck cortical bone for support. Bone density studies of cadaveric femoral heads have shown that the bone in the middle and superior femoral head is superior to the weaker bone of the inferior head[4,10] (Figure 4.2). These studies are consistent with the trabecular patterns. The most dense bone is in the central head, whereas the posterior inferior quadrant is usually the weakest.[10]

## Clinical Relevance

The geometry of placement of fixation screws is determined by the anatomy of the femoral head and neck. The femoral neck often is a relatively

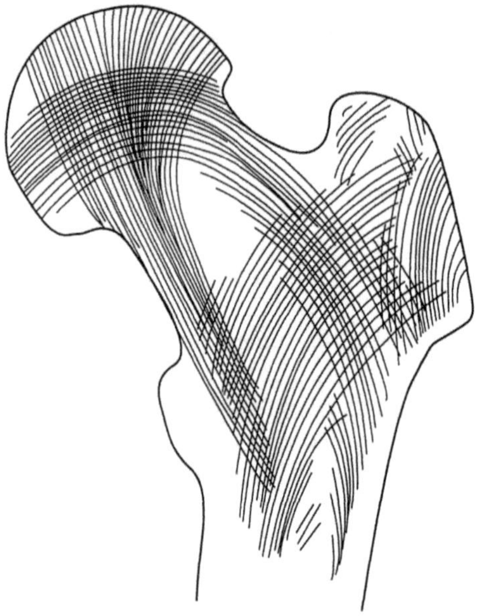

**FIGURE 4.1.** The femoral head and neck are supported by a trabecular network. The primary compressive and tension trabeculae coalesce in the center of the head giving this area the greatest bone density. The primary compression trabeculae of the superior dome of the head is second in bone density.

hollow tube in regard to bone support of the fixation device. Unlike a dynamic compression hip screw and side plate, cannulated screw heads buttress against the femoral cortex and threads lock in the femoral head. If forces are applied to direct the head fragment inferiorly or posteriorly and the screw shafts are away from the endosteal cortical femoral neck, the femoral head and screws may drift until a screw's shaft comes against the endosteal cortex[11,12] (Figure 4.3). Screw thread fixation in the head is dependent on the density of the trabecular bone. Screw threads placed in the middle and superior head have superior holding power to those in an inferior position.

## Vascular Anatomy

Crock[13,14] has given a clear description to the arterial supply to the femoral head. There are three major groups of vessels: (1) an extracapsular ring located at the base of the femoral neck, (2) ascending cervical branches on the surface of the femoral neck, and (3) arteries of the ligamentum teres or foveal arteries (Figure 4.4). An extracapsular arterial ring at the base of the femoral neck is formed by a large branch of the medial circumflex artery posteriorly and branches of the lateral circumflex artery anteriorly. From this ring arises the ascending cervical branches that are anatomically described as the anterior, posterior, medial, and lateral groups. The lateral ascending cervical arteries appear to supply most of the blood supply to superior femoral head and lateral neck. The ascending cervical vessels then go into a less-distinct vascular ring at the articular cartilage-neck junction referred to as the subsynovial

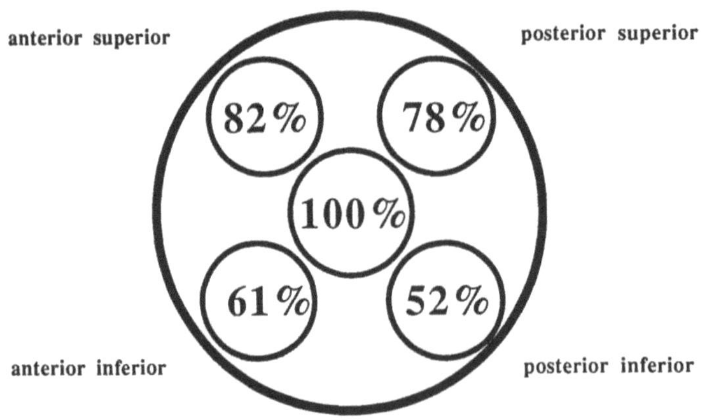


**FIGURE 4.2.** Bone density of cadaveric femoral heads. The middle and superior femoral head is denser than the inferior head. (From the data of Crowell et al.[10])

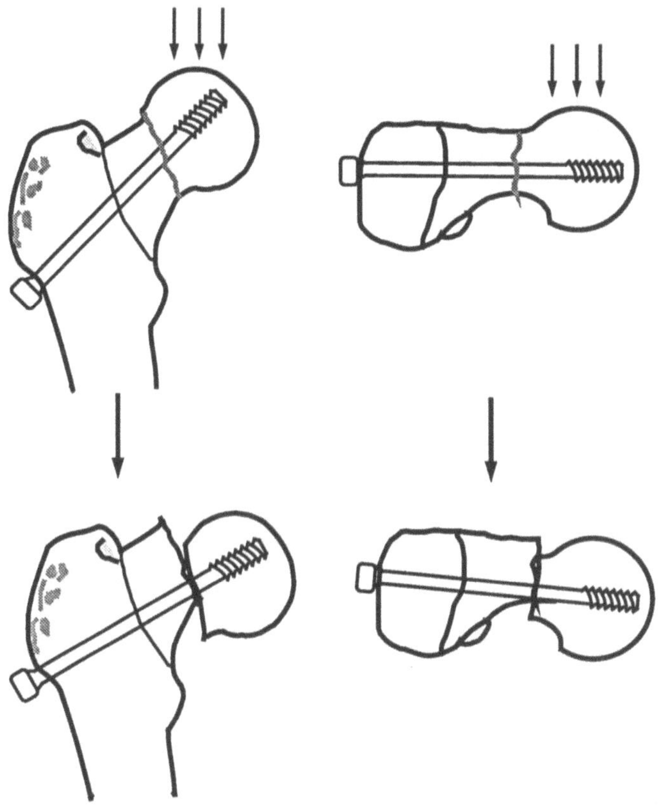

**FIGURE 4.3.** If forces are applied to direct the head fragment inferiorly or posteriorly and the screw shafts are away from the endosteal cortical femoral neck, the femoral head and screws may drift until a screw's shaft comes against the endosteal cortex.

intraarticular arterial ring.[15] From this ring vessels penetrate the femoral head and are then referred to as the epiphyseal arteries. The lateral epiphyseal artery is thought to supply most of the blood to the weight-bearing area of the femoral head. The lateral epiphyseal artery system passes within the posterior retinaculum of Weitbrecht.[14,16–19] More simply and probably as clinically relevant and accurate, Swiontkowski[20] describes the lateral epiphyseal artery as the terminal branch of the medial circumflex artery supplying the weight-bearing surface of the femoral head in 90% of adults. The terminal branch of the lateral circumflex artery supplies the inferior portion of the femoral head. The artery of the ligamentum teres is a branch of the obturator or medial circumflex artery. Only one third of patients are thought to have a substantial portion of the femoral head supplied by these vessels.[21] These vessels, however, may be important in revascularization of the femoral head after fixation. A very limited supply of blood is supplied through intraosseous vessels that come directly from the marrow below.

## Clinical Relevance

In a nondisplaced fracture there is far less chance of direct damage to epiphyseal arteries. Bleeding into a capsule that has not been disrupted may cause increased pressure and decreased blood supply by tamponade. The benefits of aspiration and capsulotomy during the procedure are still debated.[22–26] The displaced fractures are likely to have direct arterial injury by disruption or kinking. The Garden stage III and Garden stage IV fractures my differ here. The Garden stage IV fracture is thought to tear the posterior retinaculum of Weitbrecht and thus sustains a greater vascular insult. Early reduction

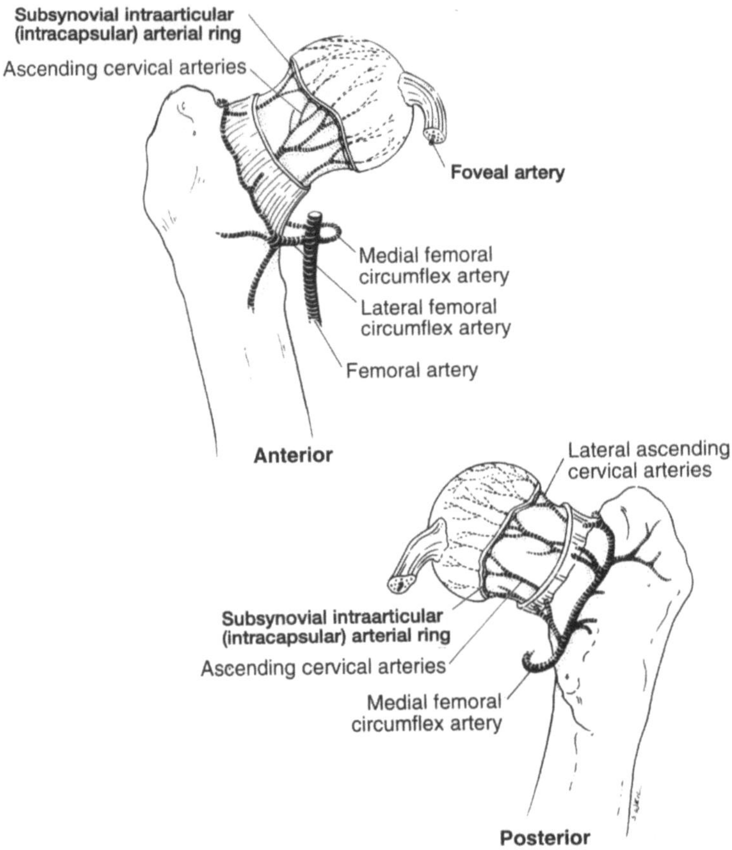


**FIGURE 4.4.** The arterial supply of the femoral head. The lateral epiphyseal vessels as terminal branches of the medial circumflex artery supply blood to the majority of the weight-bearing surface of the femoral head in most adults.

and fixation may have a positive role by unkinking intact vessels, but this is still speculative.

# Classification

Although there are several classifications for femoral neck fractures, two will be described. The Pauwels's classification[27] divides fractures into three types based on the angle formed with the horizontal plane on radiographs. Type I is a fracture 30° from the horizontal, type II is 50°, and type III is 70°. Garden[28] stated that the fracture line was actually remarkably constant in the range of 50° from the horizontal in the frontal radiograph. He found that the radiographic projection of the spirally disposed femoral neck changes with different degrees of rotation and hence the vertical appearance of the fracture. The obliquity projected on the radiograph varied with the rotation of the distal fragment more than the fracture line itself. Garden's classification[28–30] is based on the degree of displacement of the fracture (Figure 4.5). It is functional and appears to be the classification most widely used today. A Garden stage I fracture is an incomplete or an impacted fracture. A Garden stage II fracture is a complete fracture without displacement. A Garden stage III fracture is a complete fracture with displacement. The retinaculum of Weitbrecht remains intact and maintains continuity between the proximal and distal frag-

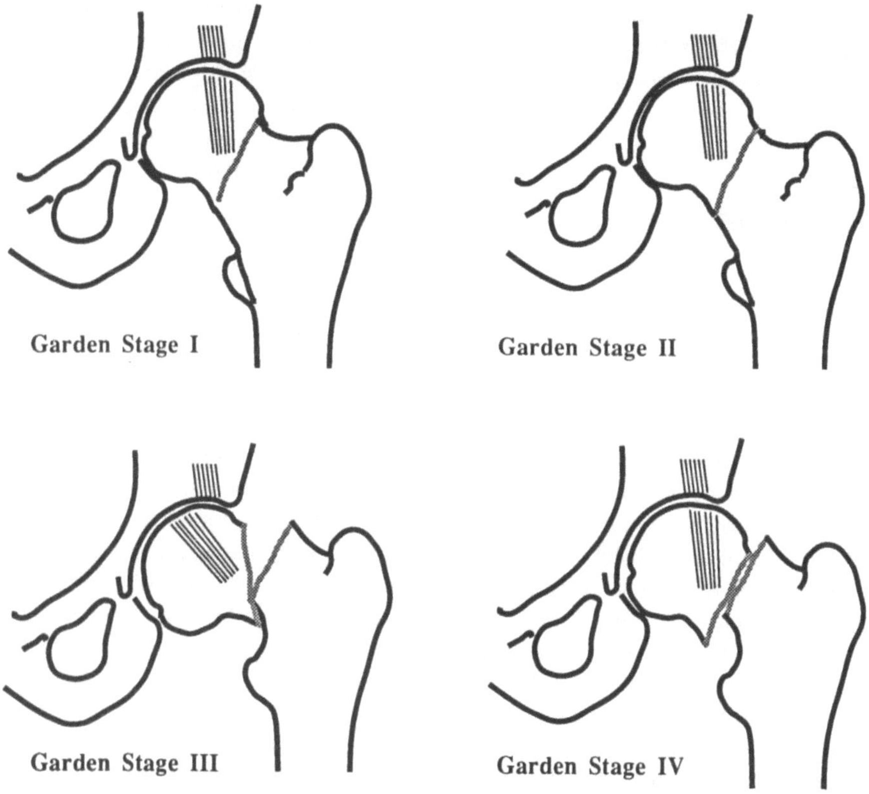


**FIGURE 4.5.** Garden's classification is based on the degree of displacement of the fracture.

ments. By being displaced and yet tethered by the retinaculum, the femoral head becomes tilted in the acetabulum and thus the trabecular pattern of the femoral head does not line up with that of the acetabulum. A Garden stage IV fracture is a completely displaced fracture with all continuity between the proximal and distal fragments disrupted. The femoral head is able to spin free and usually has its trabecular pattern line up with that of the acetabulum. Many surgeons find it difficult to differentiate between the Garden stage III and Garden stage IV fractures. The Garden stage IV fracture my have the femoral head rotated in the acetabulum because of the impingement of the distal fragment on the proximal fragment by the way the subject is lying during the radiograph. Several surgeons have simply combined the Garden stage I and II fractures into nondisplaced fractures and the Garden stage III and IV into displaced fractures.

## Clinical Relevance

The nondisplaced or Garden stage I and II fractures are fixed in situ. The valgus-impacted fractures are left in place and fixed. A capsulotomy may be considered for tamponade. Weight bearing is usually immediate after fixation. The incidence of nonunion is rare and since the vessels are intact the occurrence of avascular necrosis should be low. The displaced or Garden stage III and IV fractures can be expected to have a higher complication rate. Theoretically the Garden stage III fracture has a better prognosis for two reasons: the posterior retinaculum of Weitbrecht is intact and the lateral epiphyseal artery system is more likely to be intact. A good reduction is also more readily obtainable. With the patient in traction and the posterior retinaculum intact, internal rotation reduces the fracture. The posterior retinaculum acts like the binding of a book as it is closed. In the displaced fracture in the elderly patient with osteoporosis, the decision between fixation and arthroplasty becomes an issue.

## Treatment Controversy

The displaced intracapsular hip fracture can be treated in two ways: immediate prosthetic replacement or internal fixation. Although prosthetic replacement is a more-definitive mode of treatment, some studies have shown a higher morbidity and mortality rate than with internal fixation[31–35] and in the more-active individual this may require conversion to a total hip replacement.[36,37] Immediate total hip arthroplasty has been shown to have a far higher morbidity and mortality rate when performed for an acute fracture than in the patient with chronic arthritis. Franzen et al.[38] found the age- and sex-adjusted risk of prosthetic failure in total hip arthroplasties performed for femoral neck fracture had complication rates 2.5 times higher than after primary arthroplasty performed for osteoarthritis ($p = 0.012$). Coates and Armour[39] followed 85 patients with primary total hip replacements for displaced femoral neck fractures and found a much higher complication rate than that found for elective joint replacements. There was a 7% mortality within the first postoperative month, 7% bacteriologic-proven infections, and an 8% dislocation rate. Many other studies have found that the dislocation rate is significantly higher in the group of fracture patients.[40–43] Prosthetic survival has also been found to be shorter in fracture patients than in replacements performed for arthritis.[44,45] Nilsson et al.[46] compared one group of patients 4 to 12 years after a primary hemiarthroplasty with another group that had secondary total hip replacement as a salvage procedure for complications of reduction and fixation of intracapsular fractures. Function was classified and the Nottingham Health Profile questionnaire was applied. The two groups were comparable in regard to age, sex, and social status. The secondary total hip replacement group used walking aids to a lesser extent and experienced fewer problems in several aspects of life. The authors concluded that secondary total hip replacement in patients with healing complication following primary osteosynthesis gave better long-term functional capacity than that obtained with a primary hemiarthroplasty.

Reduction and fixation of the intracapsular hip fracture with multiple pins or screws has been reported as a procedure of much lower morbidity and mortality than prosthetic arthroplasty.[31,34,35,47,48] With improved methods of fixation and a tendency toward earlier weight bearing, internal fixation becomes a more attractive mode of treatment, especially in younger, more active patients. Patients with healed fractures have been found to have fewer problems with sleep and housework, and they generally function better than patients with a total hip replacement following their injury.[45] Those patients who develop the complication of nonunion or osteonecrosis can undergo total hip arthroplasty as a delayed elective procedure with very low morbidity and mortality.[38,39]

### Clinical Relevance

Internal fixation of displaced intracapsular hip fractures has several advantages in many patients. Although statistics vary, it appears that the risks of death or major complication is lower following internal fixation than immediate prosthetic replacement. For the 70% to 75% of patients who heal their fracture without later developing osteonecrosis, their own femoral head functions as well as, or better than, a prosthesis. For those who have a problem with union or later develop osteonecrosis, a well-planned elective total hip arthroplasty is usually a safe procedure. The risks of medical complications appear far lower at a delayed time than immediately after the fracture. In the more-active individual a primary arthroplasty does not perform as well as a total hip replacement. Primary total hip arthroplasty right after fracture has a higher complication rate and may not function as well as a delayed total hip procedure, which is required only in those patients who have complications after internal fixation.

## Indications for Internal Fixation

The authors' indication for cannulated screw fixation includes all nonpathologic nondisplaced or Garden stage I and II fractures. Age is not a factor. The displaced or Garden stage III and IV fractures can be treated by reduction and internal fixation or total or hemiarthroplasty. The authors favor reduction and fixation for all patients other than those in whom a primary prosthetic replacement is required. Prosthetic replacement is indicated for (1) failure to achieve a satisfactory reduction other than in the younger patient, (2) fracture of the femoral head or dislocation of the femoral head with fracture of the femoral neck, (3) fractures more than 5 days old, (4) pathologic fractures, (5) fractures in an abnormal hip, i.e., rheumatoid or osteoarthritis, (6) fractures with significant femoral neck comminution with a butterfly fragment of 1 cm or more, and (7) a Garden stage IV fracture in a patient over 75 years of age and a Singh classification of III or less.

In the younger patient, i.e., under 55, all attempts are made to obtain a satisfactory reduction. If this is not possible or there is posterior neck comminution, then open reduction and a bone grafting procedure should be considered.[50]

## Potential Complications of Internal Fixation

### Problems in Healing

Multiple cannulated parallel screws were introduced for the fixation of intracapsular hip fractures in 1980 in an attempt to increase the accuracy of fixation and decrease the complications following intracapsular fracture.[51,52] It appears that the rate of successful osteosynthesis has improved significantly with this technique; however, the incidence of osteonecrosis may be unchanged. In our long-term follow-up study of 141 patients treated with cannulated screws, only five had a loss of position or nonunion.[51] This gave a 96% chance of successful osteosynthesis. It must be emphasized, however, that the internal fixation of the displaced intracapsular hip fracture in not a simple procedure. A stable reduction is essential and the fixation screws must be placed accurately.

### Osteonecrosis

Osteonecrosis remains the main complication following the internal fixation of intracapsular fractures. A displaced intracapsular fracture has a devastating effect on the blood supply of the femoral head. Following autoradiograms on femoral head specimens of patients given $^{32}P$ prior to prosthetic arthroplasty for acute intracapsular fractures, Calandruccio and Anderson[53] reported that 22% of the femoral heads were completely vascular, 33% completely avascular, and 47% were partially avascular. Catto's[54,55] meticulous histologic studies of whole femoral heads obtained at least 16 days after transcervical fracture showed 34% of the femoral heads were completely vascular, 55% were partially avascular, and 11% were totally avascular.[55] Sevitt's[56] arteriographic and histologic necropsy of the femoral heads with intracapsular fractures showed total or partial necrosis in 84% of the specimens. It is apparent that the great majority of patients sustain a significant vascular injury at the time of the fracture, yet only approximately 20–30% of patients who undergo internal fixation develop roentgenographic evidence of avascular necrosis with clinical segmental collapse.

It is likely that the majority of displaced femoral neck fractures undergo significant revascularization following internal fixation. During this period, the fracture heals and most patients function well even though a significant area of the femoral head may still be partially avascular. Many of the original studies on intracapsular fractures gave rates of osteonecrosis based on the false assumption that most segmental collapse would be evident by 2 years. It appears that revascularization for the femoral head is a very slow process and in some patients never complete. In our long-term follow-up study of 141 patients treated with cannulated screws, there was an 11% rate of avascular necrosis at

2 years and an overall 22% incidence after an average follow-up of 8 years (minimum follow-up 5 years); three patients first developed clinical symptoms and segmental collapse after 5 years.[51] Segmental collapse may develop long after the initial fracture; however, function of the patient is the primary goal of treatment. It appears that many patients have no symptoms and excellent function even though their femoral head is partially avascular. Frequently symptoms appear only after the ultimate development of segmental collapse. Once the symptoms do appear, elective total hip arthroplasty appears safe and extremely effective, with results equivalent to those of total hip replacements for patients with primary osteoarthritis.

## Reduction

The most important objective in the treatment of the displaced intracapsular hip fracture is to obtain stable bony support of the femoral head on the femoral neck. The fixation is used to increase stability by compressing the fracture and then maintaining the reduction by neutralizing forces acting on the hip. Even if a patient is non–weight bearing, going from a sitting to a standing position creates three times as much force across the hip as does weight bearing.[57] The factors that decrease stability are comminution of the posterior femoral neck and poor reduction. Rubin et al.[58] designed an in vitro mechanical fracture model fixed with Knowles pins that evaluated several factors including anatomically good and poor reductions with and without posterior comminution. The most important factor producing instability was femoral neck comminution, followed by the quality of reduction.[58] Major comminution of the femoral neck is a contraindication for reduction and fixation and hemiarthroplasty usually becomes the preferred treatment; however, in the younger patient an open reduction and bone graft should be considered.[50] The goal of reduction is a position as close to a Garden index of 160/180 (AP/lateral) as possible.[28–30] On the anteroposterior radiograph the primary compression trabeculae should ideally be at an angle of 160° to the longitudinal axis of the femoral shaft, whereas on the lateral radiograph these compression trabeculae should lie in a straight line or 180° with the femoral shaft axis (Figure 4.6). The Garden index is an expression of the angle of the compression trabeculae on the anteroposterior radiograph over (/) the angle of the compression trabeculae on the lateral radiograph. A perfect anatomic reduction is therefore expressed as 160/180. A good reduction has the medial femoral head-neck fragment well supported by the medial neck of the femur. This should be either anatomic or with the head-neck fragment in slight lateral translation in relation to the supporting femoral neck. Slight valgus is acceptable, varus is not. Slight valgus with the superior femoral neck impacted beneath the subchondral bone of the superior femoral head usually provides a very stable configuration (Figure 4.7a).[5] On the

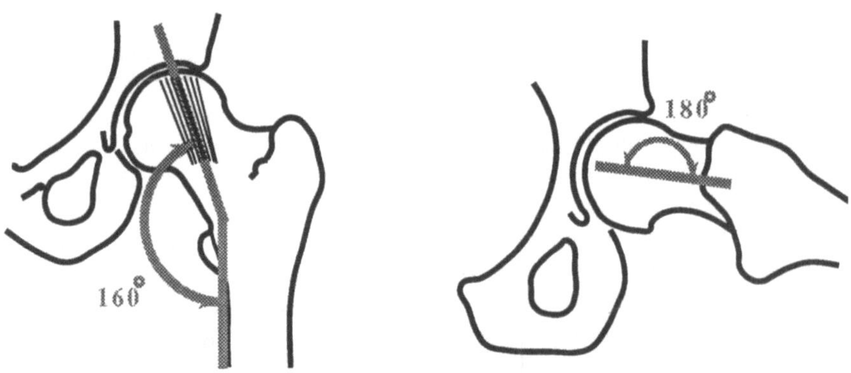


**FIGURE 4.6.** Garden index. On the anteroposterior radiograph the primary compression trabeculae should ideally be at an angle of 160° to the longitudinal axis of the femoral shaft, whereas on the lateral radiograph these compression trabeculae should lie in a straight line or 180° with the femoral shaft axis.

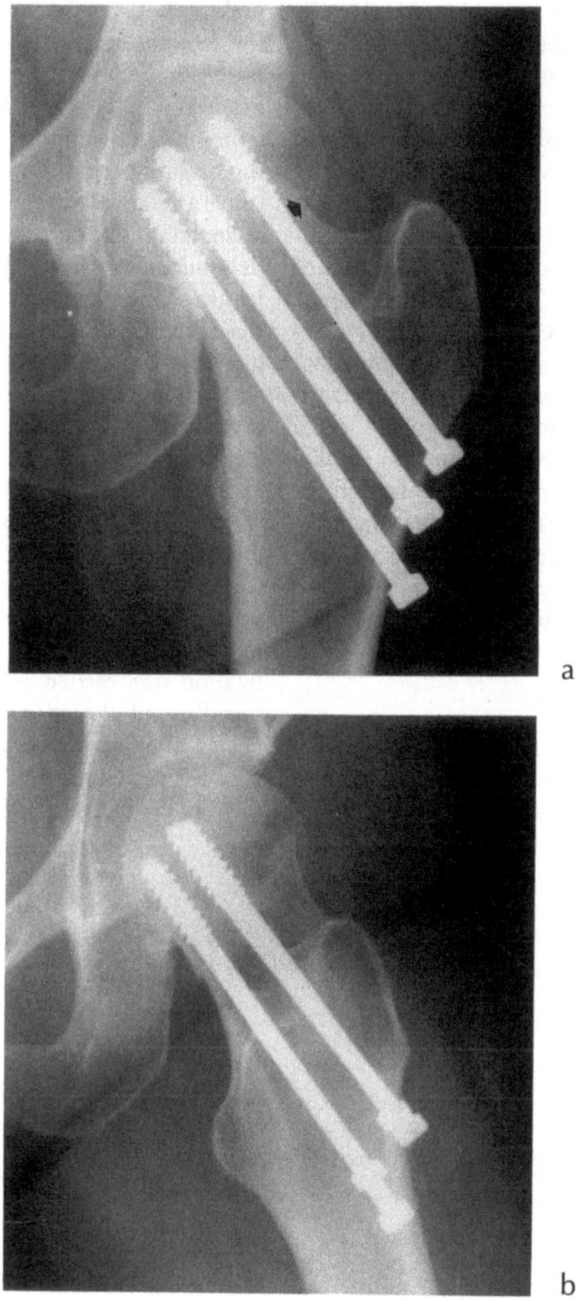

**FIGURE 4.7.** A Garden stage IV fracture was reduced on the fracture table and fixed with four 6.5-mm cannulated screws placed in a diamond configuration. (a) This AP radiograph of the hip shows the support of the femoral head by the medial femoral neck. The arrow depicts the impaction of the superior femoral neck beneath the subchondral bone of the superior femoral head. This is referred to as the "hat hook" position and often represents a very stable configuration. The most distal screw shaft lies along the medial neck, preventing the femoral head from falling into varus. (b) The lateral radiograph demonstrates the posterior neck of the distal fragment supporting that of the head-neck fragment. The posterior screw lies along the posterior femoral neck preventing the head from displacing posteriorly. (Reprinted with permission from Asnis and Wanek-Sgaglione.[51])

lateral view alignment is again important, with the posterior neck of the distal fragment supporting that of the head-neck fragment[59] (Figure 4.7b).

The authors accomplish reduction with traction on a fracture table with the leg in neutral flexion, neutral rotation, and 10° of abduction. The leg is then internally rotated as far as possible; then the leg is backed off into a position of 15° of internal rotation. The medial neck spike of the fragment should be well supported by the femoral neck of the femur. With a cannulated screw system some overdistraction is permissible since the fracture can later be guided into a good position and compressed once the parallel guide pins are in place or with the lag of the parallel cannulated screws. In the great majority of cases without major femoral neck comminution this maneuver will yield a satisfactory and stable position. In very rare cases an open reduction may be necessary prior to fixation.

## Fixation

The purpose of the fixation screws are (1) to lock the fracture in a position in which the femoral neck gives bone-against-bone support to the femoral head-neck fragment, (2) to prevent posterior and varus migration of the femoral head, and (3) to be parallel so as to maintain bone-on-bone support as the fracture settles in the healing period. There are several reasons for using a cannulated screw system: (1) the smaller-diameter guide pins can be used to accurately determine the screw position as well as the length, (2) cannulated screw systems improve the accuracy of screw placement by supplying jigs that can very accurately place guide pins, and (3) with parallel screws excellent compression can be produced atraumatically by the lag effect of the screws.

Strömqvist et al.[60] studied 22 patients with femoral neck fractures with $^{99m}$Tc-MDP scintimetry performed before and again shortly after surgery. Of eight patients with an intermediate uptake before operation, six showed a decrease in the femoral uptake after surgery. Fracture fixation was carried out by impaction with the four-flanged Rydell nail. It appeared that vascular damage could be produced by fracture fixation with a device that was impacted into place. Gentle, controlled compression with lag screws

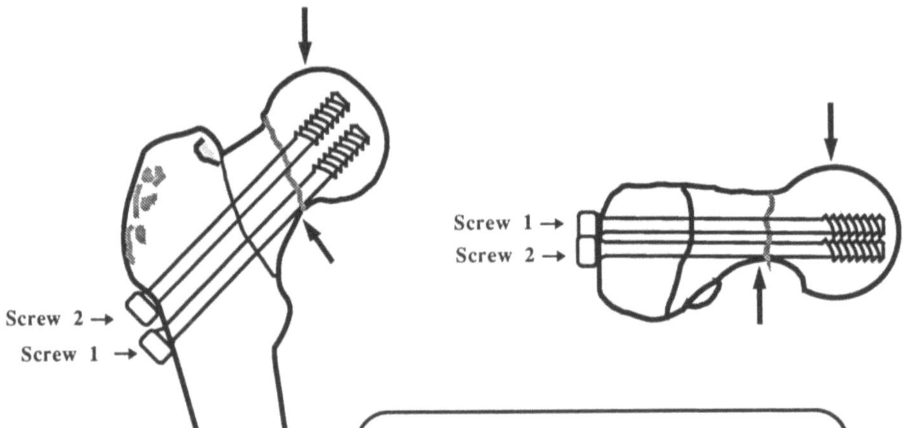


| | AP position | Lateral position |
|---|---|---|
| Screw 1 | Inferior | Midline |
| Screw 2 | Midneck | Posterior |

**FIGURE 4.8.** Screw positioning. In the AP plane the most distal screw's shaft (Screw 1) rests on the medial femoral neck. A second screw (screw 2) should be at the mid-head level on the AP projection and should rest on the posterior femoral neck in the lateral plane.

may be safer in protecting the vascular status of the femoral head.

## Geometry of Screw Position in the Femoral Neck and Head

To prevent femoral head migration, screw positioning is critical (Figures 4.7, 4.8, and 4.9). The most distal single screw passes through the femoral cortex, its shaft rests on the supporting medial neck, and its threads fix the inferior femoral head. For the femoral head to fall into varus, this screw's threads must first cut through the femoral head. In the lateral plane a second screw should be placed posteriorly so that it rests on the posterior neck of the distal fragment at the mid-head level on the anteroposterior plane. For posterior head migration to occur, its threads must cut through the head. The positions of these two screws are crucial.

Martens et al.[11] showed that internal fixation using multiple Knowles pins had a high rate of failure unless the most distal screw rested on the cortical bone of the medial aspect of the femoral neck (Figure 4.3). Lindequist[12] evaluated 87 patients who had internal fixation of intracapsular fractures with two von Bahr screws. He found that the posterior placement of the proximal screw and the inferior placement of the distal screw improved the rate of fracture union. Studies in Sweden utilizing fixation with only two hook pins in these two key locations gave fair clinical results.[61–64] Strömqvist et al.[64] reviewed 300 cases of femoral neck fractures fixed with two hook pins. In nondisplaced fractures, 95% healed with satisfactory osteosynthesis, whereas in the displaced fractures there was a 26% redisplacement or nonunion.

Deyerle[65] found that multiple pins placed around the periphery of the femoral neck compressing the fracture gave rotatory stability. He believed that this method would yield improved osteosynthesis. Three or four parallel cannulated screws placed peripherally around the femoral neck compressing the fracture are as atraumatic and also yield excellent rotatory stability. In Garden stage I and II fractures, a third screw at

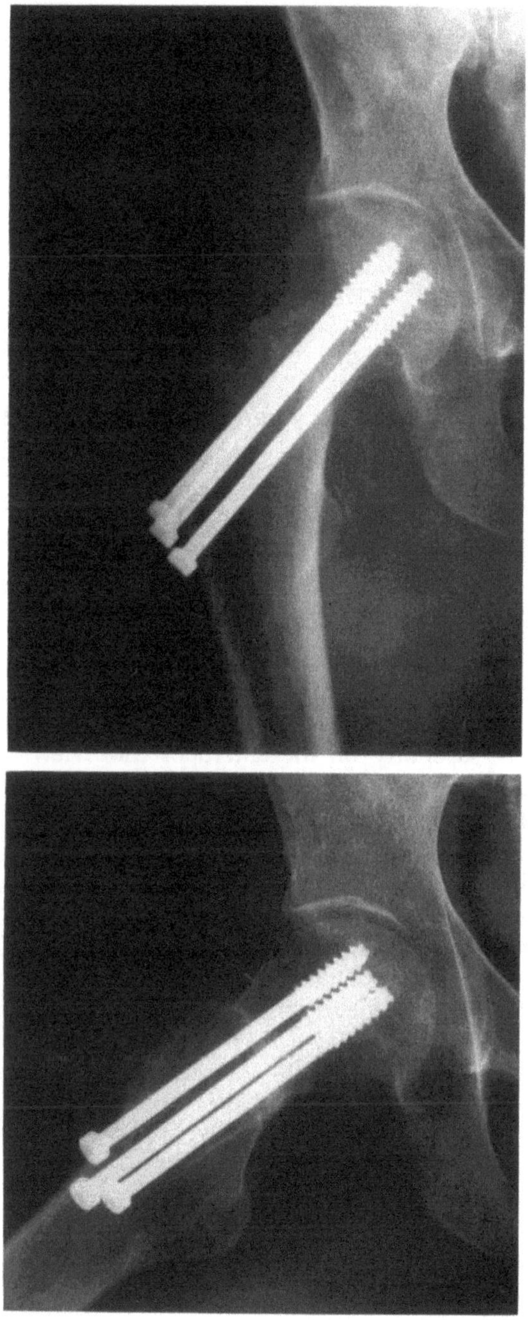

a

b

**FIGURE 4.9.** A Garden stage II fracture in a renal dialysis patient was fixed with three 6.5-mm cannulated screws placed in an inverted triangle configuration. (a) The distal screw's shaft is placed close to the medial femoral neck. The proximal two screws are placed at or slightly above the mid-femoral head level. (b) The posterior screw's shaft rests close to the posterior femoral neck.

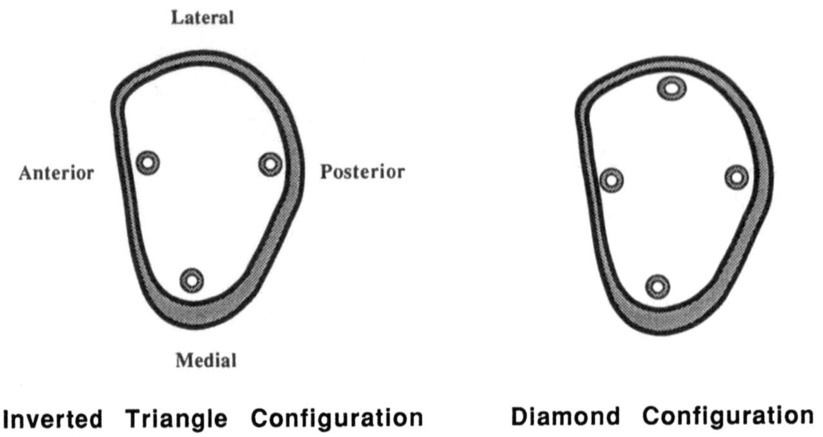


**FIGURE 4.10.** Position of screws in the femoral neck. The cross section of the femoral neck shows the three-screw inverted triangle and the four-screw diamond configurations.

the mid-head level on the anteroposterior view and in an anterior position on the lateral view gives this additional stability (Figure 4.9). In the Garden stage III and IV fractures a fourth screw superiorly on the anteroposterior view and midline in the lateral view further supplements fixation (Figures 4.7 and 4.10). Studies by Swiontkowski et al.[66] and Springer et al.[67] have suggested that the fourth screw added little in additional fixation; however, both of these authors used models that represented a Garden stage II fracture and not the Garden stage III or IV fracture with some comminution. The inverted triangle and diamond patterns of screw placement also fit well into the shape of the femoral neck. Although most mechanical models show the head loaded in the standing position, studies have shown that there is three times more force on the hip when going from sitting to standing than when walking.[57] The triangle and diamond patterns adapt well to the different forces applied to the hip in different body positions.

The distal screw should not enter the femoral cortex below the level of the lesser trochanter. No additional holes should be made at the level of the lesser trochanter. Since there is no side plate, weakness at this level can lead to a subtrochanteric fracture.[68] Two distal screw holes at the level of or distal to the lesser trochanter must be used with caution. Iatrogenic fractures can occur at this level propagating from a crack between the distal holes. There were no subtrochanteric fractures in our series of 141 patients.[51]

## Femoral Head Bone Density and Fixation Geometry

Fixation of the femoral head is also dependent on the holding power of the screw threads in the trabecular bone of the femoral head. Crowell et al.[10] and Benterud et al.[4] designed screw pullout models in which they found the previous recommendations of screw placement in the inferior and posterior-medial portions of the femoral head for better stability to be incorrect. In each of these studies screws were placed in different quadrants of femoral heads collected at autopsy and pullout tests performed (Figure 4.2). The inferior portion of the femoral heads was consistently the less dense, with significantly lower screw pullout strength ($p < .05$). The increased trabecular density of the central and superior femoral head gave far better fixation. Their data strongly favor the inverted triangle and diamond patterns for improved fixation. The trabecular patterns in the femoral head and neck go along with their data. We have found this also to be evident when reviewing patient radiographs. The center of the head where the tension and compression trabeculae both pass appears most dense, followed by the compression trabeculae in the superior femoral head. In a fracture patient with osteoporosis and/or osteopenia, the inferior head often clearly demonstrates the lack of trabeculae and minimal cancellous bone density.

# Authors' Preferred Procedure

## Cannulated Screw Systems

When choosing a cannulated screws system for fixation of the intracapsular fractures several features should be considered (also see Chapter 2).

### *Material*

Most cannulated screws systems offered today are made of titanium or stainless steel. Titanium offers a material that after fixation allows less artifact if diagnostic studies such as magnetic resonance imaging (MRI) or computed tomography (CT) scanning is later necessary about the hip. In its pure form titanium is highly resistant to corrosion but its drawback is a low yield and ultimate tensile strength. For this reason titanium "six four" alloy is usually used in trauma implants. This alloy has 5.5–6.5% aluminum and 3.5–4.5% vanadium with less than 0.01% impurities.[69] This material when properly heat treated or forged gives excellent mechanical properties. It is extremely resistant to corrosion. Titanium, however, is more notch sensitive than stainless steel and may require more force in removal after fracture healing.

Stainless steel has been the standard in trauma fixation devices throughout the years. The most popular form has been 316L, which has 17–20% chromium, 10–14% nickel, 2–4% molybdenum, less than 0.08% carbon, and the rest iron.[69] Forged 316L steel has excellent mechanical properties but is less resistant to in vivo corrosion than titanium. Recently 22-13-5 stainless steel has been used for strength, and it is superior to 316L steel. Cannulated screw systems are available in 316L or the stronger 22-13-5 alloys. These materials have all proven satisfactory in intracapsular hip fixation.

### *Guide Pin*

The guide pin should be stiff enough to maintain its position after passing through an alignment jig and passing through the dense bone of the femoral head. Its stiffness is dependent on the pin's outer diameter and material of construction. The threads at the end of the guide pin are present to maintain position and deter forward migration as a cannulated screw is passed over it. The junction of the thread and the shaft should be strong enough not to allow fatigue and breakage as the cannulated screw is passed. The guide pins should allow for easy and accurate depth measurements either directly from the pin or a direct reading depth gauge.

### *Screw Head*

Both round heads with a recessed hexagonal socket for the driver or heads with an outer hexagonal shape that use an external driving wrench are available. Although the outer wrench gives excellent mating and strength when mated with the driver, it has several disadvantages. The system is more bulky. Later removal of screws can be difficult with the outer hexagonal head. If there is any bony overgrowth around the head, the screw is locked in place and the wrench cannot be applied until an adequate amount of bone is removed. If there is some settling in healing and two heads come together, they become locked and again bone must be removed from around one screw to move the heads apart enough to apply the wrench. The round head with the recessed hexagonal socket is more readily removable with the round head spinning out of the bone or spinning off a neighboring head.

### *Screw Shaft*

The smooth screw shaft allows the screw to lag and compress the fracture. Its outer diameter must be strong enough to give adequate strength while still allowing a large enough cannulation for a guide pin of adequate dimension to make it of adequate strength and stiffness.

### Screw Thread

The length of the screw threads should be long enough to gain adequate holding power and short enough to fit in the femoral head without crossing the intracapsular fracture site. A thread length of approximately 20 mm has proven satisfactory. Because of the cancellous nature of the femoral head, a cancellous buttress thread is most commonly used. A self-cutting and -tapping tip is advantageous (see Figure 2.24). Pretapping over the guide pin other than at the femoral cortex reduces the ultimate holding power of the screw. The length of the cutting tip should be minimized to allow as much thread as possible for holding power. This can be obtained by cutting flutes with a positive rake. The back of the buttress thread may offer a reverse cutting flute to facilitate removal once the fracture has healed and the femoral cortex has reconstituted around the smooth shaft.

## Authors' Preferred Operative Technique

### Equipment

#### System 1

*Drill*: A 230-mm (9-inch) long 3.2-mm ($\frac{1}{8}$-inch) steel drill that can be used directly with a direct-reading 9-inch depth gauge. *Guide pin*: A 230-mm long 3.2-mm guide pin with a threaded tip and tapered root diameter (see Chapter 2). *Screw head*: Round head with an internal hexagon. *Screw thread*: Outer diameter—6.5 mm; pitch—2.5 mm; reverse cutting flutes; self-cutting, self-tapping positive rake tip. *Material*: 22-13-5 stainless steel. *Washers* (optional): 6.5-mm system washers.

#### System 2

*Drill*: A 3.2-mm ($\frac{1}{8}$-inch) steel drill. *Guide pin*: A 3.2-mm guide pin. *Screw head*: Round head with an internal hexagon. *Screw thread*: Outer diameter—6.5 mm; reverse cutting flutes; self-cutting, self-tapping tip. *Material*: Ti-6Al-4v. *Washers* (optional): 6.5-mm system titanium washers.

### Procedure

The patient is placed in a supine position on a fracture table. If the fracture is displaced, traction is applied with the leg in neutral flexion, 10° of abduction, and neutral rotation. The leg is then internally rotated as far as possible with moderate force, then backed off to a position of 15° of internal rotation. The reduction is confirmed by fluoroscopy. If good alignment but some distraction is present, proceed with the internal fixation and impact the fracture with the parallel guide pins in place or with the lag of the screws.

An 8-cm straight lateral incision is made starting at the flare of the greater trochanter and extending distally. The fascia lata and fascia of the vastus lateralis are cut in line with the incision and the vastus lateralis is bluntly split. The lateral femoral cortex is visualized. The most distal guide pin is to be placed first. A drill hole is made with a 3.2-mm drill 3 cm to 4 cm distal to the vastus externus tubercle, usually at the level of the lesser trochanter, and midway between the anterior and posterior femoral cortices. This is the only hole that is predrilled for the guide pin, because the cortex may be very dense at this location. The 3.2-mm guide pin is then passed through this hole, along and almost resting on the medial femoral neck, across the fracture and into the femoral head. On the lateral view this pin should stay in the midline of the femoral neck and head. Pin position is confirmed by fluoroscopy. If a correction is to be made, try to use the same cortical hole. Extra holes at this level of the femoral shaft may weaken the femur at the subtrochanteric level.

A fixed guide with a selection of triangles or diamonds is then used (Figure 4.11). The appropriate size diamond or triangle can be determined with preoperative radiograph stenciling. If there is a question between two sizes, the smaller pattern is used. The authors prefer using three screws in an inverted triangle configuration for Garden stage I and II fractures and four screws in a diamond configuration for Garden stage III and IV fractures. The fixed jig is placed over the already-positioned guide pin and the remaining two or three guide pins are placed

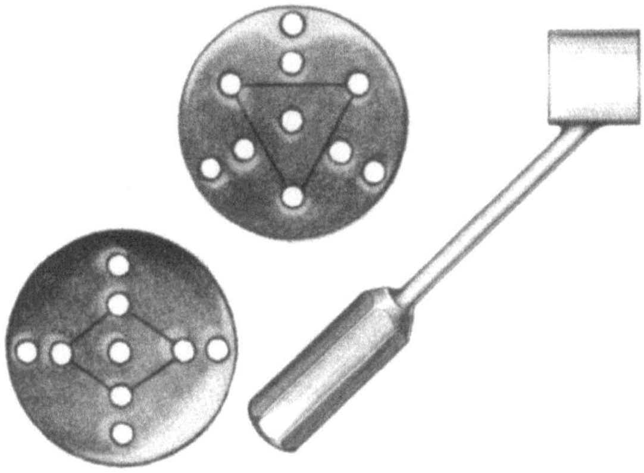

FIGURE 4.11. Fixed guides for triangle or diamond patterns. (Reprinted with permission from Asnis.[70])

(Figure 4.12). These guide pins are driven by power and predrilling is usually not necessary.

The direct reading depth gauge is then used to determine screw length. If in between sizes, use the shorter length. If the fracture is to be compressed, choose a screw 5 to 10 mm shorter than measured. This will leave room for the threads to advance in the femoral head as the screw lags and fracture compresses. An appropriate-sized self-cutting, self-tapping cannulated screw is then placed over its guide pin and driven through the cortex and across the fracture with the cannulated power screwdriver. When the head is 10 to 20 mm from the femoral cortex, the power driver is removed. The screw is then driven the remainder of its path with the hand screwdriver (Figure 4.13). The remaining screws are placed and the guide pins removed. Compression can be obtained by gently tightening the screws. When the screws are tightened, occasionally the inferior screw will spin in the osteoporotic patient. This is because the bone in the inferior head is the weakest. The remaining screws in the middle and upper portions of the head will achieve excellent hold of the femoral head. The lower screw will still deter inferior motion of the head fragment as the screw rests on the endosteum of the femoral neck.

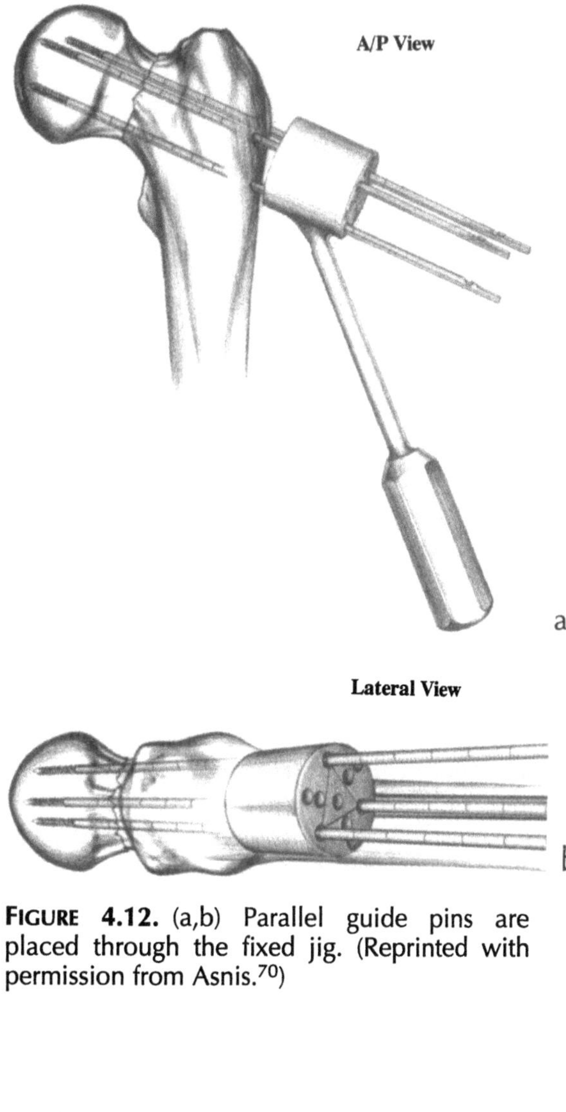


FIGURE 4.12. (a,b) Parallel guide pins are placed through the fixed jig. (Reprinted with permission from Asnis.[70])

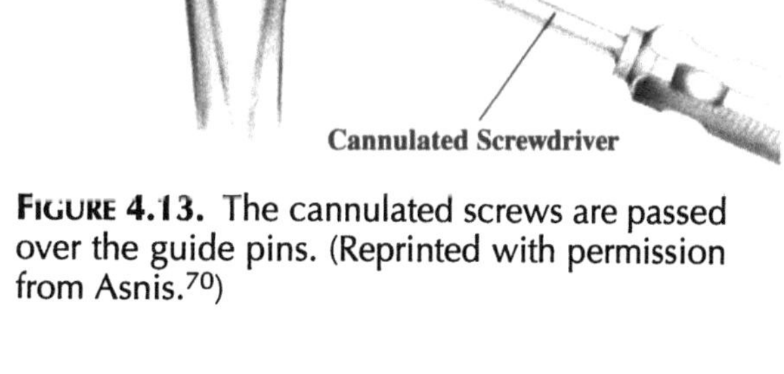


FIGURE 4.13. The cannulated screws are passed over the guide pins. (Reprinted with permission from Asnis.[70])

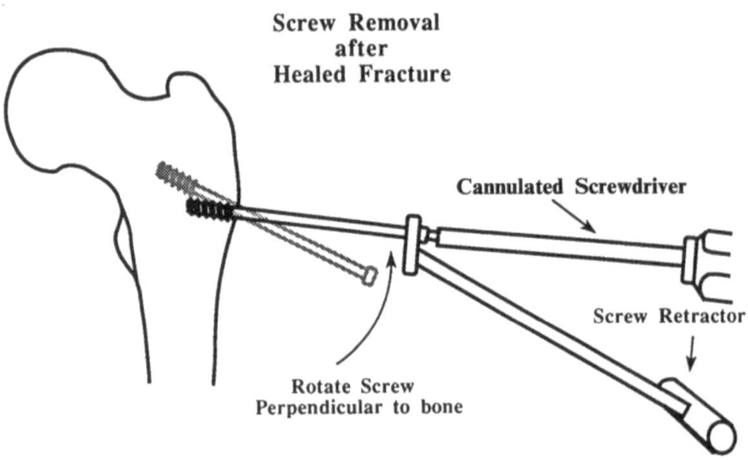


**FIGURE 4.14.** When the thread meets the endocortex, the screw can be pulled into a perpendicular position to the bone with a screw head retractor, thus permitting the reverse cutting flutes to position themselves properly and facilitate screw removal.

## Screw Removal

In the removal of a screw after fracture healing, the screw thread must recut its way through the healed femoral cortex. Reverse cutting flutes are present on many types of cannulated screws for this purpose. If the oblique angle (approximately 135°) of the screw to the femoral shaft is not changed, the reverse cutting flutes are not in an optimal position to cut into the cortex. When the thread meets the endocortex, the screw can be pulled into a perpendicular position to the bone with a screw head retractor, thus permitting the reverse cutting flutes to position themselves properly and facilitate screw removal (Figure 4.14). A worn or damaged screwdriver should never be used for fear of stripping the recess socket.

# Clinical Results of a Long-Term Follow-Up of the Parallel Cannulated Screw for Intracapsular Fractures

A retrospective study of the results of stabilizing nonpathologic intracapsular hip fractures with parallel cannulated screws in 141 patients was conducted from 1980 through 1985.[51] Fifty patients (35%) had nondisplaced fractures (Garden stage I and II), whereas 91 (65%) had displaced fractures (Garden stage III and IV). The patients had a median age of 68 (range: 24 to 95). There were 112 white women (79%) with a median age at the time of fracture of 67 years (range: 30 to 90); and 29 white men (21%) with a median age of 69 years (range: 24 to 95). The proportion of displaced and nondisplaced fractures was approximately equal by gender ($p = .32$) and side of fracture ($p = .23$). There were no deaths or wound infections during the fracture hospitalization. The mean follow-up was 8 years.

Eleven patients, six men and five women, (median age: 75) died within the first postoperative year. Twenty-nine patients (median age: 75) died within 5 years. Fifty percent of the entire group of patients had at least one major concomitant disease. Of the 29 patients who died, only three had no major initial disorder. Mortality related more to the medical condition of the patient than to the fracture episode itself. The mortality rate of this patient group was compared with a control cohort group matched for age, sex, and race. This group was from the population at large and did not account for medical illness. The survival curve of the cohort group remained within the 95% confidence limit of the fracture group for the entire length of the

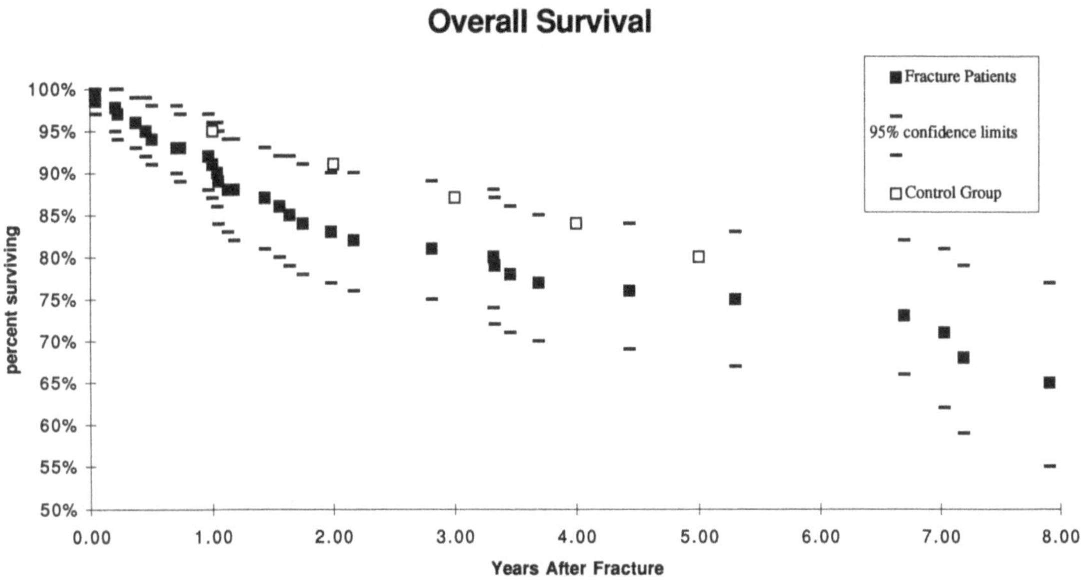


**FIGURE 4.15.** The survival curve of the cohort group matched for age, sex, and race remained within the 95% confidence limit of the fracture group for the entire length of the study. (Reprinted with permission from Asnis and Wanek-Sgaglione.[51])

study (Figure 4.15). Although there was a trend of increased mortality for the first 2 years following fracture, this was not significant. The men and women were separated and compared with each other as well as each with his or her own control cohort group. The women's survival curve followed that of their control cohort group. The survival curve for the men showed a much poorer prognosis than that for the women ($p < .0001$) (Figure 4.16), and the survival curve

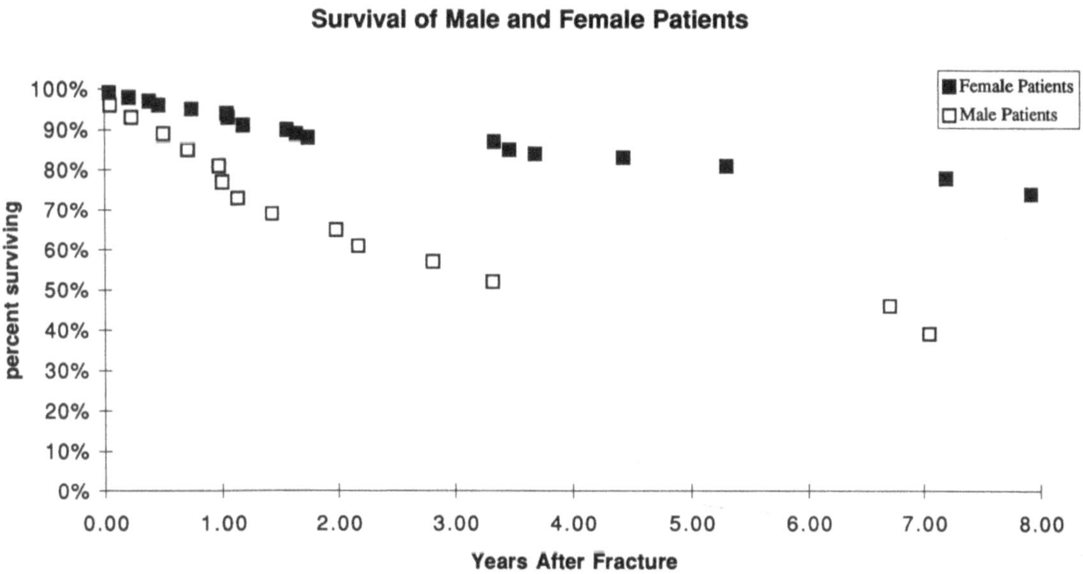


**FIGURE 4.16.** The survival curve for the males shows a much poorer prognosis than that for the females. (Reprinted with permission from Asnis and Wanek-Sgaglione.[51])

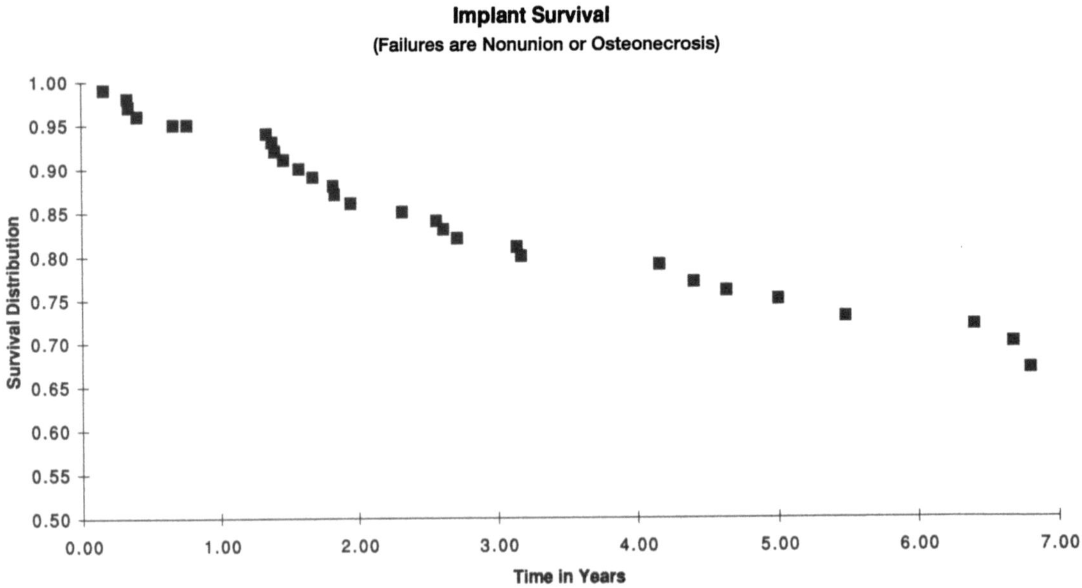


**FIGURE 4.17.** This study demonstrated more than a 71% implant survival 7 years following the fracture. (Reprinted with permission from Asnis and Wanek-Sgaglione.[51])

for the men was significantly poorer than their control cohort group.

Five of the 141 patients (4%) (two Garden stage III and three Garden stage IV) experienced a loss of position or nonunion by 6 months after surgery. All five patients were women. Two of the five patients underwent total hip replacement and one a hemiarthroplasty.

Thirteen patients were found to have histologic or roentgenographic evidence of osteonecrosis within 2 years of treatment (11% ± .03). Ten of these patients had initially displaced fractures. Another 13 cases of osteonecrosis were diagnosed after 2 years, eight being initially displaced fractures. Twenty-five of the 26 patients were females. Four of these patients first developed segmental collapse 5 to 8 years after their fracture. The prevalence of osteonecrosis was therefore 22% ± .04 with a mean follow-up of 8 years. Osteonecrosis was present in 8 of 39 patients with a Garden stage II, 6 of 30 patients with a Garden stage III, and 12 of 40 patients with a Garden stage IV fracture. Sixteen of the 26 patients with osteonecrosis underwent a total hip replacement at a mean time of 2 years following their fracture.

By a minimum 5-year follow-up period 30 patients were lost to follow-up. Fifty-five patients healed their fractures free of complications and were found to be functioning well after 5 years (average follow-up: 8 years). Using Kaplan-Meer survival rates, this study demonstrated more than a 71% implant survival 7 years following the fracture (Figure 4.17). Forty-four of these patients underwent Harris hip scoring with an average score of 94 (range 58–100) from 5 to 11 years after their procedure.

In this series, multiple cannulated screw fixation represents a procedure with low operative mortality and morbidity and a very high rate of fracture union (96%). An increased mortality rate was found for the male patients; however, this appeared to be related to the concomitant medical disorders rather than the surgery. The male patient has a poorer survival rate following hip fracture than the female. Osteonecrosis remains the major surgical complication following the fixation of the intracapsular hip fracture and continues to present itself years after fracture healing. The female patient has a far higher incidence of nonunion or osteonecrosis than the male. Segmental collapse can be treated with a well-planned elective total hip replacement at a medically safer time. Those patients who heal their fractures without osteonecrosis maintain excellent function long after their injury.

## Authors' Philosophy

Following internal fixation and fracture healing, patient function has been found to be as good as or better than prosthetic replacement and with a much lower initial risk to the patient. The goal of the internal fixation device is to obtain fracture healing and allow function for the remainder of the patient's life. Multiple cannulated screw fixation is a highly effective way to obtain this goal. Those patients who later do develop symptoms from osteonecrosis and segmental collapse can undergo a well-planned elective total hip replacement.

## References


1. Praemer A, Furner S, Rice D. *Musculoskeletal Conditions in the United States*. Park Ridge, Illinois. AAOS, 1992.
2. Cummings S, Kelsey J, Nevitt M, et al. Epidemiology of osteoporosis and osteoporotic fractures. *Epidemiol Rev* 1985;7:178–208.
3. Melton L III, Wahner H, Richelson LS, et al. Osteoporosis and the risk of hip fracture. *Am J Epidemiol* 1986;124:254–261.
4. Benterud J, Husby T, Graadahl O, et al. Implant holding power of the femoral head. *Acta Orthop Scand* 1992;63(1):47–49.
5. Brunner C, Weber B. *Special Techniques in Internal Fixation*. Berlin: Springer-Verlag, 1982; 34.
6. Hoaglund F, Low W. Anatomy of the femoral neck and head, with comparative data from Caucasians and Hong Kong Chinese. *Clin Orthop* 1980;152:10–16.
7. Pankovich A. Primary internal fixation of femoral neck fractures. *Arch Surg* 1975;110:20–26.
8. Ward F. *Human Anatomy*. London: Renshaw, 1838.
9. Singh M, Nagrath A, Maini P. Changes in the trabecular pattern of the upper end of the femur as an index of osteoporosis. *J Bone Joint Surg* 1970;52A:457.
10. Crowell RR, Edwards W, Hayes W. Pullout strength of fixation devices in trabecular bone of the femoral head. Proc of the 21st Annual Orthopaedic Research Society, 1985:189.
11. Martens M, Van Audekercke R, Mulier J, et al. Clinical study on internal fixation of femoral neck fractures. *Clin Orthop* 1970;141:199–202.
12. Lindequist S. Cortical screw support in femoral neck fractures. A radiographic analysis of 87 fractures with a new mensuration technique. *Acta Orthop Scand* 1993;64(3):289–293.
13. Crock H. A revision of the anatomy of the arteries supplying the upper end of the human femur. *J Anat* 1965;99:77–88.
14. Crock H. An atlas of the arterial supply of the head and neck of the femur in man. *Clin Orthop* 1980;152:17–27.
15. Chung S. The arterial supply of the developing end of the human femur. *J Bone Joint Surg* 1976; 58A:961–970.
16. Claffey TJ. Avascular necrosis of the femoral head—an anatomical study. *J Bone Joint Surg* 1960;42B:802–809.
17. Harty M. Blood supply of the femoral head. *Br Med J* 1953;2:1236–1237.
18. Sevitt S, Thompson R. The distribution and anastamoses of arteries supplying the head and neck of the femur. *J Bone Joint Surg* 1965;47B:560–573.
19. Tucker F. Arterial supply to the femoral head and its clinical importance. *J Bone Joint Surg* 1949;31B: 82–93.
20. Swiontkowski M. Intracapsular hip fractures. In: Browner B, Jupiter J, Levine A, eds. *Skeletal Trauma*, vol. 2. Philadelphia: Saunders; 1992; 1370.
21. Wertheimer L, Fernandez Lopes S. Arterial supply of the femoral head. *J Bone Joint Surg* 1971; 53A:545–556.
22. Crawfurd E, Emery R, Hansell D, et al. Capsular distention and intracapsular pressure in subcapital fractures of the femur. *J Bone Joint Surg* 1988;70B: 195–198.
23. Drake J, Meyers M. Intracapsular pressure and hemarthrosis following femoral neck fracture. *Clin Orthop* 1984;182:172–176.
24. Holmberg S, Dalen N. Intracapsular pressure and caput circulation in nondisplaced femoral neck fractures. *Clin Orthop* 1987;219:124–126.
25. Strömqvist B, Nilsson L, Egund N, et al. Intracapsular pressures in undisplaced fractures of the femoral neck. *J Bone Joint Surg* 1988;70B:192–194.
26. Wingstrand H, Strömqvist B, Egund N, et al. Hemarthrosis in undisplaced cervical fractures: tamponade reversible femoral head ischemia. *Acta Orthop Scand* 1986;57:305–308.
27. Pauwels F. *Der Schenkenholsbruck, em mechanisches Problem. Grundlagen des Heilungsvorganges. Prognose und kausale Therapie*. Stuttgart: Ferdinand Enke, Beilageheft zur Zeitschrift fur Orthopaedische Chirurgie, 1935.
28. Garden RS. Reduction and fixation of subcapital fractures of the femur. *Orthop Clin North Am* 1974;5:683–712.
29. Garden RS. Malreduction and avascular necrosis in subcapital fractures of the femur. *J Bone Joint Surg* 1971;53B:183–197.
30. Garden RS. Low-angle fixation in fractures of the

femoral neck. *J Bone Joint Surg* 1961;43B:647–663.
31. Arnold W, Lyden J, Minkoff J. Treatment of intracapsular fracture of the femoral neck. *J Bone Joint Surg* 1974;56A:254–262.
32. Eiskjaer S, Ostgard S. Risk factors influencing mortality after bipolar hemiarthroplasty in treating fractures of the femoral neck. *Clin Orthop* 1991;270:295–300.
33. Holmberg S, Conradi P, Kalen R, et al. Mortality after cervical hip fracture: 3002 patients followed for 6 years. *Acta Orthop Scand* 1986;57:8–11.
34. Hunter G. A comparison of the use of internal fixation and prosthetic replacement for fresh fractures of the neck of the femur. *Br J Surg* 1969; 56:229–232.
35. Hunter G. Should we abandon primary prosthetic replacement for fresh displaced fractures of the neck of the femur? *Clin Orthop* 1980;152:158–161.
36. Gebhard J, Amstutz H, Zinar D, et al. A comparison of total hip arthroplasty and hemiarthroplasty for treatment of acute fracture of the femoral neck. *Clin Orthop* 1992;282:123–131.
37. Salvati E, Artz T, Aglietti P, et al. Endo-protheses in the treatment of femoral neck fractures. *Orthop Clin North Am* 1974;5:757–777.
38. Franzén H, Nilsson L, Strömqvist B, et al. Secondary total hip replacement after fractures of the femoral neck. *J Bone Joint Surg* 1990;72B:784–787.
39. Coates R, Armour P. Treatment of subcapital fractures by primary total hip replacement. *Injury* 1979;11:132–135.
40. Dorr L, Glousman R, Sew A, et al. Treatment of femoral neck fractures with total hip replacement versus cemented and noncemented hemiarthroplasty. *J Arthroplasty* 1986;1:21–28.
41. Gregory R, Gibson M, Moran C. Dislocation after primary arthroplasty for subcapital fracture of the hip. *J Bone Joint Surg* 1991;73B:11–12.
42. Johnsson R, Bendejelloul H, Ekelund L, et al. Comparison between hemiarthroplasty and total hip replacement following failure of nailed femoral neck fractures focused on dislocations. *Arch Orthop Trauma Surg* 1984;102:187–190.
43. Sim F, Stauffer R. Management of hip fractures by total hip replacements. *Clin Orthop* 1980;152: 191–197.
44. Greenough C, Jones J. Primary total hip replacement for displaced subcapital fracture of the femur. *J Bone Joint Surg* 1988;70B:639–643.
45. Nilsson L, Franzen H, Strömqvist B, et al. Function of the hip after femoral neck fractures treated by fixation or secondary total hip replacement. *Int J Orthop* 1991;15:315–318.
46. Nilsson L, Pekka J, Franzen H, et al. Function after primary hemiarthroplasty and secondary total hip arthroplasty in femoral neck fracture. *J Arthroplasty* 1994;9(4):369–374.
47. Garcia AJ. Displaced intracapsular fractures of the neck of the femur—mortality and morbidity. *J Trauma* 1961;1:128–132.
48. Holmberg S, Kalen R, Thorngren K. Treatment and outcome of femoral neck fractures: an analysis of 2418 patients admitted from their own homes. *Clin Orthop* 1987;218:42–52.
49. Nilsson L, Strömqvist B, Thorngren K. Nailing of femoral neck fracture: clinical and sociologic 5-year follow-up of 510 consecutive hips. *Acta Orthop Scand* 1988;59:365–371.
50. Meyers M, Harvey J Jr, Moore T. Treatment of displaced subcapital and transcervical fractures of the femoral neck by muscle-pedicle bone graft and internal fixation. *J Bone Joint Surg* 1973;55A: 256–274.
51. Asnis S, Wanek-Sgaglione L. Intracapsular fractures of femoral neck: results of cannulated screw fixation. *J Bone Joint Surg* 1994;76A:1793–1803.
52. Asnis S. The guided screw system in intracapsular fractures of the hip. *Contemp Orthop* 1985;10:33–42.
53. Calandruccio R, Anderson W. Post-fracture avascular necrosis of the femoral head: correlation of experimental and clinical studies. *Clin Orthop* 1980;152:49–84.
54. Catto M. The histological appearances of late segmental collapse of the femoral head after transcervical fracture. *J Bone Joint Surg* 1965;47B: 777–791.
55. Catto M. Histological study of avascular necrosis of the femoral head after transcervical fracture. *J Bone Joint Surg* 1965;47B:749–776.
56. Sevitt S. Avascular necrosis and revascularization of the femoral head after intracapsular fractures. A combined arteriographic and histological necropsy study. *J Bone Joint Surg* 1964;46B:270–296.
57. Hodge W, Fijan R, Carlson K, et al. Contact pressures in the human hip joint measured in vivo. *Proc Natl Acad Sci USA* 1986;83:2879–2883.
58. Rubin R, Trent P, Arnold W, et al. Knowles pinning of experimental femoral neck fractures: a biomedical study. *J Trauma* 1981;21:1036–1039.
59. McElvenny R. The importance of the lateral x-ray film in treating intracapsular fracture of the femur. *Am J Orthop* 1962;212–215.
60. Strömqvist B, Hansson L, Ljung P, et al. Preoperative and postoperative scintimetry after femoral neck fracture. *J Bone Joint Surg* 1984;66B: 49–54.
61. Bauer G, Hansson L, Lidgren L, et al. Comprehensive care of hip fractures. Scientific exhibit at the Annual Meeting of the American Academy of Orthopaedic Surgeons, Las Vegas, Jan. 24–29, 1985.
62. Nilsson L. *Primary Osteosynthesis for Femoral Neck Fractures*. Lund, Sweden: Lund University Department of Orthopedics, 1989;16:28–30.
63. Strömqvist B, Nilsson L, Thorngren K. Femoral neck fracture fixation with hook-pins. *Acta Orthop Scand* 1992;63(3):282–287.
64. Strömqvist B, Hansson I, Nilsson L, et al. Hook-

pin fixation of femoral fractures: a two year follow-up study of 300 cases. *Clin Orthop* 1987;218: 58–62.

65. Deyerle W. Impacted fixation over resilient multiple pins. *Clin Orthop* 1980;152:102–122.
66. Swiontkowski M, Harrington R, Keller T, et al. Torsion and bending analysis of internal fixation techniques for femoral neck fractures: the role of implant design and bone density. *J Orthop Res* 1987;5:433–444.
67. Springer E, Lachiewicz P, Gilbert J. Internal fixation of femoral neck fractures: comparative biomechanical study of Knowles pins and 6.5-mm screws. *Clin Orthop* 1991;267:85–91.
68. Howard C, Davies R. Subtrochanteric fracture after Garden screw fixation of subcapital fractures. *J Bone Joint Surg* 1982;64B:565–567.
69. Radin EL, Rose RM, Blaha JD, Litsky AS. *Practical Biomechanics for the Orthopaedic Surgeon.* New York: Churchill Livingstone, 1992;75–79.
70. Asnis SE. The Asnis 2 Guided Screw System: Howmedica Surgical Techniques, Rutherford, New Jersey: 1991;1–9.

# 5
# Slipped Capital Femoral Epiphysis

Stanley E. Asnis

Slipped capital femoral epiphysis (SCFE) can result from acute trauma or can be spontaneous. A spontaneous slipped epiphysis can occur secondarily to epiphyseal disturbances such as sepsis, severe rickets, renal rickets, achondroplasia, radiation and chemotherapy, or dysplasia epiphyseal multiples. Clinical endocrinopathies that have been associated with SCFE include hypothyroidism, hypogonadism, and panhypopituitarism.[1,2] In the absence of an epiphyseal abnormality, spontaneous epiphyseal displacement can occur at the proximal femoral epiphysis and much more rarely at the proximal humeral epiphysis.

Spontaneous slipped proximal femoral epiphysis occurs in the general population at approximately 2 cases per 100,000 (range, 0.2 to 10.0 per 100,000).[1,3] It is two to five times more common in males than females. The usual age of onset is between 10 and 18 years; however, the age of onset of symptoms in boys is usually between 13 and 16 years, and in girls it is between 11 and 14 years. It is clinically bilateral in 20% to 30% of patients. Billing and Severin[4] have shown that the rate of bilaterality may be as high as 80% when radiograms are repeated 5 years later and carefully measured for epiphyseal plate change. Hagglund et al.[5] studied the frequency of slipping and osteoarthritis of the contralateral hip in 260 patients between 1910 and 1960. Nine percent (23 patients) had bilateral slipping, 12% (32 patients) had a contralateral slip diagnosed later during adolescence, and 40% (104 patients) had signs of contralateral slipping at follow-up 16 to 66 years later, giving a total of 61% (159 cases) with bilateral slips. The authors suggest that prophylactic contralateral pinning be performed to avoid slipping and reduce the risk of osteoarthritis. Canale[6] found that bilateral incidence was higher in blacks (32%) than in whites (27%). Bilateral hip involvement was found in 70–100% of patients with endocrinopathies.[2] It is more common in children who are abnormally heavy in proportion to their relative height or who are tall and thin.[7] There has been an association with overweight children with underdeveloped genitals and in some cases obvious Fröhlich's adiposogenital dystrophy. The clinical relevance of the SCFE is its relation to osteoarthritis in the adult. Many treated SCFEs, even when mild, will show significant signs of osteoarthritis in the seventh and eighth decades. It is even possible that asymptomatic and unrecognized slipped epiphysis may have the same result[8]; however, minimizing the amount of slippage and maintaining as anatomically normal a hip as possible seems to be the best deterrent for later degeneration.

## Clinical Relevance

Slipped capital femoral epiphysis is not an uncommon disorder. It has a high frequency of bilaterality, and in the patient with an endocrinopathy bilaterality can approach 100%. There is a definite correlation of increased osteoarthritis in patients who have had a slipped epiphysis. An adolescent with SCFE should undergo fixation as soon as possible on the affected hip to maintain as close to an anatomically normal hip as possible. With bilateral slips both hips are fixed. In patients with unilateral slips Hagglund et al.[5] suggest prophylactic pinning, whereas Morissy and Selman[1] and Canale[6] recommend closely following these patients for slippage of the opposite hip. Adolescents with endocrinopathies should be specifically examined for slipped epiphyses. If found, one should consider bilateral epiphyseal fixation.

This chapter describes and classifies slipped epiphyses and discusses which are suitable for fixation with a cannulated screw technique. Open reductions, osteotomies, and reconstructive procedures are beyond the scope and purpose of this text on cannulated screw fixation.

# Pathology

At the microscopic level, a cleft or fracture develops in the growth plate through the layer of hypertrophic cartilage cells just adjacent to the zone of provisional calcification.[3,7,9] This leaves the proliferating and palisade cells with the head, and the calcified cartilage with the femoral neck. Ponsetti and McClintock[10] believe that this is due to an abnormality in protein metabolism, causing a loss of cohesion of the cartilage matrix. Harris[7] studied the shear strength in the upper tibial epiphysis in rats and found that pituitary growth hormone decreased the shearing strength, whereas sex hormone increased it. Anterior pituitary hormone appears to stimulate the proliferation of cartilage in the epiphyseal plate, whereas sex hormones, estrogen and testosterone, depress this proliferation and decrease the thickness of the epiphyseal plate. It can be speculated that slippage in the adiposogenital syndrome may be due to a lack of sex hormone, whereas the tall thin child's problem may be due to an increase in growth hormone. Although the actual etiology is still not well understood, most authors agree that there is a weakness in the growth plate.

Key,[11] however, speculates that the thinning periosteum in the adolescent femoral neck, which helps to hold the epiphysis in place, is stretched and weakened in times of rapid growth. With the weakened or torn periosteum, the epiphysis may slip without major shear forces. This may also be enhanced by the increase in the vertical alignment of the epiphysis during adolescence. There is an increase in the slope or inclination of the proximal femoral epiphysis during normal development of the proximal femur.[12,13] This represents a change in the axis of the epiphyseal plate from a horizontal to a more vertical orientation relative to the axis of weight bearing. Speer[14] has found this progression in slope to be 13.7° between the ages of 1 and 18 with a maximal increase between 9 and 11 years of age. In patients with a unilateral SCFE, there was a 15° and 5° higher slope on the affected and unaffected sides, respectively, when compared with controls. Mirkopulos et al.[12] support these findings with a 14° increase in slope between 1 and 18 years (correlation coefficient 0.803, $p < .0001$), with a maximal increase between 9 and 12 years ($p < .005$). The slip side had an 8.0° ($p < .005$) higher slope than age-matched controls, whereas the nonslip side showed an average 4.0° ($p < .001$) increase over controls. Chung et al.[13] have found that the vector of weight bearing giving a shear force to the epiphysis during walking could be in the range of 4,800 pounds/in$^2$. This could even be increased by the added effect of obesity and excessive body mass and could lead to displacement of the susceptible growth plate.

Whatever the etiology or predisposing factors, mechanically the femoral neck moves anteriorly and upward while the femoral head slips posteriorly and downward. The periosteum and vessels over the front of the neck are stretched. Because the major blood supply of the superior femoral head comes from an end vessel of the medial circumflex artery, which is in the posterior retinaculum of Weitbrecht, avascularity is uncommon without marked displacement. It is very rare to develop avascular necrosis without surgical intervention. It is thought that without treatment, displacement may be a process of progressive acute-on-chronic slippage. The dominant action of the short external rotator muscles of the proximal femur, especially the iliopsoas, may be responsible for rotating the neck of the femur anteriorly and laterally relative to the head. Clinically, this disorder should be treated by internal fixation of the epiphysis as soon as it is recognized.

## Vascular Anatomy

The structural anatomy of the adult hip was discussed in Chapter 4. The developmental anatomy of the child and adolescent hip becomes important in relationship to SCFE. Chung[15] has carefully described the vascular anatomy as he found it in autopsy studies in 150 hip specimens in fetus and children ranging from 26 weeks of gestation to 14 years 8 months of age. Arterial perfusions were performed with either rubber latex, Batson's compound, or barium sulfate paste followed by Spalteholz clearing. Both the medial and lateral circumflex arteries originated from the femoral or profunda arteries and then formed an extracapsular ring surrounding the base of the femoral neck (Figure 5.1). The medial, posterior, and lateral parts of this ring were a continuation of the medial circumflex artery, thus giving the medial, posterior, and lateral ascending cervical arteries. The lateral portion of the arterial ring, which was essentially the termination of the medial circumflex artery, provided most of the arterial supply to the femoral head, neck, and trochanter. Therefore, the major portion of the femoral head is supplied from a single arterial stem that crosses the capsule at the posterior trochanteric fossa. The lateral femoral circumflex artery made up the anterior portion of the ring and was the source of the ascending cervical branches to a smaller area of the anterior femoral neck and head. In only approximately 8% of specimens did the lateral circumflex artery actually join the terminal branch of the medial circumflex artery at the trochanteric fossa and form a complete ring.

The ascending cervical arteries, also known as retinacular arteries, traverse the articular capsule along its femoral attachment, and pass beneath the synovium to supply the metaphysis and epiphysis. The ascending cervical arterial group (anterior, medial, posterior, and lateral) form a fine anastomotic subsynovial ring on the surface of the neck at the margin of the articular cartilage. The epiphyseal branches cross the epiphyseal plate on the surface of the head-neck junction, pass through the peripheral perichondrial fibrocartilaginous complex, then supply the secondary ossification center. The cartilaginous epiphysis forms a vascular barrier and at no age did arteries penetrate the central portion of the epiphyseal plate.

The artery of the ligamentum teres or foveal artery, a branch of the obturator artery, was studied in 123 specimens.[16] No artery was present in the ligament in 10 specimens, the artery was present in the ligament but not the femoral head in 78 specimens, it profused and provided one deep vessel to the center of the head in 20 specimens, and gave two or more deep vessels to the head in 15 specimens. In the great major-

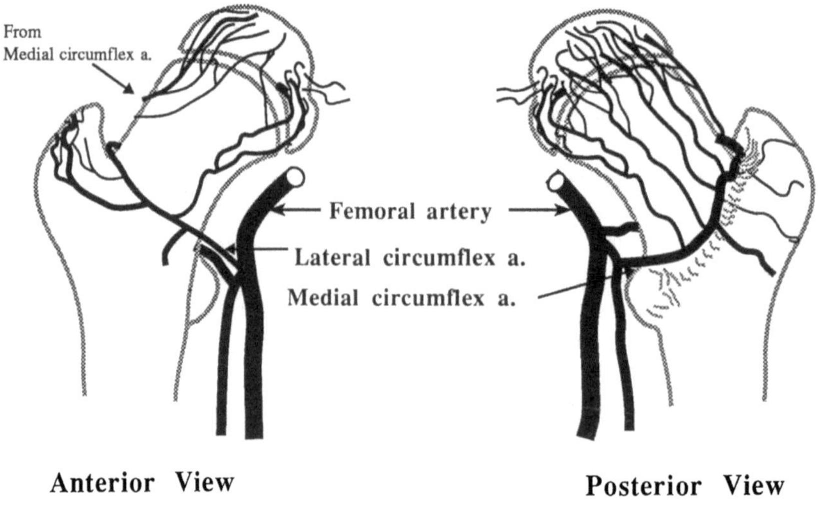


FIGURE 5.1. The vascular anatomy of the adolescent proximal femur.

ity of specimens there was little or no contribution of femoral head circulation from the artery of the ligamentum teres. Even in the 15 specimens with two vessels to the femoral head, the majority of circulation was supplied by the retinacular vessels. There was no significant age, sex, or race differentiation in the femoral head circulation. The vascular studies by Trueta[17] found that the lateral epiphyseal vessels were responsible for the blood flow of almost the entire femoral capital epiphysis until the age of 6 to 8, and afterward the vessels from the round ligament supplied a variable segment of the medial femoral head.

### Clinical Relevance

All of the epiphyseal and metaphyseal branches of the most important lateral ascending cervical artery originate from a single stem that lies along the posterior capsule at its femoral attachment and then crosses the capsule at the trochanteric notch. All drills, guide pins, and screws should not be placed along the lateral (superior) femoral neck, and must avoid the trochanteric fossa and penetration of the posterior femoral neck. Placement of a single screw in the middle area of the femoral neck and epiphysis is safest. If two screws are used, avoid the superior epiphysis.

For in situ fixation of a moderate or severe slip, the screw may enter the anterior neck, probably with little direct mechanical disturbance to the vascular supply of the epiphysis.

## Clinical Symptoms

The classical symptoms of a slipped capital femoral epiphysis are pain and limp. The pain is usually in the groin or the anteromedial thigh but may be entirely in the medial area of the knee. There may be an antalgic limp and a positive Trendelenburg's sign. The patient may stand or walk with the leg externally rotated. On physical examination there is often some loss of internal rotation, abduction, and flexion. As the hip is flexed the leg often externally rotates. Some shortening may be evident depending on the degree of epiphyseal displacement. Laboratory work is normal other than in patients with an endocrinopathy. The diagnosis is confirmed radiographically.

## Classification and Radiologic Appearance

In the earliest stages only a widening and irregularity of the epiphyseal plate is evident on radiographs. Early displacement can be demonstrated as a posterior migration of the epiphysis on the femoral neck on the lateral radiograph. The anteroposterior projection demonstrates a downward displacement of the epiphysis so that a line drawn along the superior femoral neck no longer intersects the ossification of the femoral head but lies above it (Figure 5.2).

The degree of slippage is generally classified as:

*Pre-slip*—a widening of the epiphysis and rarefaction of the epiphyseal plate without any actual displacement of the epiphysis;
*Minimal slip*—the maximal displacement of the epiphyseal head is less than 1 cm;
*Moderate slip*—the displacement of the epiphyseal head is more than 1 cm but less than two thirds of the femoral neck diameter;
*Severe slip*—the displacement is greater than two thirds of the femoral neck diameter.

Southwick[18] and Canale[6] prefer the use of an *epiphyseal line femoral shaft angle* on both the anteroposterior and lateral radiographs (Figure 5.3). This angle is measured and compared with the contralateral hip. A mild slip is less than 30°, a moderate slip is 30° to 60°, and a severe slip is more than 60°.

The differentiation between acute and chronic is usually a duration of 2 weeks (Canale[6] feels that SCFE usually can be reduced within the first 2 weeks):

*Acute slip*—the symptoms and radiographic changes are less than 2 weeks old;
*Chronic slip*—the symptoms and radiographic changes are more than 2 weeks old;
*Acute-on-chronic slip*—there has been a new change (within 2 weeks) in the slippage of an epiphysis that shows evidence of a precedent chronic slip.

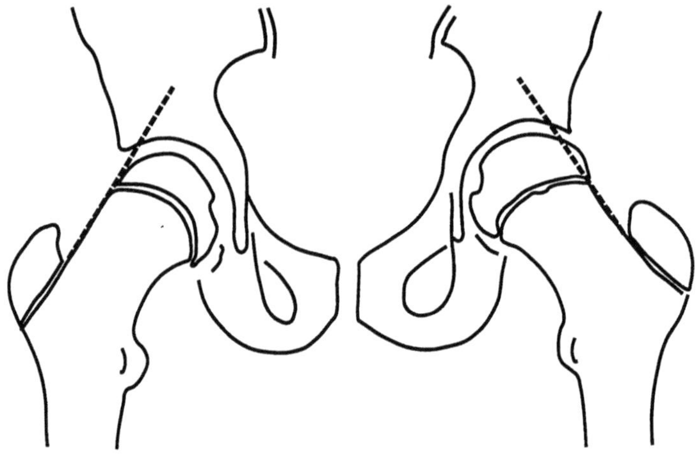

**FIGURE 5.2.** The anteroposterior projection demonstrates a downward displacement of the right epiphysis so that a line drawn along the superior right femoral neck no longer intersects the ossification of the femoral head but lies above it.

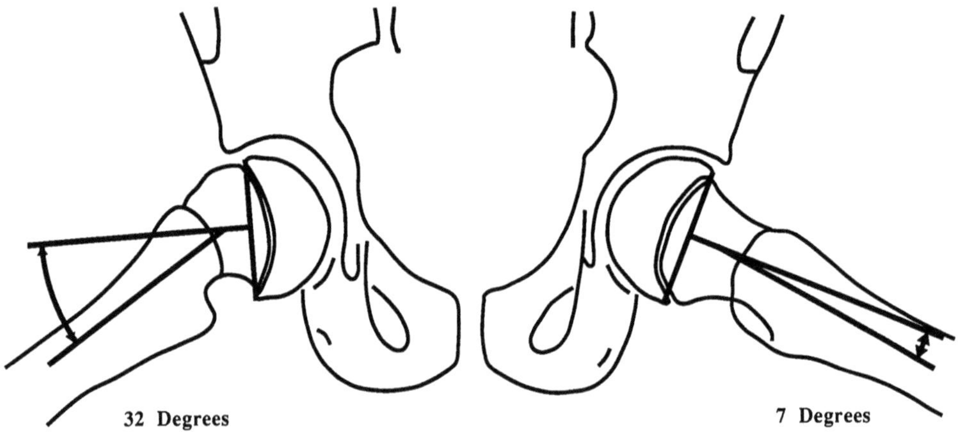


**FIGURE 5.3.** The epiphyseal line femoral shaft angle.

## Clinical Relevance

The disability caused by the slipped capital femoral epiphysis is related to the deformity it creates. The objective is to minimize this deformity by fixation of the slipping epiphysis at its earliest stage. The objective of the fixation is to hold the femoral epiphysis in as close to an anatomic position as possible until the epiphysis fuses and there is no longer a chance of slippage. If there is an acute slip or an acute-on-chronic slip, a *gentle* closed reduction can be attempted at the time of surgery. The debate of reduction or fixation in situ is still undecided and may vary at the surgeon's discretion.

## Slipped Capital Femoral Epiphysis Versus Femoral Neck Fracture in the Adult

Many physicians look at the slipped capital femoral epiphysis as a type of adult femoral neck fracture. In reality, the two disorders are very different. In the adult patient with a displaced femoral neck fracture, comminution is frequently present. The bone in the femoral neck is often very osteoporotic and fixation requires multiple screws, some of which should be supported by the endosteal side of the cortex of the femoral neck. The intracapsular hip fracture is almost always more distal than the epiphyseal scar, leaving a much larger proximal head-neck fragment. The SCFE has more dense trabecular bone on either side of the epiphyseal plate. The femoral epiphysis is much smaller and thinner than the head-neck fragment of the adult. In the intracapsular hip fracture, the head should be almost anatomically aligned with the shaft after the reduction, whereas the slipped capital femoral epiphysis may have to be fixed with some posterior alignment of the head on the neck.

Following internal fixation of the slipped capital femoral epiphysis, the child may develop chondrolysis. This is a rapidly developing stiffening of the hip with loss of motion but usually without pain. This condition can progress to fibrous ankylosis or a very limited range of motion, frequently with a flexion and adduction deformity of the hip. Gross findings show an intense synovitis, denudation of articular cartilage on both sides of the joint, and absence of subchondral bone collapse.[19] Radiographs demonstrate a progressive narrowing of the joint cartilage space without any change in the osseous structures and is no association with avascular necrosis of the capital epiphysis.[20] The incidence of this disorder is related to racial ancestry, acuteness of slipping, severity of slipping, and the methods of treatment.[21,22] The etiology of chondrolysis still remains unclear; however, unrecognized pin penetration into the joint may be the single most important iatrogenic factor, especially with the multiple pin technique.[23,24] This again demonstrates the need for the accurate placement of the internal fixation screw(s) without joint penetration.

## Clinical Relevance

The slipped epiphysis can usually be satisfactorily fixed with one or at most two screws crossing the epiphyseal plate.[25] Due to the dense bone on both sides of the plate, this can be done with a screw in the center of the epiphyseal plate, as cortical femoral neck support is not necessary. The screw threads should cross the epiphyseal plate because the object of treatment is to obtain closure of the plate without further slippage. Fusion of the epiphysis is enhanced by the compression caused by the screw threads crossing the plate as the bone tries to grow, not by the lag of the screw (Figure 5.4). Due to the thin shape of the epiphyseal plate, the target for the screw threads is much smaller than in an adult fracture. The plate is thickest in its center, thus this is the preferred target. A screw crossing the epiphyseal plate in its center also has the least chance of joint penetration and does not interfere with the blood supply of the femoral epiphysis. The direction of the screw may have to enter the femoral cortex or even the femoral neck anteriorly, depending on the degree of slippage, and be aimed posteriorly to pass into the center of the epiphysis.

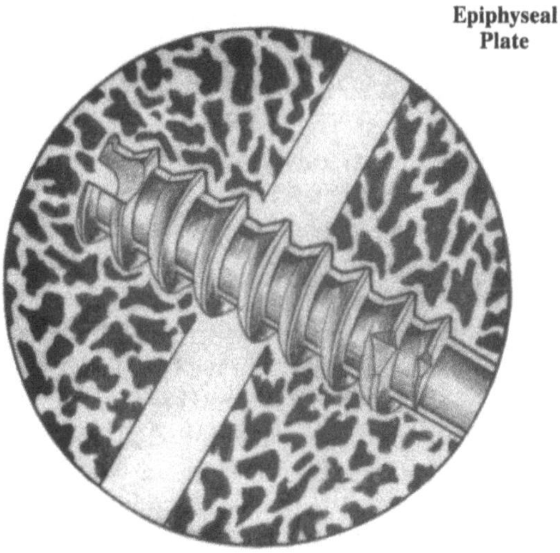


**FIGURE 5.4.** Fusion of the epiphysis is enhanced by the compression caused by the screw threads crossing the plate as the bone tries to grow. (Reprinted with permission from Asnis.[32])

## Advantages of Cannulated Screws

Herndon[26] states, "The objective in treating a patient with a minimally slipped upper femoral epiphysis is to stabilize the epiphysis, thus preventing further displacement until solid bony fusion has occurred." If this objective is achieved without complication, an essentially normal hip should be obtained. The fixation device locks the epiphysis in place and encourages epiphyseal plate fusion as atraumatically as possible.

Many pinning devices are available for such a procedure including Knowles pins, Steinmann pins, Haggie pins, Moore pins, Goufan pins, and AO screws, just to name a few. The number of screws or pins thought to be necessary also has varied. In a review by Swiontkowski[23] of the complications related to internal fixation at the Children's Orthopaedic Hospital in Seattle, in 56 patients treated with in situ pinning there were four cases (7%) of avascular necrosis, ten cases (18%) of a mild loss of motion (loss of 10° to 20° of internal rotation), and two cases (3.5%) of chondrolysis. Five pins were inserted in one case, four pins in 20, three pins in 41, and two pins in four. The cases of avascular necrosis all occurred in acute slips that had been managed with closed reduction prior to pinning. Seventeen of 56 cases (30%) had pin penetration with more than 2 mm of pin penetrating the femoral head on a single radiographic view. Haggie and Moore pins were more difficult to remove than the other pins used. In their award-winning paper, Walters and Simon[24] enlightened the orthopaedist about the devastating sequelae and chondrolysis caused by undetected pin penetration into the joint. Their study revealed that a penetrating pin can appear well within the femoral epiphysis on two mutually perpendicular x-rays. The chances of this undetected penetration increase as the pin is more peripheral in the femoral head. Chances of pin penetration also increase along with the number of pins used.

The cannulated screw systems offer a technique of more accurate screw placement. With the aid of jigs, guide pins (or drills used as guide pins) can be accurately placed and if not ideal, removed and repositioned with minimal disturbance to the host bone. The guide pin also can be used to establish the ideal screw's length prior to screw placement. The cannulation in the screw can be used to inject Renografin to confirm that there is no joint penetration.[27,28] I have used this technique in the adult fractured hip, where peripheral screws are placed, by injecting the dye with a large angiocath pressed firmly into the cannulation. An arthrogram reveals communication with the joint and clearly outlines the articular cartilage surface. I have chosen not to do this with the slipped epiphysis. After drilling and tapping the screw channel, some debris could be present that dye could flush into the joint during the study. Since the etiology of chondrolysis is still not fully understood, the effect of this possible intraarticular debris is uncertain. The merits of this technique are left to the discretion of the surgeon.

Cannulated screws are usually stronger than classic, solid 6.5-mm AO cancellous screws. Even though these screws are cannulated, the root diameters of the threads are usually in the range of 4.5 to 5.0 mm (4.5 mm Synthes; 4.6 mm Richards; 4.8 mm Howmedica; and 5.0 mm Ace and Zimmer), or much larger than the 3.0-mm root diameter of the solid 6.5-mm cancellous screw. This more than makes up for the weakness created by the cannulation (see Chapter 2). Titanium six-four alloy and 22-13-5 stainless steel are also significantly stronger than 316L stainless steel of the classic solid screws. Cannulated screws used today are significantly stronger than $\frac{5}{32}$-inch stainless steel Knowles pin.[23] The shank diameter of the cannulated screw is the same as the root diameter of the thread, avoiding a potential weakness at this junction. The screw thread has reverse cutting flutes to facilitate later removal of the screw.

## Clinical Relevance

The cannulated screw systems offer certain major advantages in the fixation of the slipped epiphysis. The operation is relatively atraumatic, and only one or two screws can give excellent fixation. Accurate screw placement is easier to obtain with the screw in the safest portion of the epiphysis, its center. Placement of threaded devices directly into the femoral epiphysis can be difficult due to the hard bone in the adolescent. With a cannulated screw system, a drill can be used as a guide pin. This can be controlled easily with power equipment, thus neutralizing the increased stress of the hard bone and making accurate placement easier.

# Author's Preferred Technique

## Equipment

*Drill*: 230 mm (9-inch-long) 3.2-mm ($\frac{1}{8}$-inch) steel drill, which can be used directly with a direct reading depth gauge. *Guide pin* (optional): A 230-mm guide pin with a threaded tip and tapered root diameter. *Screw head*: Round head with an internal hexagon. *Screw thread*: Outer diameter—6.5 mm; pitch—2.5 mm; reverse cutting flutes; self-cutting, self-tapping positive rake tip. *Material*: 22-213-5 stainless steel.

## Technique

The fracture table is used with biplane fluoroscopy. With the patient lying supine, a gentle reduction or in situ pinning is performed at the surgeon's discretion.

With the hip placed in 20° internal rotation, a 5-cm incision is made over the lateral thigh, approximately 4 cm distal to the prominence of the greater trochanter. The fascia lata and vastus lateralis are split the length of the wound, exposing the lateral femoral cortex.

Because of the often very dense bone in the adolescent proximal femur, a 230-mm-long, 3.2-mm drill bit is driven with a power drill through the lateral femoral cortex, up the center of the neck, across the epiphyseal plate, and into the epiphysis (Figure 5.5). Every effort is made not to penetrate the joint. If any posterior slippage (acute or chronic) is present, the drill hole should be made toward the anterior aspect of the femoral shaft and directed more posteriorly so as to come across the posteriorly sloped epiphyseal plate in a more perpendicular direction. In a moderate or severe slip, the anterior femoral neck may have to be exposed for the entrance site of the screw to approach the epiphysis in the proper direction. To facilitate the procedure, the leg in such cases is often externally rotated on the fracture table. This makes the anterior entrance easier to visualize. It also brings the epiphyseal plate of the posteriorly displaced epiphysis into a more vertical position on the lateral fluoroscopic view. The position of the drill is confirmed by fluoroscopy.

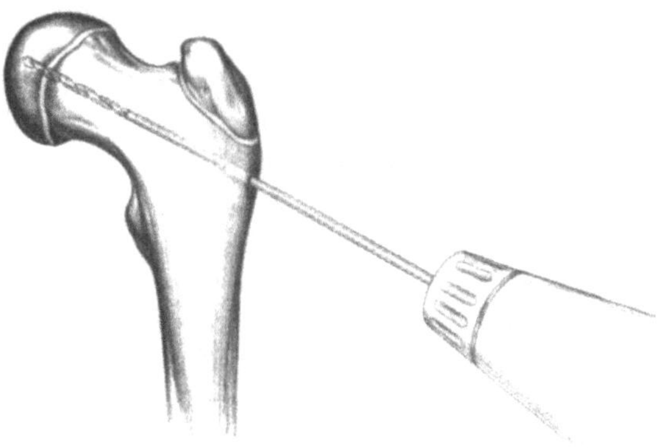

**FIGURE 5.5.** The placement of a 3.2-mm drill used as a guide pin. (Reprinted with permission from Asnis.[32])

If two screws are to be placed, a second drill is passed. The drills do not have to be parallel, as they should be in the adult intracapsular fracture, since there is no later settling of the epiphysis with healing.[29]

The drill is measured for length with a direct reading depth gauge. In the system used here, the 3.2-mm drill and 3.2-mm guide pin are of equal length. A screw approximately 5 to 8 mm longer than the measured length is selected. A tap may optionally be used to enter the femoral cortex only. As per the surgeon's discretion, a self-cutting, self-tapping screw can be used immediately in most patients. Once the cannulated screw threads pass halfway up the femoral neck, the drill may be removed. When the drill bit is removed, an optional guide pin can be placed in the hole in the position of the previous drill. If the surgeon has made only one pass with the drill, the guide pin is no longer necessary; the screw should follow the hole even without a guide.

The appropriate-length cannulated screw or screws are placed (Figure 5.6). The screw threads should cross the epiphyseal plate, yet the screw tip should not perforate subchondral bone. The preferred position of the head of the screw is 5 to 8 mm proud of the femoral cortex. This makes later finding and removal of the screw easier. Screw heads left against the femoral cortex may become partially or wholly covered by cortical bone as the child matures. Again unlike the fixation of an adult's femoral neck fracture, the lag of the screw is nonfunc-

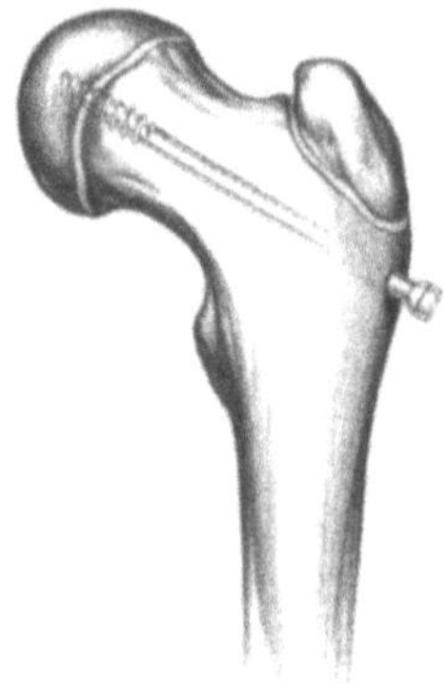

**FIGURE 5.6.** The appropriate length cannulated screw is positioned with its threads across the epiphyseal plate. The screw head is left 5 to 8 mm proud of the femoral shaft. (Reprinted with permission from Asnis.[32])

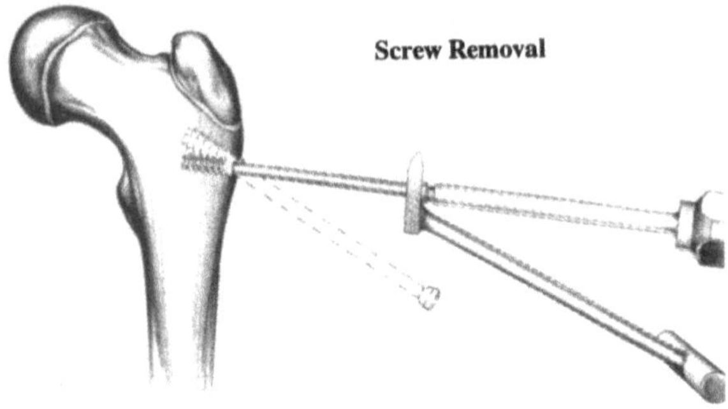


**FIGURE 5.7.** The screw is pulled into a 90° position to the shaft with a screw retractor that fits around the screw neck in order to place the reverse cutting flutes at their proper position for screw removal. (Reprinted with permission from Asnis.[32])

tional in the slipped epiphysis. Compression is obtained by the screw threads as the epiphysis attempts to grow, not by the lag of the screw itself (Figure 5.4). The leg is then rotated carefully under fluoroscopy in the AP and lateral positions to confirm no joint penetration.

## Screw Removal

Screw removal is recommended after the fusion of the epiphyseal plate. It is often performed approximately 18 months after the original procedure. Bone growing around the head of the screw makes removal more difficult. For this reason the original screw head is left 5 to 8 mm proud. Bone growing around a round head with an inner recess hexagon is much less of a problem than one with an outer hexagon. Here the bone must be removed to allow the fitting of the external wrench. Before attempting removal, the screwdriver must be carefully examined. The screwdriver tip must show no signs of wear to ensure a good fit into the hexagonal socket. A system with a hexagonal wrench or screwdriver that converts into a wrench (a rod passing through its handle) is advantageous. A screw with reverse cutting flutes is also advantageous. The screw must cut its way back through the bone in the femoral neck and the femoral cortex. When the femoral endocortex is reached, the screw is pulled into a position of 90° to the shaft with a screw retractor that fits around the screw neck (Figure 5.7). Reverse cutting flutes do not perform well at oblique angles to the cortex but do function well in this perpendicular position.

The construction of the screw may also be a factor. Vresilovic et al.[30] found a significant difference between titanium and stainless steel screws. Pin or screw breakage or stripping was significantly higher with titanium than with stainless steel ($p < .001$).

## Case 1

A $9\frac{1}{2}$-year-old African-American girl presented with 3 days of discomfort in both hips and a limp on ambulation. Family history revealed her father to have had a unilateral SCFE. Her radiographs revealed bilateral *mild* slipped capital femoral epiphyses (Figure 5.8a,b). This is best demonstrated on the lateral radiograph with widening of the epiphyseal plate and posterior slippage. A line drawn up the cortex of the anterior femoral neck of either hip would not intersect but lie above the femoral head ossification (Figure 5.8b). She underwent bilateral 6.5-mm cannulated screw fixation of her hips. The screws are well placed in the centers of the epiphyses (Figure 5.8c,d). The screw threads are centered over the epiphyseal plate and encourage fusion of the plate by the compression produced as the plate tries to continue growth.

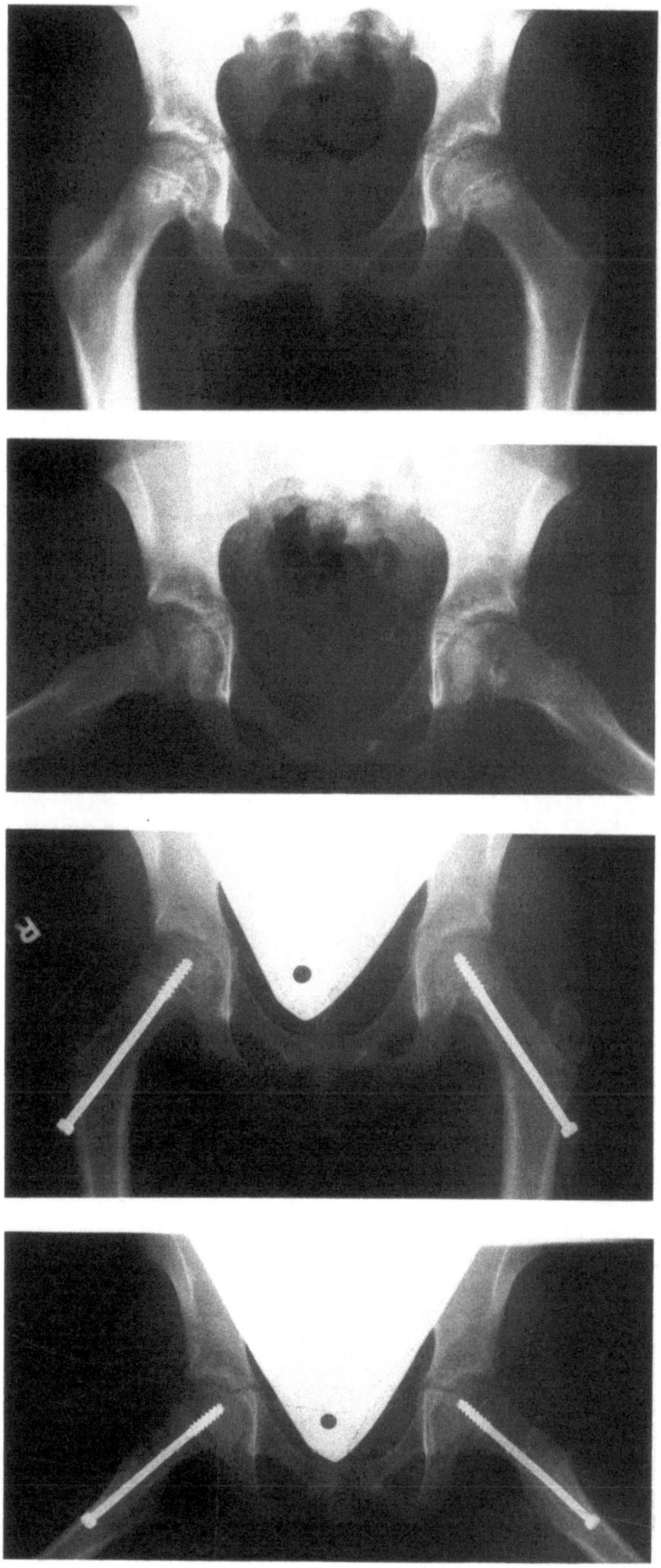

a

b

c

d

**FIGURE 5.8.** The anteroposterior radiograph of a (a) $9\frac{1}{2}$-year-old African-American girl with bilateral mild slipped capital femoral epiphyses. (b) The frog lateral view: A line drawn up the cortex of the anterior femoral neck lies above the femoral head ossification center. (c) Anteroposterior radiograph showing screws in centers of the epiphyses. (d) Frog lateral demonstrating single cannulated screws.

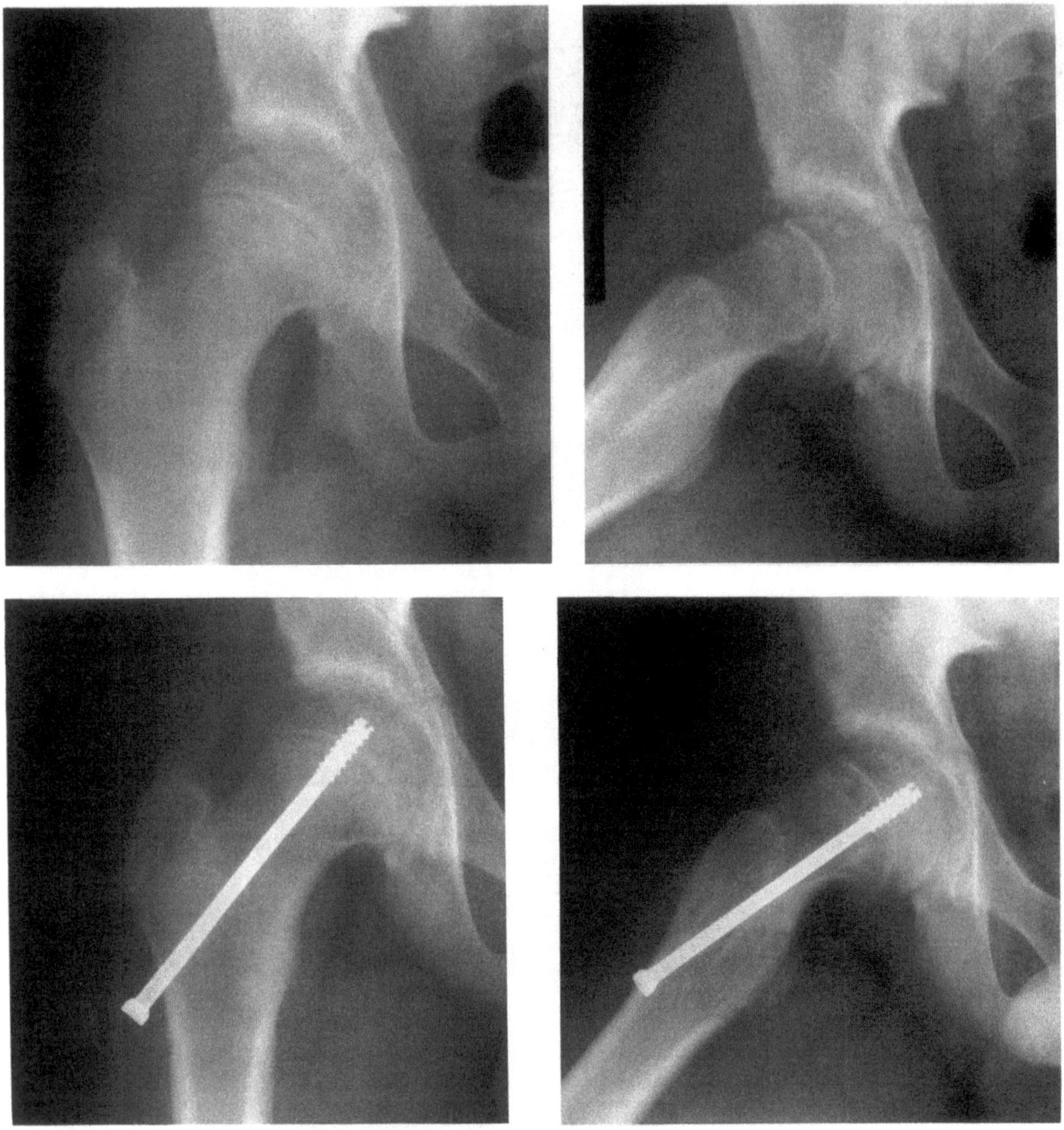


**FIGURE 5.9.** A 12-year-old white boy with a mild SCFE of his right hip. (a) Anteroposterior radiograph. (b) Frog lateral radiograph. (c) The anteroposterior radiograph shows the single cannulated screw (left) 5 mm proud of the lateral femoral cortex. (d) The single cannulated screw toward the center of the epiphyseal plate as seen on the lateral radiograph.

**FIGURE 5.10 (a,b).** The anteroposterior (a) and frog lateral radiograph (b) of a 15-year-old large African-American boy with an acute-on-chronic SCFE of his left hip. (c,d) Two cannulated screws were used because of his weight and degree of slippage.

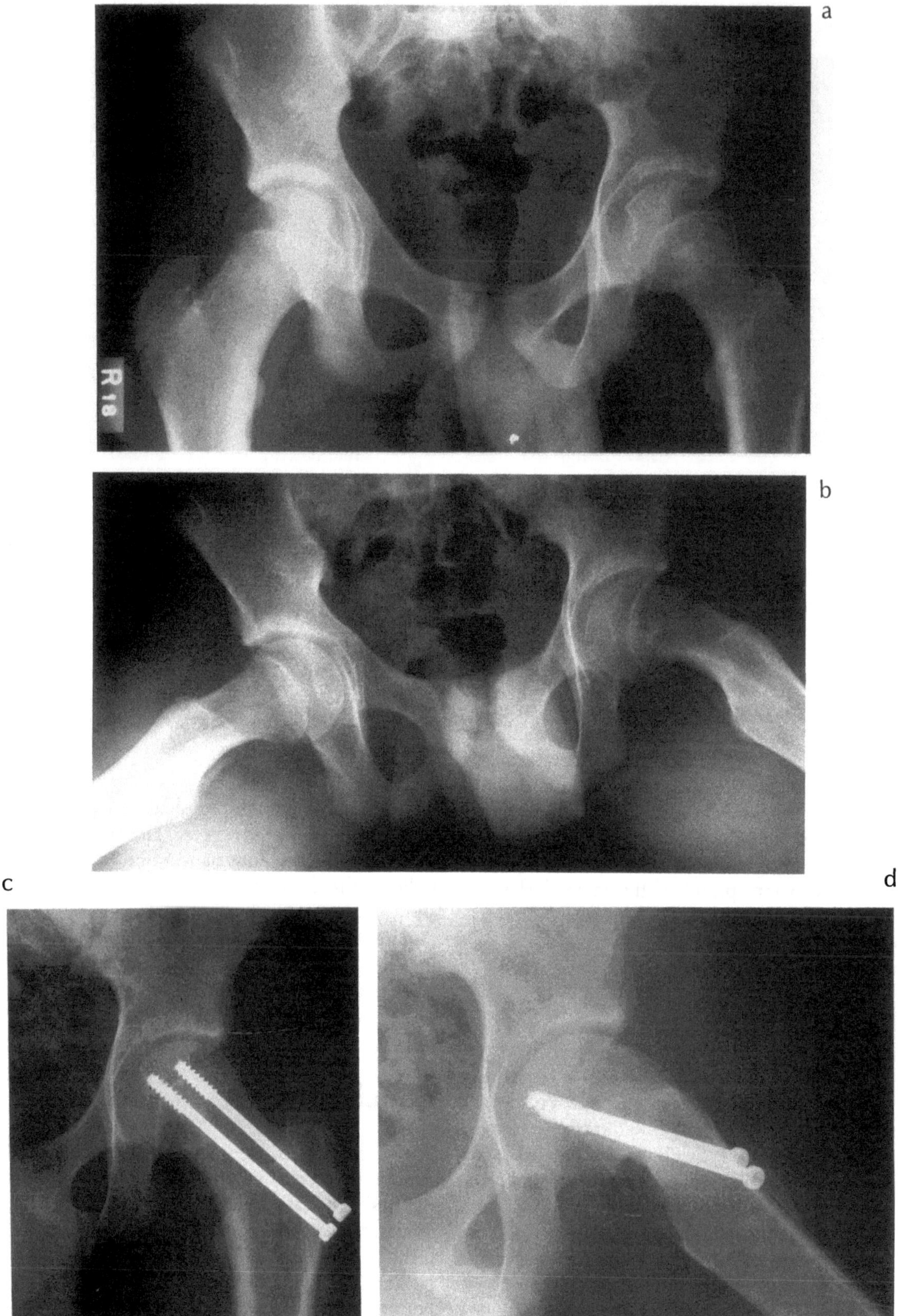
a
R 18
b
c
d

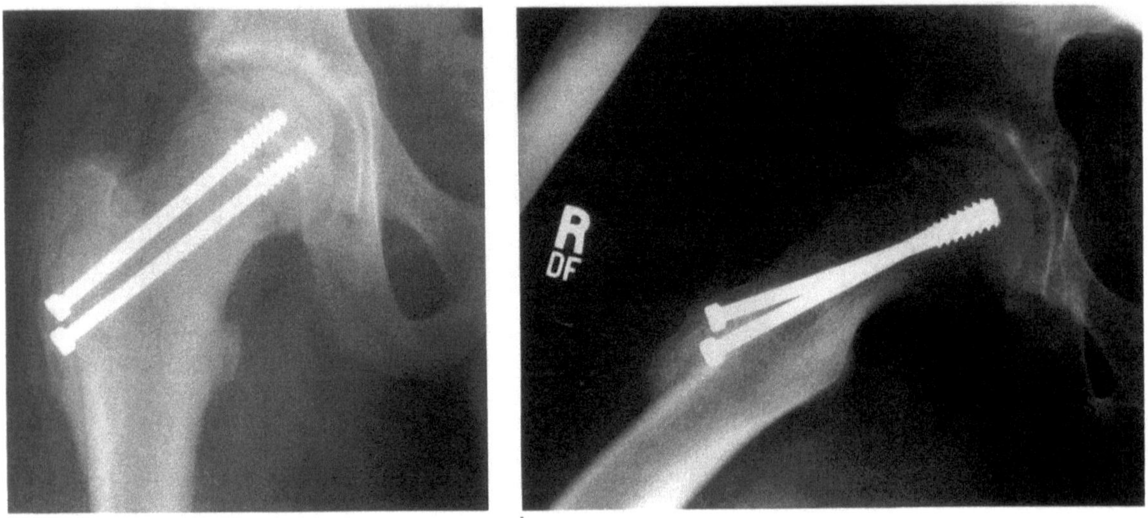


a b

**FIGURE 5.11.** Anteroposterior and lateral radiographs taken seven months after cannulated screw fixation of the SCFE of the right hip. Cortical bone has overgrown the screw heads.

## Case 2

A 12-year-old white boy started having left hip pain after playing tennis. This persisted over the ensuing 3 weeks. He walked with an antalgic gait and had a loss of internal rotation and extension. The lateral radiograph best demonstrated the *mild* SCFE of his right hip (Figure 5.9a,b). He underwent fixation with a 6.5-mm cannulated screw (Figure 5.9c,d). The screw was left 5 to 8 mm proud of the femoral shaft to make it more accessible for later removal.

## Case 3

This 15-year-old large African-American boy gave a history of intermittent pain in his left hip for over 5 months. Physical examination showed a loss of internal rotation. Radiographs showed an acute-on-chronic SCFE with a rounded hump on the anterior femoral neck on the lateral radiograph (Figure 5.10a,b). He had fixation with two 6.5-mm cannulated screws. Two screws were used because of his size and degree of slippage (Figure 10c,d). The screws do not have to be parallel. The entrance sites for the screws are along the anterior femoral shaft to allow them to stay within the neck and still pass through the epiphyseal plate toward the center of the femoral head ossification (Figure 5.10d).

## Case 4

A 12-year-old white boy had a right SCFE fixed with cannulated screws. The slippage was arrested and the epiphysis went on to fuse. The radiographs done 7 months after his surgery showed the screw heads overgrown by bone (Figure 5.11). The author now recommends leaving the screw heads 5 to 8 mm proud of the lateral femoral shaft so that after epiphyseal fusion screw removal is facilitated.

## Conclusion

In situ pinning of the minimally slipped upper femoral epiphysis has been used widely during the past 40 years. Even in the treatment of the moderately displaced epiphysis, many surgeons feel that if the epiphysis does not reduce readily, in situ pinning is the treatment of choice.[21,31] For the traumatic or acute moderate to severe slipped epiphysis a gentle reduction may be attempted. The goal of in situ fixation of the slipped epiphysis is to obtain fusion of the epiphyseal plate without further slippage as atraumatically to the joint as possible. When a cancellous bone screw thread is placed across the epiphyseal plate, it causes the plate to compress itself as it attempts to grow and encourages fusion.

Cannulated screw fixation of the slipped capital femoral epiphysis gives excellent fixation with instrumentation that facilitates accurate placement. The strength of the modern cannulated screw and the cancellous thread offer excellent fixation of the epiphysis and encourage fusion of the epiphyseal plate. One centrally placed screw has the least chance of occult pin penetration. It also is in the position for best fixation in that the epiphysis is widest in its center. Two screws can be used in the large or obese patient. All drills, guide pins, and screws should avoid penetrating the superior (lateral) or posterior portion of the femoral neck to prevent injury to the medical circumflex artery, which supplies the circulation to the majority of the femoral head. The hip should be rotated under the fluoroscope in both the AP and lateral positions at the end of the procedure to assure that there is no penetration of the screw into the joint.

## References


1. Morissy R, Selman S. Slipped capital femoral epiphysis. *Orthop Nursing* 1991;10(1):11–20.
2. Wells D, King J, Roe T, et al. Review of slipped capital femoral epiphysis associated with endocrine disease. *J Pediatr Orthop* 1993;13:610–614.
3. Bush M, Morissy R. Slipped capital femoral epiphysis. *Orthop Clin North Am* 1987;18(4):637–647.
4. Billing L, Severin E. Slipping epiphysis of the hip: a roentgenologic and clinical study based on a new roentgen technique. *Acta Radiol Suppl (Stockh)* 1959;174.
5. Hagglund G, Hansson L, Sandstrom S, et al. Bilateral slipped capital femoral epiphysis. *J Bone Joint Surg* 1988;70B:179–181.
6. Canale S. Problems and complications of slipped capital femoral epiphysis. *Instr Course Lect* 1989; 38:281–290.
7. Harris R. The endocrine basis for slipping of the femoral epiphysis. *J Bone Joint Surg* 1950;32B(1): 5–11.
8. Stulberg S, Cordell L, Harris W, et al. Unrecognized childhood hip diseases: a major cause of idiopathic osteoarthritis of the hip. In: *The Hip: Proceedings of the Eighth Open Meeting of the Hip Society*. St. Louis: Mosby, 1975;112.
9. Harris W, Hobson K. Histological changes in experimentally displaced upper femoral epiphyses in rabbits. *J Bone Joint Surg* 1956;38B(4): 914–921.
10. Ponsetti IV, McClintock R. The pathology of slipping of the upper femoral epiphysis. *J Bone Joint Surg* 1956;38A:71.
11. Key J. Epiphyseal coxa vara or displacement of the capital epiphysis of the femur in adolescence. *J Bone Joint Surg* 1926;8:53–117.
12. Mirkopulos N, Weiner D, Askew M. The evolving slope of the proximal femoral growth plate relationship to slipped capital femoral epiphysis. *J Pediatr Orthop* 1988;8:268–273.
13. Speer D. Collagenous architecture of the growth plate and perichondral ossification groove. *J Bone Joint Surg* 1982;64A:399–407.
14. Speer D. Experimental epiphysiolysis: an etiologic mode of slipped capital femoral epiphysis. *Trans Orthop Res Soc* 1978;3:47–55.
15. Chung S, Batterman S, Brighton C. Shear strength of the human femoral capital epiphyseal plate. *J Bone Joint Surg* 1976;58A:94–103.
16. Chung S. The arterial supply of the developing proximal end of the human femur. *J Bone Joint Surg* 1976;58A:961–970.
17. Trueta J. The normal vascular anatomy of the human femoral head during growth. *J Bone Joint Surg* 1957;39B:358–394.
18. Southwick W. Osteotomy through the lesser trochanter for slipped capital femoral epiphysis. *J Bone Joint Surg* 1967;49A:807–835.
19. Jacobs B. Laminar coxitis and associate lesions. In: Delohef MJ, ed. *Societe Internationale de Chirurgie Orthopedique et de Traumatologie*. Paris: Imprimerie des Sciences, Bruxelles, 1966;78–79.
20. Wilson P. Laminar coxitis and associate lesions. In: Delohef MJ, ed. *Societe Internationale de Chirurgie Orthopedique et de Traumatologie*. Paris: Imprimerie des Sciences, Bruxelles, 1966;76.
21. Carney B, Weinstein S, Noble J. Long-term follow-up of slipped capital femoral epiphysis. *J Bone Joint Surg* 1991;73A(5):667–673.
22. Maurer R, Larsen I. Acute necrosis of cartilage in slipped capital femoral epiphysis. *J Bone Joint Surg* 1970;52A(1):39–50.
23. Swiontkowski M. Slipped capital femoral epiphysis: complications related to internal fixation. *Orthopaedics* 1983;6:705–712.
24. Walters R, Simon S. Joint destruction: a sequel of unrecognized pin penetration in patients with slipped capital femoral epiphysis. In: *The Hip: Proceedings of the Eighth Open Scientific Meeting of the Hip Society*. St. Louis: Mosby, 1975;145–164.
25. Asnis S. The guided screw system in slipped

capital femoral epiphyses. *Contemp Orthop* 1985; 11(1):27–33.
26. Herndon C. Treatment of minimally slipped upper femoral epiphysis. *Instr Course Lect* 1972;21:188–195.
27. Lehman W, Grant A, Rose D, et al. A method of evaluating possible pin penetration in slipped capital femoral epiphysis using a cannulated internal fixation device. *Clin Orthop* 1984;186:65–70.
28. Shaw J. Preventing unrecognized pin penetration into the hip joint. *Orthop Rev* 1984;13:142–152.
29. Asnis SE. The guided screw system in intracapsular fractures of the hip. *Contemp Orthop* 1985;10(6):33–42.
30. Vresilovic E, Spindler K, Robertson JWW, et al. Failures of pin removal after in situ pinning of slipped capital femoral epiphyses: a comparison of different pin types. *J Pediatr Orthop* 1990;10: 764–768.
31. Boyer D, Mickelson M, Ponsetti I. Slipped capital femoral epiphysis: long-term follow-up and study of one hundred and twenty-one patients. *J Bone Joint Surg* 1981;63A:85–95.
32. Asnis SE. The Asnis 2 Guided Screw System: Howmedica Surgical Techniques: Rutherford, New Jersey: 1991;4–5.

# 6

# Acetabular Reconstruction with Allografts Utilizing Cannulated Screws

Bruce A. Seideman and Stanley E. Asnis

The acetabulum in revision total hip arthroplasty frequently demonstrates bone stock deficiency secondary to prior surgical technique and bone resorption due to loosening. Dysplasia of the hip and degenerative arthritis may be associated with acetabular bone stock deficiencies as well. These defects in the acetabulum may be small, such as those from prior cement anchoring holes, and only require minor particulate grafting. Alternatively, the defect may be massive and complex, requiring extensive acetabular reconstruction with allograft bone. It is these latter defects that present a significant challenge to the orthopaedic surgeon performing revision total hip arthroplasty.

## Preoperative Planning

Medial wall perforation (acetabular protrusion) enclosed cavitary and segmental rim defects may all require acetabular grafting. Complex combinations of these defects may exist as well.[1] A detailed classification system of these deficiencies has been created by the American Academy of Orthopaedic Surgeons (AAOS) Committee on the Hip.

## Classification of Acetabular Deficiencies

Type I—Segmental deficiencies
- A. Peripheral
  1. Superior
  2. Anterior
  3. Posterior
- B. Central (medial wall absent)

Type II—Cavitary deficiencies
- A. Peripheral
  1. Superior
  2. Anterior
  3. Posterior
- B. Central (medial wall intact)

Type III—Combined deficiencies
Type IV—Pelvic discontinuity
Type V—Arthrodesis

Segmental deficiencies are characterized by a complete loss of bone in a portion of the acetabulum. Cavitary deficiencies represent bone loss with the maintenance of a supporting bony rim. The deficiencies may be located in various quadrants of the acetabulum and in combination (type III).

Use of this classification system helps with preoperative planning and choice of surgical exposure. In addition to standard and oblique plain radiographs of the pelvis, more complex evaluation may be required. Computed tomography (CT) with three-dimensional reconstruction is a useful addition to preoperative planning. With large medial wall defects and component migration into the pelvis, angiography can disclose the proximity of major vessels to the proposed operative areas. Consideration of infection as the cause of implant failure must always be addressed. Appropriate hematologic testing, nuclear medicine scans, and preoperative aspiration arthrogram are performed as indicated. If considerable doubt exists concerning the possibility of infection, then a staged reconstruction is performed allowing for final results of deep culture specimens.

Reconstruction of the deficient acetabulum utilizing allograft bone allows for potential long-term biologic augmentation of these deficiencies. The use of large cement masses is avoided and the acetabular implant can potentially be placed in a more appropriate anatomic position. By avoiding high placement of the acetabular component the hip center of rotation is not directed superiorly above the true acetabulum. In addition, the ilium above the acetabulum thins out and becomes insufficient for adequate support of an acetabular component due to the lack of adequate anterior and posterior bone stock. Recently, Paprosky et al.[2] have reported a 6-year follow-up of 147 press-fit acetabular revisions with allograft, with only six failures. All of the failures occurred in the type 3B class (massive superior rim defects extending into the anterior and posterior columns), in which proximal femoral "arc" grafts were utilized with pelvic reconstruction plates for fixation. Of note, the grafts did not fail, but rather the cups migrated due to lack of adequate ingrowth.

Isolated medial wall defects, whether segmental or cavitary, can be treated by packing with a mixture of cortical and cancellous allograft, autograft, or a combination of both. The peripheral intact rim is reamed to support an acetabular component that is larger than the defect. Porous ingrowth acetabular components are utilized. The inserted component is generally 2 mm larger than that of the last utilized reamer. The acetabular component is supported by the intact peripheral rim and acts as a mold to the graft. Acetabular fixation is augmented with screws, if thought to be indicated. Isolated cavitary defects with adequate surrounding bone may be treated in a similar fashion by packing them with bone and placement of an acetabular component in an appropriately reamed acetabulum.[1]

Peripheral rim defects are reconstructed utilizing a structural allograft. They may be isolated or in association with other defects. Their location and extent will determine the type of allograft required and the method of fixation necessary to provide rigid fixation of the allograft to the acetabulum.

Harris[3] originally fixed allograft femoral heads to the pelvis utilizing screws with bolts. Several authors have described the use of cancellous lag screws to secure the allograft.[4–6] Most isolated superior rim defects and those associated with a cavitary defect can be reconstructed utilizing an allograft femoral head fixed to the pelvis with screws. More complex deficiencies may require the use of proximal femoral, distal femoral, proximal tibia, or pelvic allografts. These may require both plate and screw fixation for adequate support. It is beyond the scope of this book to detail each of these situations and the reader is referred to several excellent publications for further information concerning these more complex reconstructions.[7,8]

## Advantages of Cannulated Screws

There are several advantages of the use of cannulated screws in the fixation of the bone graft in acetabular reconstruction:

1. Guide pins provide temporary fixation of the graft during preliminary shaping to conform with the host acetabulum.
2. Guide pins can be placed in the ideal site in the graft, allowing for temporary fixation while working on the graft without loss of bone stock necessary for the final screw fixation.
3. Guide pins allow for the determination of the ideal position for the final fixation screws.
4. Guide pins allow for the determination of the ideal screw length prior to final fixation.

The large bone graft is first cut and shaped to fit into its bed in the pelvis utilizing a saw and high-speed power burr. The graft is then initially placed in the pelvis utilizing a drill followed by a guide pin. The site of optimal position for the graft may be modified as required without loss of significant graft or host bone. Additional guide pins can be used for temporary fixation. Some or all of these pins can later be used to guide screws for final fixation. The acetabular surface of the graft is then shaped to conform with the remainder of the host acetabulum. This is performed with a power burr system followed by the acetabular reamers. If the final fixation screws are used before the final shaping of the graft, the forces and motion of the burring and reaming may loosen and compromise the final fixation. The use of guide pins as preliminary fixation avoids this potential problem.

# Authors' Preferred Technique

Guided screws allow for the accurate fixation of allografts to the pelvis for acetabular reconstruction. The technique utilized by the authors for a combined superior rim and intraacetabular defects is described.

## Equipment

The authors suggest a screw system with a 6.5-mm outer diameter over a 3.2-mm guide pin for firm fixation of the graft; however, this is occasionally mixed with some smaller cannulated screws of 5.0 mm over 2.0-mm guide pins. The strong and stiff 3.2-mm guide pin best supports the bone graft as it is positioned and shaped. Although the acetabular shells utilized are titanium, the acetabular screws are not in contact with the shell, and stainless steel screws can be safely utilized. The threaded tip of the steel screw has excellent holding power. The tip has a positive rake cutting surface, which makes it sharp only when turning clockwise (see Chapter 2). As an alternate some surgeons may use primarily 6.5-mm self-tapping titanium screws with a 3.2-mm stainless steel guide pin. These screws allow better visualization if a postoperative CT or magnetic resonance imaging (MRI) is to be performed; however, these tests are not commonly used in arthroplasty situations because of the interference caused by the materials of the arthroplasty itself. Some of the presently available 6.5-mm titanium screws have a sharper tip, which may be positioned just through the inner pelvic wall. There is also less holding power of the thread tip in some of these titanium screws due to the type of cutting flutes used.

### *The 6.5-mm Stainless Steel Screw System*

*Drill*: A 9-inch-long, 3.2-mm steel drill, which can be used with a direct-reading 9-inch depth gauge. *Guide pin*: A 9-inch-long, 3.2-mm guide pin with a threaded tip and tapered root diameter (Chapter 2). *Screw head*: Round head with an internal hexagon. *Screw thread*: Outer diameter—6.5 mm; pitch—2.5 mm; reverse cutting flutes; self-cutting, self-tapping positive rake tip. *Material*: 22-13-5 stainless steel. *Washers*: 6.5-mm system washers.

### *The 5.0-mm Stainless Steel Screw System*

*Drill*: A 2.0-mm steel drill, which can be used with a direct-reading depth gauge. *Guide pin*: A 2.0-mm guide pin with a threaded tip. *Screw head*: Round head with an internal hexagon. *Screw thread*: Outer diameter—5.0 mm; self-cutting, self-tapping positive rake tip. *Material*: 316LVM stainless steel. *Washers*: 5.0-mm system washers.

### *Alternate: Titanium 6.5-mm Screw System*

*Drill*: A 3.2-mm steel drill. *Guide pin*: A 3.2-mm guide pin. *Screw head*: Round head with an internal hexagon. *Screw thread*: Outer diameter—6.5 mm; reverse cutting flutes; self-cutting, self-tapping tip. *Material*: Titanium 6Al 4V alloy. *Washers*: 6.5-mm system titanium washers.

## Technique

The authors prefer to utilize a modification of the Hardinge[9] direct lateral approach for revision total hip arthroplasty, extending the dissection distally along the femur to elevate the anterior half of the quadriceps. If the defect is anticipated to require greater exposure, particularly posteriorly, then a trochanteric slide as described by Glassman et al.[10] is utilized. The acetabulum is exposed with appropriate retraction after removal of the prior components, cement, and soft tissue.

The defect is assessed for size and configuration. An appropriate femoral head allograft is utilized. We have initially fashioned the graft in the "number 7" configuration described by Paprosky et al.[8] for these defects as it allows for reconstruction of the superior rim and intraacetabular defect and for extraacetabular screw fixation of the graft. Gross fashioning of the

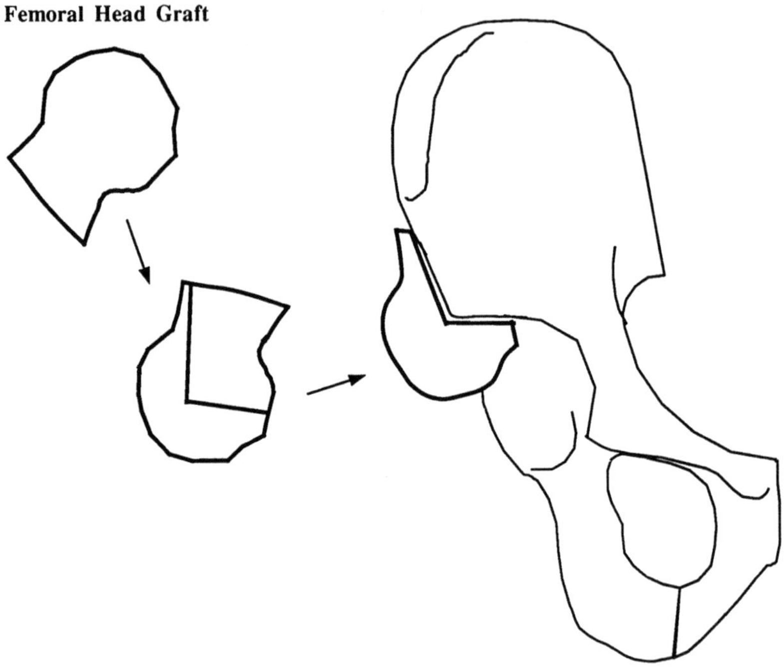


**FIGURE 6.1.** The femoral head is fashioned in the "number 7" configuration to fit the acetabular defect.

graft is performed utilizing a high-speed drill. Consideration is given to cut the graft so that the axis of the weight-bearing trabeculae of the graft will align with that of the reconstructed hip after placement of the allograft (Figure 6.1). The graft bed is lightly abraded with a high-speed burr and the graft is placed in the appropriate line of axis onto this bed. Further modeling of the graft may be necessary in order to achieve the best contact between the graft and its bed.

Once the graft has been placed in the ideal position, it is held in place with at least two 3.2-mm guide pins placed in the line of weight bearing (Figure 6.2). The guide pins are placed in the position that will most likely be used for the permanent screws.

Great care is taken to not drill beyond the opposite cortex of the pelvis due to risk of neurovascular damage. The guide pins can be placed directly, or a preliminary drill technique may be utilized. A 3.2-mm drill is driven through the dense bone of the graft material, then slowly

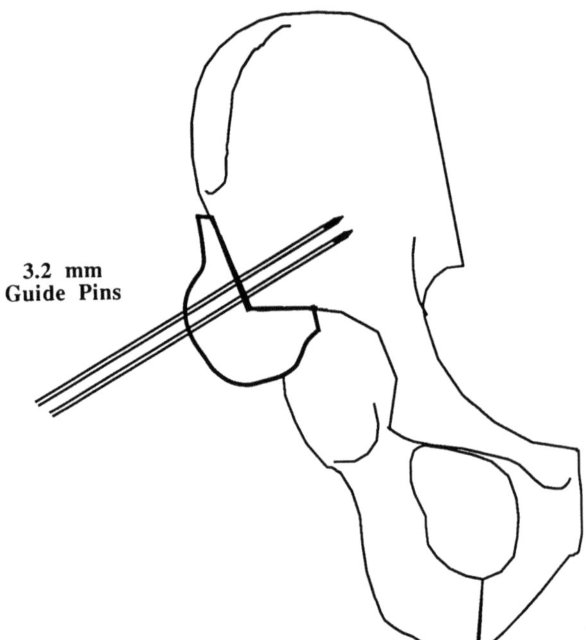


**FIGURE 6.2.** The allograft is secured to the pelvis with guide pins.

advanced through the cancellous bone of the pelvis to the opposite cortex. To better feel the opposite cortex (inner pelvic wall) and not penetrate it, the drill can be put in *reverse* and advanced so that the tip is blunt, or it can be left on *forward* and advanced with a gentle to-fro motion to feel the inner pelvic cortex. Once the inner pelvic cortex is felt, a depth gauge measurement is made. If guide pins are used directly, they are now carefully advanced to or through the inner cortex. If drills are first used, two are initially placed. When the inner cortex is felt with the drills, one drill is removed while the other holds graft position. The first drill is replaced with a guide wire and the guide wire advanced through the inner cortex. The second drill is then likewise exchanged for its guide wire.

Guide pins and screws should avoid the anterior quadrants where damage to neurovascular structures is most possible[11] (Figure 6.3). The external iliac vessels, the obturator vessels, and obturator nerve are at risk from damage secondary to screws placed beyond the bone in these zones. Screws placed in the posterior superior quadrant may be directed toward the sciatic nerve and superior gluteal vessels and nerve. In an intact acetabulum Wasielewski et al.[12] have recommended that screws up to 25 mm in length can be safely placed in the poster superior quadrant. In a similar fashion, screws up to 25 mm in length are safely recommended in the posterior inferior quadrant, avoiding damage to the inferior gluteal and internal pudendal nerves and vessels. A small zone in the posterior superior quadrant allows for placement of screws longer than 35 mm between the tables of the ileum toward the sacroiliac joint.[12] When using these guidelines for screw placement during revision total hip replacement, it must be realized that these estimated measurements were made from intact acetabulae and that bone loss must be taken into account when considering screw length and structures at risk. It must be made clear, however, that these measurements represent the depth that the *threaded end* of the screw can be placed in the host pelvic bone. A cannulated screw with a *thread length* of 20 mm has proven to fit very well within the ilium. The width of the allograft must be taken into account when determining final total screw length. Generally cannulated screws of approximately 50 mm or greater are needed to span both the allograft and pelvic bone. A drill and depth gauge technique can readily be utilized prior to pin placement to assure that plunging beyond the inner cortex does not occur and that a screw of appropriate length is used.

With the graft held in place by the provisional pins, further gross modeling of the graft is undertaken with a high-speed bur and acetabular reamers (Figure 6.4). The dense bone of the allograft may be tapped by placing a cannulated tap over the first guide pin. The first cannulated screw is loaded with a washer, if desired, and passed over the first guide pin. The second site is then tapped around the guide pin and the second screw with washer placed. With a self-cutting and self-tapping thread, the screw may be used directly without tapping. The graft is now rigidly fixed to the pelvis with the cannulated screws, and the guide pins are removed. Final reaming of the acetabulum and graft is now carried out sequentially until appropriate bone contact has been achieved with the reamers (Figure 6.5). A porous ingrowth acetabular component is impacted in place and supplemental screw fixation of the acetabular component is undertaken with the regular acetabular shell fixation screws, if desired (Figure 6.6). A bone slurry is made by using the acetabular reamers on the unused portion of the femoral head allograft. This is utilized to fill any gaps around the host-graft junction.

Postoperatively the patient is restricted from full weight bearing for a period of approximately 3 months. Modification of this program may be undertaken depending on the reconstruction.

# Clinical Examples

## Case 1

A 62-year-old woman had severe degenerative joint disease secondary to long-standing avascular necrosis of the femoral head. The preoperative radiograph shows significant superior-lateral acetabular bone stock loss with lateral subluxation of the femoral head (Figure 6.7). At the

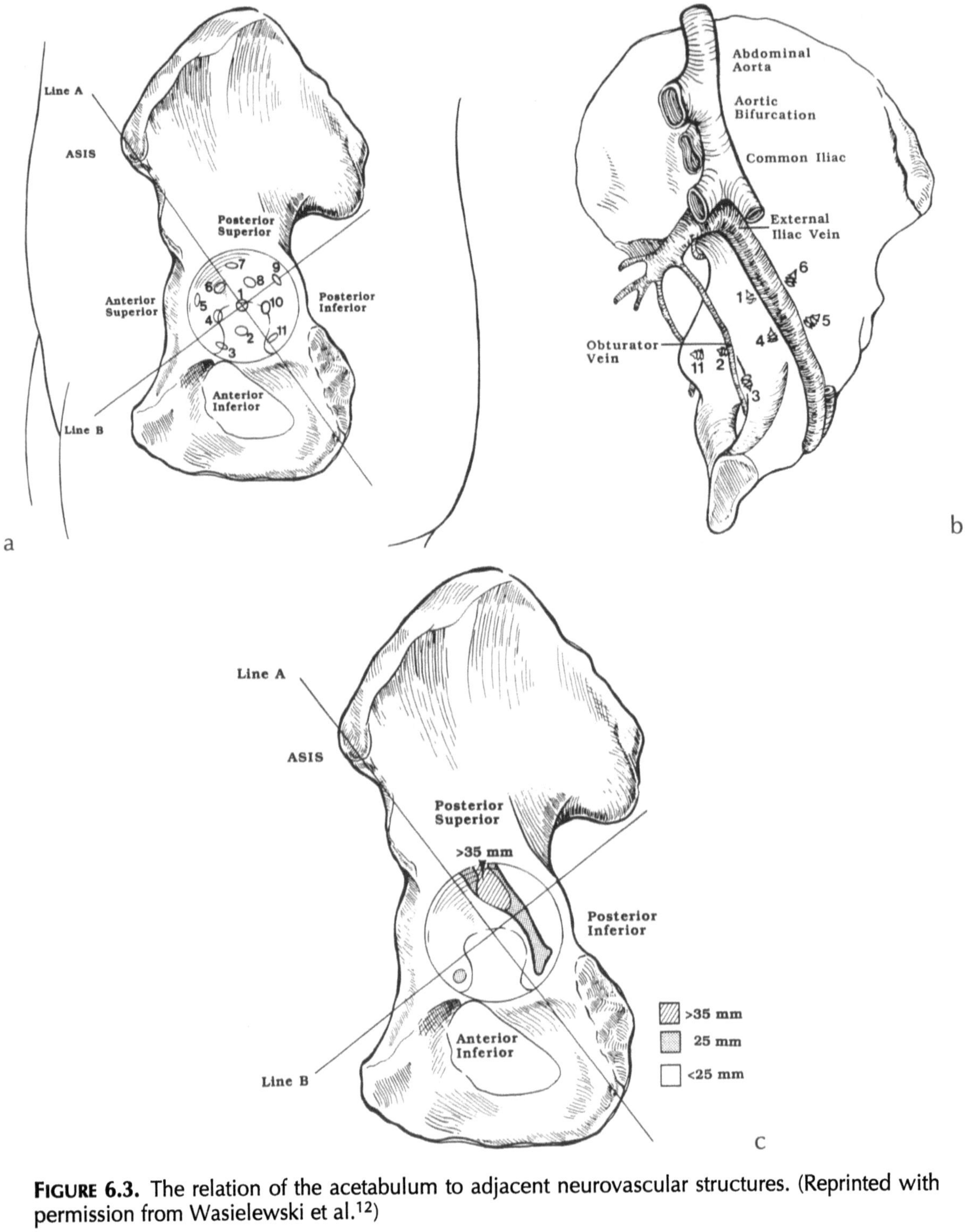


**FIGURE 6.3.** The relation of the acetabulum to adjacent neurovascular structures. (Reprinted with permission from Wasielewski et al.[12])

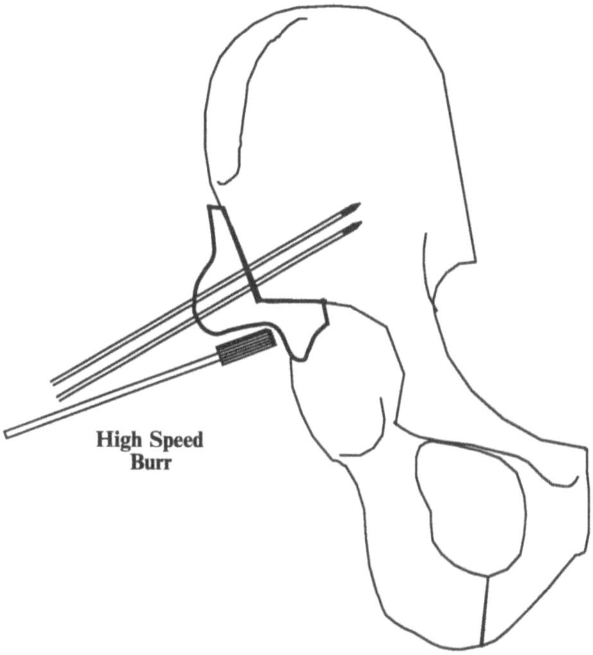


FIGURE 6.4. The graft is contoured with a high-speed burr.

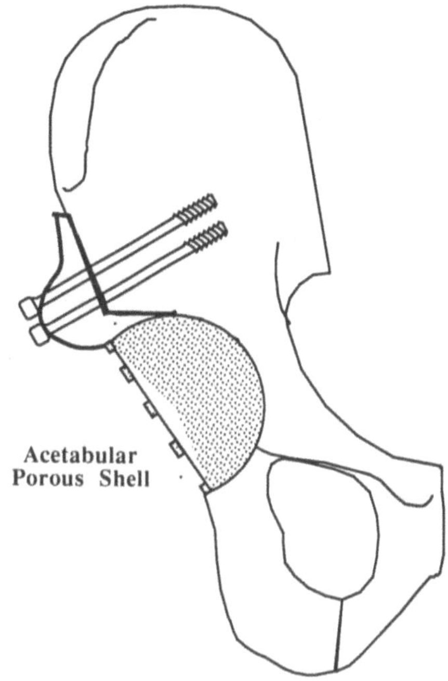


FIGURE 6.6. The porous ingrowth acetabular shell is impacted in place.

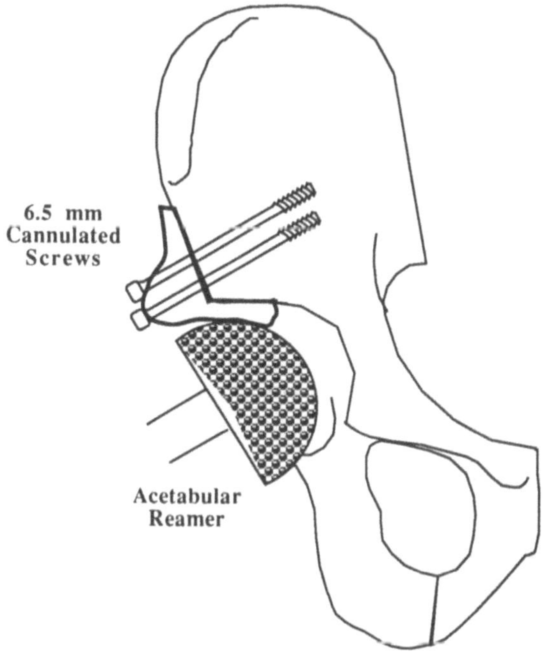


FIGURE 6.5. The final reaming of the graft is performed after it is firmly fixed with the cannulated screws.

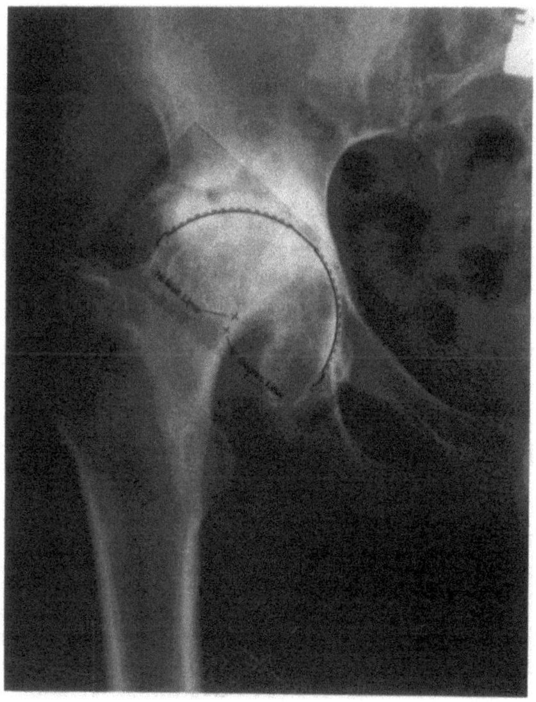

FIGURE 6.7. Severe degenerative arthritis of the right hip with superior-lateral acetabular deficiency. The acetabular template is used in preoperative planning.

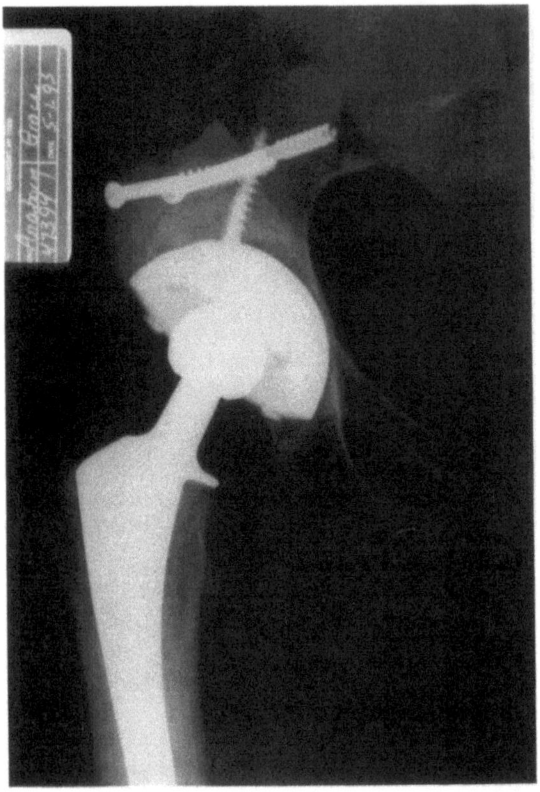

**FIGURE 6.8.** The superior-lateral acetabular deficiency was reconstructed with a femoral head allograft using the technique described.

time of surgery the acetabulum demonstrated superior-lateral and posterior deficiency. This was reconstructed with a femoral head allograft secured to the pelvis with screws as described in the operative technique (Figure 6.8).

## Case 2

An 80-year-old man had undergone a total hip arthroplasty for osteoarthritis 11 years prior to our initial evaluation. His radiographs reveal a loose femoral and acetabular component with associated superior lateral acetabular bone loss and severe myositis ossificans (Figure 6.9). Both components were revised for aseptic loosening with a porous ingrowth prosthesis. A femoral head allograft was utilized to reconstruct a combined superior rim and intraacetabular defect (Figure 6.10).

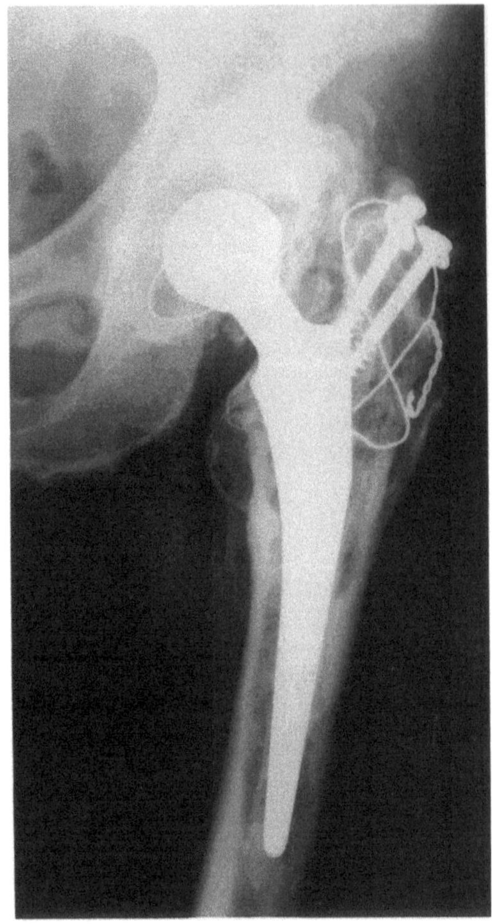

**FIGURE 6.9.** The radiograph demonstrates loosened femoral and acetabular components with a superior-lateral acetabular deficiency.

## Case 3

A 45-year-old man presented with degenerative joint disease of the hip secondary to dysplasia. Radiographs reveal joint space loss associated with a superior segmental rim defect (Figure 6.11). A porous ingowth total hip arthroplasty was performed with an autograft utilizing the patient's femoral head (Figure 6.12).

Acetabular grafting has allowed for the reconstruction of deficiencies in complex primary and revision total hip replacement surgery. The use of allografts allows for this reconstruction without large cement masses and provides for a true biologic reconstruction of the acetabulum with

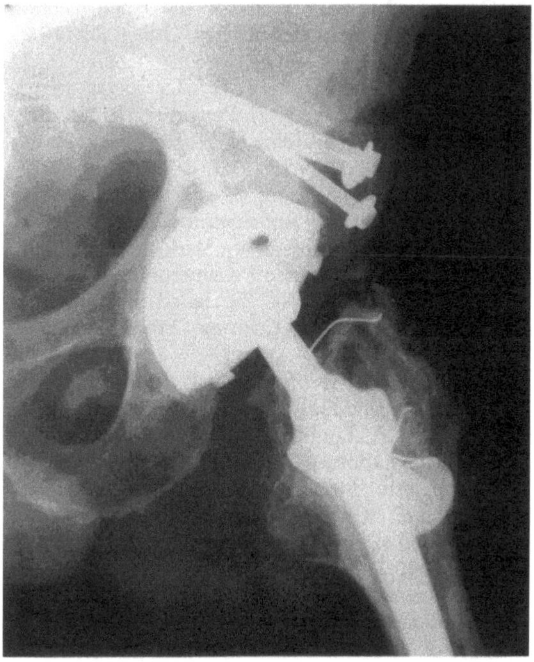

FIGURE 6.10. A femoral head allograft was used to reconstruct the intraacetabular defect and superior acetabular rim.

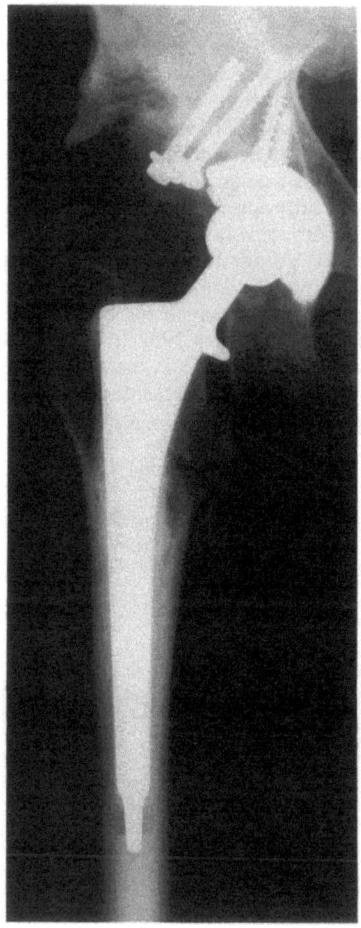

FIGURE 6.12. The patient's femoral head was used as an autograft to reconstruct the acetabular deficiency during the total joint replacement.

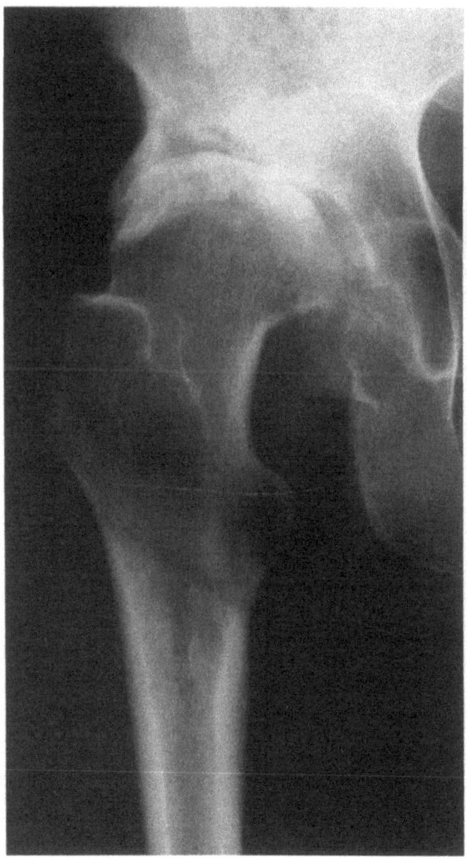

FIGURE 6.11. This degenerative dysplastic hip demonstrates a superior segmental rim defect with lateral pseudosubluxation of the femoral head.

the potential for long-term acetabular augmentation. Improved positioning of acetabular components in more anatomic sites is achieved as well. Guided screws allow for accurate placement and rigid fixation of the allograft to the pelvis.

## References


1. Chandler H. Use of allografts and prosthesis in the reconstruction of failed total hip replacements. *Orthopaedics* 1992;15(10):1207–1218.
2. Paprosky W, Perona P, Lawrence J. Acetabular defect classification and surgical reconstruction in revision arthroplasty. A six year follow-up evaluation. *J Arthroplasty* 1994;9(1):33–44.
3. Harris W. Allografting in total hip arthroplasty: in adults with severe acetabular deficiency including a surgical technique for bolting the graft to the ilium. *Clin Orthop* 1982;162:150–164.
4. Barrack R, Newland C. A technique of acetabular reconstruction for uncemented total hip replacement. *Orthop Rev* 1990;19(9):807–817.
5. Cameron M. Four methods for reconstruction of acetabular floor deficiencies. *Orthop Rev* 1985; 14(9):71–75.
6. Chandler H, Penenberg B. Acetabular reconstruction. In: Chandler H, Penenberg B, eds. *Bone Stock Deficiency in Total Hip Replacement.* Thorofare, NJ: Slack, 1989;55.
7. Chandler H, Penenberg B, eds. *Bone Stock Deficiency in Total Hip Replacement, Classification and Management.* Thorofare, NJ: Slack, 1989:
8. Paprosky W, Lawrence J, Cameron H. Classification and treatment of the failed acetabulum: a systematic approach. *Contemp Orthop* 1991;22(2): 121–129.
9. Hardinge K. The direct lateral approach to the hip. *J Bone Joint Surg* 1982;67B:17–19.
10. Glassman A, Engh C, Bohyn J. A technique of extensile exposure for total hip arthroplasty. *J Arthroplasty* 1987;2(11):17–19.
11. Keating E, Ritter M, Faris P. Structures at risk from medial placed acetabular screws. *J Bone Joint Surg* 1990;72A(4):509–511.
12. Wasielewski R, Cooperstein L, Kruger M, et al. Acetabular anatomy and the transacetabular fixation of screws in total hip arthroplasty. *J Bone Joint Surg* 1990;72A(4):501–508.

# 7
# Pelvic and Acetabular Fractures

Dana C. Mears

Significant or displaced fractures of the pelvic ring and acetabulum constitute a diverse group of skeletal injuries that usually result from motor vehicular accidents, industrial trauma, or falls from great heights. The typical pelvic ring disruption requires the application of immense forces to the patient, who thereby is likely to present with other serious or life-threatening injuries involving the musculoskeletal (85%), respiratory (60%), central nervous (40%), gastrointestinal (30%), urologic (12%), and cardiovascular (6%) systems.[1] The management of a pelvic ring fracture, therefore, requires a concomitant diagnosis and treatment of the other systemic and musculoskeletal injuries. About 50% of acetabular fracture patients have sustained associated injuries, and about 30% have experienced injuries to three or more organ systems. As McMurtry et al.,[2] Tile,[3] and others[4] have emphasized, a meticulous diagnostic protocol is needed that prioritizes the evaluation of diverse organ systems by the degree of urgency. From a recent report by Dalal et al.,[5] a correlation of the pelvic injury pattern with the statistical likelihood for particular patterns of associated visceral injuries may facilitate the application of diverse diagnostic procedures.

Historically, the stabilization of the pelvic ring was deemed to be of secondary importance after the preliminary resuscitative phase of management had been completed. In the patient who is hemodynamically unstable, acute stabilization of the pelvic ring provisionally by resort to a pneumatic anti-shock garment, and more definitively by an external frame or comparable pelvic clamp, assists in the provision of hemostasis.[1,6] Such a method can facilitate the elimination of enforced recumbency with the associated predilection for thromboembolic problems, decubitus ulcers, urinary retention, urinary tract infections, and atelectasis. External fixation is biomechanically inadequate to effectively immobilize many injury patterns, especially those with a major disruption or bilateral disruption of the posterior pelvic ring or associated acetabular fractures.[7] In common with other intraarticular disruptions, an acetabular fracture is exceedingly vulnerable to progress to posttraumatic arthritis unless an accurate reduction is achieved. During the past 20 years, extensive clinical and biomechanical research has focused upon attempts to devise operative approaches, reduction strategies, and fixation methods that are appropriate for a broad spectrum of pelvic and acetabular fractures.[8] The application of cannulated screws has become an attractive form of fixation that is applicable for certain injury patterns. The assets include a minimally invasive insertional mode combined with radiographic targeting of a preliminary guide wire. Lag screw fixation is a particularly impressive form of stabilization for the ring like pelvis, where bending movements are relatively low and frictional properties of interdigitating fracture fragments are outstanding.[9]

As a supplementary clinical problem and one of ever-increasing presentation, insufficiency fractures of the elderly are complicated by the pathologically osteoporotic bone.[10] Historically, these problems were managed by primary care physicians and rheumatologists who were under the mistaken hypothesis that conservative methods were uniformly successful. Currently, orthopaedists are requested to assist in the management of a small percentage, but ever-increasing number of such patients who experience chronic pain and progressive subsidence of their pelvic fractures that follow a trivial fall or other mishap. Usually the fractures are stabilized in situ so that an extensile surgical approach is unnecessary. For an insufficiency fracture, cannulated screw fixation is a particularly attractive form of stabilization.

This chapter focuses on the role of cannulated screws for the fixation of many types of pelvic and acetabular fractures.

## Structural Anatomy of the Pelvis

Upon inspection of the front of the pelvis and torso, the most prominent features are the symmetrical iliac crests, anterosuperior iliac spines, and the symphysis pubis. In a lean individual, the inguinal ligament visibly spans from the anterosuperior iliac spine to the ipsilateral pubis tubercle in a cord-like fashion. If the iliac crest is traced posteriorly, the palpating finger courses from the crest to the posterosuperior iliac spine and continues obliquely in a medial and distal direction to the tip of the sacrum and coccyx. Anterior or posterior scrutiny of the torso is notable for the lateral prominence of the greater trochanter and the allied abductor musculature that originates along the iliac crest and adjacent lateral ilium. Upon initial inspection of the patient who has sustained a major disruption of the pelvic ring or an acetabular fracture, a careful scrutiny and palpation of these bony landmarks may indicate an asymmetrical disposition, instability, or other abnormality.

The pelvic girdle is a ring-like structure comprising two innominate bones, which articulate anteriorly in a direct fashion at the symphysis and posteriorly by an interposed sacrum (Figure 7.1). In turn, the sacrum articulates superiorly with the lumbar spine and inferiorly with the coccyx. The pelvic ring is subdivided into an upper or false pelvis, a clinical extension of the abdomen, and an inferior or true pelvis. The dividing line, the pelvic inlet, is an oblique plane that passes through the upper symphysis pubis, and the iliopectineal lines to the sacral promontory. In an erect posture, weight-bearing forces are transmitted from the spinal column through

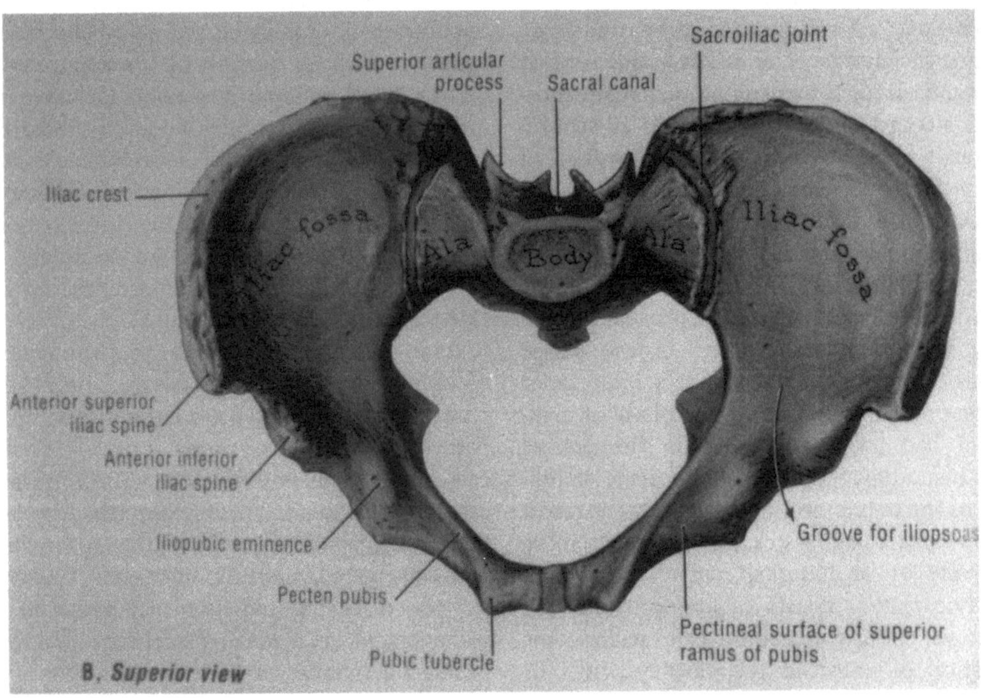


**FIGURE 7.1.** Bony anatomy of the pelvis. (Reprinted with permission from Agur.[12])

the sacrum and sacroiliac joints, along the thick sections of ilia, to the acetabulae and, thereby, to the proximal femora. While this femorosacral arch is crucial for weight transmission in an erect posture, in a sitting position weight-bearing forces pass through the sacroiliac joints into the ilia with a progression into the ischial tuberosities via either ischiosacral arch. To a lesser degree, weight-bearing forces are transmitted around the anterior portions of the pelvic ring. With the limited mobility of the pelvic articulations at the sacroiliac and sacrococcygeal joints and the symphysis pubis, the muscles originating on the pelvis provide locomotion for the lower extremities or postural support for the torso. There is no demonstrable motion of the articulations of the pelvic ring itself, apart from that associated with childbirth.

Letournel and Judet[11] redefined the innominate bone as a bony support for the acetabulum. The acetabulum is perceived as a socket contained within two arms of an inverted Y formed by a stout posterior column, the ilioischial component, and a longer anterior column that extends from the anterior extension of the superior iliac crest to the pubic symphysis (Figure 7.2). The internal surface of the acetabulum constitutes the quadrilateral surface on the inner aspect of the body of the ischium. The posterior border of the ilioischial column is formed superiorly by the ilium and inferiorly by the greater and lesser sciatic notches separated by the ischial spine. The iliopubic column is subdivided into iliac, acetabular, and pubic segments. The iliac segment is notable for a lateral pillar or gluteal ridge that extends superiorly from the roof of the acetabulum to the gluteus medius tubercle. Its anterior border possesses two thick projections, the anterior superior and anterior inferior iliac spines separated by the interspinous notch. The acetabular portion continues medially with a thickened segment of anterior wall, the iliopubic eminence, that attaches to the pubic ramus. In fact, the anterior wall is dwarfed by the larger posterior wall, thereby creating the relative acetabular anteflexion of about 20°.

The sacrum is a large, irregular pyramid with five surfaces (Figure 7.3). Its embryological origin is five fused vertebrae of progressively diminishing size from superior to inferior. The principal component, the first sacral vertebra, is tilted forward in the erect posture to an angle of about 30° to 40°. The slightly convex posterior surface possesses a thickened medial crest as a modification of the spinous processes. The slightly concave anterior surface forms the posterior pelvic wall. Matching pairs of sacral foramina are evident on both the anterior and posterior surfaces. A lateral mass of bone, the ala, affords a thickened buttress for the articular portion of either sacroiliac joint with a corresponding iliac buttress. The sacrum is positioned about 3 cm anterior to the posterior superior spines and the adjacent posterior iliac crests. The recessed position of either sacroiliac joint compromises the view realized by a posterior approach and thereby hampers the assessment of accuracy achieved with an open reduction.

The bony pelvis is notable for thickened condensations of bone that provide attractive sites for the application of internal fixation to the innominate bone (Figure 7.4). Screws can be inserted into drill holes prepared in the anterior and posterior iliac spines, the gluteal tubercle, the gluteal ridge, the pubic ramus, and along the iliopubic and ilioischial columns. Screws also can be inserted across the sacroiliac joint and the symphysis pubis. For immobilization of a longitudinal sacral fracture (Figures 7.3d and 7.5), iliosacral screws can extend from the ipsilateral ilium into the first or second sacral body. In the presence of a bilateral sacral fracture, lengthy screws can be used that extend from one ilium and across the sacrum into the other ilium. As an alternative, bilateral iliosacral screws can be used, or as another option, screws can be inserted horizontally that extend from one posterior superior spine to the other with a pathway that is similar to that of a sacral bar and behind the sacral bodies.

Dense ligaments anchor the sacroiliac joints, especially the posterior interosseous ligaments. The corresponding anterior sacroiliac ligaments are relatively attenuated. Two crucial supplementary ligaments afford rotational stability to the hemipelvis. The strong sacrotuberous ligament is a fan-shaped band that extends from the lateral portion of the dorsum of the sacrum and the adjacent iliac spines to the ischial tuberosity. A supplementary sacrospinous ligament is a

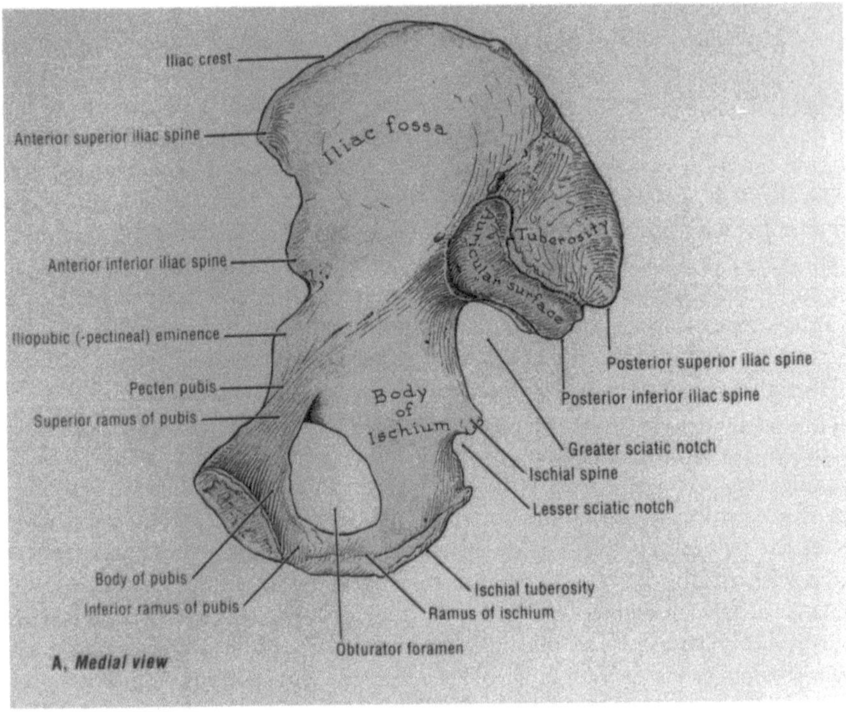


a

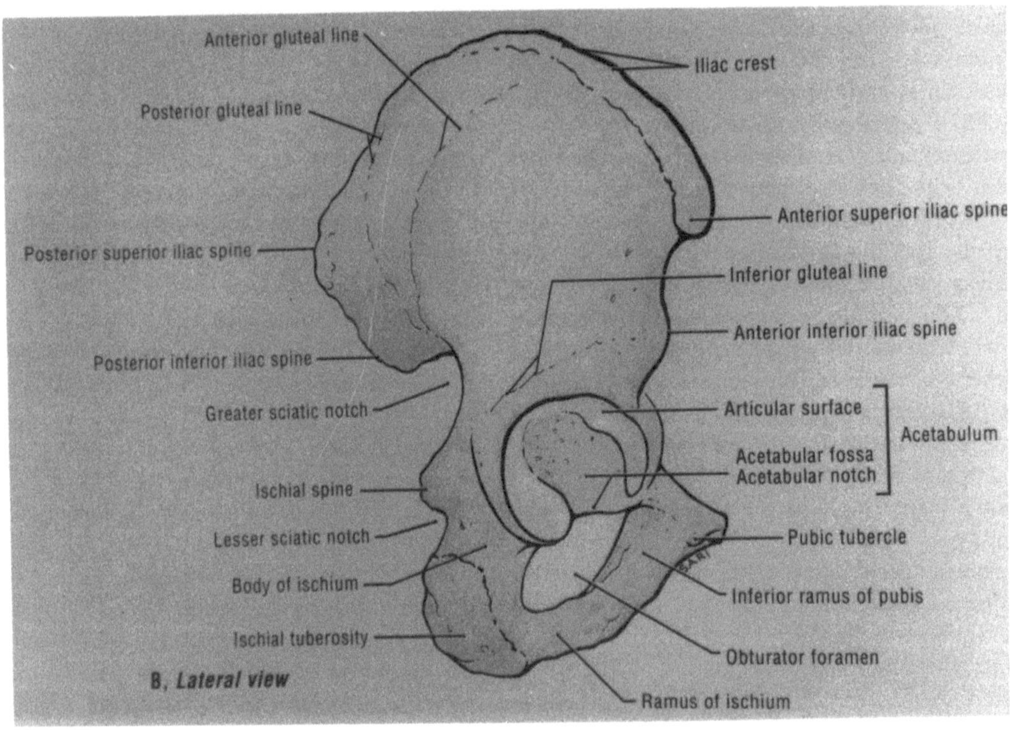


b

**FIGURE 7.2.** Bony anatomy of the acetabulum. (a) Medial view. (b) Lateral view. (Reprinted with permission from Agur.[12])

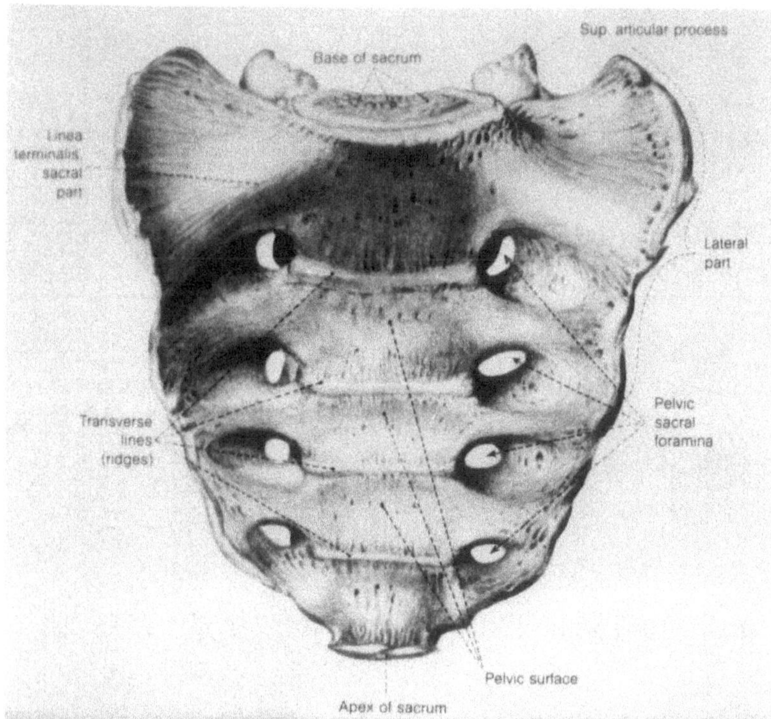

a

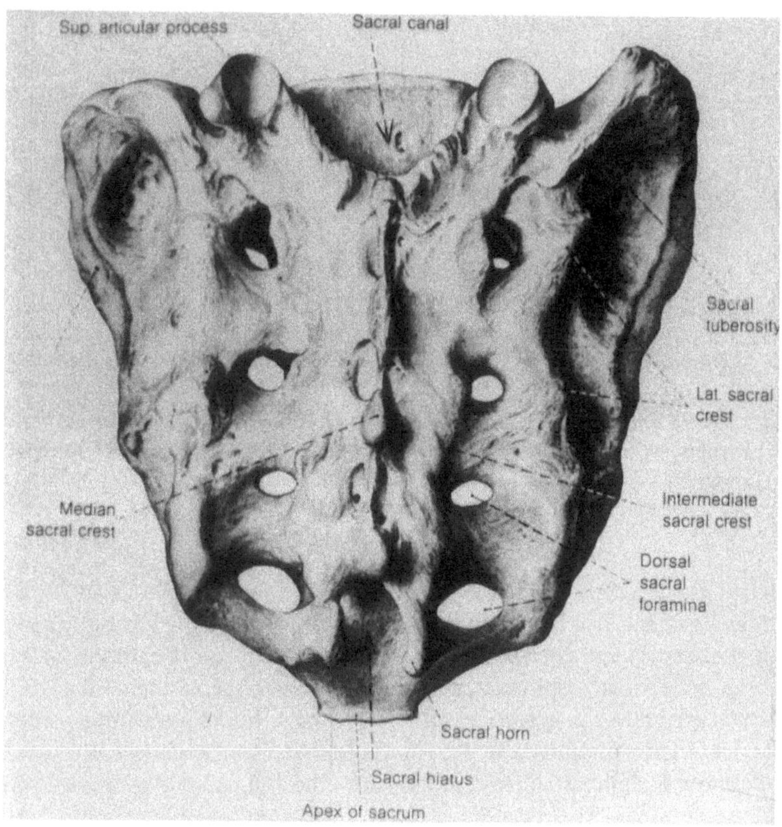

b

**FIGURE 7.3.** Bony anatomy of the sacrum. (a) Anterior view. (b) Posterior view.

*continued*

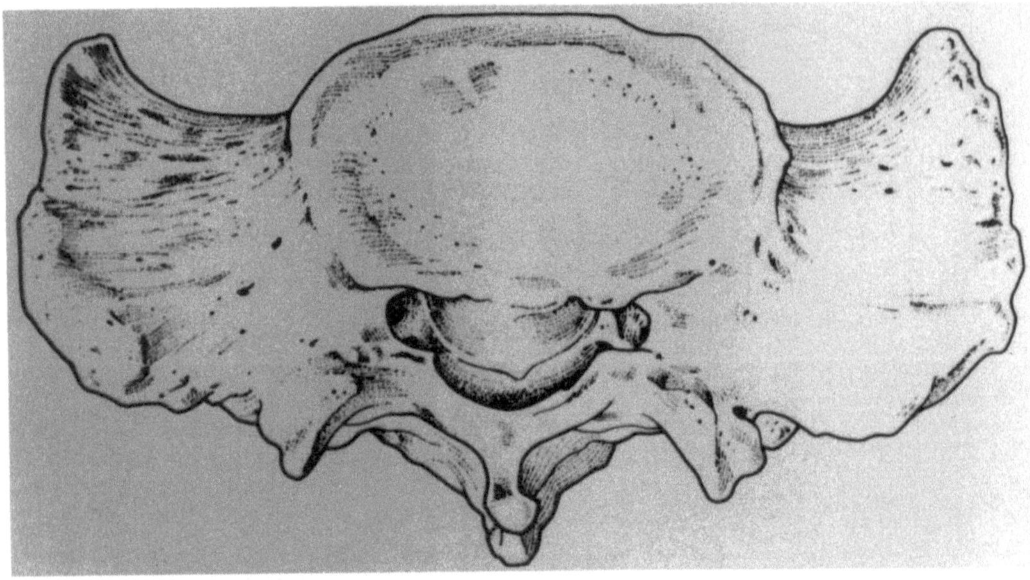

c

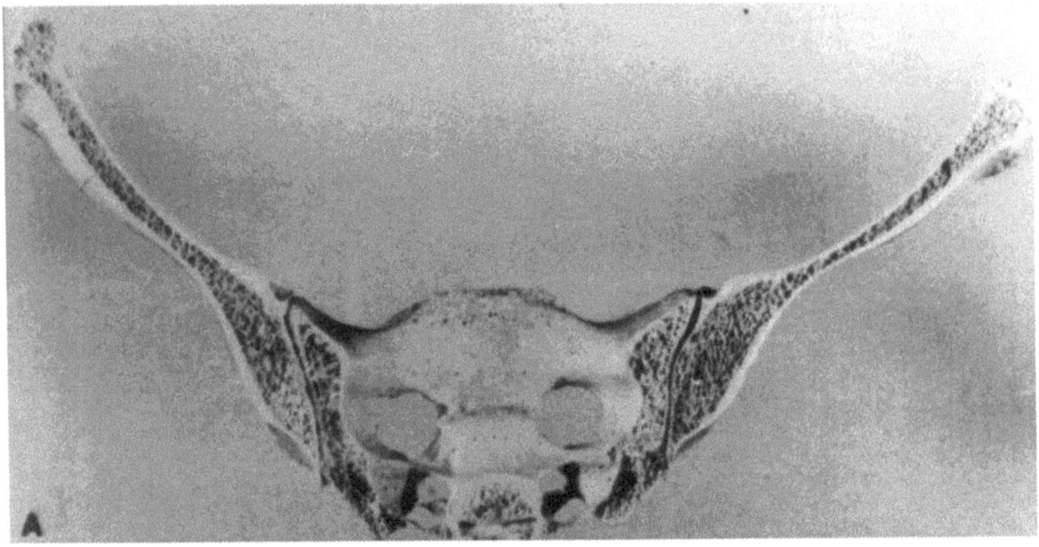

d

**FIGURE 7.3** (*continued*) (c) Superior view. (d) Transaxial view through S-1 body. (a & b reprinted with permission from Ferner and Staubesand.[49] c & d reprinted with permission from Rockwood and Green.[50])

dense triangular sheet that is deep to the sacrotuberous ligament. It arises from the lateral margin of the sacrum and coccyx and inserts on the ischial spine. The sacrospinous ligament divides the ischial area into the greater sciatic notch and the lesser sciatic foramen. At the lumbosacral articulation, iliolumbar ligaments secure the axial skeleton to the pelvis and thereby supplement the strong intervertebral disk complex. All of the posterior pelvic ligaments constitute a tension band that resists rotational and longitudinal shearing forces. With its wedge-shaped configuration, the sacrum is suspended by the ligaments as a self-locking system.

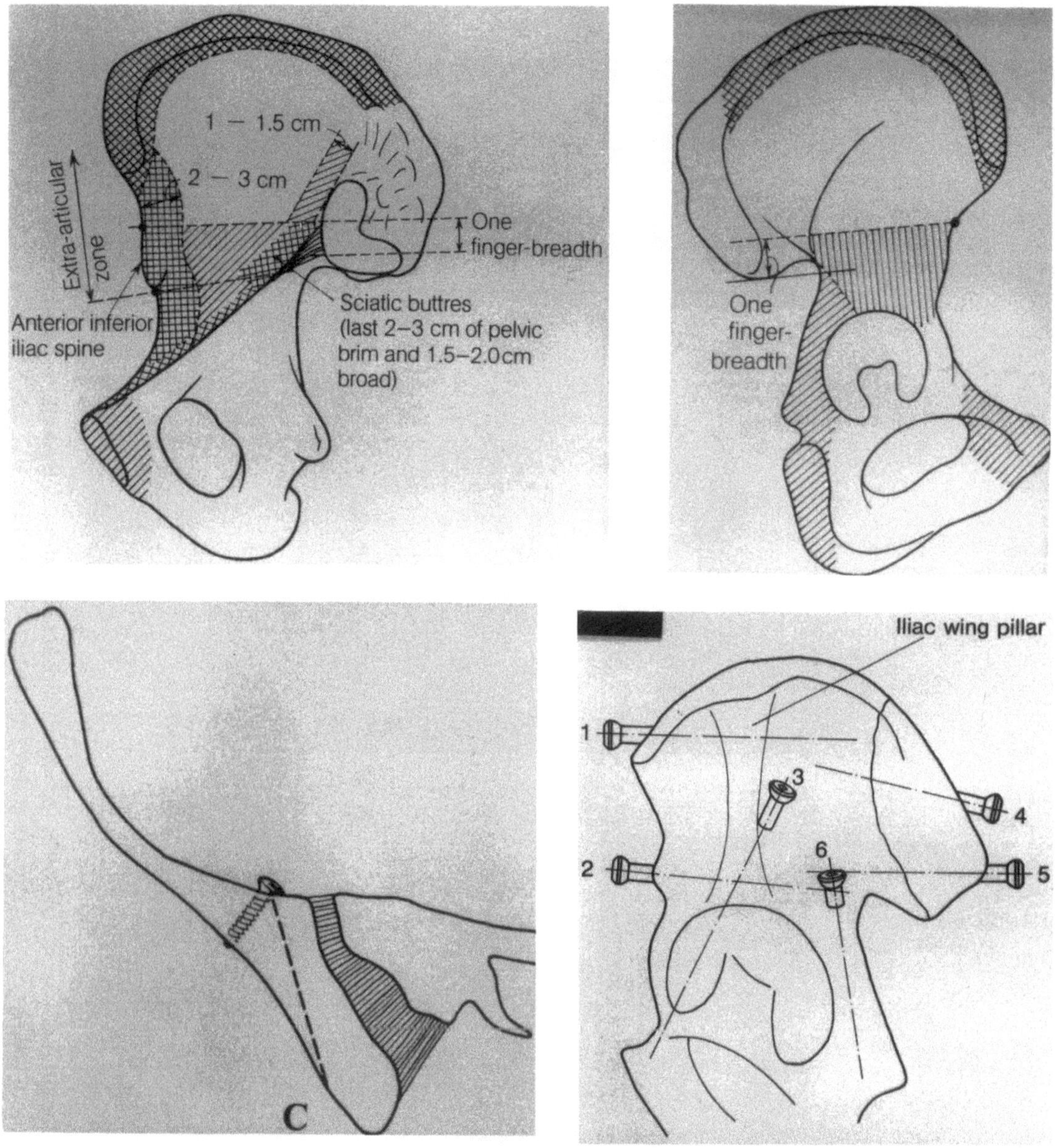


a b c d

**FIGURE 7.4.** Pelvic bony condensations as suitable sites for insertion of lag screws. Vertical or oblique striations the thickest zones. Cross-hatched areas correspond to dense areas. (a) Inner view. (b) Outer view. (c) Transectional view. From the same starting point, screws of very different length can be inserted. (d) Standard pathways for lag screw insertion: 1, Anterior iliac crest; 2, Anterior inferior spine to greater sciatic buttress; 3, Anterior column; 4, Posterior iliac crest; 5, Posterior spine to greater sciatic buttress; 6, Posterior column. (a–c reprinted with permission from Letournel and Judet.[11] d reprinted with permission from Letournel.[51])

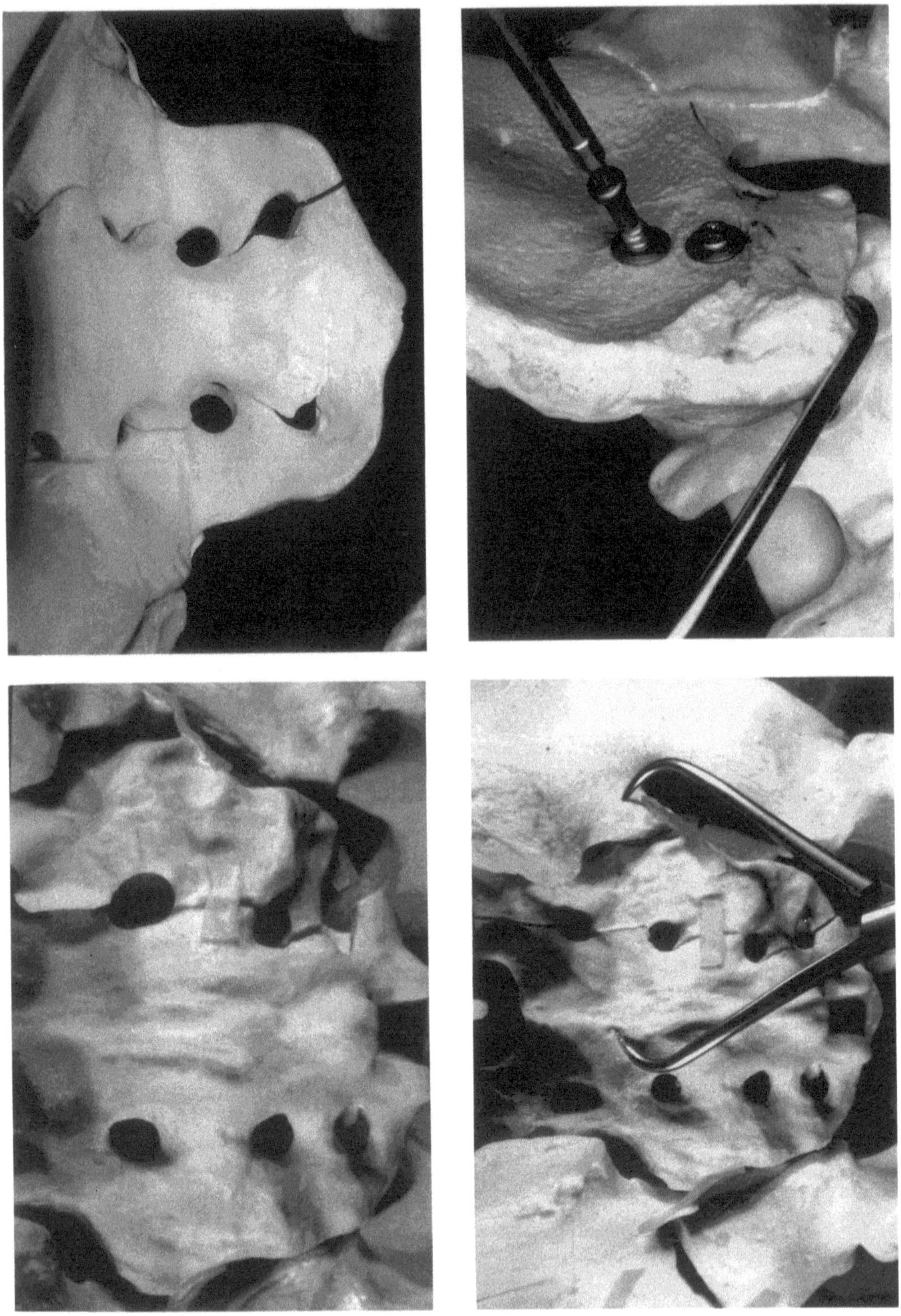

**FIGURE 7.5.** Uni- and bilateral longitudinal sacral fractures for which iliosacral fixation is feasible. (a) Posterior view. (b) Anterior views. (c) Reduction with tenaculum forceps. (d) Insertion of screws in posterolateral ilium.

## Vascular Anatomy of the Pelvis

A knowledge of the vascular supply of the pelvic region is crucial for the recognition of sites of potentially massive hemorrhage accompanying a pelvic disruption, for potential iatrogenic injury to major pelvic vessels, and for compromise of the nutrition of the pelvis with surgical reconstruction.[12] In the false pelvis, the common iliac vessels divide into the internal and external iliac branches. With severe pelvic trauma, that nevertheless is consistent with a viable patient, these major vessels rarely are damaged. When the common, internal, or external iliac vessels are disrupted, urgent identification and a direct surgical repair of the vascular disruption provides the only likelihood for survival. At the pelvic brim, the internal iliac artery divides into anterior and posterior divisions. Typically, the latter subdivides into the superior gluteal, iliolumbar, and lateral sacral arteries. With posterior displacement of the hemipelvis, an injury to the posterior division and/or superior gluteal artery is likely to ensue with the potential for major hemorrhage and compromise of the viability of the gluteus medius and minimis. The anterior division possesses many branches including the internal pudendal, inferior gluteal, and obturator arteries. Injury to these 3-mm vessels, likewise, can be followed by significant hemorrhage. An extensive venous plexus, accompanying the pelvic arteries, also is vulnerable to injury with a pelvic disruption.

At the time of surgical reconstruction of a pelvic or acetabular fracture, preservation of the blood supply of each major bony fragment is crucial to facilitate healing and afford resistance to infection. On the inner surface of the anterior ilium and iliac crest, nutrition is provided by the deep circumflex iliac artery, a branch of the external iliac artery. A still larger nutrient foramina is situated in the internal iliac fossa, 1 cm anterior to the surface of the sacroiliac joint and 1 cm superior to the iliopectineal line, where it receives a branch from the iliolumbar artery. On the external surface of the bone, a large nutrient foramen is observed in the middle of the gluteal area of the iliac wing, which receives a branch from the superior gluteal artery. Supplementary vascular supplies include multiple nutrient vessels around the acetabular margin, which form a complete vascular circle arising from the obturator and the superior and inferior gluteal arteries. The sciatic buttress receives numerous branches from the superior gluteal artery.

## Major Nerves Adjacent to the Pelvis

Virtually all portions of the lumbosacral and coccygeal plexuses may be injured by pelvic trauma. The lumbosacral and coccygeal nerve plexuses are derived from the anterior rami of the T-12 to S-4 spinal nerves.[13] The L-4 to S-1 segments are particularly prone to injury including the femoral nerve (Figure 7.6). After the lumbosacral trunk and the first sacral root unite anterior to the sacroiliac joint, they join with S-2, S-3, and S-4 anterior to the piriformis. The common outflow divides into two terminal branches, the sciatic and pudendal nerves, and supplementary branches including the superior and inferior gluteal nerves. Many branches pass through the greater sciatic notch, notably the sciatic nerve, which forms the largest branch of the sacral plexus. The sciatic nerve exits the pelvis between the inferior border of the piriformis and the ischial border of the greater sciatic notch. It possesses two divisions, the tibial and peroneal, which are loosely bound together. The nerve is vulnerable to injury, especially with a posterior dislocation of the hip or a posterior acetabular fracture. The peroneal division is particularly susceptible to injury and less likely to recover. The principal L-5 root contribution to the peroneal division is vulnerable to injury at the root level, both behind the hip joint and where it exits the greater sciatic notch. The superior gluteal nerve (L-4 to S-1) is susceptible to injury with posterior approaches to the hip and acetabulum. Typically, such a traction injury is associated with the insertion of a retractor or a lengthy plate on the posterior column. With anterior or ilioinguinal approaches, the lateral femoral cutaneous nerve of the thigh is vulnerable to a laceration or to a traction injury. When an ilioinguinal incision is used to expose an extensive acetabular fracture, typically some

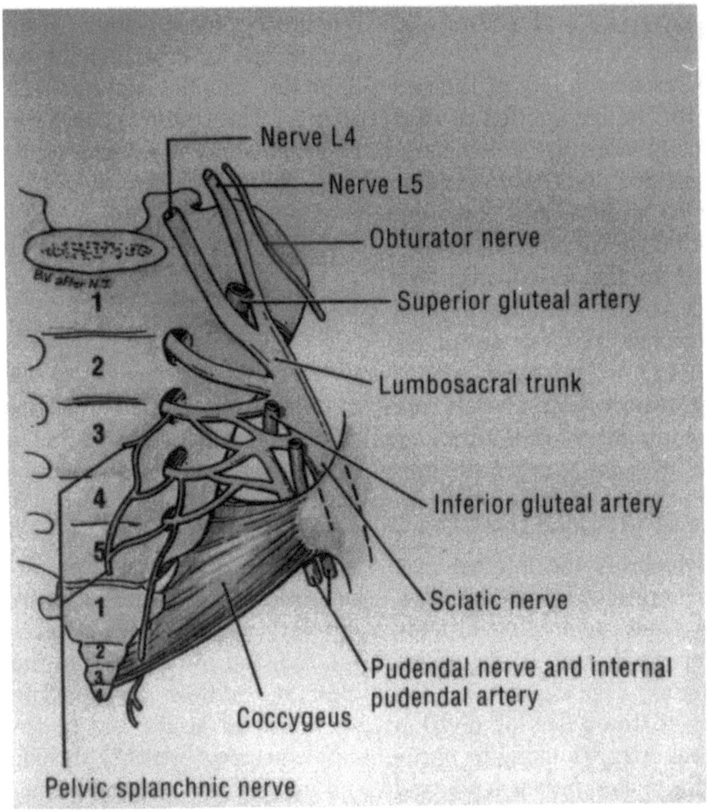


**FIGURE 7.6.** The sacral plexus and origin of the sciatic nerve. (Reprinted with permission from Agur.[12])

degree of hypesthesia of the anterior thigh ensues.

# Assessment

Before definitive treatment of a pelvic or acetabular fracture is initiated, the injury is rigorously characterized by its clinical and radiographic features.[14,15] The direction of the provocative forces may be obtained from the history of an alert patient and from clinical inspection for sites of contusion or ecchymosis. The history of a motor vehicular or industrial accident should alert the surgeon to the high likelihood for the presence of a major unstable pelvic injury and the potential for concomitant visceral or neurovascular insults. The pelvic region is examined for evidence of asymmetry, instability, or the presence of an open wound. A laceration in the groin, scrotum, or peroneal region or of the vagina and rectum is highly suspicious of an open pelvic fracture. An apparent deformity of the lower extremity in the absence of a fracture in the lower limb may indicate a pelvic fracture

In the presence of hemodynamic instability, the initial radiographic assessment of the pelvis may be limited to an anteroposterior view. Subsequently, precise characterization of the injury necessitates a minimum radiographic protocol of anteroposterior, inlet, and outlet views. For the inlet view of the supine patient, the x-ray beam is directed from the head to the mid-pelvis at about 45° with respect to the radiographic table.[15,16] Such a projection is perpendicular to the pelvic brim and illustrates the true pelvic inlet, as well as the anteroposterior displacement of the pelvic fracture. To obtain an outlet projection of a supine patient, the beam is directed from the foot to the pubic symphysis at 45° with respect to the radiographic plate. The outlet projection highlights superior displacement of the posterior half of the pelvis, as well as superior or inferior displacement of the rami. Apparent limb length discrepancy secondary to a sagittal malrotation of a hemipelvis is highlighted, along with avulsion fractures of the transverse processes of the lower lumbar vertebrae or ramus fractures. For an acetabular disruption, special Judet or obturator and iliac oblique views are obtained by rolling the injured patient carefully from one side to the other to provide a transverse axis of the pelvis of 45° relative to the radiographic table. Supplementary computed tomography (CT) is indispensable to document sites of pelvic disruption, displacement, and comminution.[17] A sacral fracture that is virtually invisible on plain radiographs is readily documented by resort to computed axial tomography. The degree of separation and instability of a sacroiliac joint or sacral fracture is evident.

Five standard coronal sections are taken at intervals of about 2 cm. The most superior section projects the iliac wings and the adjacent sacroiliac joints. The second highlights the principal part of the sacrum and adjacent sacroiliac joints. The third displays the dome of the acetabulum with a circular cross section. The fourth transects the mid-acetabular region and includes a midpolar view of the femoral head, whereas the fifth documents the inferior pubic ramus and the ischial tuberosity at the level of the greater trochanter. Where surgical reconstruction of a comminuted and displaced pelvic or acetabular fracture is anticipated, an accurate three-dimensional (3D) radiographic perspective is extremely valuable to define the optimal surgical approach, the strategy for the open reduction, and the preferred method of fixation. When reviewing the conventional two-dimensional radiographs and CT scans, even an experienced surgeon has difficulty with the extensive mental integration needed to achieve an accurate three-dimensional image of the injury. Typically, the displacement of the major fracture fragments is primarily a rotational distortion that further complicates the mental imaging. Computer programs are available to produce three-dimensional surface reformations from sets of contiguous axial computed scans of the pelvis.[18,19] The images can be obtained within 1 to 12 hours after the arrival of the patient in the radiographic suite. While the 3D CT images can be created from virtually any angle of scrutiny, a standard pelvic series comprises the anterior, posterior, superior, and inferior orthogonal views and the inlet and outlet 45° oblique projections. Also, the 45° oblique views comprising the iliac and obturator oblique projections display the internal and external surfaces of the acetabulum. A special "dome view" is obtained from a projection approximating 20° inferior and 20° anterior to the true lateral view. After a subtraction, or so-called disarticulation, of the femoral head, the last view presents the acetabulum as a true hemispherical recess and provides a clearer view of the acetabular dome, as well as the medial, anterior, and posterior walls.

# Classification of Injuries

## Pelvis

Pennal, Tile, and associates[20] classify the principal pelvic ring disruptions based upon the direction of the provocative force and the degree of pelvic disruption. Injuries may result from provocative blows that impose anterior-posterior or lateral compressive forces on the pelvis or from falls or other unusual injuries that exert vertical shearing forces on the pelvic ring. This classification provides insight into the nature of the injury, the morbidity, the potential sites of disruptions, the degrees of pelvic instability, and recommendations for treatment. An anterior posterior compression injury, also known as an external rotation deformity, results from a blow that strikes the posterior ilium or the anterior pelvis to disrupt the symphysis and the anterior sacroiliac ligaments of one or both sacroiliac joints. Usually, the crucial posterior sacroiliac complex is spared so that the injury is vertically stable. Not infrequently the ipsilateral floor of the hemipelvis, including the sacrospinous and sacrotuberous ligaments, is compromised so that a modest sagittal malrotation of the hemipelvis ensues.

A lateral compression injury arises from a direct blow to the lateral ilium, typically to provoke an extremely unstable impacted fracture of the sacrum. Most typically, an accompanying anterolateral rotational force provokes an inward rotation of the ipsilateral hemipelvis, so that the ipsilateral pubic rami, or occasionally all four rami, are disrupted with some overlapping of the fracture fragments.

A vertical shear injury is a highly unstable disruption with complete posterior ligamentous instability of one or both sacroiliac joints. Most of the patients are victims of falls from a great height or of high-speed crashes. Usually, the associated anterior disruption is a diastasis of the symphysis pubis. Supplementary radiographic findings include avulsion fractures of the sacrospinous and sacrotuberous ligaments from the ischial spine or the adjacent sacrum, as well as avulsion fractures of the transverse processes of the fourth and fifth lumbar vertebrae.

## Acetabulum

Currently, the most widely employed classification scheme of acetabular fractures is that devised by Letournel and Judet.[11,21] These workers identified two major categories of elementary and associated fractures. In an elementary fracture, all or part of one column is involved to provoke a posterior wall, posterior column, anterior wall, or anterior column fracture. One other elementary pattern is a transverse fracture in which the superior acetabulum is separated from the inferior portion. The associated fracture patterns include any two of the elementary forms. The five principal examples are a fracture of the posterior column and posterior wall, a transverse and posterior wall fracture, a T-type fracture, a fracture of the anterior column and anterior wall associated with a hemitransverse fracture posteriorly, and a complete both-column fracture. The last example is where all of the articular surface is disrupted to create at least three major fracture fragments. Characterization of the injuries by these patterns provides insight into the optimal surgical approach and a guideline to prognosis with or without surgical reconstruction.

# Acute Management

The management of a patient with a pelvic ring or acetabular disruption is logically divided into two principal phases.[22] During the first phase of acute resuscitation, diagnostic and therapeutic measures are initiated. A multidisciplinary protocol is needed to define the priorities of diagnosis and therapy involving the general surgical, orthopaedic, urologic, and neurosurgical members of the trauma team. Quantitative assessment of the extent and severity of the injuries using an injury-severity scale is strongly advised. The conventional priorities of acute therapy are repair of respiratory, cardiovascular, central nervous system, urologic, gastrointestinal, and musculoskeletal systems. In the presence of hemodynamic instability, a definitive diagnosis and stabilization of the pelvis is deferred. In the other patients, a complete diagnostic survey of the pelvis can be undertaken soon after admission. In either event, the goals of management include anatomical restoration of the pelvis with sufficient stability so that the patient can be mobilized to at least a bed to chair existence, if not a partial weight-bearing gait. Surgical reconstruction should provide substantial alleviation of fracture pain and sufficient mobilization to facilitate pulmonary toilet, general patient care, and expeditious discharge from the hospital. Acute stabilization of a displaced injury minimizes the likelihood for a catastrophic late problem such as a painful nonunion or malunion of the pelvis.

# Definitive Stabilization

The preferred techniques for stabilization of the pelvis and acetabulum remain controversial in a field that is evolving very rapidly. While diverse therapeutic protocols are available, certain features of any acceptable format can be clearly defined. An algorithm for pelvic stabilization should outline a suitable technique for the fixation of virtually any type of pelvic ring disruption or acetabular fracture.[23] Such an algorithm needs to provide viable therapeutic options, depending upon the sites of open pelvic wounds, a diversion colostomy or a urinary drainage, as well as the diverse injury patterns, the varying amounts of comminution, and the degree of osteopenia. For the pelvic ring, historically external fixation evolved as the first definitive method to address a variety of disruptions with moderate instability of the posterior pelvic ring. During the past decade, a rapid increase in the clinical application of techniques of internal fixation has occurred as surgeons recognized the superior mechanical stability afforded by internal fixation of unstable injury patterns. Also, the availability of percutaneous lag screws has created a stable method of internal fixation that necessitates minimal surgical exposure. As the number of pelvic injury sites increases, the need for rigorous internal fixation rapidly accelerates. Ironically, the most complicated cases have the greatest absolute indication for technically demanding surgical reconstruction. Especially in a community hospital or a tertiary center with limited experience in pelvic reconstruction, many of the complicated cases merit referral to a regional trauma center where the appropriate surgical training and instrumentation are available.

## Indications for Internal Fixation of the Pelvic Ring

Currently, the indications for the application of internal fixation to an unstable pelvic ring disruption remain highly controversial. Most surgeons agree that stable injuries with minimal instability and minimal pelvic deformity merit conservative treatment. Once the pelvic ring is traumatically rendered unstable and deformed, the questions arise about the degree of instability and deformity that constitute indications for internal fixation. The enthusiasm for surgical reconstruction has to be tempered by the potential for surgical complications and the 40% incidence of late posterior pelvic and low back pain that ensues even when an accurate stable internal fixation is achieved without a surgical or iatrogenic complication. For unstable pelvic injuries that are managed by external fixation, Riemer and Miranda[24] report that the results documented at late outcome, in terms of the amount of pain, functional incapacity, and return to gainful employment, are equivalent to those documented after the use of internal fixation. Where the least doubt about the role of internal fixation exists is with respect to bilateral unstable posterior injuries and other complex injury patterns where isolated external fixation has no potential to stabilize the pelvic ring with respect to the spine.

Probably at least half of the patients who sustain a pelvic injury present with a minimally displaced fracture, especially following a low-velocity lateral compressive force. Another example is a diastasis of the symphysis with less than 2 cm of displacement. In these instances, temporary bed rest followed by partial weight bearing for a few weeks is usually sufficient treatment. Another large subcategory includes a diastasis with greater than 2 cm of displacement of the symphysis, when surgical stabilization is recommended. Plate fixation of the symphysis through a limited anterior exposure is the method of choice. While plate fixation can be applied to anterior ramus fractures, the surgical approach across the inguinal region is moderately difficult and potentially hazardous. Generally, external fixation is preferred to manage an anterior injury with multiple displaced ramus fractures. One exception is the presence of displaced rami in a young female. In this instance, a persistent nonunion or malunion of the rami often leads to dyspareunia or the need for a cesarean section at the time of delivery. With an open reduction, an accurate reconstruction of the anterior pelvic ring can provide a minimal risk for the late obstetric and gynecological complications.

A second category of displaced pelvic disruptions with posterior instability follows a dislocation of the sacroiliac joint or a fracture of the neighboring portions of the posterior ilium or sacrum. Typically, an anterior accompanying injury involves a diastasis of the symphysis or ramus fractures. In such an example, the pelvic ring can be perceived as having three supportive columns of bone.[25] The anterior column refers to the symphysis and the adjacent superior pubic rami. The middle column refers to the body of the sacrum, the adjacent portions of sacroiliac joints, and the allied posterior ilium. The posterior column refers to the posterior elements of the sacrum and the neighboring portions of posterior ilia via the posterior superior spine. Two of the three columns are immobilized with internal fixation. Typically, the anterior column injury is surgically exposed, reduced, and plated. This maneuver generally provides a satisfactory reduction of the posterior injury. As an alternative, anterior column fixation can be afforded by a simple external frame that spans from half pins inserted into either anterior iliac crest. Subsequently, either the middle column is stabilized with lag screws or anterior plates, or the posterior column is immobilized with a plate. In osteopenic individuals, and especially the elderly, usually the rami afford insufficient structural integrity to merit plate fixation. In such an instance, the middle and posterior columns are immobilized as the preferred strategy of fixation.

A third major category of pelvic fracture is a complex ring disruption. The largest group is a family of bilateral posterior unstable injuries with a combination of sacroiliac dislocations or unstable fractures involving the sacrum or posterior ilium. Another pattern is where an unstable posterior fracture dislocation is accompanied by an acetabular fracture as well as an anterior injury. Still other cases involve multiple combinations of posterior, unstable injuries and bilateral acetabular fractures. All of these injuries may have various combinations of anterior disruption. Typically, each unstable site merits an open reduction and internal fixation. With ipsilateral superior and inferior ramus fractures, however, generally only the superior ramus is immobilized. By resort to a bilateral ilioinguinal surgical exposure, the rami and symphysis, as well as the lateral ilium and sacroiliac joint, can be exposed for the reduction and fixation. As part of the procedure, percutaneous lag screws can be utilized to stabilize the sacral body. A supplementary surgical approach may be necessary to expose an accompanying fracture of the posterior acetabular wall or column or a displaced sacral fracture

## Indications for Acetabular Fixation

Currently, for most displaced acetabular fractures in young adults or children, an open reduction with internal fixation is recommended.[26] Posterior fracture dislocations and transverse fractures have a particularly poor outlook unless an accurate reduction is achieved. Certain both-column fractures possess so-called secondary congruity, whereby the fracture fragments rotate around the femoral head to maintain a spherical bearing surface. Of the significant displaced acetabular fractures, this injury pattern possesses the best outcome following the application of nonoperative methods. Particularly in the elderly with marked comminution, osteopenia, and associated medical problems, conservative management of such an injury may be preferred. A small spectrum of acetabular fractures are notable for marked impaction or abrasive damage to the bearing surfaces or occasionally other problems such as late presentation, morbid obesity, and concomitant medical problems, where conservative management is doomed, and yet an open reduction and internal fixation is impractical or impossible. An acute total hip joint replacement may be the best current option for those uncommon cases.[27] For the acetabular component, an associated metal cup with an outer porous coating for bony ingrowth and with the capability for the insertion of multiple screws serves as a hemispherical plate. The femoral head can be morselized for bone graft, or it can serve as a structural graft for augmentation of the posterior wall or dome. The major acetabular fragments can be reduced through a relatively limited and conventional total hip exposure. Supplementary lag screws can be used to immobilize large extraarticular fragments such as a large portion of the anterior ilium and iliac crest. Usually, such screws are inserted through small additional incisions, frequently superficial to the anterior superior and anterior inferior iliac spines.

## Contraindications for Internal Fixation of the Pelvis and Acelabulum

In the presence of an unstable pelvic fracture, most contraindications to internal fixation are of a transient nature. With hemodynamic instability or other acute medical problem, deferral of a major pelvic reconstruction may be necessary. In the presence of an open pelvic fracture, especially with fecal contamination, transient external fixation may be preferred while diversion of the bowel and cleansing of the wound are undertaken. Typically, within a few days, internal fixation of the pelvic ring, by resort to cannulated lag screws, especially of the critical posterior portion, can be undertaken by the use of a limited surgical exposure somewhat remotely situated with respect to the colostomy or an open wound. In cases of late presentation. assessment referable to the assets and practicality of surgical reconstruction merits special consideration. Factors under review will include the acceptability of the deformity, the potential for spontaneous union and stability of the pelvic ring, the degree of technical difficulty and, especially, the presence or risk of complicating features such as massive heterotopic bone.

## Complications of Internal Fixation of the Pelvis and Acetabulum

A principal source of complications of internal pelvic fixation is related to the particular surgical exposure. The juxtaposition of major neurovascular structures, as well as the intraabdominal viscera, combined with most orthopaedic surgeons' limited familiarity with the pelvic region, provides a special likelihood for allied complications. This problem is further aggravated if the surgery is undertaken after a delayed presentation. Scarified boundaries, the presence of heterotopic bone, and abnormalities such as traumatically induced urinary diverticula create particularly hazardous conditions. A second family of complications is related to the surgical reduction. A traction injury to the sciatic nerve is perhaps the best-known problem following a posterior fracture dislocation of the hip. Where the sciatic nerve is contused at the time of the traumatic injury, subtle features of nerve deficit, including mild hypesthesia of the second and third toes or a corresponding mild weakness of the extensor digitorium longus, may be the only sign of the potential impending catastrophe.[28] With even a limited surgical manipulation of the nerve or limited retraction, it is susceptible to frank deterioration in function to culminate in a complete foot drop, with hypesthesia of the foot and a potential for late dysesthetic pain in the lower leg and foot. The use of intraoperative somatosensory evoked potential monitoring permits the recognition of such a susceptible nerve and the potential for rapid correction of the provocative surgical maneuver.[29,30]

The third family of complications is related to the application of the fixation devices. The guide wires or drill bits that are used in conjunction with cannulated screws are particularly hazardous, especially if the far cortex of bone is breached. Many columns of pelvic bone, such as the superior pubic ramus, are relatively small so that the target area is limited. Alternatively, in the sacrum, the presence of nerve roots in the foramina provides a source of neurological hazard that is in close proximity to the limited available bone stock. A fourth category pertains to a postsurgical problem such as problematic wound healing, heterotopic bone around the acetabulum after a lateral surgical exposure, avascular necrosis of the femoral head or acetabulum, and a late nonunion or malunion.[31] Many of these problems represent complications that follow excessive stripping of soft tissue and devascularization of the bone fragments. To minimize the risk of heterotopic bone, several strategies are available. When an anterior ilioinguinal approach is used, the risk of significant heterotopic bone is minimal. For a high-risk patient, especially a large obese male who has sustained an accompanying closed head injury, an extended lateral surgical approach to the acetabulum should be avoided if at all possible. From the time of surgery, indomethacin can be given as a prophylactic agent. Alternatively, postoperative irradiation therapy of 700 to

1,000 C Gy can be given as a single pulse or in subdivided doses.[32]

## Intraoperative Imaging Techniques

Currently, intraoperative imaging of the pelvis and acetabulum is a critical part of most reconstructive procedures. The accuracy of a reduction can be assessed. Minimally invasive fixation, especially by resort to cannulated lag screws, can be utilized. The presence of a screw violating the hip joint or a foramen can be documented so that a timely corrective measure follows. To facilitate the intraoperative imaging, the use of the Jackson graphite composite operating table is strongly preferred. The completely radiolucent table is supported at the top and the bottom so that the central region beneath the pelvis is totally accessible for a C-arm. The newest version of the table permits the application of longitudinal or lateral traction. In conjunction with the table, a modern C-arm image intensifier with a 9-inch field size is recommended. The Siemens and O.E.C.-Toshiba models possess a high resolution and large field size for satisfactory visualization. Once the patient has been anesthetized and positioned on the tables and prior to draping the patient, a trial rehearsal of the relevant imaging techniques is performed. Where the x-ray technician possesses less than optimal training, this rehearsal period enables the surgeon to educate the technician, while the position of the patient is clearly evident. When necessary, the position of the patient can be modified somewhat to optimize the field for imaging.

Where high-resolution imaging is needed, towel clips are secured where they will not compromise the field of imaging. Typically, the clips are positioned sufficiently superior and inferior so that they are out of the radiographic field. Within the surgical field, supplementary skin staples or sutures are used to secure the drapes. As a third method, plastic adhesive barrier drapes are used to anchor the cloth drapes. After the patient has been draped, another scout image with the C-arm image intensifier is obtained to ensure the absence of the towel clips and other artifact from the field of interest. During the surgery, the anterior-posterior, inlet, and outlet views, as well as the Judet views, are obtained. For the documentation of an iliosacral screw, a supplementary direct lateral sacral view is necessary.

## Mechanical Criteria for Pelvic Fixation Devices

The optimal mechanical behavior of fixation devices for use on the pelvis is quite different from the criteria for devices that are designed for application on the appendicular skeleton. With its ring-like nature, the pelvis is not subject to bending stresses that rival loads imposed upon long bones and the allied fixation.[9] When plates are applied to the curved surfaces of the innominate bone, contouring of the plate to fit accurately to the osseous surface becomes a major concern. If a plate is rigid, even a minor error in the contour will provoke a displacement of an anatomically reduced fracture when the corresponding screws are tightened. Flexibility of the plate, thereby, represents a significant attribute. As with all fracture fixation hardware, an ability to tolerate fatigue forces imposed by the presence of a delayed union is valuable. After surgery, the use of standard transaxial CT or 3D CT for the scrutiny of the reduction and the position of the hardware is very helpful, especially for cases where a screw approximates the hip joint or a foramen. From all of these points of view, a titanium alloy, such as 6% aluminum and 4% vanadium, is the optimal material for plates and screws, and possesses a marked superiority over surgical grade stainless steel. Reconstruction plates with oval holes or slots permit the optimal deviation of the screw away from the axis of the plate. For most applications of a plate around the acetabulum, a 3.5- or 3.7-mm size in terms of adequate strength and ductility is preferred. The screws are of 3.5- or 3.7-mm cortical or 4.0-mm fully threaded cancellous designs and ideally of a self-tapping configuration. Lengthy screws of up to 120 mm are needed. Particularly for longer screws, power insertion is recommended. For application in deep wounds consistent with pelvic incisions, special long drill bits and drill sleeves are needed. For the immobilization of the posterior portion of the pelvic ring, 4.5-mm reconstruction plates are preferred, along with 4.5-mm cortical or 6.5-mm cancellous screws. Such a plate can be contoured to fit across the back of the sacrum and adjacent ilia as a tension-plate configuration.[33] For fixation of the front of the sacroiliac joint, 4.5-mm screws can be inserted through 4.5-mm or ideally 3.5-mm plates of two holes. The plates are directed across the alar region of the sacroiliac joint with the screws oriented parallel to the axis of the joint. With the 3.5-mm plates, the screws are closer together and tend to be directed along the narrow juxta-articular region of the thick bone that is free of a neural foramen. In contrast, a 4.5-mm plate possesses a wider interspace between the holes. Either the medial end of the plate is liable to injure the L-5 nerve root or the lateral end is situated above the thin portion of lateral ilium. In the latter case, the fixation is significantly compromised by the corresponding short screws (Figure 7.4c). Special anterior sacroiliac plates are available that effectively link two short conventional plates in an H-like design. With their added cost and limited utility, probably the H-plates are not cost-effective.

For the thin portions of the posterior and anterior wall of the acetabulum, specialized plates have been devised that permit a buttressing of the bone with a minimal risk for a screw to penetrate the hip joint. Such a spring or hook plate design was popularized by Mast et al.,[34] and assessed biomechanically by Goulet et al.[35] A short one-third tubular plate of 3.5-mm size and typically of three holes in length is trimmed to prepare two pointed spurs at one end. The pointed ends are bent by 90° to create hooks. The plate is contoured with a gentle convexity away from the bony surface. As screws are inserted into the apex of the curve and at the end of the plate remote from the hip joint, the hooks engage the juxtaarticular wall to buttress it. Assemblies of one or more hook plates can be combined with a conventional reconstruction plate and are fashioned to immobilize comminuted segments of the posterior or anterior column and wall.

## Cannulated Screws

The 7.0- and 4.5-mm cannulated screws are particularly suitable for fixation of the posterior hemipelvis and acetabular region, respectively. The larger screws are preferred for the posterior ilium, sacroiliac joint, and sacral body, whereas the smaller ones are effective for fixation of the anterior and posterior columns and adjacent structural columns neighboring the acetabulum. In the biomechanical studies in pelvic ring and acetabular fixation performed by Sawaguchi et al.,[9] and by Rubash et al.,[36] the optimal characteristics of screws for strength and holding power were defined. As a generalization, longer screws of a small diameter are particularly effective in the pelvis. For younger adults, cortical screws realize as effective a fixation as cancellous screws. Admittedly, these studies did not evaluate cannulated screws. For lag screws, generally a thread length of 32 mm or more is preferred. For the lengthy screws of 90 to 150 mm that transfix the sacral body and occasionally both sacroiliac joints, excessive flexibility of a guide wire is potentially a great problem. A guide wire of 2.0-mm diameter is highly vulnerable to bend as it penetrates the iliac or sacral subchondral bone as it crosses the sacroiliac joint. The optimal range of guide wires is 2.8 to 3.2 mm in diameter. While the 3.2 mm is highly rigid, it presents a concern that excessive heat might be generated during its insertion so that thermal damage of an adjacent nerve root could occur. The author has assessed a 7.2-mm design with a 2.8-mm cannula. The tip of the screw is designed for self-drilling and self-tapping. Both threaded tip guide wires and small drill bits are available as a pilot for the screw. Associated tools include a depth gauge and a set of drill sleeves. A supplementary drill sleeve permits the insertion of two 7.2-mm screws in parallel, divergent, or convergent alignment. The 4.5-mm screws possess a similar collection of tools. During insertion, undulation of the smaller, but shorter guide wires has not been a problem.

## Indications For the Use of Cannulated Lag Screws in the Pelvis

The attributes of a cannulated screw for pelvic fixation pertain to a minimally invasive or percutaneous method of fixation and the preliminary insertion of a small guide wire under image intensification for penetration of a column of bone that is of a small diameter or that is adjacent to vulnerable soft tissue, especially nerves. In the latter situation, when a conventional drill bit is replaced with a screw, the screw has a potential to follow an errant pathway with possible damage to associated tissues that cannot occur when the screw is driven over a guide wire. While a cannulated screw of a given core and outside diameters is of somewhat lesser static and fatigue strength than a solid counterpart, in clinical practice, this feature is a minor liability.[37] Currently available designs of cannulated screws possess an enlarged core diameter so that breakage of screws has not been a significant problem. During the insertion of a cannulated screw, the surgeon needs to have a firm grasp of the anatomical landmarks and must obtain a variety of special radiologic views on the image intensifier that permits a documentation of a safe and appropriate insertional pathway.

## Fixation Techniques for Particular Sites

### The Sacroiliac Joint

Cannulated lag screw fixation can be undertaken for a subluxed or dislocated sacroiliac joint. In the former case, the anterior aspects of the joint are separated, possibly with a limited accompanying sagittal or coronal rotational deformity. In the latter situation, the articular surfaces are displaced in a multiplanar fashion that renders the joint highly unstable unless an accurate reduction is achieved. Where cannulated screws are selected for fixation, the crucial recognition is that the operative procedure needs to include some method for accurate reduction of the joint (Figure 7.7). Where the anterior injury is a diastasis, the open reduction of the symphysis may facilitate a corresponding reduction of the sacroiliac joint so that percutaneous fixation with cannulated screws is feasible. For a late presentation, more than a week after the injury, and where skeletal traction was not used to control the initial deformity, an open reduction by resort to an an anterior approach of the sacroiliac joint affords the optimal view to facilitate the reduction. Once reduced, direct anterior fixation with two of the two-hole plates is readily undertaken. The use of cannulated screws for fixation is particularly attractive where a minimally displaced sacroiliac joint merits fixation or where an accurate closed reduction accompanies the reconstruction of the anterior pelvic ring disruption. About 20% of transverse or T-type acetabular fractures are complicated by a subluxation of the ipsilateral sacroiliac joint. Prior to the acetabular exposure, an accurate realignment or fixation of the sacroiliac joint is needed to anatomically reduce the upper half of the acetabulum. While the amount of displacement of the ilium at the sacroiliac joint may appear to be inconsequential, nevertheless this amount is magnified greatly at the level of the acetabular articular surface. With the patient situated in a lateral decubitus position, the sacroiliac joint tends to spontaneously reduce so that cannulated lag screw fixation is feasible.

In the presence of marked displacement of the sacroiliac joint, an accurate reduction may be difficult or impossible to achieve by resort to a closed manipulation so that usually an open reduction is indicated. Initially, a closed reduction may be attempted as an effort to preserve the neighboring soft tissues and, especially in the presence of a diversion colostomy or an open wound where contamination of an open surgical wound represents a clinical concern (Figure 7.8). The patient is positioned in a lateral fashion to rest on the contralateral side of the pelvis. While a supine or even prone position can be used, typically the crucial reduction technique is less satisfactory for restoration of alignment of the sacroiliac joint. Image intensification with anteroposterior (AP), inlet, and outlet views is performed. The ipsilateral hip is flexed beyond 90° so that its rotation transmits a corresponding rotational force to the displaced hemipelvis. The extremity is draped and manip-

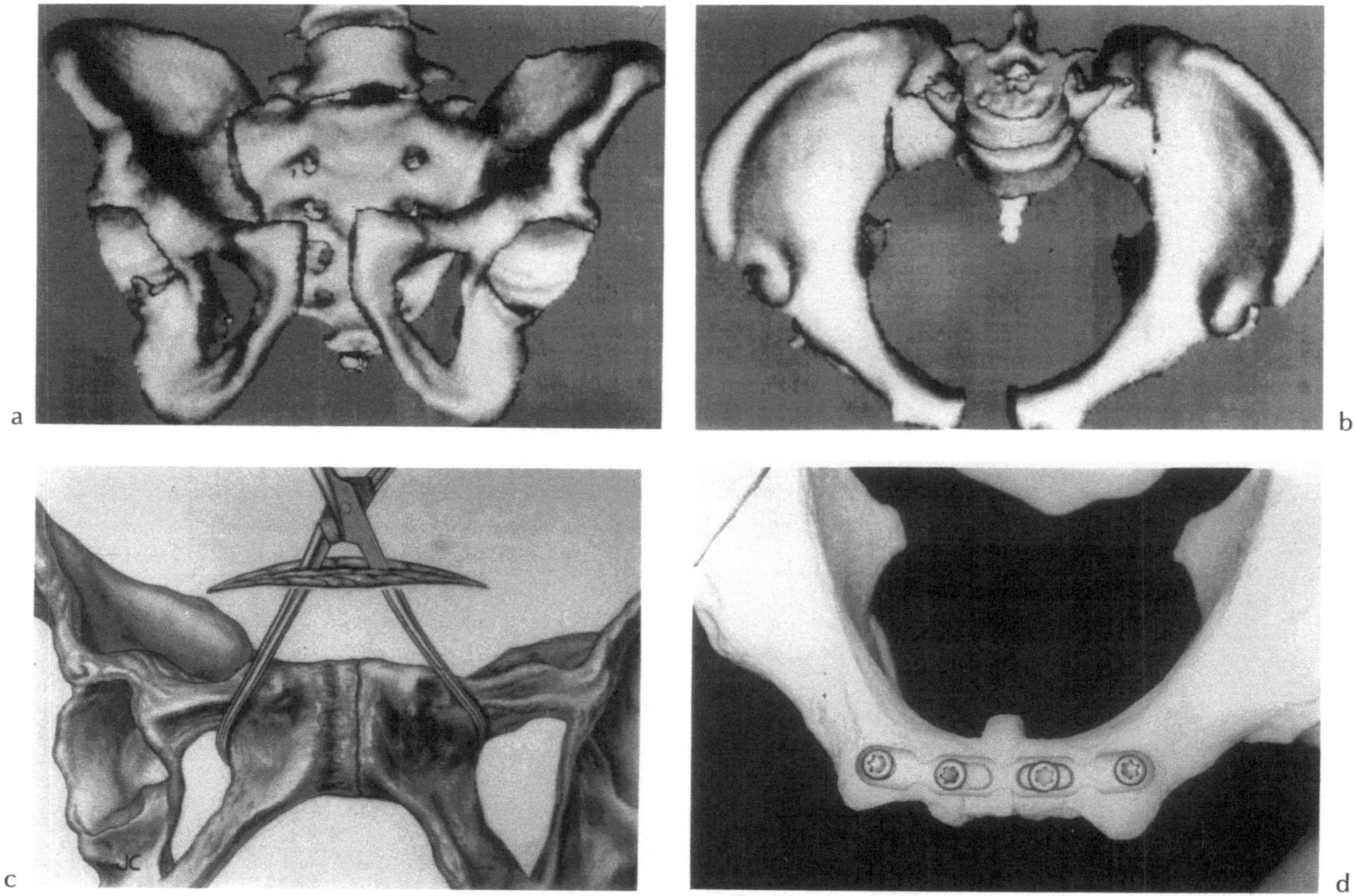


**FIGURE 7.7.** Technique for iliosacral fixation of external rotation injury by a percutaneous or limited open technique. (a) Anterior outlet 3D CT view. (b) Inlet 3D CT view. (c) Reduction of symphysis through Pfannenstiel approach. (d) Fixation of symphysis.

(*continued*)

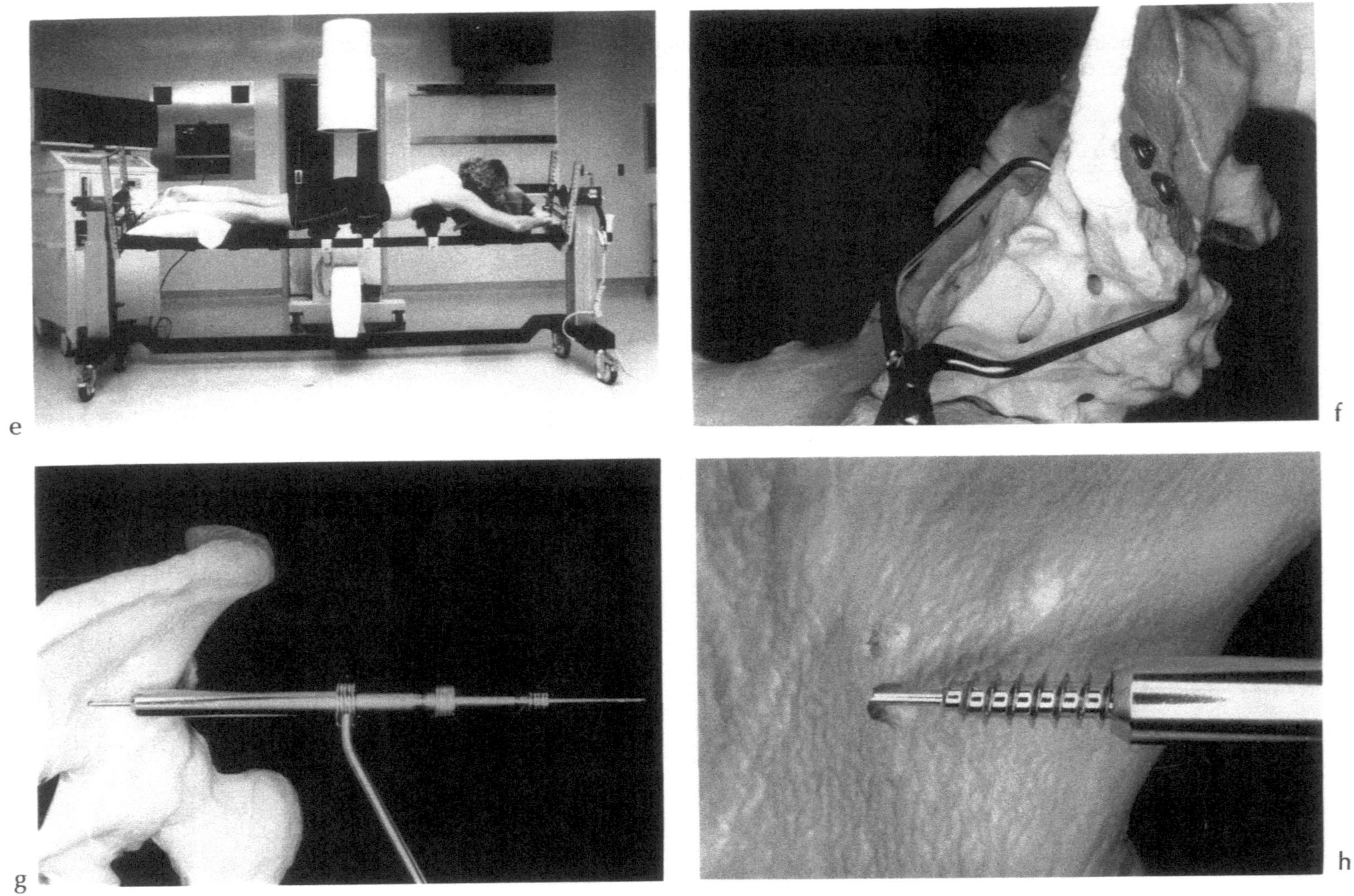

**FIGURE 7.7** (*continued*) (e) Imaging on radiolucent table for iliosacral fixation. (f) Position of tenaculum forceps accompanying a limited posterior reduction. (g) Insertion of iliosacral guide wire with drill sleeves. (h) Iliosacral screw insertion.

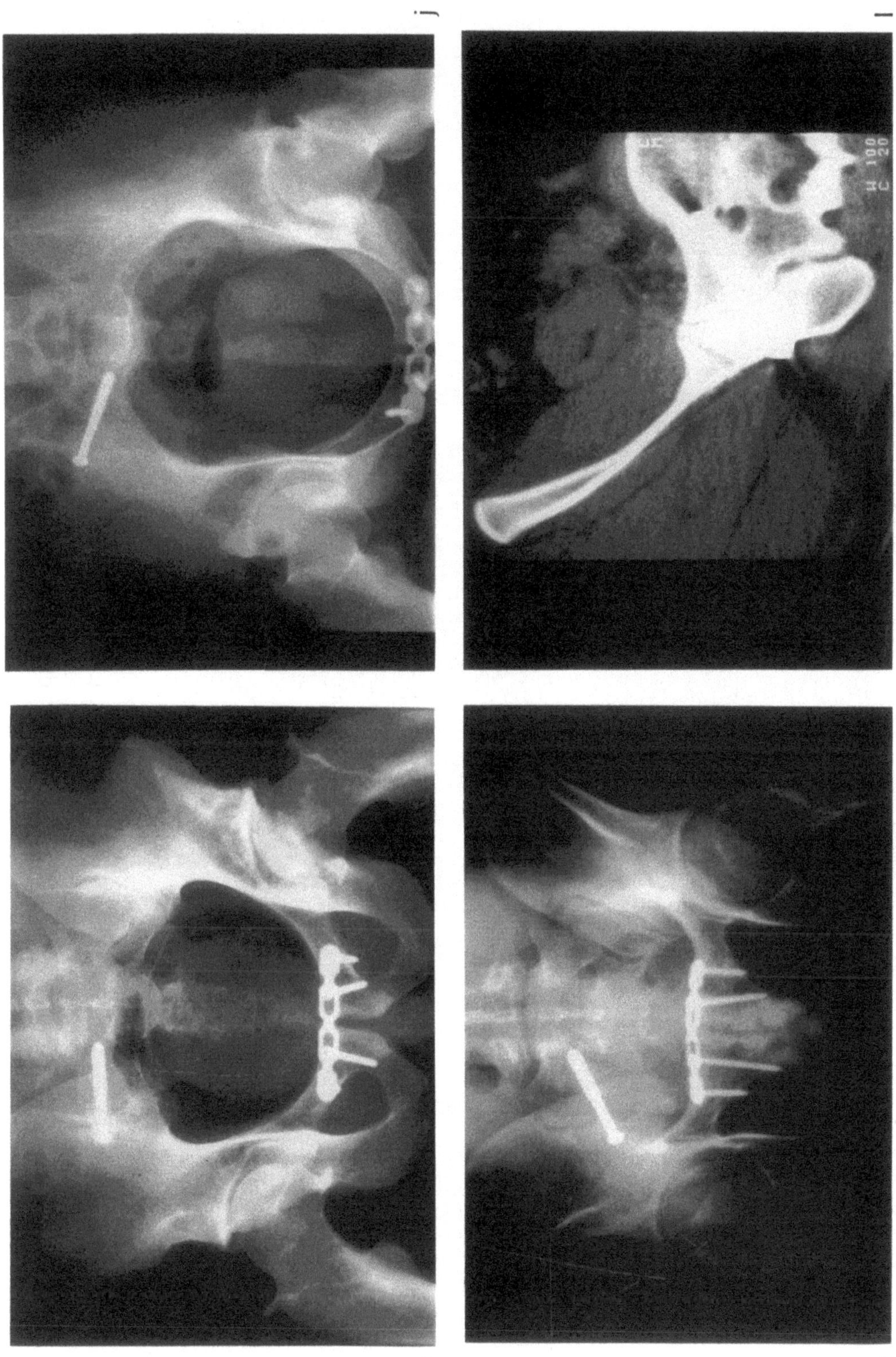

**FIGURE 7.7** (i) Postoperative AP view. (j) Postoperative inlet view. (k) Postoperative outlet view. (l) Postoperative CT iliosacral view.

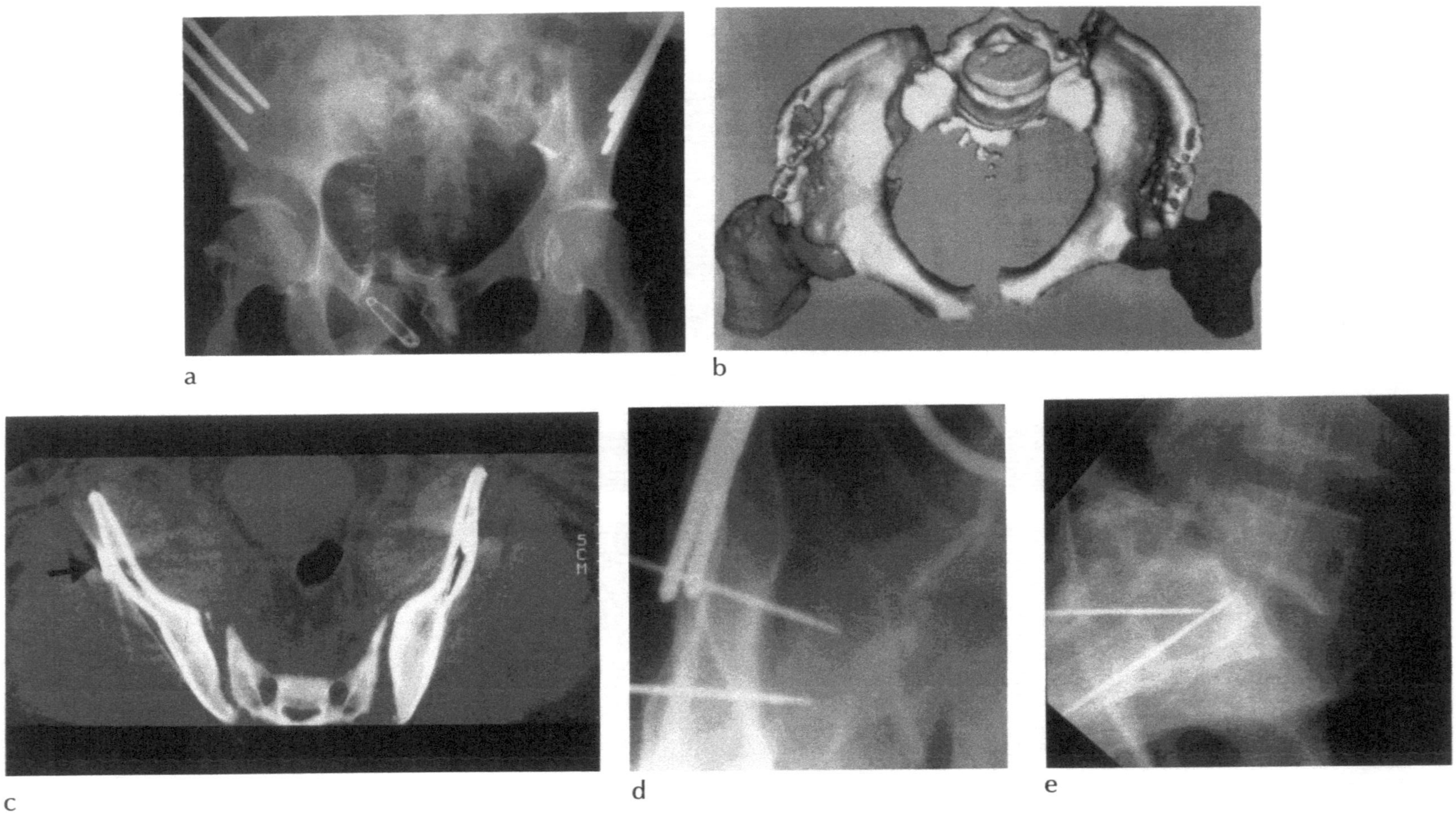


**FIGURE 7.8.** Percutaneous iliosacral screw insertion for a C-2 injury with a right SI dislocation and a left SI subluxation in a 28-year-old man with initial external pelvic fixation. A bladder rupture for which a primary repair was performed was complicated by dehiscence so that an open reduction of the symphysis was contraindicated. (a) Outlet view. (b) 3D CT inlet view. (c) Transaxial CT of posterior pelvic ring. (d) Intraoperative obturator oblique view of right SI joint after closed reduction with insertion of iliosacral guide wires. (e) Intraoperative direct lateral view of guide wires in S-1 body.

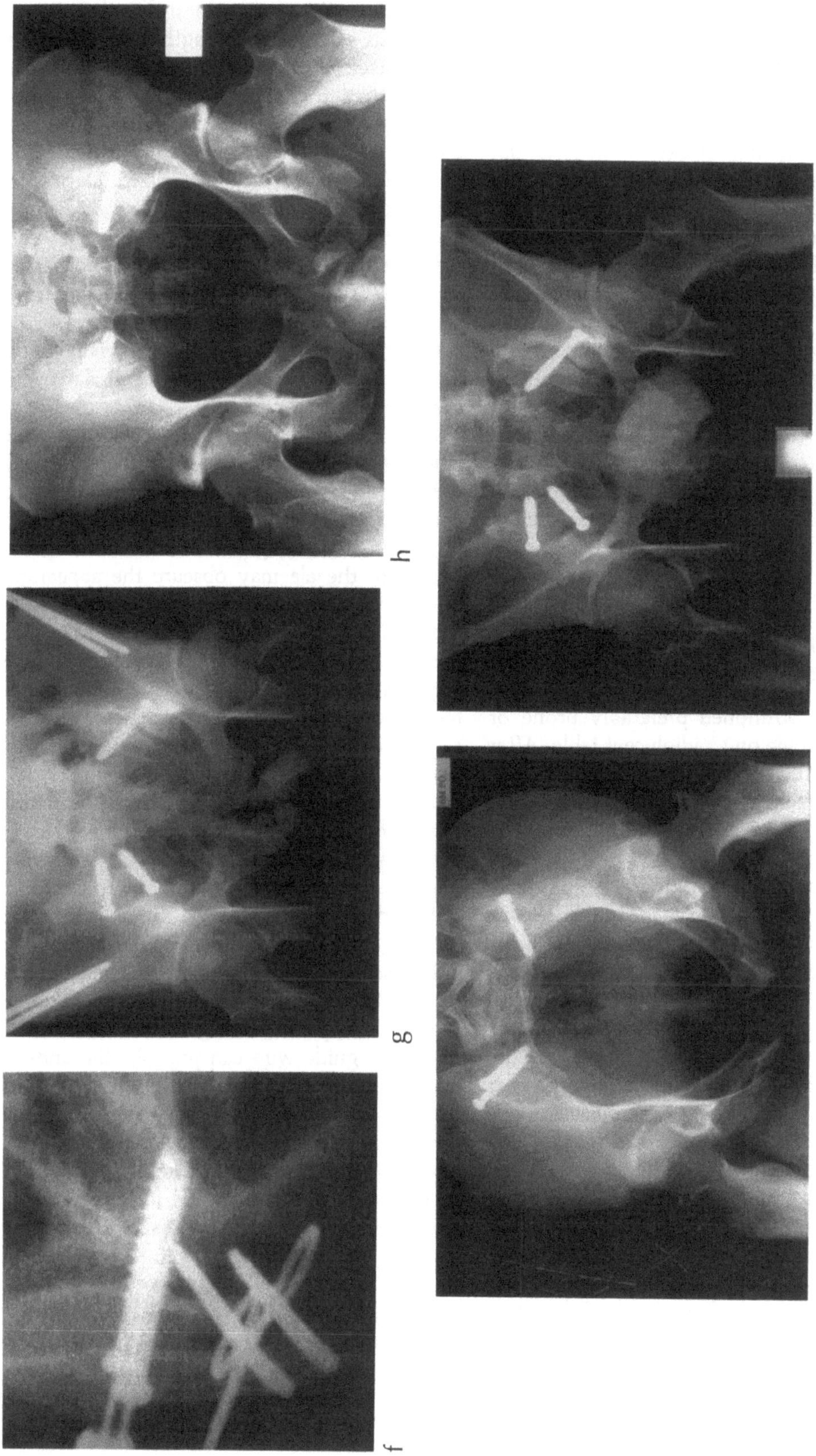

**FIGURE 7.8** (f) Intraoperative obturator oblique view after iliosacral screw insertion. (g) Initial postoperative outlet view. (h) Postoperative AP view one year later. (i) Late postoperative inlet view. (j) Late postoperative outlet view.

ulated under image intensification. Supplementary pressure can be applied on the anterior iliac crest to compress the sacroiliac joint. More effective manipulation of the hemipelvis can be achieved by the insertion of a large Schanz screw, a Steinmann pin, or external fixation pin into the anterior inferior spine, which serves as a reduction tool. Longitudinal traction can be achieved by resort to a distal femoral or proximal tibial pin. For most highly displaced sacroiliac disruptions, initially the accompanying anterior pelvic lesion, such as a diastasis of the symphysis pubis, is reduced and stabilized by an open technique. During this stage, image intensification is performed to confirm the presence of an accurate reduction of the entire pelvic ring. If the attempted anterior reduction does not reduce the sacroiliac joint, then the incision is converted into an ilioinguinal approach, and a direct open reduction and internal fixation of the sacroiliac joint is undertaken.

## Percutaneous Fixation of the Sacroiliac Joint

The patient is positioned preferably prone or alternatively supine on a radiolucent table. After block draping the surgical field, a guide wire is placed transversely across the lumbar region at the level of the posterior superior spines and an AP image is obtained (Figure 7.7).

For insertion of the guide wire, a transverse incision of 1 cm in length is made at the level of the posterior superior spine. The entry point is situated where the guide wire can be directed about 10° to 20° anterior to a transaxial plane. With this orientation, the guide wire can be advanced at a right angle with respect to the axis of the sacroiliac joint. This orthogonal relationship with respect to the sacroiliac joint is further achieved if the guide wire is advanced slightly superiorward, also by about 10° to 20°. The guide wire or corresponding drill bit is advanced through the lateral iliac cortex followed by penetration of the inner iliac table of the sacroiliac joint and the adjacent sacral subchondral table. Further advancement of the guide wire into the alar portion of the first sacral body is undertaken. In most cases, the sacral penetration continues for an additional 30 to 40 mm, although the anterior sacral cortex is not breached. In this way, a long-threaded 7.0-mm cancellous screw with a length of 45 to 60 mm can be used. By penetration of three instead of four cortices, the guide wire and screw are kept within bone so that the risk of inadvertent penetration of the anterior presacral soft tissues and of the S-1 nerve root is minimized. During the insertion of the guide wire, multiple AP, inlet, and outlet views are obtained. The AP view confirms that the guide wire is inserted parallel to the transaxial plane. The outlet view permits a recognition of undesirable penetration of the superior alar surface. The inlet view is preferred for the advancement into the sacral ala toward the anterior sacral cortex.

Once the guide wire is fully inserted, a direct lateral view is taken to confirm that the guide wire remains embedded in the sacrum.[38] Particularly in an elderly individual, a large osteophyte situated along the anterior and superior border of the ala may obscure the appearance on the inlet view of excessive penetration of the guide wire beyond the anterior cortex. This problem is recognized or prevented by taking sequential lateral views (Figure 7.8). The ideal target zone for the screw thread is within the sacral ala lateral to the S-1 nerve foramina and inferior to the L5-S1 disk space. Typically, two guide wires are inserted prior to the sequential replacement with screws of appropriate length. After the use of the depth gauge, the screws are inserted while spot radiographic views are obtained to ensure that the guide wire is not inadvertently advanced during the insertion of either screw. If the guide wire bends during its insertion by even an imperceptible amount, then a subsequent binding of the screw on the deformed guide wire can provoke the undesirable advancement of the wire. Where the bone is somewhat osteopenic, a supplementary washer can be used. After tightening of the screws, an obturator oblique view is taken that is parallel to the plane of the sacroiliac joint. This image permits confirmation that the sacroiliac joint is rigorously approximated.

### *Insertion of a Percutaneous Screw Across a Longitudinal Sacral Fracture*

Generally, the technique for insertion of a screw across a sacral fracture is similar to the method described for sacroiliac fixation.[38] The patient can be positioned in a fully prone, supine, or even a lateral decubitus position, although the crucial use of the image intensifier appears to be most readily achieved in the prone position. Imaging is most difficult in the lateral position. The target zone for the screw becomes the first sacral body, and to a lesser degree, the S-2 body. With the patient situated in a prone fashion, a guide wire is placed transversely across the middle of the S-1 body for an initial AP image (Figure 7.9). Then a transverse incision of about 3 cm in length is made at an equivalent point on the side of the injury that is about 6 cm posterior to the prominence of the greater trochanter. After spreading the incision down to the bone, with use of a small vascular clamp, the guide wire and drill sleeve assembly is introduced through the incision and advanced to bone. An AP image is taken to confirm that the second guide wire is coaxial with the first. The second guide wire is drilled into the lateral ilium for about 3 cm. An inlet view is taken to confirm that the guide wire is centrally disposed from anterior to posterior in the S-1 body. Also, the guide wire is oriented in a transverse manner so that it is not directed toward the front of the sacrum nor toward the neural canal. A supplementary outlet view is taken to ensure that the guide wire is oriented parallel to the top of the S-1 body and midway between the top and the S-1 foramen. If necessary, the guide wire is repositioned until these criteria are satisfied. In the presence of a pronounced osteophytic ridge along the anterior and superior border of the sacrum, the guide wire needs to be positioned a few millimeters more posteriorward in the S-1 body to ensure that the screw is within the bone. The guide wire is advanced so that it is embedded within the bone for about 90 mm. This distance is consistent with the screw threads of a long threaded screw being located within the S-1 body and between the ipsilateral and contralateral foramina.

After confirmatory AP, inlet, and outlet images are obtained, a supplementary direct lateral image is viewed. The position of the guide wire within the S-1 body is confirmed. If the fracture is an unstable one where displacement was documented prior to the closed or open reduction, a second iliosacral screw is inserted parallel to the first. The corresponding guide wire can be introduced into the S-1 or S-2 bodies. For a large male patient, the easier technique is the insertion of two screws into the first sacral body. In such a patient, frequently the S-1 body is large enough so that the two screws can be inserted with one in front of the other or with one superior to the other. In a small woman, the S-1 body may be too small to contain two sacral screws. Once the S-2 body is needed, the anatomical details of the sacrum need to be carefully reviewed. The S-2 body is substantially narrower than the S-1 body in the anteroposterior dimension. The anterior surface of the sacrum possesses a concavity so that the anterior surface of S-2 is considerably more posterior than the corresponding surface of S-1. In the inlet view, this curved configuration of the sacrum is radiographically obscured. Its crucial recognition is achieved by a scrutiny of the lateral image. For insertion of a second screw into S-1, the original incision can be used. For insertion of a sacral screw into S-2, a separate incision is made about 3 cm inferior to the first. The guide wire is advanced down to bone. An AP image is obtained to confirm that the second guide wire is parallel to the first and mid-axial with respect to the S-2 body. After the pin is advanced into the bone for about 3 cm, the AP, inlet, outlet, and direct lateral images are obtained. The guide wire is documented to be centered in the midportion of S-2 and to be parallel to the first guide wire. Then the guide wire is fully inserted to about 90 mm from the entry point in the lateral ilium. Once both guide wires are satisfactorily inserted, a depth gauge is applied over the guide wire. Then a 7.2-mm-long threaded cancellous screw of appropriate length is advanced over either guide pin and tightened.

## Hazards and Associated Technical Details

For insertion of iliosacral screws into the midsacral region, subtle anatomical variations, possibly combined with conditions of less than optimal imaging, can lead to conditions of marked escalation in the risk of formidable complica-

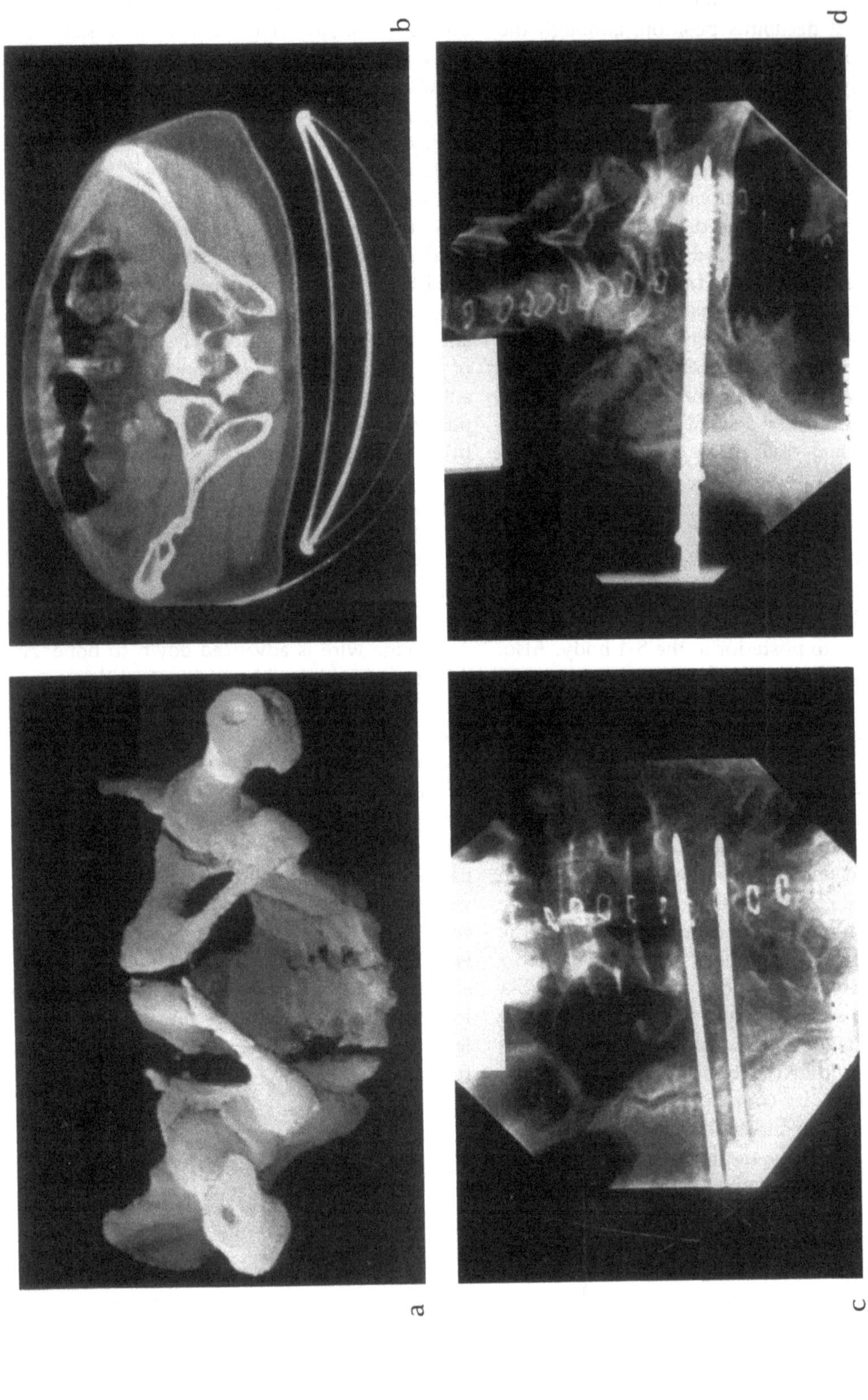


**FIGURE 7.9.** Percutaneous iliosacral fixation of a longitudinal sacral fracture. (a) Anterior outlet 3D CT view. (b) Transaxial CT view. (c) Intraoperative outlet view after guide wire insertion. (d) Intraoperative inlet view after screw insertion over guide wires.

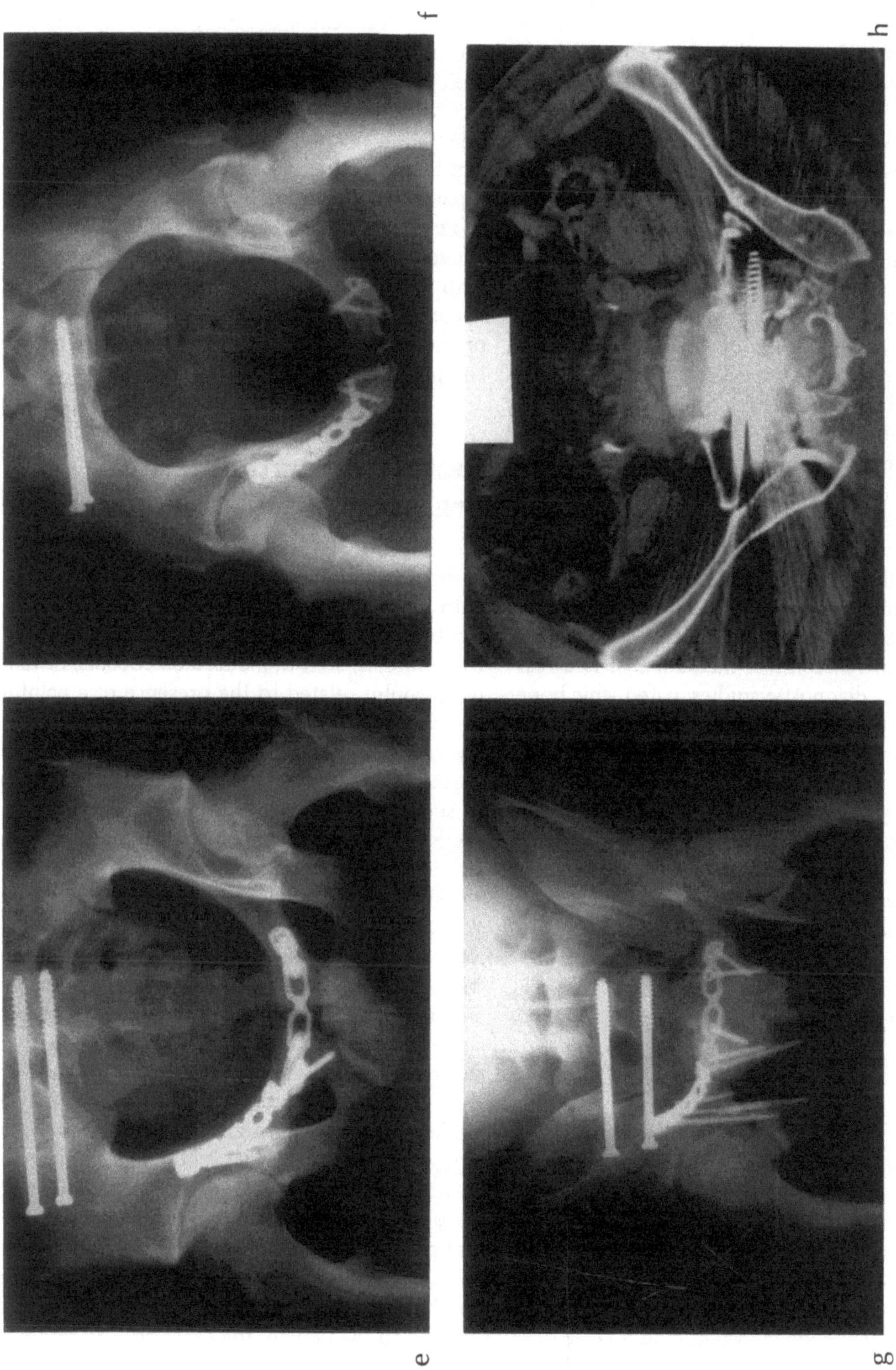


**FIGURE 7.9** (e) Postoperative AP view. (f) Postoperative inlet view. (g) Postoperative outlet view. (h) Postoperative transaxial CT view.

tions. The degree of lumbar lordosis and corresponding tilt of the sacrum influence the ideal orientation of the x-ray beam of the image intensifier that is appropriate for each patient.[38] The detailed features of the sacral anatomy vary considerably with further alterations afforded by degenerative changes. Transitional vertebra at the lumbosacral junction further complicate the imaging with the aberrant contours of the lumbarized S-1 or sacralized 1-5 vertebra. The sacral foramina possess a variable but oblique course through the bone. An appreciation of the apparent orientation of the foramina is further complicated by the degree of tilt of the sacrum. While a precursory inspection of the S-1 body might lead to an impression that a 30-mm cylindrical column of bone is available for the insertion of the two 7-mm screws, the actual space that is available is significantly compromised by the presence of the foramina. In many instances, a centrally placed screw will be surrounded by not more than 3 mm of bone at crucial sites such as the neighboring foramen. In the presence of morbid obesity, a paralytic ileus with dilated loops of bowel, contrast medium that is a residue of prior diagnostic studies, osteopenic bone, or a faulty image intensifier, inadequate resolution may necessitate abandonment of this method. The resources for open fixation of the posterior sacrum with a plate or with sacral bars should be available as an alternative. When a switch to open sacral fixation is necessary, the use of the prone position facilitates the altered surgical plan.

## Bilateral Vertical Sacral Fractures

For the bilateral injury patterns, two therapeutic alternatives exist. Iliosacral screws can be introduced from either side of the sacrum (Figure 7.10). In this instance, the method is similar to that just described. In the center of the sacral body, however, four screws have to be positioned with an overlapping of screws that is thwarted by the limits of space. In a large male, this method is entirely suitable, although in a small female it may be impractical. The other option is to introduce two lengthy screws that traverse entirely across the posterior pelvic ring (Figure 7.11). Great accuracy in the orientation and location of the screws is essential. The imaging technique is similar to that described for the ipsilateral iliosacral screw. The transverse orientation is crucial for the entire 120 to 150 mm length of the screws. For fixation of a long threaded screw within bone, the screw thread is liable to cross the sacroiliac joint. This shortcoming appears to be relatively minor compared with the other practical considerations of these uncommon and challenging cases. The presence of the screws has not been attributable to the complaint of late posterior pelvic pain.

## Iliosacral Fixation in the Presence of Osteopenic Bone

A further technical complexity of sacral fixation with iliosacral screws arises when the quality of the bone is impaired by the presence of senile osteoporosis, steroid-induced osteopenia, or disuse atrophy related to the presence of a painful nonunion or nonunion malunion. Previously, if the screw thread did not anchor securely in the weakened bone, the fixation was unsatisfactory. In such a case, the use of supplementary methyl methacrylate to augment the strength of the pelvic bone stock is complicated by the limited thickness of the bone, the juxtaposition of nerve roots in adjacent foramina, and other neurovascular structures or viscera adjacent to the bone that are vulnerable to thermal damage imposed by solidifying extravasated cement. As an alternative, a novel method of securing two adjacent 7.2-mm cannulated screws with a 2.0-mm Dall-Miles cable has been devised.[39] The cable is passed through the cannula of one screw (Figure 7.12). Then it is advanced through a two-hole 3.5-mm plate that serves as a washer. Subsequently, the cable is retrograded through the cannula of the second iliosacral screw. The two free ends of the cable are passed through the holes of a second washer plate. A sleeve is applied to the ends of the cable prior to tightening the cable with the tightening instrument. Once the cable is taut, the sleeve is crimped and excessive cable is removed with the cable cutter. The screws are selected of a length whereby they extend across the posterior pelvic ring just to the surface of their threaded tips.

# Acetabular Fixation with Cannulated Screws

The pattern of acetabular fracture dictates the type of surgical approach or approaches, the reduction strategy, and the preferred type of fixation. Historically, the posterior injury patterns including posterior wall, posterior column, posterior wall–posterior column, and posterior wall–transverse injuries have been visualized by resort to a Kocher-Langenbeck approach.[40] The anterior injury patterns include anterior wall, anterior column, anterior column or anterior wall–posterior hemitransverse, and most typical both-column fracture patterns. All of these injuries, including the last pattern which has a major constituent of posterior column that is contiguous with the quadrilateral surface, can be accurately reduced by resort to an ilioinguinal exposure. Admittedly, with delayed presentation, or in certain other complex injury patterns, a both-column injury may be best managed by the use of two approaches for anterior and posterior visualization, respectively. For transverse and T-type injury patterns, the optimal surgical approach varies depending upon certain subtle aspects of the injury. In some instances, the displacement is almost entirely posterior, where the anterior edge of the transverse fracture serves as a fulcrum. In this instance, a posterior approach may suffice. Examples would include many posterior wall–transverse fractures with minimal displacement of the transverse fracture itself, as well as some posterior T-type injuries. In other cases, the displacement is almost entirely anterior when an ilioinguinal approach may be preferred. When the entire transverse fracture is significantly displaced, then the anterior and posterior edges of the fracture need to be visualized for an accurate reduction. In this instance, an extended lateral approach, such as a triradiate or extended iliofemoral, may be necessary. For substantially displaced T-type fractures, another option is to use anterior and posterior approaches for the corresponding portions of the reduction.

For the reduction of an acetabular fracture, a broad spectrum of specialized reduction tools is available. Most of these forceps possess pointed tip jaws that are of various lengths and differing shapes. An alternative technique is to employ a Farboeuf forceps applied to screw heads after a screw is embedded in either principal fracture fragment.[40] This technique affords robust temporary fixation, although the time required for its application with insertion of the screws is somewhat longer than that required for the use of a tenaculum-type forceps. A special family of acetabular reduction forceps, identified as the king, queen, and prince tong, are particularly useful for spanning from the inside to the outside of the pelvis. The prince tong is a so-called eccentric forceps with jaws of differing lengths. It is perhaps the most satisfactory design for the reduction of the quadrilateral surface or of the posterior wall by resort to an ilioinguinal approach.

Most of the fractures are suitably immobilized by standard 3.5- or 4.5-mm cortical screws and highly flexible reconstruction plates. For immobilization of especially thin bone, such as the posterior and anterior wall, a hook or spring plate is fashioned from a 3.5-mm one-third tubular plate.[34] This method permits the fixation of thin sections of bone with a buttressing technique, whereby the screws are remote from the joint surface. For acetabular fixation, cannulated screws have a limited but valuable role for two special applications. Around the acetabulum, limited columns of bone, typically with a maximum diameter of 7 to 9 mm, provide the principal source of bone stock for fixation (Figure 7.4a). Log screw fixation of these columns by resort to conventional screws was popularized by Letournel.[21] With such a limited cross-sectional area for immobilization, the screw is highly vulnerable to extend beyond the surface of the bone prematurely, either to compromise fixation or to jeopardize adjacent soft tissues. With the use of a cannulated screw, the guide wire can be inserted initially for radiographic confirmation of appropriate position. Also, the guide wire ensures that the screw follows

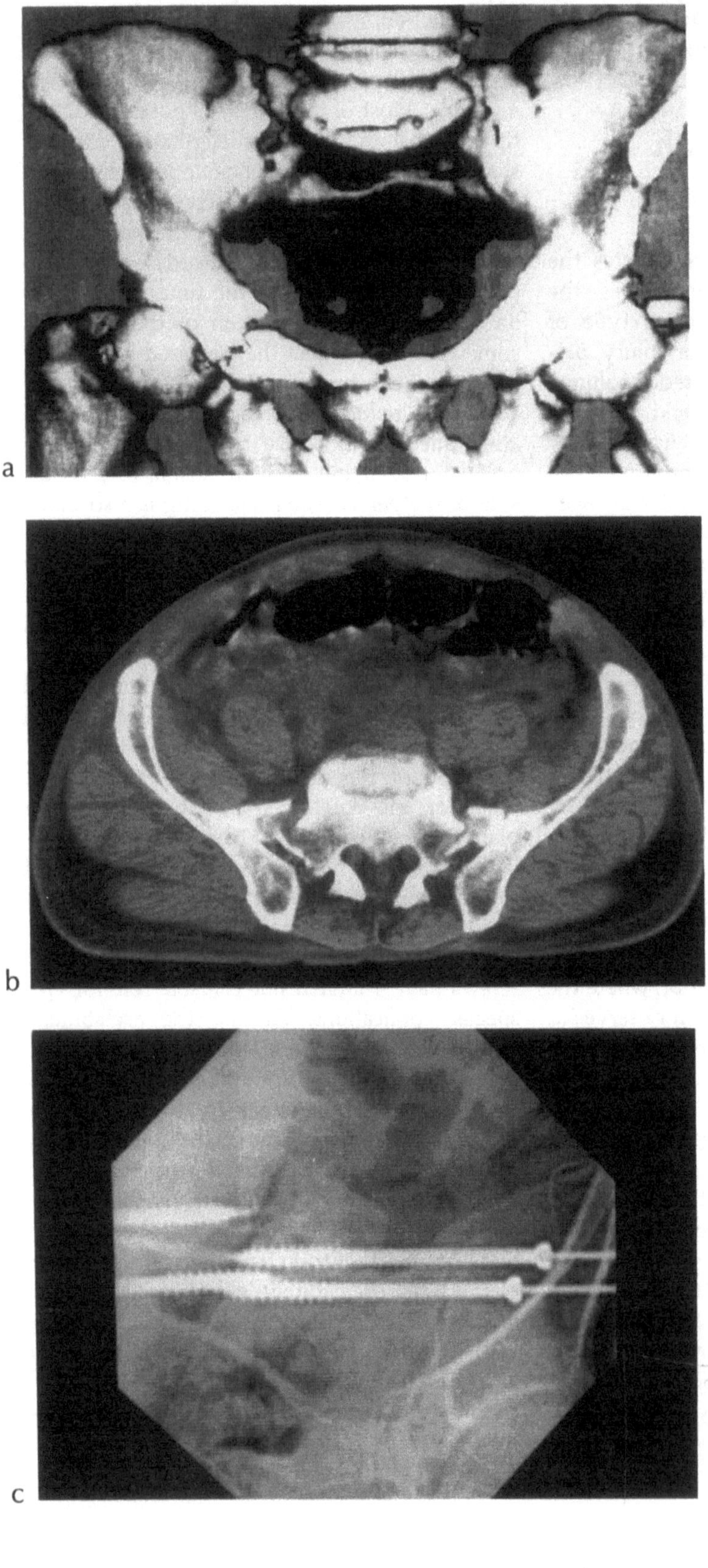


**FIGURE 7.10.** Bilateral longitudinal fractures with percutaneous iliosacral screw insertion for a C-3 injury in a 43-year-old man. (a) Initial 3D CT. (b) Transaxial CT view of S-1 body. (c) Intraoperative outlet view.

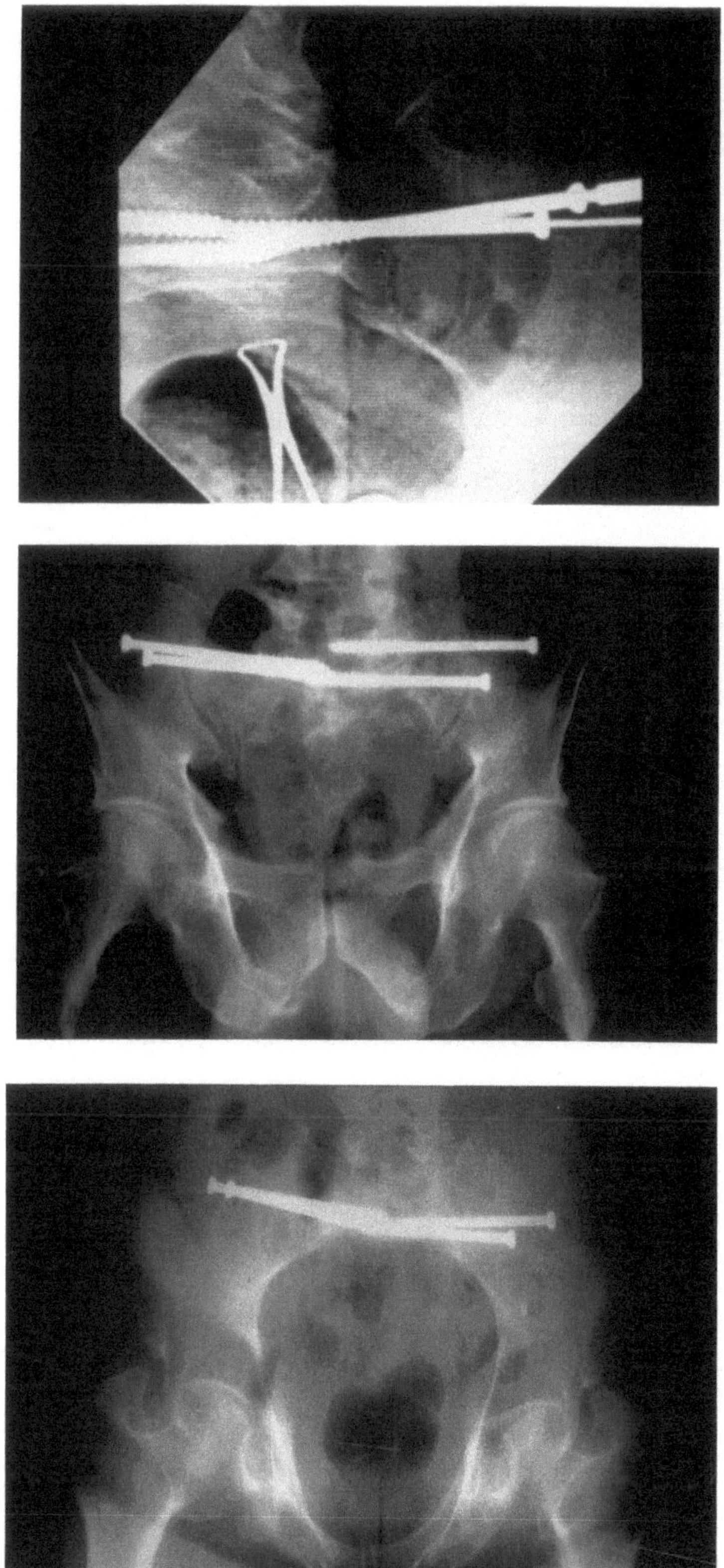


**FIGURE 7.10** (d) Intraoperative inlet view. (e) Postoperative AP view at one year. (f) Postoperative inlet view.

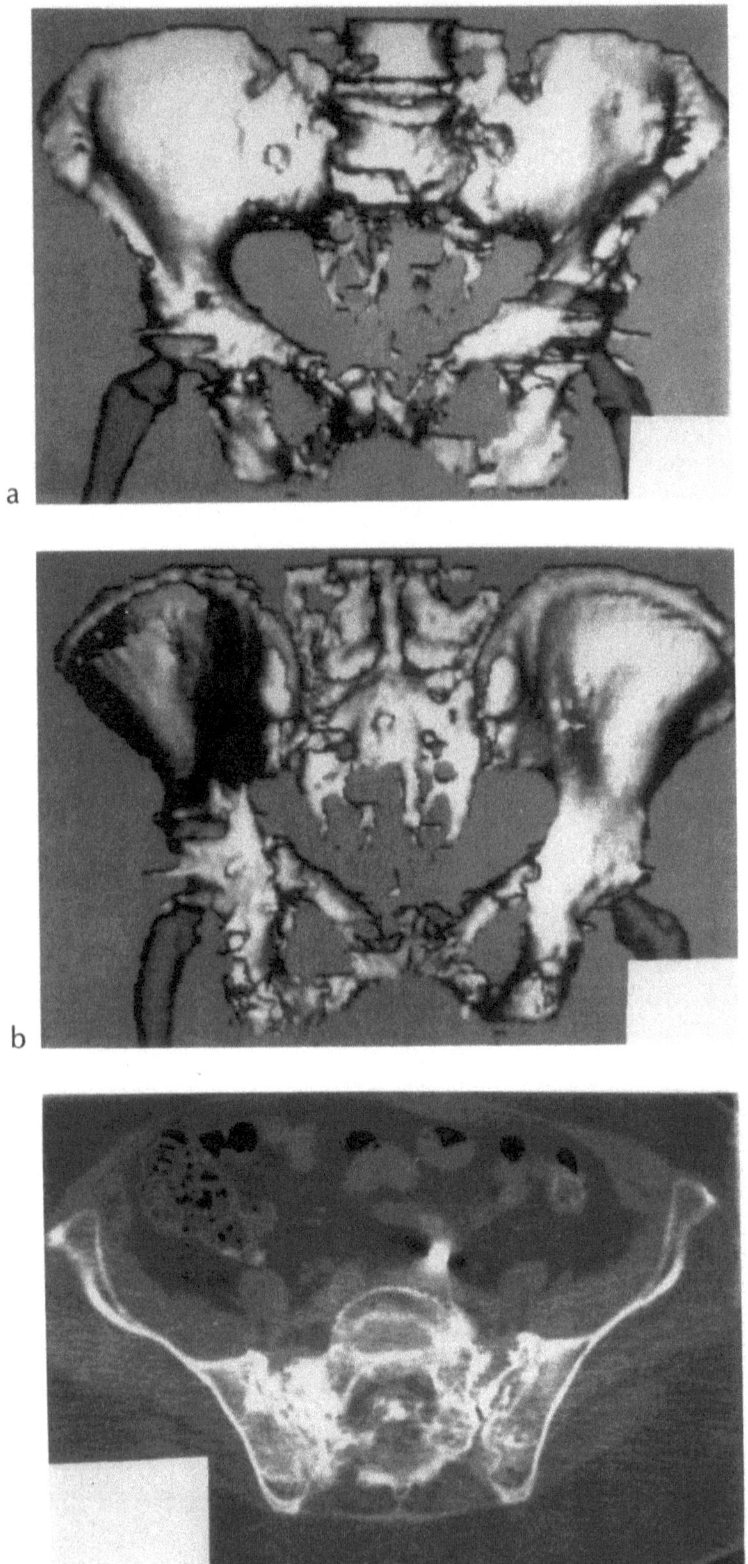

**FIGURE 7.11.** Percutaneous iliosacral screw fixation and posterior plate fixation in a 72-year-old woman with bilateral sacral alar insufficiency fractures secondary to irradiation therapy for uterine carcinoma. The lengthy iliosacral screws were inserted through the left ilium. (a) Initial anterior 3D CT view. (b) Posterior 3D CT view. (c) Transaxial CT view of posterior pelvis.

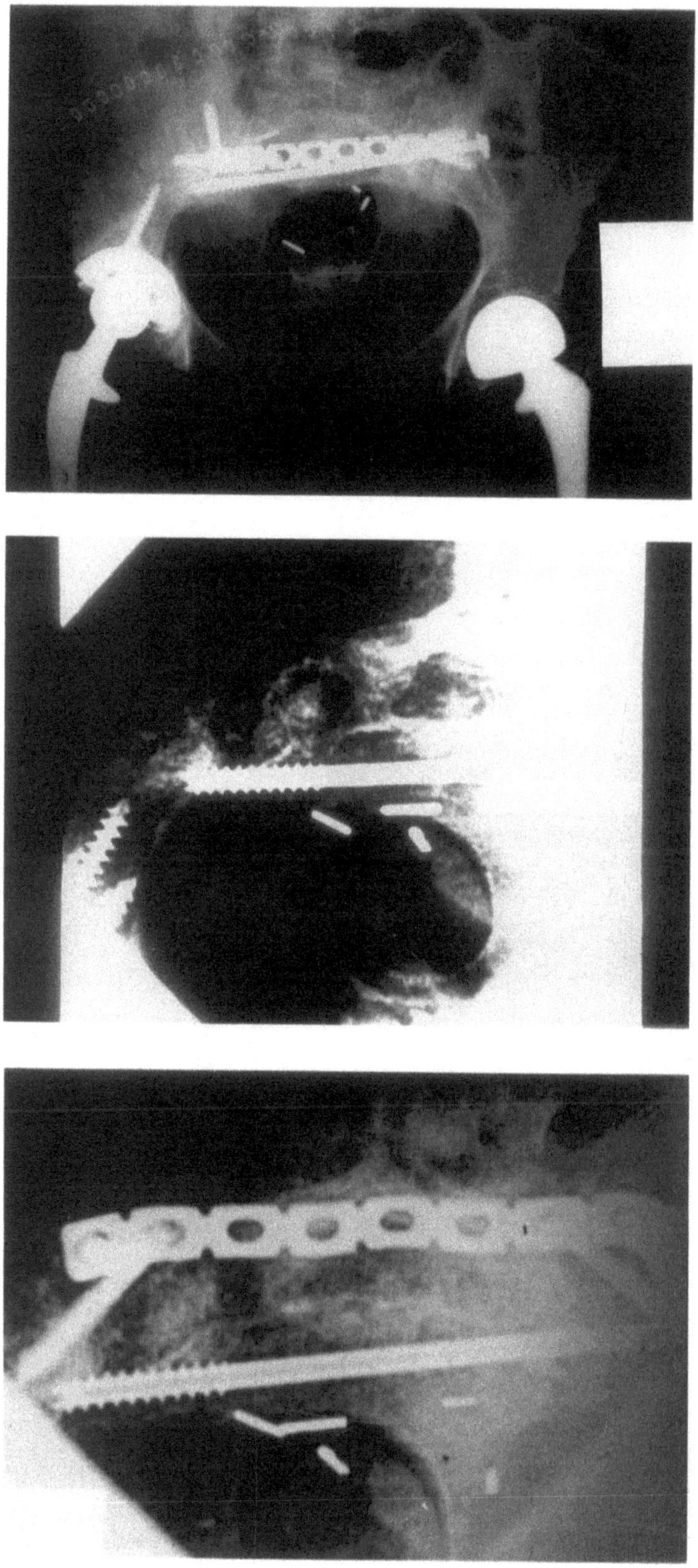

d

e

f

**FIGURE 7.11** (d) Postoperative AP view. (e) Intraoperative inlet view. (f) Intraoperative outlet view.

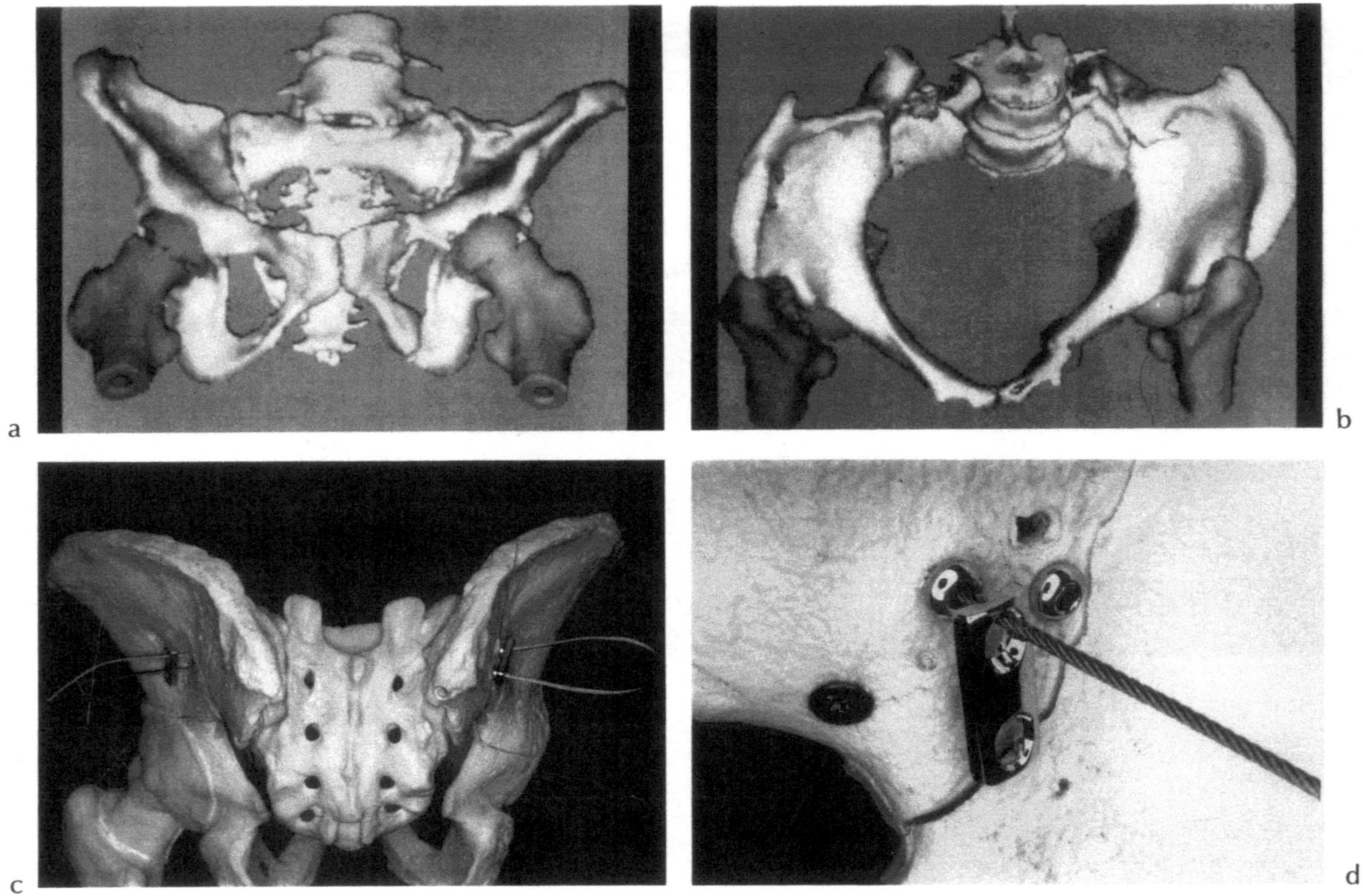


**FIGURE 7.12.** Augmentation of cannulated iliosacral screws with 2.0-mm cable in a 63-year-old woman with posterior insufficiency sacroiliac disruptions secondary to extensive harvesting of bone graft. (a) Anterior 3D CT outlet view. (b) Inlet views. (c) Cable threaded through two cannulated screws. (d) Use of a two-hole plate as a washer.

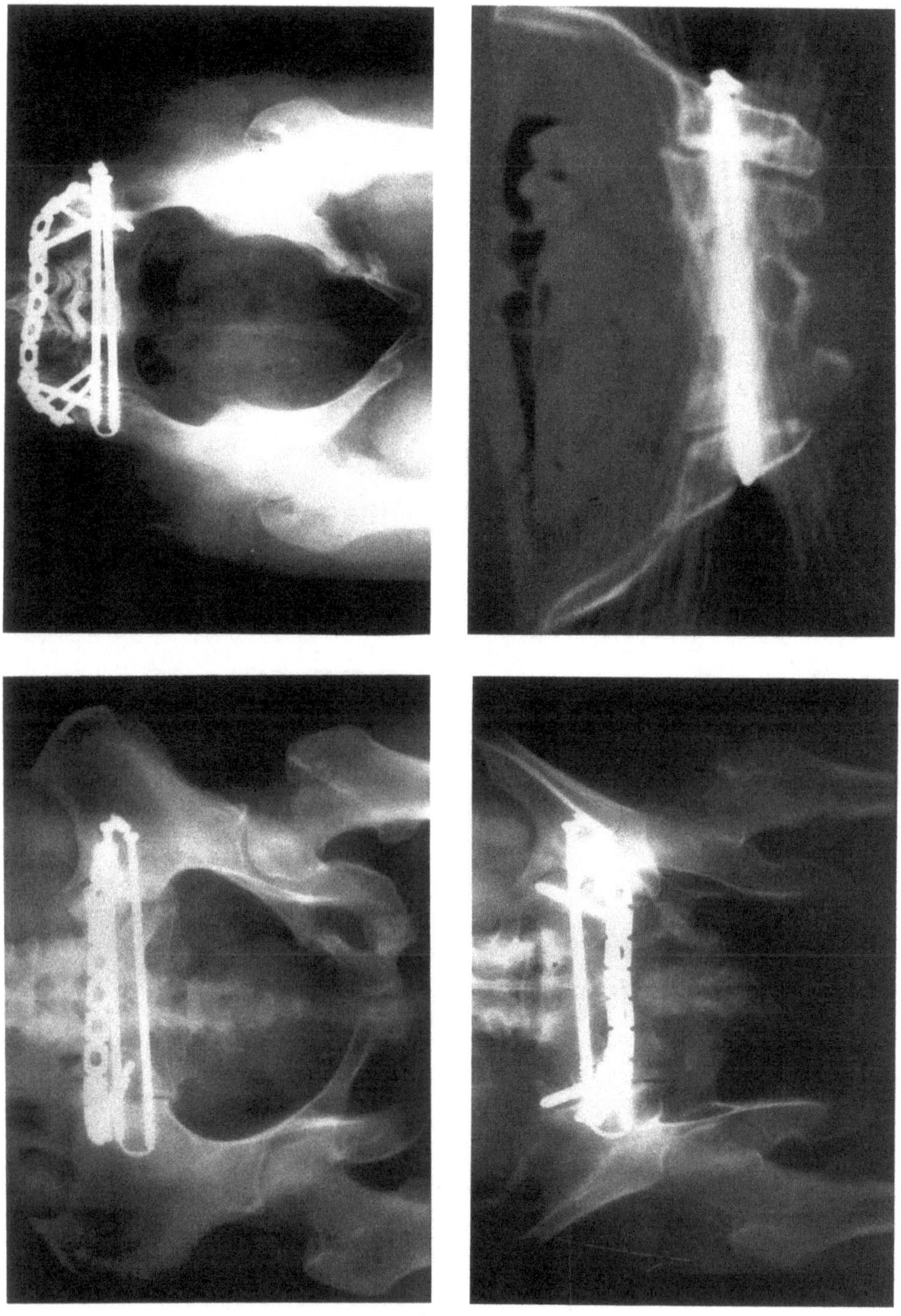

e f g h

**FIGURE 7.12** (e) Postoperative AP view one year later. (f) Postoperative inlet view. (g) Postoperative outlet view. (h) Postoperative transsacral CT views.

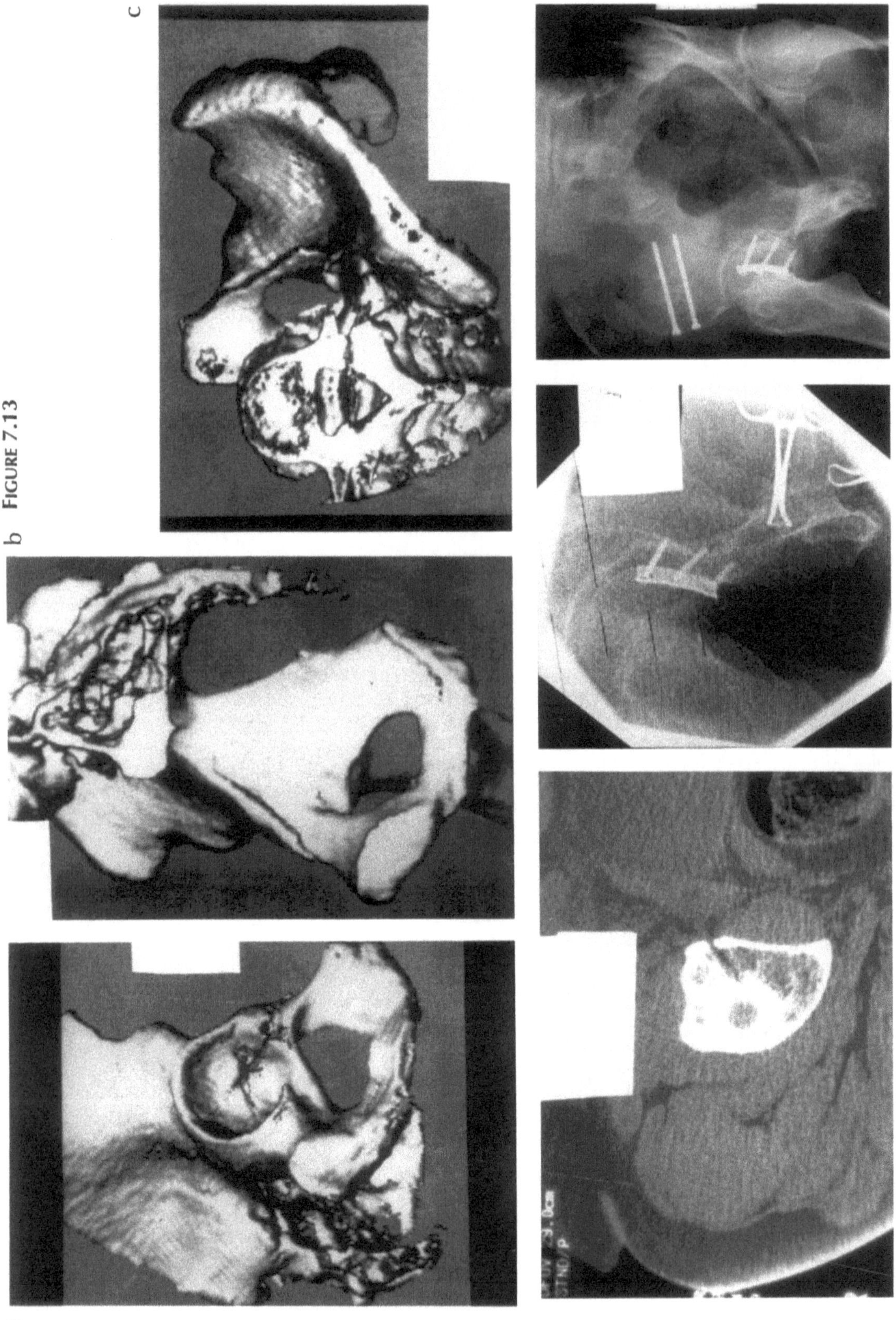


FIGURE 7.13

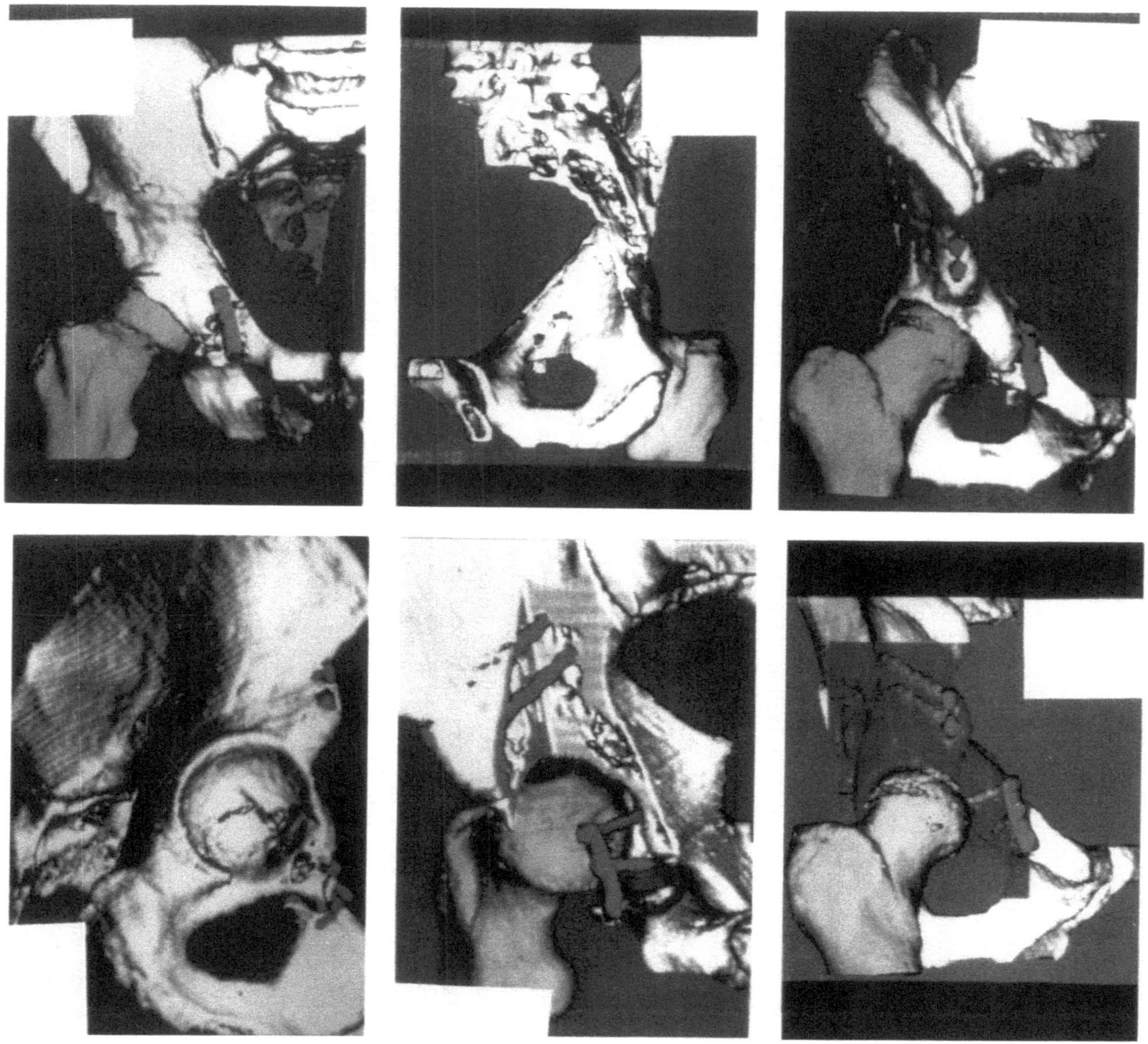


**FIGURE 7.13.** Percutaneous fixation of the anterior column in a 51-year-old man where a limited ilioinguinal approach to the medial eminence was undertaken to stabilize the quadrilateral surface. (a) Disarticulated 3D CT of acetabulum. (b) 3D CT of quadrilateral surface. (c) Superior 3D CT views. (d) CT view of dome. (e) Intraoperative iliac oblique view of plate on medial eminence. (f) Iliac oblique view highlighting percutaneous screws. (g) Postoperative anterior 3D CT view. (h) Postoperative 3D CT view of quadrilateral surface. (i) Postoperative obturator oblique view. (j) Postoperative disarticulated acetabular view. (k) Postoperative 3D CT with partial acetabular subtraction to confirm sagittal congruency. (l) Postoperative 3D CT with translucency of acetabulum to highlight fixation screws.

exactly the same course as the guide wire. Alternatively, when a conventional screw is employed, occasionally, where the corresponding column of bone is curved, the initial drill bit may follow the course of the cancellous bone, although the larger screw may follow a different pathway, either to exit through the fracture or through relatively thin cortex. The other application of cannulated screws around the acetabulum is to achieve fixation with a minimally invasive or percutaneous technique. Certain acetabular fractures, especially of a transverse nature or as a pathologic variant, are minimally displaced but potentially unstable. Percutaneous screw fixation is a highly attractive method for immobilization. Other acetabular fractures merit approach by an acetabular exposure that is selected for the optimal visualization of the fracture and reduction. Nevertheless, that approach may be inappropriate for insertion of lag screws. In this instance, a cannulated lag screw may be inserted percutaneously, either as a principal or supplementary source of fixation (Figure 7.13). Perhaps the best example is fixation of the anterior column of a transverse fracture with a screw that courses through the superior gluteal ridge and along the superior pubic ramus, a so-called anterior column screw.

A 4.5-mm-diameter cannulated screw is preferred for acetabular fixation. The principal sites for insertion of such screws include the anterior, superior, and inferior spines, the posterior, inferior and superior spines, the superior gluteal ridge, and the posterior and anterior columns (Figure 7.4d). In practice, some of these sites of bony condensation are appropriate for either acetabular or pelvic ring fixation (Figure 7.14). Apart from the anterior column screw, the remaining sites for fixation are of sufficient size so that the 4.5-mm-diameter screw can be inserted with relative ease provided that image intensification with a high resolution is available. For the anterior column screw, a detailed scrutiny of the hemipelvis is necessary (Figure 7.15). The screw has to follow a pathway that is coaxial with the superior pubic ramus along its innermost aspect. The entry site is between 4 and 5 cm superior to the lateral acetabular margin. The screw enters the posterior aspect of the superior gluteal ridge. In some instances, the guide wire is best inserted prior to the reduction of the transverse fracture. In this way, the tip of the guide wire exiting in the fracture surface permits a confirmation of the appropriate site of the guide wire through a column of about 40 mm in length. Once the fracture is reduced, then the column of bone becomes 80 to 100 mm in length, whereby the assessment of the target zone is much more difficult. During the insertion of the guide wire, the image intensification confirms the appropriate pathway by viewing the AP, inlet, and Judet views. The inlet view permits a confirmation that the screw follows the course of the pelvic brim. The obturator oblique view permits a documentation that the screw is consistent with the position of the acetabular roof.

For a both-column fracture with the typical high anterior fracture fragment, screws inserted into the anterior aspect of the anterosuperior spine and through the anteroinferior spine permit effective fixation with little prominence of the fixation device (Figure 7.4d). The former screw passes immediately along the course of the iliac crest through the corresponding thickened ridge of bone. The latter screw is inserted slightly to the lateral aspect of the most prominent tip of the anterosuperior spine. The screw continues parallel to the course of the sacroiliac joint as documented on the obturator oblique view. A supplementary iliac oblique view permits documentation that the screw is directed superior to the roof of the greater sciatic notch into the so-called greater sciatic buttress. The use of this screw is also appropriate for a high transverse fracture. In this case, however, the screw is directed more inferiorly toward the greater sciatic notch. Here the guide wire is assessed on the iliac oblique view to ensure that it does not extend beyond the confines of the posterior column where impalement of the sciatic nerve would become a possibility. Again, the obturator oblique view permits documentation that the screw follows the course of the roof of the acetabulum.

For a both-column fracture complicated by a large posterior wall fracture fragment, initially most of the injury is reduced and stabilized by resort to an ilioinguinal approach. For immobilization of the posterior wall, and potentially the

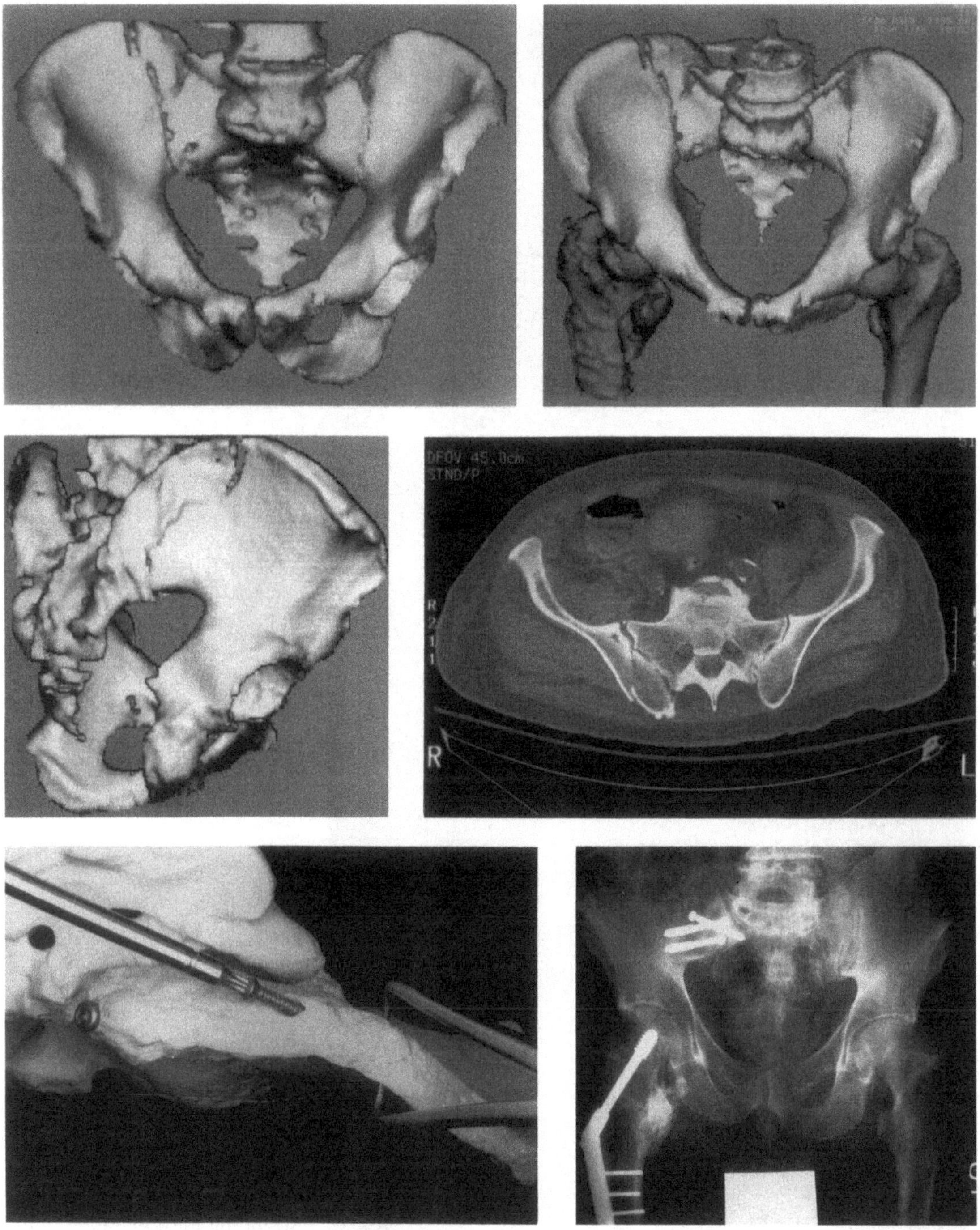

a b c d e f

**FIGURE 7.14.** Example of posterior iliac fixation with percutaneous screws inserted into postero-superior and -inferior spine for an insufficiency fracture in a 78-year-old man. (a) 3D CT anterior view. (b) 3D CT inlet view. (c) 3D CT external iliac view. (d) Transaxial CT view. (e) Direction of screws inserted through the posterior spines. (f) Postoperative AP view with two posterior iliac screws and one iliosacral screw.

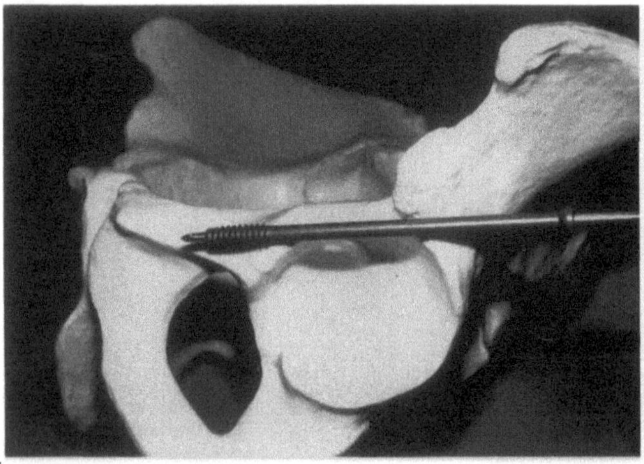

a

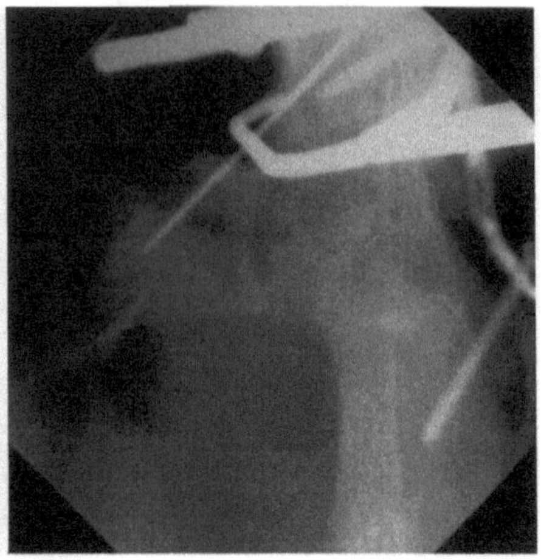

b

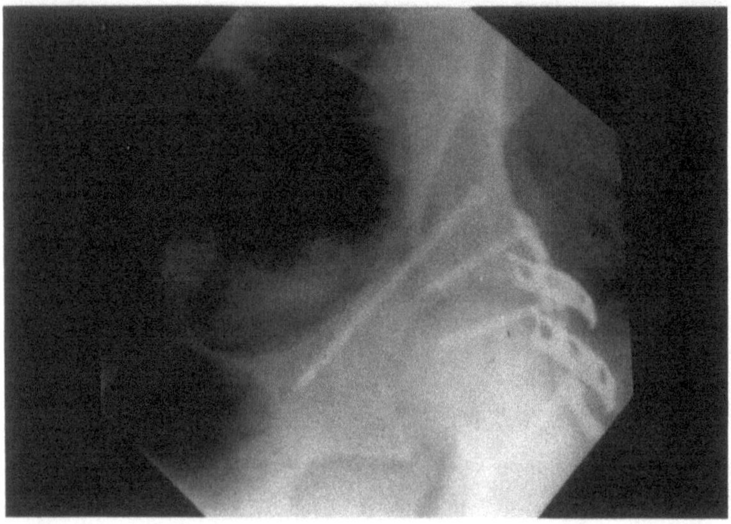

c

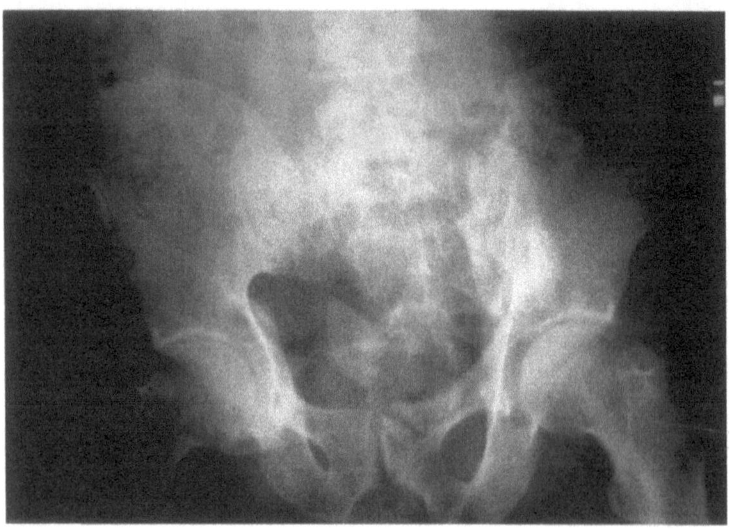

d

**FIGURE 7.15.** Insertion of an anterior column lag screw including clinical case with nonunion of anterior column and sacral ala in a 39-year-old man. (a) Position of cannulated screw. (b) Corresponding intraoperative obturator oblique view with guide wire. (c) Subsequent insertion of 3.5-mm cannulated screw. (d) Preoperative AP view with nonunions of the sacrum and anterior column.

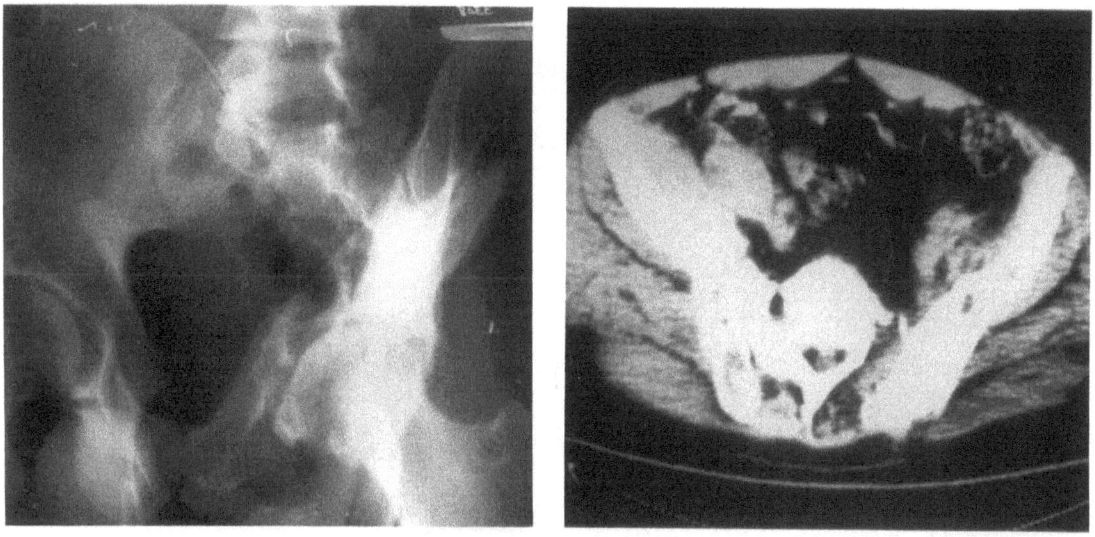

e f

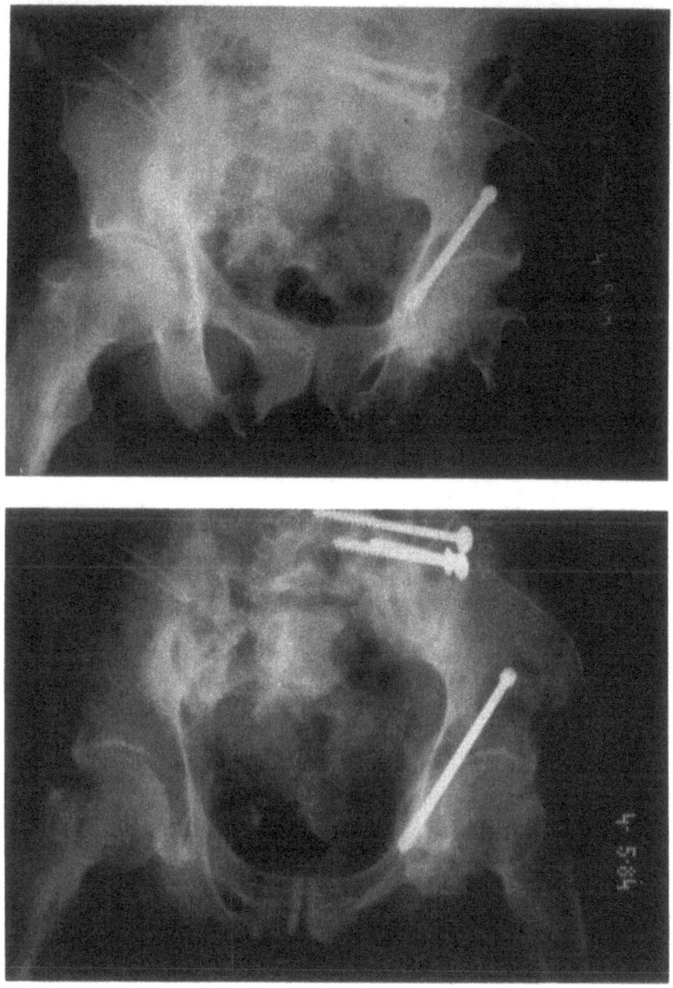

g

h

**FIGURE 7.15** (e) Preoperative obturator oblique view. (f) Preoperative CT view. (g) Postoperative AP view. (h) Postoperative inlet view.

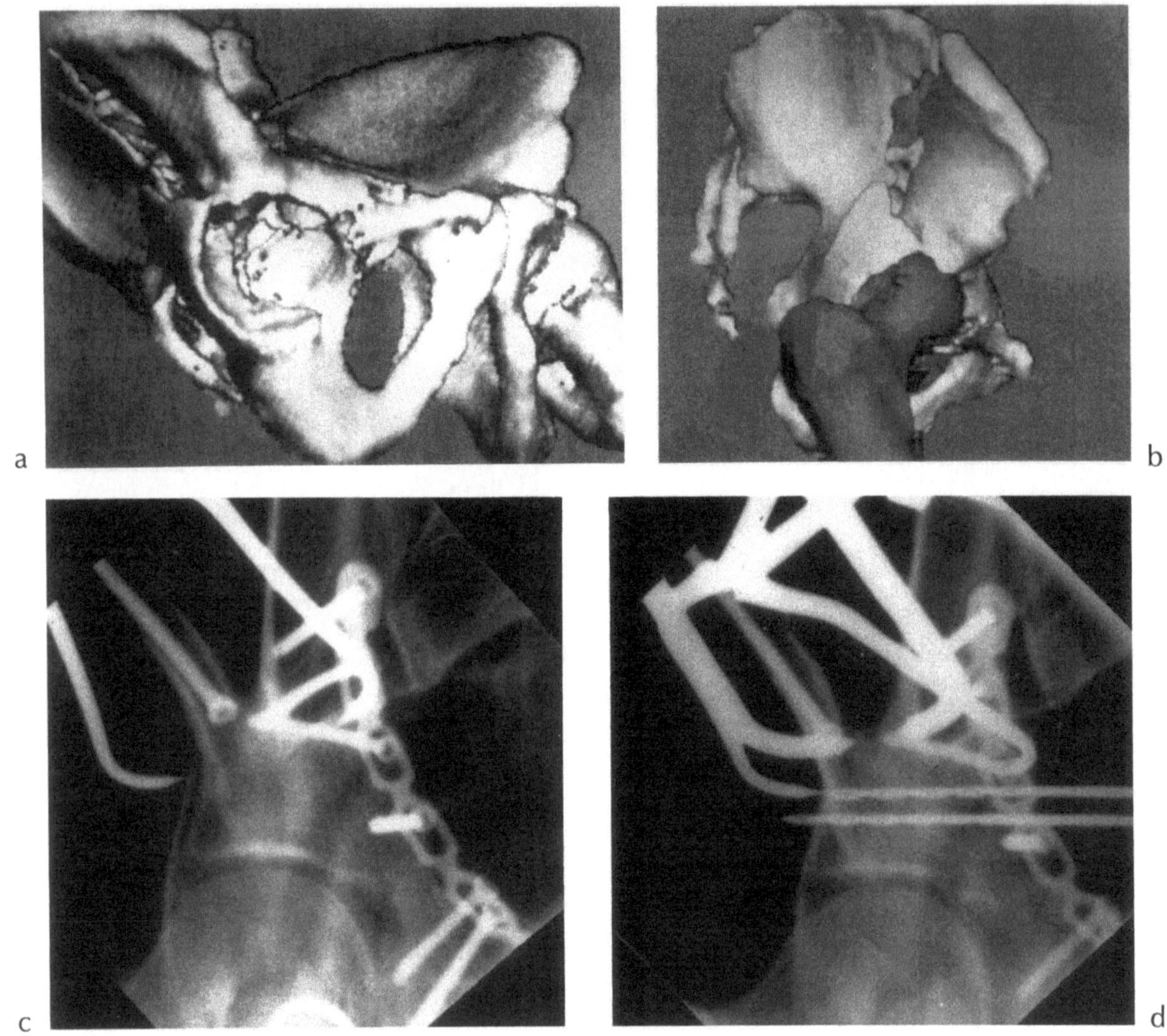

**FIGURE 7.16.** An open reduction, internal fixation of a both-column posterior wall fracture by resort to an ilioinguinal incision. After an open reduction of the anterior and posterior columns, the posterior wall fragment is immobilized with a pointed forcep and cannulated screws are inserted from the pelvic rim into the fragment. (a) Disarticulated 3D CT acetabular view. (b) External iliac 3D CT view. (c) Intraoperative obturator oblique view with reduction of posterior wall fragment. (d) Intraoperative obturator view with insertion of guide wires for cannulated screws.

associated posterior column, two methods are feasible. A second Kocher-Langenbeck incision can be used for the posterior exposure. Certainly this is the preferred method for a fracture of belated presentation.[41] Another possibility is to use solely an ilioinguinal approach (Figure 7.16). After fixation of the anterior and posterior columns, the posterior wall is immobilized. A limited pathway is developed between the anterior superior and inferior spines that follows the outer table of the pelvis to the posterior wall. The longer jaw of the prince tong forceps is passed along the outside of the acetabulum to impinge upon the posterior wall fragment. Under image intensification, the wall fragment is reduced. Immobilization can be achieved with

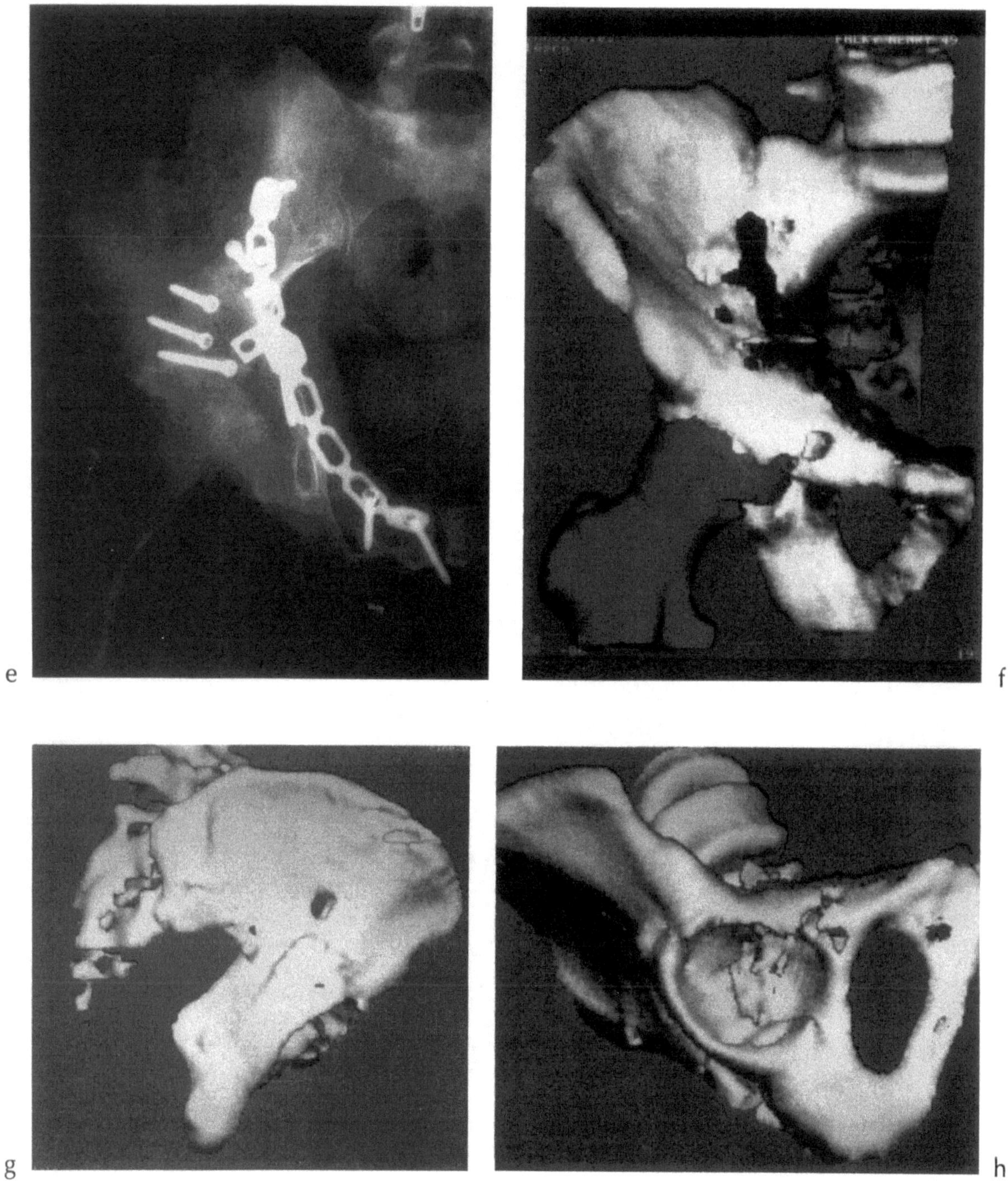


**FIGURE 7.16** (e) Postoperative AP view. (f) Postoperative anterior 3D-CT view. (g) Postoperative iliac 3D-CT view. (h) Postoperative disarticulated view.

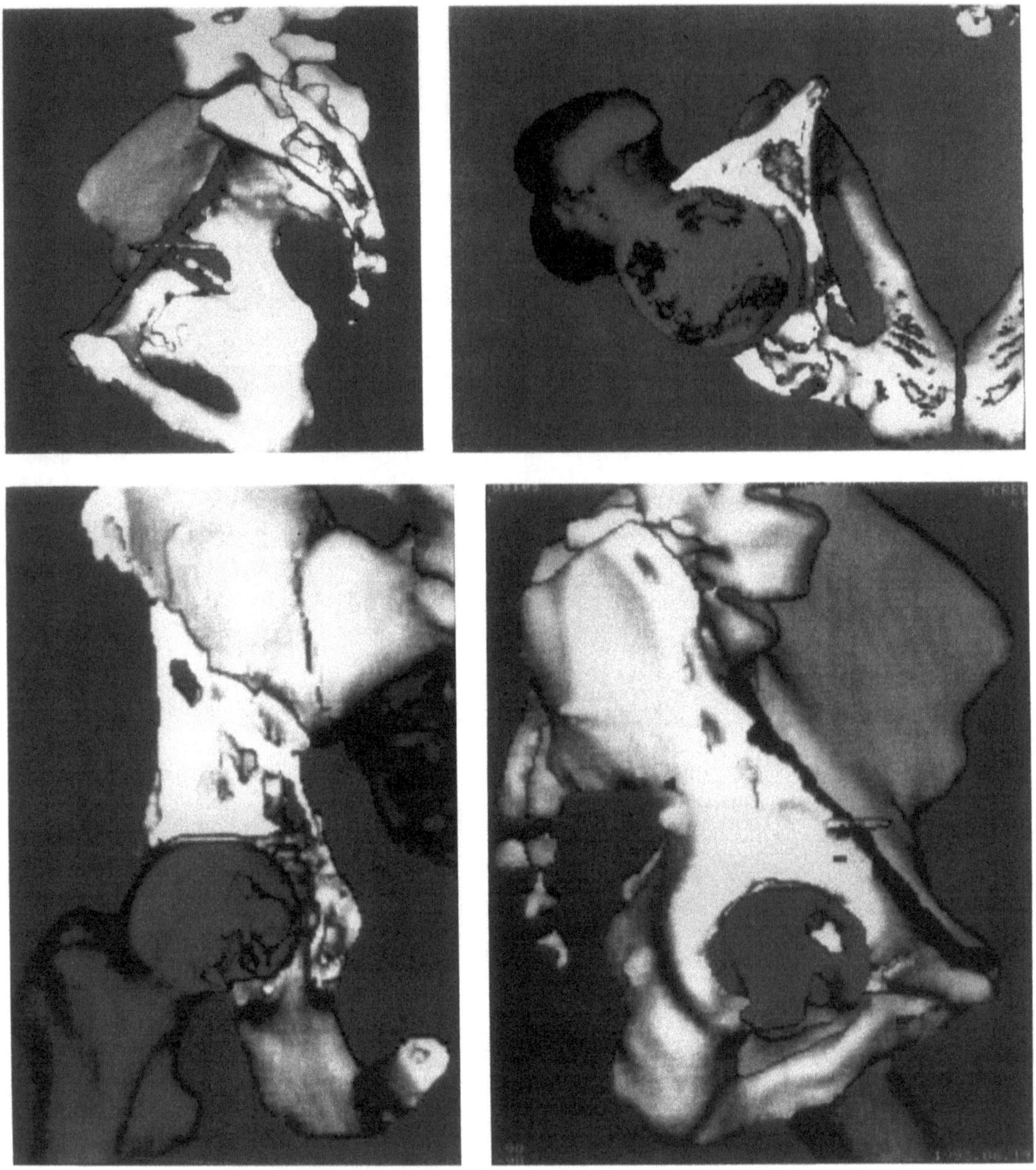

i j k l

**FIGURE 7.16** (*continued*) (i) Postoperative inner view. (j) Postoperative transaxial view. (k) Postoperative sagittal view. (l) Postoperative coronal view.

two of the 4.5-mm cannulated screws that are inserted near the pelvic brim and directed toward the posterior wall. This retrograde fixation eliminates the need for the second surgical approach. The entry site is slightly medial and posterior to the prominence of the medial eminence.

Another site for immobilization of the anterior column is insertion of the cannulated screw medial to the pubic tubercle and directed along the superior pubic ramus.[42] The screw is inserted between 2 and 3 cm from the symphysis pubis. The pathway of the guide wire is primarily followed in the obturator oblique view and the inlet view. Meticulous documentation of the pathway of the screw is necessary to ensure that the screw does not penetrate the hip joint. In essence, this method, which was popularized by Routt et al.,[43] represents a retrograde insertion of an anterior column lag screw.

## Intraoperative Imaging

Once the fixation has been inserted, careful imaging of the hemipelvis is needed to ensure that the reduction and fixation are satisfactory. The reduction is assessed for its accuracy with respect to the amount of persistent displacement and the restoration of congruity of the joint. Even under ideal intraoperative conditions, it is unlikely that the accuracy can be assessed with a resolution of better than 2 to 4 mm. Restoration and documentation of congruency of the acetabular surface with respect to the femoral head is critical. Multiplanar imaging is necessary with respect to the assessment of congruency and residual displacement. The presence of fixation plates may greatly hamper the quality of the imaging. The other critical documentation is the absence of a screw from the hip joint. Such confirmation can be surprisingly difficult. It is not unusual for meticulous intraoperative imaging to be undertaken with an apparent acceptable appearance when a postoperative CT scan confirms the penetration of the hip joint by a screw. In addition to the various multiplanar views, a supplementary image is taken in a plane that is coaxial with the course of a high-risk screw. Once the screw has been inserted, a screwdriver for use in a power tool is inserted into the corresponding recess of the screw head. The x-ray beam is aligned so that it is coaxial with the course of the screw and the screwdriver. The shaft of the screwdriver provides an aligning guide to assist in the adjustment of the x-ray tube. The highest risk is the anterior acetabulum where a plate is positioned along the true pelvic brim and an associated screw is directed parallel to the quadrilateral surface.

## Postoperative Imaging Following Surgery

After completion of an acetabular reconstruction, a complete standard radiographic series and a CT scan are strongly recommended. As a bare minimum, postoperative AP, inlet, and outlet views are necessary, while supplementary inlet and outlet views are recommended. Nevertheless, a standard CT scan with 2.0- to 3.0-mm cuts across the acetabulum greatly assists in an assessment of accuracy of the reduction. The author prefers to obtain a supplementary postoperative 3D CT scan with supplementary images that disarticulate the femoral head (Figures 7.5, 7.13, and 7.16). Typically, even in the presence of a very accurate reduction as assessed by conventional radiographs, an associated CT scan and 3D CT scan will confirm the presence of imperfections in the reduction that otherwise would be unrecognized. If the accuracy of the reduction is a major aspect of prognostication for prolonged function of the hip, the CT affords the most critical assessment of the reduction with sobering recognition of postoperative malreduction. A surgeon is liable to become much more critical of his reduction strategy on subsequent acetabular reconstructions.

## The Use of Computed Tomographic Guidance For the Insertion of Cannulated Screws

### Insertion of Iliosacral Screws to Immobilize the Sacroiliac Joint and Sacral Fractures

Prior application of the image intensifier to facilitate percutaneous insertion of cannulated screws for pelvic and acetabular fixation has been compromised by the limited resolution that is attainable with this method. Under ideal conditions, the resolution suffices to provide efficacious guidance for the procedure. In the presence of a paralytic ileus, morbid obesity, or osteopenic bone, the use of the image intensifier may become difficult or unrealistic. Recently, several attempts have been made to employ CT guidance for insertion of the percutaneous pelvic screws.[44,45] The method has been employed in the radiographic suite where typically epidural anesthesia is used. The method is particularly suitable for unstable but well-aligned fractures that are immobilized in situ. The technique can be performed with the patient situated in a supine or lateral position. A scout CT scan is obtained to permit the determination of the ideal center axis for the screw. The entry point thereby is predetermined, along with the angulation of the screw with respect to the horizontal axis. The computer assists in determination of the distance of the cutaneous surface to the outer cortex of bone and the optimal length of the screw. A small incision is made for insertion of a guide wire with drill sleeves. After determination of depth, a cannulated drill is employed prior to insertion of the 6.5- or 7.0-mm cannulated screw. Ebraheim et al.[44] employed the method for insertion of iliosacral screws. Duwelius et al.[45] also described the insertion of posterior iliac screws that extended transversely from one posterior superior spine to the other. The latter method was employed for immobilization of sacral fractures. Clinical experience has documented the superb accuracy of the CT guidance. The authors have acknowledged the potential compromise to the sterile field that is consistent with completion of such a procedure in the radiographic suite. Where the pelvic fracture is displaced, some supplementary procedure may be needed to achieve an accurate reduction. The ancillary procedure might include an open reduction of the symphysis or insertion of an external fixation pin into the anterior superior spine, or the application of supplementary skeletal traction. Undoubtedly, with the difficulties to achieve an accurate reduction, a potential shortcoming of the method would be acceptance of a malaligned fracture where inadequate reduction techniques were utilized. In a review of the clinical cases submitted for publication by Ebraheim et al. and Duwelius et al., a notable feature of most of the cases is a marked malreduction that at least for many surgeons would be considered unsatisfactory. The target zone for safe insertion of iliosacral screws is markedly reduced in the presence of a malaligned fracture. The risks for impalement, especially of a sacral nerve root, thereby are markedly increased. Clearly, implementation of the method would be greatly enhanced by the availability of a CT scanner in the operating room.

More recently, Kahler[46] has reported the application of CT guidance for percutaneous fixation of acetabular fractures. The methodology was very similar to that described for pelvic ring fixation. To date, the principal problem has been attainment of a satisfactory closed reduction of the fracture. Where an acetabular fracture is truly undisplaced, probably the injury is significantly stable so that the need for fixation is relatively limited. Once the fracture is displaced, the restoration of an anatomical reduction is greatly hampered by the percutaneous methodology and the presence of the CT scanner gantry. Kahler has devised a radiolucent lateral traction frame as a means to achieve an accurate reduction in this constraining environment. While a reported pilot study provides encouraging results, further clinical documentation will be needed to validate the assets of the method.

## Clinical Results with Percutaneous Cannulated Screw Fixation of the Pelvic Ring

Recently, Routt et al.,[47] reported the results of iliosacral screw fixation in 66 patients managed for posterior pelvic ring disruptions. For this group, 100 iliosacral screws were employed. Of the 34 male and 32 female patients, the range of age was from 11 to 33 years. The source of the injury was a motor vehicle accident in 36 patients, motorcycle trauma in 12 patients, pedestrian insults in 8 cases, with 5 crush injuries and 5 cases of a fall from a great height. The sacroiliac joint was disrupted in 59 patients, and a sacral fracture was documented in 31 patients, and combined or bilateral injury patterns were present in 24 patients. While all of the screws were placed percutaneously, 96 were inserted into the first sacral body and 4 into the second sacral body. For the reduction of the pelvic ring, an open anterior approach, the fixation of an associated acetabular fracture, the application of longitudinal skeletal traction, the insertion of an iliac crest pin or screw, or a femoral distractor was employed. Intraoperative imaging was hampered in 18 patients by the presence of significant flatus or intraabdominal contrast media related to prior imaging studies. In nine other patients, morbid obesity complicated the imaging and screw placement. Also, the standard instruments for cannulated screw insertion were of insufficient length for routine screw placement in all nine cases. Ten of the patients possessed features of sacral dysplasia that altered the typical site for optimal screw placement. In two of these cases, hazardous insertion of the screws ensued. One of the patients sustained an L-5 neuropraxia related to problematic screw placement. In another patient, a screw exited from the contralateral ala. There were no infections, wound problems, and no cases of significant blood loss. In two patients, the screws failed at approximately 6 months following surgery. Both of the cases' were notable for highly unstable sacral fractures. One of the patients progressed to a symptomatic nonunion so that a supplementary bone graft was necessary. Two other patients progressed to failure of fixation. These cases were complicated by craniocerebral trauma with spasticity and combativeness.

In a separate report by Keating,[48] 40 unstable pelvic fractures were managed with iliosacral screw fixation. Twenty-nine of the cases were highly unstable injury patterns. In the retrospective analysis, six of the screws were misplaced, typically with an unacceptable anterior position. The initial reduction was judged to be satisfactory in 33 patients, while ultimately 19 patients (48%) developed a malunion, irrespective of the type of the anterior fixation. At the time of the final assessment of 1 to 4 years after the time of the injury, 33 patients complained of low back or posterior pelvic pain, of which three cases had severe and disabling symptoms. Half of the patients returned to their original employment, although 33% progressed to long-term disability. Sixty-eight percent of the cases failed to return to a former level of recreational activity. The authors felt that the results of iliosacral fixation for highly unstable pelvic ring disruptions were consistent with low mortality and morbidity but with disappointing long-term anatomical and functional results.

In a separate analysis, Routt et al.[43] reported the results of 24 patients in whom 28 retrograde superior pubic ramus screws were inserted under biplane image intensification. Fifteen of the screws were inserted percutaneously in 15 patients following a closed manipulation of the fracture. In nine other patients, 13 screws were inserted as part of an open reduction of the ramus fracture by resort to a Pfannenstiel exposure. Four of the patients were managed with bilateral screws for bilateral ramus fractures. Of these cases, 11 screws were inserted so that they passed cephalad to the acetabulum and exited from the lateral ilium. None of these screws violated the acetabulum. There were no nonunions or infections, while all of the fractures healed uneventfully. There was no screw breakage evident in any of these cases. In five of the patients, however, errant screw placement was documented only in postoperative plain radiographs. or in two cases, a postoperative CT scan. In all of these cases, intraoperative image intensification had been employed and was apparently satisfactory. This technical shortcoming highlights the difficulties in the application of the image intensifier in the operating room, even in highly experienced hands.

## Author's Philosophy

Percutaneous fixation and the use of cannulated screws for immobilization of the pelvic ring and acetabulum remain a highly attractive method that is still in a preliminary stage of clinical application. The attributes include minimal surgical invasiveness, combined with the potential for rapid and stable fixation. This method is especially suitable for minimally displaced but potentially highly unstable fractures. The technique has a potential for application during the early resuscitative phase as an alternative to external pelvic fixation. Nevertheless, the technique has considerable potential for surgical hazards, and it utterly depends upon the availability of high-quality image intensification. Perhaps the biggest shortcoming to date has been the difficulty to achieve adequate closed or open reductions, so that the method was not feasible. Unless an accurate pelvic or acetabular reduction can be achieved, the fixation of a mal-aligned fracture with percutaneous screws is contraindicated. With respect to the pelvic ring, an open reduction or the application of a fixation pin in the iliac crest or other indirect method may well suffice to obtain an accurate reduction of the posterior pelvic injury. With respect to acetabular fractures, currently the potential for closed methods to achieve an accurate reduction is highly limited. As an exception, the pathologic acetabular fractures of the elderly with minimal displacement are particularly suitable for fixation with cannulated screws. In the future, CT guidance may become a viable alternative to the image intensifier. Undoubtedly, the availability of a high-speed CT scanner in the operating room would immeasurably increase the role for this type of guidance for percutaneous screw insertion.

## References


1. Mears DC. Fracture-dislocation of the pelvic ring. In Chapman MW, ed. *Operative Orthopaedics*. Philadelphia: J.B. Lippincott, 1983;505.
2. McMurtry R, Walton D, Dickinson E, et al. Pelvic disruption in the polytraumatized patient: a management protocol. *Clin Orthop* 1980;151:22–29.
3. Tile M. *Fractures of the Pelvis and Acetabulum*. New York: Springer-Verlag, 1995.
4. Bosch U, Pohlemann T, Hoas N, Tscherne H. Klassifikation und Management des Komplexen Beck en Traumos. *Unfallchirurg* 1992;4:189–196.
5. Dalal SA, Burgess AR, Siegel SH, et al. Pelvic fractures in multiple trauma: classification by mechanism is key to pattern of organ injury, resuscitation requirements and outcome. *J Trauma* 1989;29:981–988.
6. Pohlemann T, Krettek C, Hoffman R, Colemann U, Gansslen A. A biomechanical comparison of various emergency stabilization measures of the pelvic ring. *Unfallchirurg* 1994;97:503–510.
7. Rubash HE, Mears DC. External fixation of the pelvis. *Instr Course Lect* 1983;32:329–348.
8. Mears DC, Rubash HE. *Pelvic and Acetabular Fractures*. Thorofare, NJ: Slack, 1986;45.
9. Sawaguchi T, Brown TD, Rubash HE, Mears DC. Stability of acetabular fractures after internal fixation, a cadaveric study. *Acta Orthop Scand* 1984; 55:601–605.
10. Gotis G, McGuigan L, Diamond T, Portek I, Quinn R, Sturgess A, Tulloch R. Sacral insufficiency fractures in the elderly. *J Bone Joint Surg* 1994;76B:882–886.
11. Letournel E, Judet R. *Fractures of the Acetabulum*. Berlin: Springer-Verlag, 1993;17.
12. Agar AMR. *Grants Atlas of Anatomy*, 9th ed. Baltimore: Williams & Wilkins, 1991.
13. Basmajian JV, Slonecker CE. *Grant's Method of Anatomy*, 11th ed. Baltimore: Williams & Wilkins, 1989.
14. Schatzker J, Tile M. *The Rationale of Operative Fracture Care*. Berlin: Springer-Verlag, 1987.
15. Mears DC. Pelvic fractures. In Edlich RF, Spyker DA, eds. *Current Emergency Therapy*. Norwalk, CT: Appleton-Century-Crofts, 1984;124.
16. Tile M. Pelvic ring fractures: should they be fixed? *J Bone Joint Surg* 1988;70:1–12.
17. Hansen ST Jr. Computerized axial tomography for pelvic fractures. *Am J Radiol* 1982;138:592–597.
18. Fishman EK, Magid D, Ney DR, Drebin RA, Kuhlm WW. Advanced three-dimensional evaluation of acetabular trauma: volumetric image processing. *J Trauma* 1989;29:214–218.
19. Mears DC, Ward AJ, Wright MS. The radiological assessment of pelvic and acetabular fractures using three-dimensional computed tomography. *Int J Orthop Trauma* 1992;2:196–209.
20. Pennal GF, Tile M, Waddell JP, Garside H. Pelvic disruption: assessment and classification. *Clin Orthop* 1980;151:12–21.
21. Letournel E. Acetabular fractures: classification and management. *Clin Orthop* 1980;151;81–106.
22. Browner BD, Cole JD. Initial management of pelvic ring disruptions. *Instr Course Lect* 1988;37: 129–138.
23. Mears DC, Rubash HE. External and internal fixation of the pelvic ring. *Instr Course Lect* 1984;33: 144–151.
24. Riemer B, Miranda MA. Late functional results of unstable pelvic fractures managed with acute external fixation. Presented at Surgery of the Pelvis and Acetabulum: The Second International Consensus, Pittsburgh, PA, 1994.
25. Mears DC. The results of treatment of two hundred pelvic malunions and nonunions. *Clin Orthop* 1996, in press.
26. Letournel E. Surgical management of fractures of the acetabulum. In Laurin CA, Riley LH, Roy-Camille R. eds. *Atlas of Orthopaedic Surgery*. St. Louis: C.V. Mosby, 1992.
27. Mears DC, Ward AJ, Hardy SL. Acute total hip arthroplasty for acetabular fractures. Presented at Surgery of the Pelvis and Acetabulum: The Second International Consensus, Pittsburgh, PA, 1994.
28. Jacobson G, Tew J Jr. Intra-operative evoked potential monitoring. *J Clin Neurophysiol* 1987;4: 145–176.
29. Vrahas M, Gordon RG, Mears DC, Kregor P, Sclabassi RS. Intra-operative somatosensory

evoked potential monitoring of pelvic and acetabular fractures. *J Orthop Trauma* 1992;6:50–58.
30. Helfet D, Kovalik J, Hosa D, Patterson S, DiPasquale T, Sanders R. Intra-operative somatosensory potential monitoring during acute pelvic fractures. *J Orthop Trauma* 1995;9:28–34.
31. Mayo KA. Open reduction and internal fixation of the acetabulum: results in 163 fractures. *Clin Orthop* 1994;305:31–37.
32. Wilson FB. Post-operative irradiation decreases ectopic bone formation after an extended iliofemoral surgical exposure. Presented at Surgery of the Pelvis and Acetabulum: The Second International Consensus, Pittsburgh, PA, 1994.
33. Mears DC, Capito CP, Deleeuw H: Posterior pelvic disruptions managed by the use of the double cobra plate. *Instr Course Lect* 1988;37:143–152.
34. Mast J, Jakob R, Ganz R. *Planning and Reduction Techniques in Fracture Surgery*. Berlin: Springer-Verlag, 1989.
35. Goulet JA, Mason DL, Roubeau JP, Goldstein SA. Comminuted posterior wall acetabular fractures. A biomechanical evaluation of fixation methods. *J Bone Joint Surg* 1994;76A:1457–1463.
36. Rubash HE, Brown TD, Nelson DD, Mears DC. Comparative mechanical performances of some new devices for fixation of unstable pelvic ring fractures. *Med Biol Eng Comput* 1983;21:657–663
37. Leggon R, Lindsey RW, Doherty BS, Alexander J, Woble P. The holding strength of cannulated screws compared with solid core screws in cortical and cancellous bone. *J Orthop Trauma* 1993; 7:450–457.
38. Routt MLC Jr, Meier MC, Kregor P, Mayo KA. Percutaneous ilio sacral screws with the patient supine technique. *Operative Tech Orthop* 1993;3: 35–45.
39. Mears DC, Henry JL. The use of cable fixation for pelvic and acetabular fractures. Presented at Surgery of the Pelvis and Acetabulum: The Second International Consensus, Pittsburgh, PA, 1994.
40. Matta JM, Bray TJ. Operative Treatment of Acetabular Fractures. In: Chapman MW, ed. *Operative Orthopaedics*. Philadelphia: J.B. Lippincott, 1993.
41. Moroni A, Caja VL, Sabato C, Zinghi G. Surgical treatment of both column fractures by staged combined ilio inguinal and Kocher-Langenbeck approaches. *Injury* 1995;26:219–224.
42. Simonian PT, Routt ML Jr, Harrington RM, Tencer AF. Internal fixation of the unstable anterior pelvic ring: a biomechanical comparison of standard plating techniques and the retrograde medullary superior pubic ramus screw. *J Orthop Trauma* 1994;8:476–482.
43. Routt MLC Jr, Simonian PT, Grujic L. Preliminary report. The retrograde medullary superior pubic ramus screw for the treatment of anterior pelvic ring disruptions: a new technique. *J Orthop Trauma* 1995;9:35–44.
44. Ehraheim NA, Rusin JS, Coombs RJ, Jackson WT, Holiday B. Percutaneous computed-tomography-stabilization of pelvic fractures. *J Orthop Trauma* 1987;1:197–204.
45. Duwelius PJ, VonAllen M, Bray TJ, Nelson D. Computer tomography guided fixation of unstable posterior pelvic ring disruptions. *J Orthop Trauma* 1992;6:420–426.
46. Kahler DM. CT guided fixation of minimally displaced acetabular fractures. Presented at Surgery of the Pelvis and Acetabulum: The Second International Consensus, Pittsburgh, PA, 1994.
47. Routt MLC Jr, Kregor PJ, Simonian PT, Mayo KA. Early results of percutaneous iliosacral screws placed with the patient in the supine position. *J Orthop Trauma* 1995;9:207–214.
48. Keating J. Early fixation of the vertically unstable pelvis—the role of iliosacral screw fixation of the posterior lesion. Presented at Surgery of the Pelvis and Acetabulum: The Second International Consensus, Pittsburgh, PA, 1994.
49. Ferner H, Staubesand J, eds. *Sobotta Atlas of Human Anatomy*. Baltimore: Urban and Schwarzenberg, 1983.
50. Rockwood CA Jr, Green DP, Bucholz RW. *Rockwood and Green's Fractures in Adults*. New York: J.B. Lippincott, 1991.
51. Letournel E. *Fractures of the Pelvis and Acetabulum*. Selzach, Switzerland: Osteo, 1986.

# 8
# Cannulated Screws for Pelvic Fractures

David L. Helfet and Neel Anand

## Anatomy

To better understand the classification and the rationale of management of pelvic fractures, some knowledge of pelvic anatomy and biomechanics is essential.

### Ring Structure of the Pelvis

The pelvis is a true ring structure. For a ring to be broken in one area and displaced there must be a fracture or dislocation in another portion of the ring. Gertzbein and Chenoweth,[1] in a series of patients with undisplaced anterior pelvic fractures, noted that a technetium polyphosphate bone scan of the posterior sacroiliac complex gave a positive reading in every case, indicating the definite presence of a posterior lesion. This was further confirmed by Bucholz,[2] who found posterior lesions at autopsy even when the radiograph revealed only an anterior lesion.

The anterior pelvic lesion may be through the symphysis pubis or through the pubic rami unilaterally or bilaterally. A symphysis disruption may also occur with pubic rami fractures. The posterior lesion may be a fracture of the ilium, often in the coronal plane, a dislocation or fracture-dislocation of the sacroiliac joint, or a fracture through the sacrum. The most common lesion is a sacral fracture followed by a combined injury, that is a fracture-dislocation of the sacroiliac joint, usually with a portion of the ilium remaining attached to the main sacral fragment.

The degree of displacement of the posterior sacroiliac complex is more important than the site of posterior lesion. Posterior pelvic disruption is best identified on the inlet and outlet pelvic radiographs and confirmed by computed tomography (CT) scan. The posterior lesion, although present, may be nondisplaced with intact posterior ligaments, most often a lateral compression injury associated with a sacral crush. Alternatively the posterior lesion may be displaced with a major osseous-ligamentous disruption of the posterior pelvic complex.

### Stability of the Pelvis

Stability may be defined as the ability of the pelvis to withstand physiologic forces without significant displacements.[3] It is dependent not only on the bony structures, but also on the strong ligamentous structures binding the three bones of the pelvis together (sacrum and the two iliac bones). This stability is dependent predominantly on the integrity of the posterior weight-bearing sacroiliac complex. The major posterior ligaments are the sacroiliac, the sacrotuberous, and the sacrospinous. The intricate posterior sacroiliac complex is a masterly biomechanical structure able to withstand the transference of weight-bearing forces from the spine to the lower extremities. The ligaments have a major role as posterior stabilizers. The posterior sacroiliac interosseous ligaments have been described as being the strongest in the body.[4] The iliolumbar ligaments join the transverse processes of L-5 to the iliac crest and the intervening transverse fibers of the interroseous sacroiliac ligaments further enhance the suspensory mechanism. The entire complex looks and functions as a suspension bridge.

The sacrospinous ligament resists external rotation of the pelvic ring, whereas the complex sacrotuberous ligament, positioned in the vertical plane, resists vertical shearing forces applied to the hemipelvis. Therefore, these two supplementary ligaments oriented at right angles to each other are well adapted to resist the two major deforming forces acting upon the pelvis.

The anterior sacroiliac ligaments also resist external rotation and shearing forces but do not have the strength of the post-sacroiliac ligaments.

# Surgical Anatomy of the Sacrum

## Bony Anatomy

The adult sacrum consists of five vertebrae that are fused to create a concavity on the anterior pelvic surface.[5] The lateral portions of the upper two or three sacral vertebra form the auricular surface, which articulates with the ilium bilaterally. The most important feature of the anterior sacral surface is the four pairs of foramina through which pass the ventral rami of the sacral nerves into the pelvis. Lateral to the pelvic foramina is the pars lateralis. It is marked by grooves traversing laterally and caudally from each foramen. These grooves mark the passage of the ventral roots.

Classically the sacrum has been described as trumpet shaped, and gross differences in foraminal patterns have been described. Significant variations in the angles have also been noted. If the superior surface of the sacrum is being used as a reference point, the angle of the first sacral foramen, in the sagittal plane, ranges from 0° to 45°. With the midsagittal line as the reference point, the angle of the first sacral foramen in the axial plane ranges from 0° to 60°.

## Neural Anatomy

The spinal nerves emerge from the dorsal root ganglia, course a few millimeters, and then split into ventral and dorsal rami. The ventral sacral rami turn in a slightly anterior direction and emerge from the anterior sacral foramina, whereas the dorsal rami pass through the dorsal foramina. The first three ventral sacral roots emerge from the sacral foramina and travel laterally in their sacral grooves contributing, in part, to the sacral plexus.

The obturator nerve emerges on the medial border of the psoas muscle and travels in a caudal direction, where it runs along the superior surface of the sacroiliac joint. From there it runs laterally to the pelvic brim. Just medial to the obturator nerve on the superior aspect of the sacral ala lies the lumbosacral trunk. It receives its major contribution from the fifth lumbar root and, to a lesser degree, the fourth lumbar root.

A marked variability in the position of the fifth lumbar root has been described. It has been found well lateral to the ala close to the sacroiliac joint, while at other times the fifth lumbar root has been found positioned more medially, overlying the first sacral pedicle.

Each of the large first four ventral sacral rami is closely adherent to the anterior surface of the sacrum and covers almost all of the sacrum lateral to the foramina from the second sacral foramen in a distal direction.

The sympathetic chains (superior hypogastric plexus) are also closely adherent to the anterior surface of the sacrum running just medial to the pelvic foramina and meeting on the surface of the coccyx as the ganglion impar.

The cauda equina occupying the central spinal canal of the sacrum forms the most important neural structure relevant to the sacrum, and its position cannot be overemphasized. The lumbar nerve roots exit the thecal sac at a mean angle of 36° to 42°. The takeoff angle of the first sacral root is significantly smaller, the angles becoming progressively even smaller at lower sacral levels.

## Vascular Anatomy

Just proximal to the bifurcation of the aorta is the origin of the middle sacral artery, which travels down the midline over the sacrum. It runs posterior to the venous system and anastomoses with the lateral sacral arteries. This anastomosis sends branches into each of the pelvic sacral foramina.

The common iliac arteries arise from the bifurcation of the aorta and run caudally and laterally to the level of the inferior edge of the lumbosacral disk lateral to the sacroiliac joint, where they divide into internal and external iliac arteries. On the right side, the common iliac artery crosses over the right common iliac vein so that at its bifurcation, it lies lateral and slightly anterior to the vein. On the left side, the artery lies lateral and anterior to the vein, but it travels parallel with it (Figure 8.1).

The first branch of the internal iliac artery is the iliolumbar artery, which for part of its course overlies the superior aspect of the sacroiliac joint.

The second branch is the lateral sacral artery, and there may be two of them for each internal iliac artery. The superior lateral sacral artery crosses the sacroiliac joint near the level of the first or second anterior sacral foramen and runs in an inferior direction on the sacrum lateral to the foraminal edges. It then anastomoses with the middle sacral artery and it is this anastomosis that sends branches to the superior sacral foramen. If there is an inferior lateral sacral artery, it arises of the internal iliac in a more distal direction and traverses the sacroiliac joint near the level of the lower foramen to anastomose with the middle sacral artery.

The superior gluteal artery is the largest

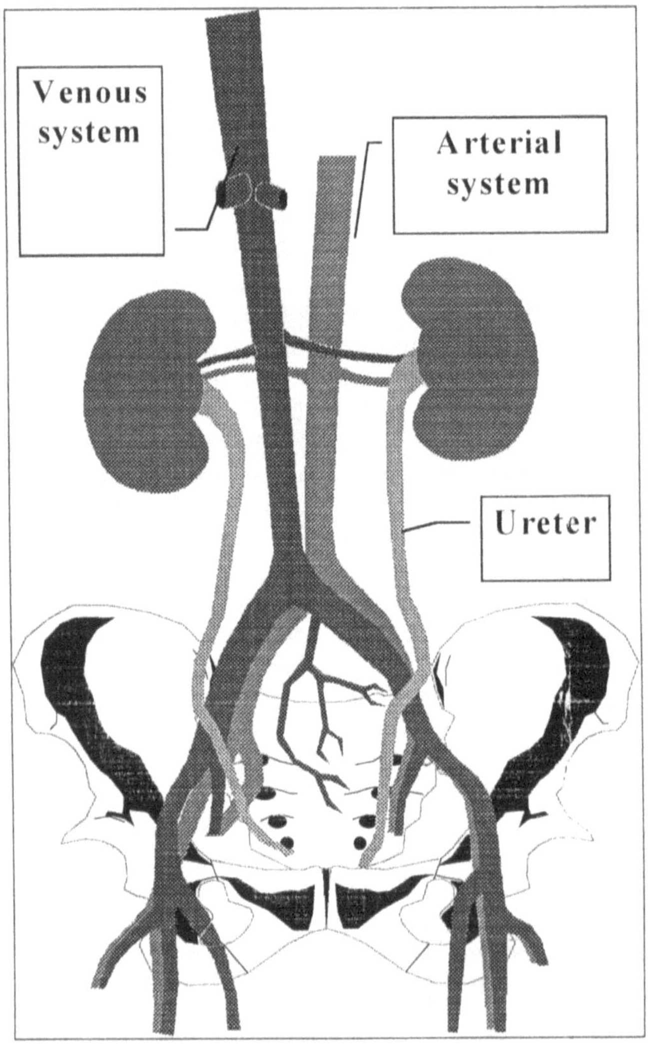


**FIGURE 8.1.** Vascular anatomy anterior to the sacrum.

branch of the internal iliac. It usually passes between the branches of the fourth and fifth lumbar anterior rami, proximal to where they join to form the lumbosacral trunk. At times it passes between the lumbosacral trunk and the first sacral nerve. It travels lateral to the sacrum, superior to the piriformis muscle, and exits the plexus through the greater sciatic foramen.

As a broad generalization, it can be said that the venous anatomy is analogous to the arterial anatomy. There are, however, a few important exceptions. The middle sacral vein, which is often double, drains into the left common iliac vein rather than into the inferior vena cava because the latter structure lies to the right of the spine. The right common iliac vein is shorter than the left, and it lies directly posterior to the artery with the same name. The iliolumbar vein drains into the posterior part of the common iliac vein. This vein can be quite large, and it's important to note its posterior position at the level of the common iliac vein.

## Direction and Guidelines for Screw Insertion

Preoperative assessment of the sacral morphology is important in deciding optimal screw placement. CT scanning provides an accurate means of evaluating the curved surface of the sacrum as well as the position of the sacral foramina. It is a simple means of unveiling potentially disastrous anatomic aberrations in the highly variable, transitional lumbosacral region. This is best performed with the scanner gantry tilted parallel to the superior sacral end plate.

The lumbosacral plexus is firmly affixed to the anterior bony sacral surface. It is not recommended that any implant be inserted that would require penetration of the anterior bony sacrum lateral to the sacral foramina. This would endanger the integrity of the sacral roots inferior to the first sacral foramen and endanger the L-5 root at the level of the first sacral foramen. In addition, an anterior sacral screw placed at or above the first sacral foramen could easily penetrate the iliac vein, particularly on the left side. Medial to the foramina is the middle sacral artery with the venous plexus and the superior hypogastric plexus.

Considering the position of the cauda equina, L-5 root, sacral roots, and the iliac vessels, the safe area for screw insertion would be one directed toward the sacral promontory, above the level of the first sacral foramen and parallel to the superior sacral end plate. It does not endanger any neurovascular structure with the exception of the middle sacral artery and vein. Screws placed through the anterior sacral cortex lateral to the sacral foramina can compromise the iliac vessels, L-5 nerve root, S-1 nerve root, and sympathetic chain. Anterior sacral cortical purchase for the screws is best avoided and is not necessary.

## Classification

At the Hospital for Special Surgery we have been using the Alphanumeric Classification[6] or the Comprehensive Classification of Fractures of the Pelvis and Acetabulum, a consensus classification adopted by the S.I.C.O.T. Commission, and by the Documentation Committee of OTA and the AO/ASIF Foundation (Table 8.1). The

**TABLE 8.1.** Classification of injuries to the pelvic ring–61.

| | |
|---|---|
| Type A | —lesion sparing the posterior arch; stable |
| A1 | —Fracture of the innominate bone; avulsion |
| A2 | —Fracture of the innominate bone; direct blow |
| A3 | —Transverse fractures of the sacrum and coccyx |
| Type B | —Incomplete disruption of the posterior arch; partially stable |
| B1 | —Unilateral, incomplete disruption of the posterior arch, external rotation ("open-book" injury) |
| B2 | —Unilateral, incomplete disruption of the posterior arch, internal rotation ("lateral compression" injury) |
| B3 | —Bilateral, incomplete lesions of the posterior arch |
| Type C | —Complete disruption of the posterior arch; unstable |
| C1 | —Unilateral, complete disruption of the posterior arch |
| C2 | —Bilateral, disruptions of the posterior arch; ipsilateral complete, contralateral incomplete |
| C3 | —Bilateral, complete disruptions of the posterior arch |

use of posterior pelvic cannulated screws as described here would be predominantly applicable to the unstable or type C pelvic injuries.

# Imaging of the Pelvis

## Plain Radiography

Since the plane of the true pelvic brim in the anatomic plane lies oblique to the axis of the trunk, the beam of the usual anteroposterior radiograph, is therefore oblique to the pelvic brim. To obtain more information on the anterior and posterior displacement of the pelvic ring and also superior or inferior displacement, 40° caudad and 40° cepahalad projections as described by Pennal et al.[7] are needed. These are easily obtained as follows:

1. Anteroposterior view: patient supine, beam directed perpendicular to the midpelvis and radiographic plate.
2. 40° caudad or inlet view: patient supine, beam is directed from the head to the midpelvis at 40° to the radiographic plate.
3. 40° cephalad or tangential or outlet view: patient supine, beam is directed from the foot to the symphysis at an angle of 40° to the plate.

The inlet view demonstrates the ring configuration of the pelvis, and narrowing or widening of the diameter of the ring is immediately apparent. In this projection the x-ray beam is parallel to the plane of the sacrum, and the sacrum is seen on end with the vertebral body situated anteriorly and the sacral lamina posteriorly. The inlet view also best demonstrates posterior translation, which occurs at right angles to the x-ray beam.

The outlet view shows the anterior ring superimposed on the posterior ring. Superior or inferior displacement of the anterior or posterior portion of the ring is best appreciated in this view. The x-ray beam in this view is perpendicular to the plane of the sacrum. The sacrum appears in its longest dimension, with the neural foramina clearly visible.

The 45° oblique views of the pelvis as described by Letournel and Judet[8] will also help in the diagnosis of associated acetabular fractures. These views are also useful in evaluating sacroiliac joint dislocations and injuries to the obturator foramen.

## Computed Tomographic (CT) Scan

This is particularly useful in assessing the posterior pelvic injury, especially in sacral fractures. Careful examination of the scan will also show the relation of the sacral nerve roots to the fracture. They also allow for a better assessment of any associated acetabular injury, especially the assessment of wall fractures, rotation of the columns, and the presence of intraarticular fragments or femoral head injuries.

### *Three-Dimensional CT Scan*

Technological advances in imaging software have led to the development of three-dimensional computed tomography (3D CT). The 3D CT scan can provide a better understanding of spatial relationships of the pelvis and the complex pathoanatomy of injuries to the pelvis and acetabulum. It also greatly assists the surgeon in characterizing a fracture pattern and in planning the surgical procedure.

# Assessment of an Unstable Pelvis

## Clinical

The majority of unstable pelvic injuries occur in the polytraumatized patient. The evaluation and management of the "whole" trauma patient is beyond the scope of this chapter.

The essence of the local (pelvic) physical examination is to inspect the patient for major bruising, any open wounds or lacerations, and any bleeding from the urethral meatus, vagina, or rectum. If these latter two areas are not carefully inspected, occult lacerations may be overlooked, with dire consequences, since these lacerations always mean an open fracture of the pelvis.

In most cases it is possible to assess the pelvis

clinically for stability by applying one's hands to the anterior superior iliac spine and moving the affected hemipelvis.[3] The completely unstable pelvis can be moved in any direction and diagnosis is easy. By contrast the stable pelvic fracture is resistant to motion in all planes. Certain fracture patterns, however, lead to relative stability and are very difficult to assess clinically for stability [open-book (B1) and lateral compression (B2) injuries].

### Radiographic

Stability is assessed using the three views as described by Pennal et al.,[7] and confirmed by the CT scan. The common signs of instability are avulsion of the ischial spine and/or the tip of the transverse process of L-5, a shearing fracture through the cancellous bone of the sacrum, a posterior gap, and the displacement itself (> 1 cm). These signs are further confirmed by CT scanning. The degree of instability is probably the most important criterion in determining the appropriate method of treatment. In rare cases, the addition of fluoroscopic pelvic stress views in the hemodynamically stable patient may be helpful.

## Cannulated Screws in Pelvic Fractures

### Indications

Peltier,[9] in studying 186 pelvic disruptions, recognized the increased mortality and morbidity resulting from fractures through the weight-bearing femoral sacral arch of the pelvic ring. Holdsworth[10] studied 50 pelvic fractures treated by nonoperative means: bed rest, slings, and traction. Of the 27 patients with sacroiliac dislocations, only 12 were able to return to heavy work and 15 had significant sacroiliac joint pain. The results were even worse in the 15 patients with sacral fractures as only 2 of 15 (13%) returned to work. Symphyseal pain, although a frequent early complaint, appeared to subside in 2 years, but the posterior pelvic pain remained. Raf[11] reported similar results in a review of 101 unstable Malgaigne fractures treated nonoperatively; 52% of the posterior pelvic fractures involving the sacroiliac joint or sacrum had persistent low back pain and discomfort. When the fracture passed through the posterior ilium, the outcome was more favorable. Not surprisingly the neurologic sequelae of pelvic fractures are most common in patients with sacral fractures. Dunn and Morris[12] demonstrated that the unstable pelvic fracture had more morbidity and mortality than the stable pelvic fracture.

Huittinen and Slatis,[13] in a classic paper on pelvic fracture treatment, reported on 407 consecutive disruptions of which 82% were the result of high-energy trauma. The mortality rate was approximately 6%. The worst results were in the double vertical fracture with significant gait abnormalities and pain in 32% and 17%, respectively. Semba et al.[14] confirmed the difficulty of treating unstable pelvic fractures nonoperatively. Only 11 of their 30 patients were free of symptoms at follow-up, whereas 8 had severe low back pain, commonly on the side of injury.

Schatzker and Tile[3] studied two groups of patients. Series A was a retrospective, multicenter study of 148 patients, and series B was a prospective group of 100 consecutive patients admitted to the Sunnybrook Trauma Unit. Four of the nine unstable fractures in group A had severe late pain, while 16 of the 25 unstable fractures in group B had the same complaint. Most of the pain was located in the sacroiliac joint area and in the lower back. The most common unsatisfactory results were in the sacroiliac dislocations with chronic late pain in 60%. The highest incidence of malunion and nonunion was also found in this group. Patients with anatomical reduction and stabilization of the pelvic ring had much better results than those in whom the pelvis was left unreduced.

Matta and Saucedo[15] treated 54 patients with unstable pelvic injuries using three different treatment modalities: skeletal traction, external fixation, and open reduction and internal fixation (ORIF); 51% of the patients treated nonoperatively suffered either a nonunion or a malunion of their fracture. Sacroiliac dislocations with associated symphysis pubis dislocations were particularly difficult to treat nonoperatively. In this series, patients treated with internal fixation had the best clinical results, as well as the highest rate of union, in a satisfactory position.

The above studies confirm the fact that the treatment of unstable pelvic fractures is dependent on the stability and adequacy of the sacroiliac reduction. The more stable the fracture pattern, the fewer and less significant are the long-term problems when compared with unstable fracture patterns with more significant long-term problems.

It is these unstable posterior pelvic injuries (type C) involving sacral fractures and sacroiliac joint disruptions that lend themselves to cannulated screw fixation.

## Advantages of Cannulated Screws

1. Can be performed percutaneously with fluoroscopy or with CT guidance as long as a reduction of the sacroiliac (SI) joint or sacrum is possible by closed techniques; or can be performed with a limited open reduction and then screw placement under fluroscopy or CT guidance.
2. Percutaneous fixation after closed or limited open reduction may obviate the need for a large surgical incision and exposure through compromised tissue and thus lower the morbidity and potential blood loss of the procedure.
3. Allows for initial placement and confirmation of the guide wire in the intended area prior to drilling and screw insertion, thereby decreasing the chance of neural or vascular injury. The ability to change the position of the guide pin prior to screw placement is an obvious advantage.
4. Measurement from a properly placed guide pin allows for the selection of the proper screw length, and hence improves accuracy.

## Potential Drawback

The flexible 2.0-mm guide wire tends to wander and does not allow a good feel of the bone due to its threaded tip. It also does not allow the use of the in-out technique as with the reciprocating drill to avoid any potential soft tissue injury. Other systems are available that utilize a larger guide pin (3.2 mm), which could obviate the above problem.

## Timing

The majority of pelvic ring internal fixations are not performed during the acute period following the injury. They are usually performed 2 to 3 days following the injury and initial stabilization of the patient. Early open operative intervention may be justified when an initial laparotomy or bladder repair is performed when the injury is open, or in select unstable pelvic fractures in trauma centers with an experienced surgical team, especially for the multiply injured patient. Goldstein et al.[16] studied 33 patients who underwent ORIF of a disrupted pelvis; 15 of these patients had surgery within 72 hours of injury. They concluded that an aggressive approach including expeditious preoperative angiography, embolotherapy, and early O.R.I.F. of the pelvis, along with other skeletal injuries, was safe and offered significant advantages in terms of postoperative recovery and rehabilitation.

## Position and Technique

Matta and Saucedo[15] performed their reductions and fixations of sacral and sacroiliac joint disruptions with the patient in the prone position on a radiolucent table. Their technique involved open reduction with exposure of the greater sciatic notch for palpation and assessment of reduction. An image intensifier was then used to place screws perpendicular to the iliac wing across the sacroiliac joint into the sacral ala. The point of entry for the screw was at the intersection of a point 15 mm anterior to the crista glutea and the midpoint between the iliac crest and the greater sciatic notch. Anteroposterior, inlet, and outlet views were obtained with the image intensifier to confirm screw position and reduction. Fixation was usually obtained with one or two screws into the S-1 vertebral body.

Routt et al.[17] reported on 68 consecutive patients with posterior pelvic ring injuries who were treated with percutaneous screw fixation.

The reduction maneuver was planned preoperatively. Reduction was achieved with distal femoral skeletal traction in eight cases. Schanz pins placed percutaneously in the iliac crest, inferior iliac spine, and proximal femur aided reduction in 20 cases. The percutaneous iliosacral screws provided the final reduction during seating in 16 patients. Anterior pelvic ring open reduction and internal fixation was used in 32 patients to simplify the closed reduction posteriorly. Seventeen complete sacroiliac disruptions required an open reduction prior to screw fixation; 99 screws were placed in the first sacral body, with four placed in S-2. The reduction was fluoroscopically guided in all cases. All screws were inserted with the patient in the supine position.

McLaren[18] recommended the addition of the lateral sacral view during fluoroscopy in addition to the inlet and outlet views of Matta. He stated that this allowed easier starting point placement and decreased the chances of exiting the ala or pedicle mass of the S-1. Duwelius et al.[19] reported 13 cases using a CT-guided technique for screw fixation of sacral fractures and sacroiliac joint disruptions. All patients had reducible but unstable pelvic fractures. Under CT guidance each patient underwent percutaneous placement of posterior iliosacral screws. An AO 7.0-mm cannulated screw system was utilized. Eleven patients were done in a prone position, with the other two in a lateral decubitus position on a scanning table. Reduction was obtained in a supine position with traction-countertraction; the patient was placed in a lateral position if reduction was not successful in the supine position. All patients had one sacral screw with a second iliosacral screw or a screw between the posterior superior spines added unless they had already undergone a stabilization of the anterior pelvis.

## Authors' Preferred Technique

### Authors' Cannulated System

*Guide pin:* 2.0-mm guide pins with a threaded tip. *Cannulated overhead, screw head:* Round head with an internal hexagon. *Screw thread:* Outer diameter—7.0 mm; pitch—2.7 mm; preferably fully threaded. *Material:* 316 stainless steel.

### Alternate Systems

Some surgeons may prefer systems that utilize a larger guide pin. This gives the advantage of increased stiffness and strength. In these systems a drill may also be used as the guide pin for the cannulated screw.

*Drill:* 3.2-mm (1/8-inch) steel drill that can be used with a threaded tip and tapered root diameter. *Screw head:* Round head with internal hexagon. *Screw thread:* Outer diameter—6.5 mm self-cutting, self-tapping tip. *Material:* 22-13-5 stainless steel or titanium alloy.

The major problem in posterior ligamentous disruptions is not the ability to manipulate and close the sacroiliac joint dislocation but rather to adequately assess the accuracy of the reduction.[20] With open reduction this is readily achieved by placing a finger gently into the greater sciatic notch and palpating the line between the greater sciatic notch and the lateral border of the sacrum, which should follow a gentle curve. Superiorly by placing a finger over the sacroiliac joint, one can generally palpate a ridge, the sacral ridge, on the ilium at the level of the superior aspect of the sacroiliac joint. This should be in continuity with the lateral portion of the ala of the sacrum if there has been an adequate reduction. By palpating inferiorly and superiorly as described, one can also control flexion and extension of the hemipelvis. This can be temporarily reduced by applying a clamp between the sacral tubercle and the iliac wing.[21] The use of the cannulated screw for fixation of posterior pelvic lesions mandates an accurate reduction of the posterior pelvic ring. Hence, if any doubt remains as to the adequacy of a closed reduction, then an open reduction and internal fixation of the posterior pelvic ring is performed. Anterior pelvic ring fixation may be performed to help in the reduction of the posterior ring. However, in general it is preferable to perform the anterior fixation after the posterior ring is stabilized. Prior anterior fixation may render inadequate posterior rotational control, thereby inhibiting one's ability to adequately reduce the posterior pelvic lesion.[21]

For sacroiliac dislocations a closed reduction is attempted with the patient supine. If successful, then percutaneous screw fixation in the supine position is carried out. If not successful, then open reduction is required and this is best done with the patient prone through the standard posterior approach to the sacroiliac joint. For transforaminal sacral fractures, we recommend removal of bony fragments within the foramen, open reduction, and internal fixation with a non-lag screw to prevent overcompression of the foramen.

Once reduction is achieved, with either position, under fluoroscopy control, the entry point for the cannulated screw is determined. This is best achieved by localizing the position required on the sacrum with the help of the inlet and outlet views.[7] One can identify the ala of the sacrum on the inlet view and the height of the drill bit on the outlet view to ensure it is above the S-1 foramen. The guide wire for the cannulated screw is then inserted across the iliac wing into the sacral ala. The direction and depth is monitored so as to place it in the safe zone above the S-1 foramen within the sacral promontory. The lateral view as described by McLaren[18] is essential to confirm placement of the guide wire in the correct location. Care should be taken to ensure the guide wire is below the profile of the variable sacral slope as seen on the lateral view. The length of the screw required is determined with the depth gauge. The 7.0-mm system's cannulated drill is passed over the guide wire and the reaming performed at least to a point past the fracture. The 7.0-mm screw of measured length is then pased over the guide wire. Confirmation of the progress of the cannulated drill and screw over the guide wire is done by intermittent fluoroscopy to assure that the guide pin itself does not advance. Final position is confirmed on the inlet, outlet, and lateral pelvic views. A second screw may be added in a similar fashion depending on the stability of the pelvis as determined by the fracture configuration. Somatosensory evoked potential (SSEP) monitoring of the lumbosacral plexus is used throughout the procedure, and if any significant changes are noted, immediate corrective measures are taken.[22]

Some surgeons may vary the technique slightly. Systems are available in both titanium alloy and 22-13-5 stainless steel that have 6.5-mm threads and a larger cannulation. This is possible without weakening the screw because of the improved strength characteristics of these alloys. In these systems overdrilling is not necessary since the screws are self-tapping. The 3.2-mm guide pins are stiffer and have increased strength over 2.0-mm pins. Some of these systems also have a tapered root diameter on the guide pin's threaded tip. This makes the junction of the guide pin and its threaded tip stronger and decreases the possibility of guide pin bending or breakage. A 3.2-mm drill bit may also be used instead of a guide pin. These are manufactured to the same length as the guide pins and therefore can be used with the direct reading depth gauges. The drill allows the to-fro technique to be used to feel the far cortex. Caution must be used, however, as the screw is advanced over a drill. The drill may advance forward more readily than a threaded tip guide pin. The disadvantages of these systems is that the cannulated screws are not presently available fully threaded. Overcompression should be avoided with a smooth shaft screw.

## Representative Cases

Representative case examples are shown in Figures 8.2 and 8.3 and the desired position of the iliosacral screw in Figure 8.4.

## Complications

Routt et al.[17] reported in their series of 68 patients with 104 percutaneous screws no nonunions or wound infections, but 12 malreductions (18%). Five screws were misplaced (4%) with one causing transient L-5 neuropraxia. They felt that obesity, abdominal gas or contrast agents, and inexperience were the major causes of difficult screw placement in 16 of their patients. Two patients had failure of fixation, one due to spasticity, and one due to poor preoperative planning.

McLaren[18] reported no complications in his series of 20 sacroiliac disruptions treated by percutaneous fluoroscopic iliosacral screw fixation with at least 3 years follow-up. Duwelius et al.,[19] in their series with an average follow-up of 12.6 months, had one sacral screw that migrated. This was attributed to the fact that the patient did not have a second screw between the posterosuperior spines as he had prior external fixation for anterior pelvic stabilization. An infected pin tract, though, necessitated early removal of the fixator, which likely led to some movement at the sacroiliac joint prior to complete healing. At 10 weeks the patient was clinically healed. No other complications were identified.

Keating et al.[20] reported on 40 vertically unstable pelvic fractures treated with iliosacral screws for the posterior element of the injury; 15 of the 40 patients had percutaneous screw insertion. They found three deep infections, 15% screw malposition, and four screws protruded through the anterior body of S-1 and S-2 and impinged on the S-1 foramen. A satisfactory reduction was obtained in only 33 patients. Loss of fixation was noted in 13 (33%) and at final follow-up 19 patients (48%) developed a malunion. Only 15% had no pain, and although half of the patients had returned to their original employment, 32% were on long-term disability and 69% failed to return to their former level of recreational activity.

Although not reported in the literature we have seen examples of all the potential inadvertent placement of iliosacral screws including:

1. anterior to the sacrum—both intra- and retroperitoneal vascular/neurologic injury.
2. sacral foramina with impingement or damage to L-5, S-1, and S-2 nerve roots.
3. Spinal canal with injury to the cauda equina.

## Conclusion

The results of posterior pelvic unstable injuries appear mutifactorial, but a direct relationship exists between the adequacy of reduction and long-term good results, especially when addressing sacroiliac joint dislocations or fracture dislocations.

Closed manipulation and percutaneous fixation of the disrupted posterior pelvic ring by screws provides stability, minimizes blood loss, and avoids wound problems. However, the essential prerequisite for such a procedure, as mentioned before, is the attainment of an anatomical reduction of the posterior pelvis. Fixation of the anterior ring disruption, preoperative planning, and experience seem to be the key in simplifying reductions. Unfortunately, in most cases of type C (unstable) pelvic injuries, unless fixation is performed within the first few days, such a closed anatomical reduction is not possible, mandating an open reduction and internal fixation. Then the advantages of cannulated screws over standard screw fixation are obviously less significant.

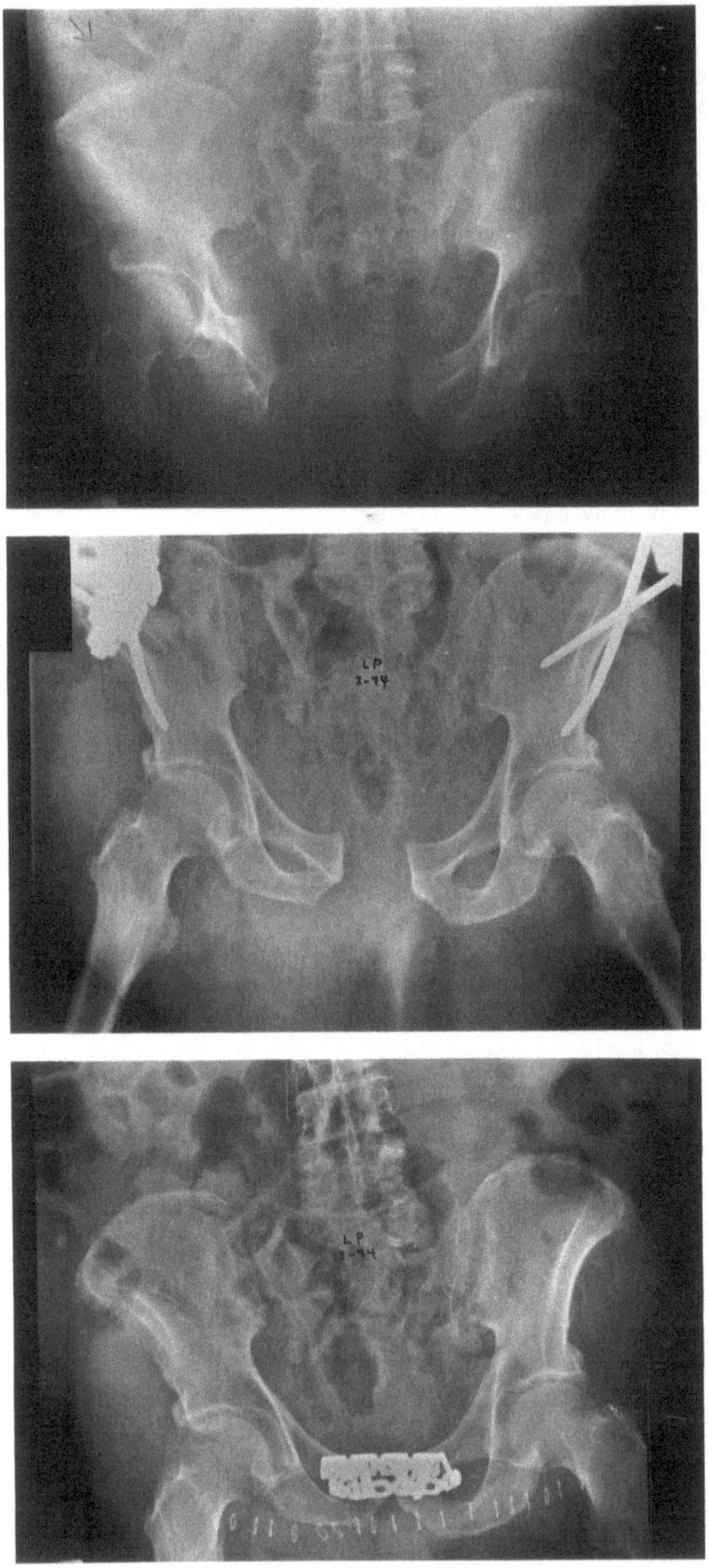


**FIGURE 8.2.** A 54-year-old man involved in a motor vehicle accident with an open pelvic injury. (a) ER anteroposterior radiograph showing a type C-3 pelvic injury. (b) Immediate external fixation to reduce the volume of the pelvis and tamponade the bleeding. Note the posterior pelvis remains unreduced. (c) Anterior pelvic fixation with double symphyseal plating.

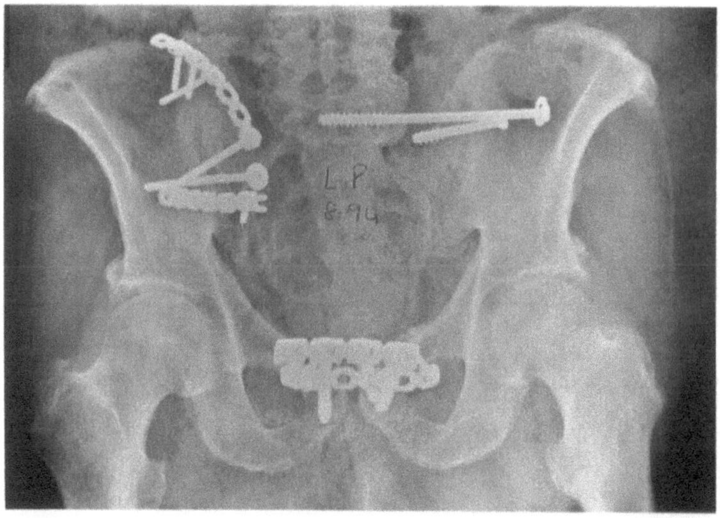


d

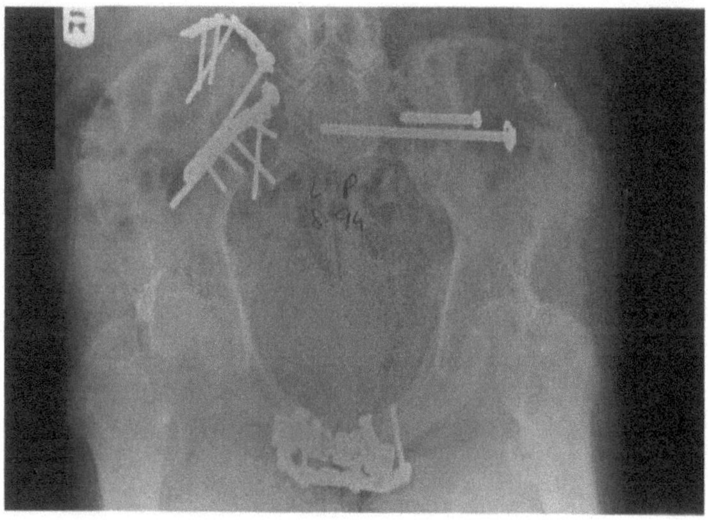


e

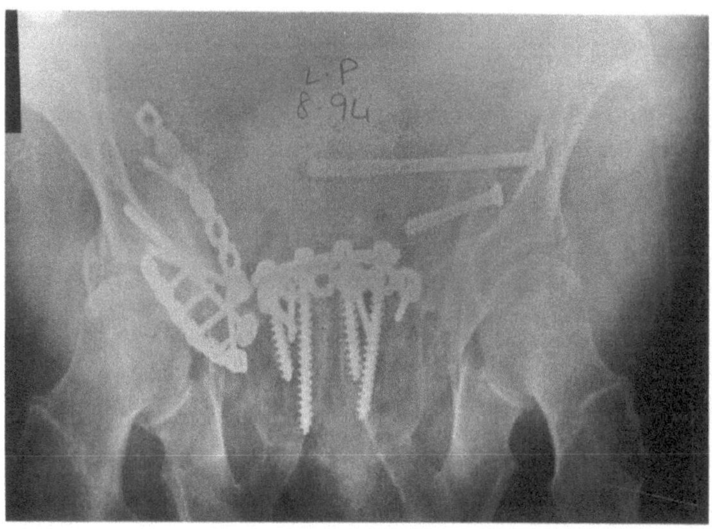


f

**FIGURE 8.2** Note: (d–f) Posterior pelvic fixation with cannulated screws on the left—(d) anteroposterior, (e) inlet, and (f) outlet views.

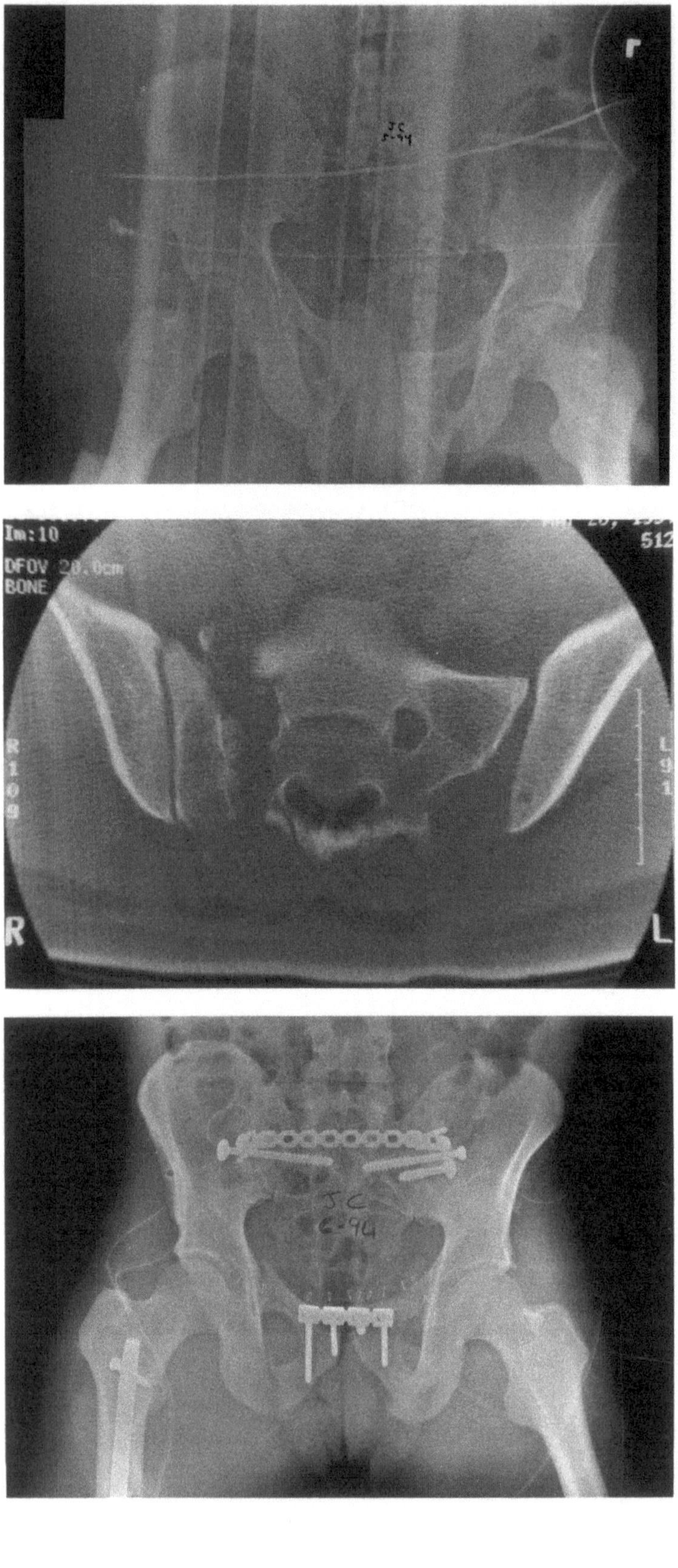


a

b

c

**FIGURE 8.3.** A 32-year-old man run over by a truck. (a) ER anteroposterior radiograph showing a type C-3 pelvic injury. (b) CT scan showing transforaminal sacral fracture on the right with sacroiliac dissociation on the left. (c) Postoperative radiograph showing symphyseal plating, bilateral iliosacral screw fixation supplemented with a posterior "tension band" plate.

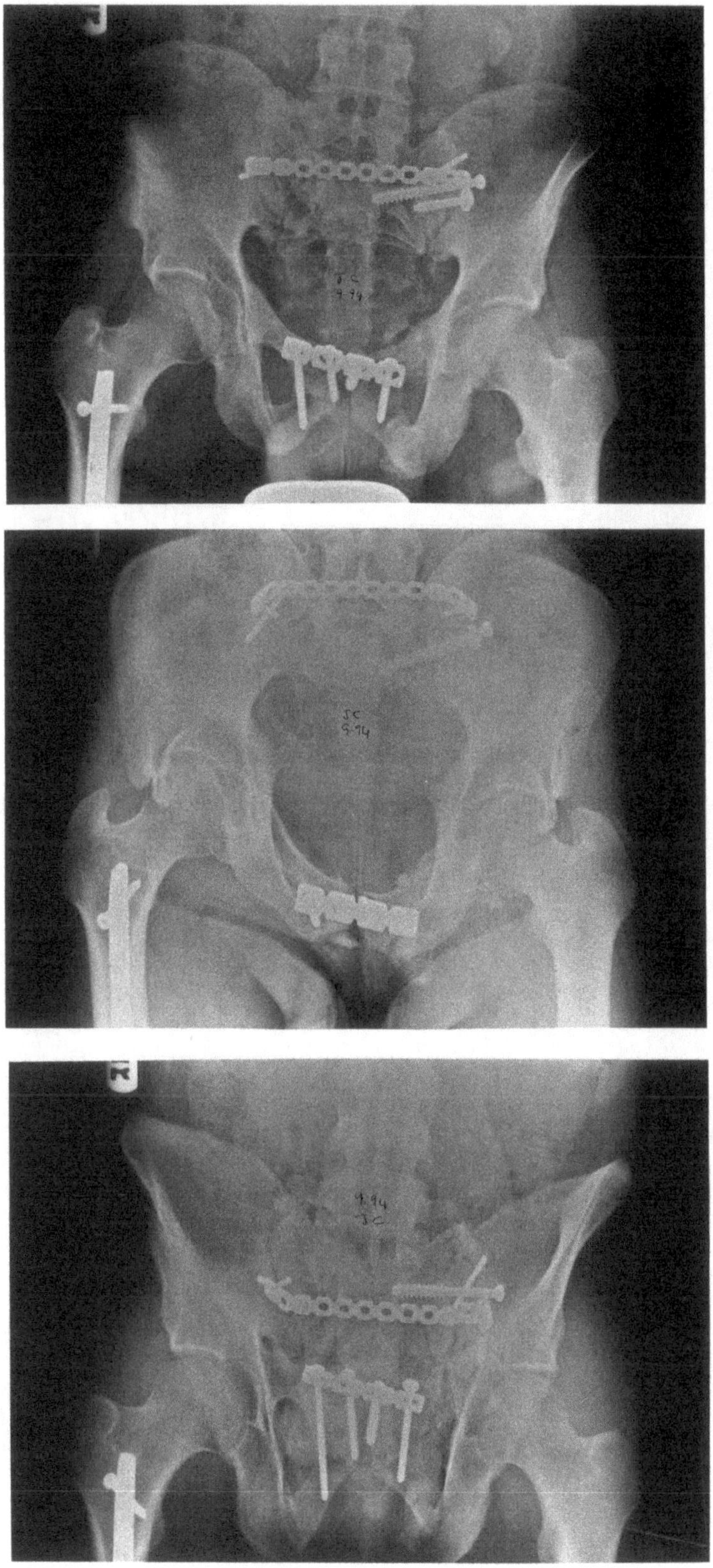

d

e

f

**FIGURE 8.3** (d–f) Three-month postoperative radiographs following removal of the iliosacral screw on the right due to persistent radiculopathy—(d) anteroposterior, (e) inlet, and (f) outlet views.

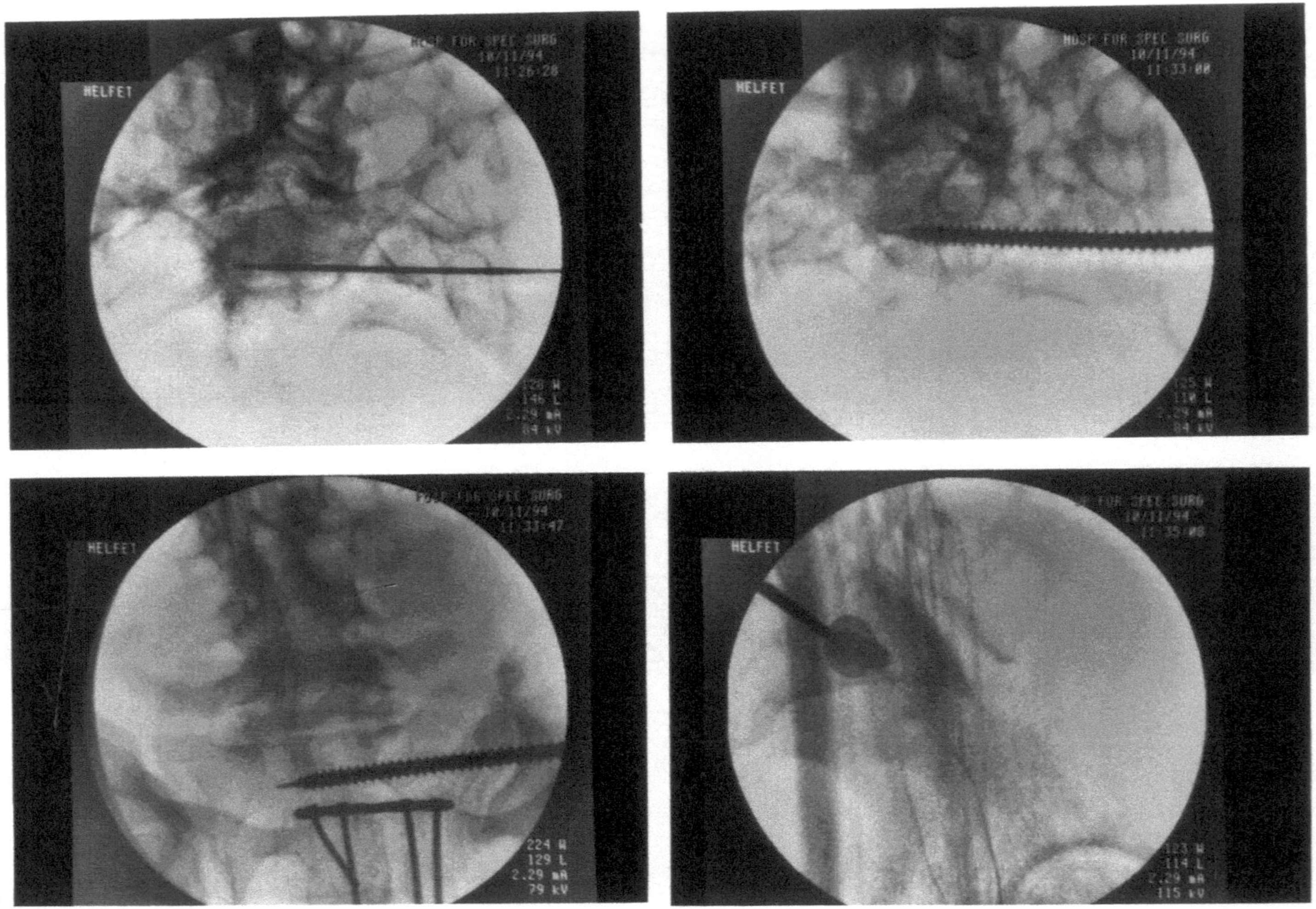


a b c d

**FIGURE 8.4.** Fluoroscopic views illustrating the screw position in iliosacral fixation. (a) Inlet view with guide wire in position. (b) Inlet view with screw in position. (c) Outlet view with screw in place. (d) Lateral sacral view confirming position within sacral safe zone.

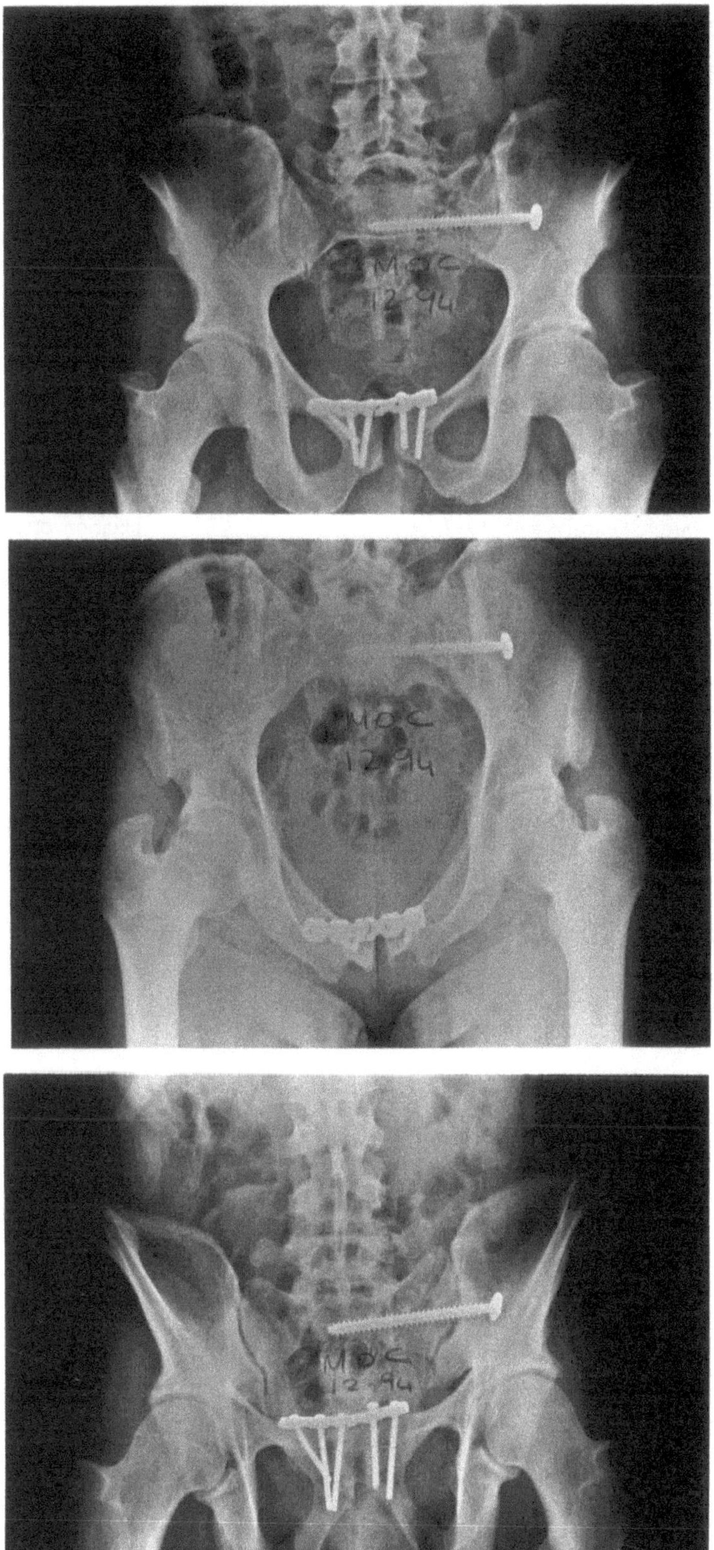

a

b

c

**FIGURE 8.5.** The result at three months postsurgery, with healing on the AP (a), inlet (b), and outlet (c) x-ray views.

## References


1. Gertzbein SD, Chenoweth DR. Occult injuries of the pelvic ring. *Clin Orthop* 128:202–207.
2. Bucholz RW. The pathological anatomy of Malgaigne fracture dislocations of the pelvis. *J Bone Joint Surg* 63A(1):400–404.
3. Schatzker J, Tile M. *The Rationale of Operative Fracture Care.* Berlin, Heidelberg, New York: Springer-Verlag, 1987.
4. Tile M. *Fractures of the Pelvis and Acetabulum.* Baltimore: Williams & Wilkins, 1984.
5. Esses SI, Botsford DJ, Huler RJ, Raushning W. Surgical anatomy of the sacrum. A guide for rational screw fixation. *Spine* 1991;16(6S):S283–S288.
6. Helfet DL. Alphanumeric classification for pelvic fractures. Presented at Surgery of the Pelvis and Acetabulum: An International Consensus, Pittsburgh, Pennslyvania, 1992.
7. Pennal GF, Tile M, Waddell JP, Garside H. Pelvic disruption: assessment and classification. *Clin Orthop* 1980;151:12–21.
8. Letournel E, Judet R. *Fractures of the Acetabulum.* Berlin, Heidelberg, New York: Springer-Verlag, 1981.
9. Peltier LF. Complications associated with fractures of the pelvis. *J Bone Joint Surg* 1965;47A:1060–1069.
10. Holdsworth FW. Fracture-dislocations of the pelvis. *J Bone Joint Surg* 1948;30B:461–466.
11. Raf L. Double vertical fractures of the pelvis. *Acta Care Scand* 1965;131:298–305.
12. Dunn AW, Morris HD. Fractures and dislocations of the pelvis. *J Bone Joint Surg* 1968;50A:1639–1648.
13. Huittinen VM, Slatis P. Fractures of the pelvis: trauma mechanisms, type of injury, principles of treatment. *Acta Care Scand* 1972;138:563–569.
14. Semba RT, Yasukawa K, Gustilo RB. Critical analysis of results of fifty-three Malgaigne fractures of pelvis. *J Trauma* 1983;23:535–537.
15. Matta JM, Saucedo T. Internal fixation of pelvic ring fractures. *Clin Orthop* 1989;242:83–97.
16. Goldstein A, Phillips T, Sclafani SJA, Scalea T, Duncan A, Goldstein J, Panetta T, Shaftan G. Early open reduction and internal fixation of the disrupted pelvic ring. *J Trauma* 1986;26:325–332.
17. Routt MLC, Kregor PJ, Mayo KA. Indirect reduction and percutaneous fixation of the disrupted posterior pelvic ring: indications, techniques, errors and results. Presented at the Annual Meeting of the American Academy of Orthopaedic Surgeons, 1993.
18. McLaren AC. Percutaneous fluoroscopic screw Fixation of the SI joint. Presented at Surgery of the Pelvis and Acetabulum: An International Consensus, Pittsburgh, Pennslyvania, 1992.
19. Duwelius PJ, Van Allen M, Bray TJ, Nelson D. Computed tomography-guided fixation of unstable posterior pelvic ring disruptions. *J Orthop Trauma* 1992;6:420–426.
20. Keating JF, Blachut PA, O'Brien PJ, Meek RN, Broekhuyse HM. Vertically unstable pelvic fractures—the outcome of iliosacral screw fixation of the posterior lesion.
21. Helfet DL. Open reduction internal fixation of the pelvis. *Tech Orthop* 1990;4(4):67–78.
22. Helfet DL. Intraoperative somatosensory evoked potential monitoring during acute pelvic fracture surgery. *J Orthop Trauma* 1995;9:28–34.

# 9
# Internal Fixation of Sacral Fractures

David C. Templeman and Paul J. Duwelius

Progress in fracture care continues to improve the treatment of the severely injured patient. Early stabilization of fractures permits patients to be moved; this reduces the risk of pulmonary complications, sepsis, and death. For many fractures, the patient's rehabilitation and final function are also improved after successful internal fixation.[1]

Operative techniques that reduce and stabilize the pelvic ring are available to treat many pelvic injuries.[2] The development of classification systems by Letournel, Bucholz, and Tile are reproducible methods of categorizing fractures; this ensures that injuries of similar severity are compared.[1,3,4] These classifications also help to differentiate injuries that will benefit from internal fixation from injuries that are successfully treated without surgery.

Letournel's system describes the anatomy of the injury.[3] Injuries to the anterior ring are usually vertical fractures of the pubic rami or diastasis of the pubic symphysis. Letournel defined the four posterior injuries that occur: iliac wing fractures, sacroiliac dislocations, fracture dislocations of the sacroiliac joint, and fractures of the sacrum. This chapter discusses fractures of the sacrum.

The widely used system of Tile and Pennal classifies the injury by deducing the deforming force and the resultant instability of the pelvic ring. Type A fractures are stable. Type B injuries are rotationally unstable but vertically stable. This is the most frequent type of ring injury seen and is usually caused by a lateral compression injury, but also includes disruption of the symphysis pubis ("open book") when the posterior sacroiliac ligaments remain intact. Type C injuries are both rotationally and vertically unstable; these are the most severe pelvic ring injuries. Type C injuries are thought to be caused by an axial load to the pelvis that causes both anterior and posterior disruption of bone and/or ligaments, leaving the hemipelvis unstable. Type C injuries are associated with the highest incidence of life-threatening hemorrhage, neurologic injuries, and pelvic deformities (Table 9.1).

Many sacral fractures are Tile type B injuries, secondary to lateral compression. These fractures usually have impaction of the sacral ala or impaction of the foraminal region. Impaction is best seen with computed tomography (CT) scans. The great majority of these fractures are stable (impacted) and do not require operative treatment. These patients should be examined to determine that leg length inequalities and rotational deformities of the lower extremities are not present. In the absence of these findings, nonoperative treatment is usually successful.

Based on cadaveric dissections that studied the pathological anatomy of the pelvic ring injury, Bucholz described a system that assessed the instability and displacement of the pelvic ring.[4] Type I injuries consist of minimal anterior and posterior displacement in which the ring is stable. Type II injuries define disruption of the anterior ring with minimal instability of the posterior ring; these are similar to the Tile type B injury where a symphysis diastasis with disruption of the anterior sacroiliac joint (intact posterior ligaments) results in rotational instability, but the hemipelvis is vertically stable. Type III injuries define unstable anterior and posterior injuries. An important contribution of this work was the recognition that the direction of displacement of the hemipelvis in type III

**TABLE 9.1.** Tile classification

| | |
|---|---|
| Type A | Stable |
| Type B | Rotationally unstable |
| | "Open book" |
| | Lateral compression |
| Type C | Rotationally and vertically unstable |

injuries was not only vertical, but also included posterior translation and external rotation.

In contrast to the Tile B and Bucholz II injuries, Tile C and Bucholz III injuries that have a sacral fracture, as described by Letournel, are inherently unstable. Leg length inequalities and deformities of the pelvic ring are frequently seen. The presence of a diastasis of the sacral fracture is best seen by CT scans and, in our opinion, indicates an unstable fracture that requires internal fixation.

## Sacral Fractures—Literature Review

It is difficult to determine from the literature the best treatment of sacral fractures. Published reports describe either a small number of fractures treated by a single method or larger numbers of fractures treated by several methods. The lack of a large series that reports a single protocol makes it difficult to determine the best way to treat sacral fractures. (See Chapter 8 for a discussion of sacral anatomy.)

Most early papers described the patterns of fractures or associated neurologic injuries.[5–7] These classifications accurately described the geometry of the fractures, but were not helpful in directing which sacral fractures required surgery.

The recent interest in the operative management of pelvic ring injuries has led to a better understanding of sacral fractures. In a study of 776 pelvic fractures, 236 patients (30%) were diagnosed as having a sacral fracture as a component of their pelvic ring injury.[8]

Neurologic injuries are the major sequelae of sacral fractures; the incidence of neurologic injury associated with sacral fractures is reported to range between 6% and 70%. The variable incidence of nerve injury is dependent upon the specific sacral fracture pattern that is being reported. For example, fractures that involve the sacral canal are expected to have a higher incidence of neurologic injuries.

In addition to injuries of $S_1$ through $S_5$, fractures of the sacrum occasionally injure the $L_5$ nerve root. $L_5$ is damaged on the anterior surface of the sacral ala, usually when there is cephalad displacement of the pelvis. $S_1$ is the major source of motor innervation to plantar flexion of the foot and $S_2$ through $S_5$ are the major components of the pudendal nerve for genital, bladder, and anorectal function. Studies of structures innervated by the lumbosacral plexus do not provide a complete understanding of the precise innervation by $S_1$ through $S_5$. However, information gathered from resection of sacral tumors indicates that continence and sexual function are at least dependent on the unilateral function of $S_2$ and $S_3$.

The vulnerability of the sacral nerve roots to injury is explained by their anatomy. Denis studied the relationship of the sacral nerve roots relative to their neural foramina and documented that: (1) the $S_1$ and $S_2$ nerve root diameters were one-third to one-fifth the diameter of their neural foramina and; (2) the $S_3$ and $S_4$ root diameters were one-sixth the diameter of their foramina.

Denis's work indicates not only the susceptibility to neurologic injury, but also the need for obtaining a precise reduction of fractures that transgress the foraminal zone of the sacrum.

Based on both his anatomical and clinical studies of 236 cases, Denis described a classification that is prognostic for the incidence of neurologic injury.[8] In the authors' experience, this is the best system to use due to its clarity, simplicity, and reproducibility:

*Zone I* injuries are fractures of the sacral ala lateral to the foramina. Denis found that injuries in this zone had a low incidence of neurologic injury (5.9%).[8] Most of these injuries involve either the sciatic nerve or the $L_5$ root and are thought to be secondary to the cephalad displacement of the hemipelvis with damage to the nerve roots that lie on the pelvic surface of the ala.

*Zone II* injuries involve the sacral foramina. Some of these injuries may not involve all five of the sacral foramina, but usually the sacral foramina of $S_1$ and $S_2$ are fractured.[8] Fractures in this zone have a 28% incidence of neurologic injury. These are manifest as sciatica and incontinence.

*Zone III* injuries transgress the central canal of the sacrum. Neurologic injury is common in this pattern and occurred in 57% of the patients reviewed by Denis. Bowel, bladder, and sexual dysfunction were observed in 76% of the patients that had a neurologic injury.[8]

## Initial Assessment

Advances in trauma delivery systems continue to improve survival after severe pelvic fractures; however, patients with pelvic fractures and associated injuries have about a 10% incidence of mortality. Leading causes of death in these patients are hemorrhage and head injuries.[1,9] Genitourinary injuries occur in up to 15% of patients, more likely when the symphysis is dislocated or multiple rami fractures are present.[10] The variety and complexity of associated injuries requires that a multidisciplinary approach be taken to the care of these patients.

All patients with sacral fractures require a detailed neurologic examination. Careful documentation of the motor examination is done in reference to the motor groups innervated by $L_5$ through $S_5$. Sensation of the dorsolateral foot and the lateral lower leg and perineum should be recorded.

The initial evaluation of the bladder is usually complicated by the placement of a Foley catheter during the patient's initial resuscitation. Therefore, many patients will not manifest incontinence or changes in bowel or bladder habits until later in their rehabilitation. Referral to a urologist and the use of electromyograms (EMGs), cystometrograms, and urodynamic studies may be needed at a later time.

## Indications for Surgery

The current indications for surgical stabilization of sacral fractures are controversial.[11,12] We believe that several factors need to be considered before deciding on operative management. First, there must be a comprehensive study of the anatomy of the sacral fracture and resultant deformity of the pelvic ring.[13] The following studies are necessary: anteroposterior roentgenogram, inlet and outlet projection, and CT scans. In complex deformities, three-dimensional CT scans of the pelvic ring assist in arriving at a complete understanding of the deformity.

The goals of the surgery include the prevention of nonunion, pelvic deformity, and leg length inequality. For example, many sacral fractures are caused by lateral compression of the pelvis that results in compression of the pelvis by impacting the sacral ala or transforaminal region. In the absence of neurologic injury, leg length inequality, and rotational deformity of the hip, many of these injuries are inherently stable and do not require operative management. In contrast, injuries that cause cephalad migration of the involved hemipelvis or have CT scan evidence of a diastasis at the sacral fracture line are inherently unstable. Matta and Semba documented that the long-term results of operative management are best when there is less than 1 cm of cephalad displacement after reduction and internal fixation.[14,15] While most authorities agree that posterior pelvic injuries with greater than 1 cm of cephalad displacement are best treated with reduction and fixation, the indications for internal fixation of lesser degrees of deformity, as well as the indications for the fixation of nondisplaced fractures to mobilize multiply-injured patients, are controversial. More studies are needed to answer these important questions.

It is also critical to state that nonoperative treatment does not mean that treatment is neglected. Careful mobilization of the patient, according to the level of pain and a period of non–weight bearing, are needed to avoid late displacement.

## Preoperative Planning

Successful treatment of displaced sacral fractures requires accurate reduction of the displaced fracture and the associated deformities of the pelvic ring. Only by arriving at a thorough understanding of the fracture anatomy is it possible to understand what maneuvers will be necessary to achieve reduction of the deformity.

## Study of X-Rays

The study of the anteroposterior, caudad, and cephalad views indicates both the magnitude and the direction of fracture displacement. Starting with the anteroposterior view, the relationship of the symphysis to a vertical line drawn through the spinous processes of the lumbar spine indicates that the film taken is a true anteroposterior view. Shifting of the symphysis from the midline indicates a rotational deformity of the ring, a finding that is confirmed by the caudal view that indicates rotational deformity of the pelvic brim, either by internal or external rotation. The caudal view also shows posterior displacement of the posterior ring. Both the caudal view and the anteroposterior view are studied to determine if the width of the sacrum from the middle of $S_1$ to the sacroiliac joint is symmetrical. Increased width of the sacrum indicates diastasis of the fracture; decreased width indicates impaction of the sacrum. Diastasis and impaction are then correlated with the CT appearance. The sacrum can be difficult to visualize on the cephalad view due to the overlap of the anterior ring. Usually, the relationship of the fracture line to the sacral foramina, particularly $S_1$ and $S_2$, can be seen. For fractures through the foraminal zone or the ala, a study of the base of the sacrum on the cephalad view indicates the extent of cephalad displacement.

A clear understanding of the deformities of translation, cephalad displacement, and rotation is necessary to determine which maneuvers will be necessary to reduce the pelvic ring and the sacral fracture.

When the injury to the anterior ring of the pelvis consists of rami fractures, the sacrum is usually reduced and fixed first. An accurate reduction of the sacrum usually reduces the rami fractures to less than 1 cm so that operative management of the anterior ring is not required.

In contrast, when the anterior injury is a symphysis diastasis, the anterior ring is usually approached first. When the entire innominate bone is intact, reduction of the symphysis can effect a partial reduction of the posterior ring. Then, open reduction and internal fixation is done as a second stage for anatomic reduction of the sacral fracture.

# Operative Technique

The patient is placed in the prone position. This is not only necessary for a posterior incision, but the prone position helps in reducing the posterior displacement of the hemipelvis. As previously noted, this displacement was diagnosed on the preoperative caudal view.

The posterior approach to the sacrum is made approximately 2 cm lateral to the posterior superior iliac spine. The incision extends proximally to the underlying iliac crest and distal to the apex of the sacrum. With scalpel dissection, the subcutaneous tissues are raised from the gluteus maximus fascia midline to the tendinous insertion of the gluteus maximus fascia. The gluteus maximus is first elevated from the crest, leaving a fascial cuff for reattachment. Dissection extends distally with great care taken to cut the tendon of the gluteus maximus from its fascial insertion on the multifidus and erector spinae. Careful preservation of the tendon allows for a secure and anatomic repair of the maximus.

The abductors are elevated laterally, exposing the greater sciatic notch and the christae glutaris. The multifidus is elevated in a medial direction exposing the sacral lamina. At this point, the fracture site is identified. Palpation of the pelvic surface of the sacrum is possible by elevating the piriformis tendon from the inferior lateral edge of the sacrum. Reduction is usually achieved with the use of either Weber or Matta pelvic reduction clamps. Close observation of the fracture site guides an anatomic reduction, which is confirmed by palpating the pelvic surface of the sacrum. In the presence of a neurologic deficit, exploration of the sacral nerve roots is possible at this time. Gentle distraction of the fracture allows inspection of the nerve roots.

Comminution of the foramina is occasionally associated with transforaminal fractures; fragments should be cleared from the foramina so the subsequent reduction does not entrap fragments within the foramina. The role of foraminotomy in cases with neurologic injury is unknown. We believe that the neural injury is determined by the displacement of the fracture at the time of injury, which stretches the nerves.

The role of intraoperative nerve monitoring during fixation of acute pelvic fractures has been advocated.[16] This may provide a method to reduce the incidence of neural injuries caused during manipulation and fixation of sacral fractures.

# Fixation

## Cannulated Systems Used

### System 1

*Guide pin*: 2.0-mm guide pins with a threaded tip. *Cannulated overdrill. Screw head*: Round head with an internal hexagon. *Screw thread*: Outer diameter—7.0 mm; thread length—16 mm; pitch—2.7 mm. *Material*: 316 L stainless steel.

### System 2

Some surgeons may prefer systems that utilize a larger guide pin. This gives the advantage of increased stiffness and strength. In these systems, a drill may also be used as the guide pin for the cannulated screw. *Drill*: 3.2-mm steel drill that can be used with a direct reading depth gauge. *Guide pin*: 3.2-mm guide pin with a threaded tip and tapered root diameters. *Screw head*: Round head with internal hexagon. *Screw thread*: Outer diameter—6.5 mm; thread length —2.0 mm; self-cutting, self-tapping tip. *Material*: 22-13-5 stainless steel or titanium alloy.

Several methods are described for the fixation of sacral fractures. These include iliosacral screws (inserted by open or closed methods); and sacral bars, posterior plates, and local osteosynthesis with small plates applied on the sacral lamina. In our opinion, more important than the type of fixation is the need to achieve an accurate reduction.

As early as 1945, Bonin[5] recognized the need to "reduce the pelvis satisfactorily by the appropriate method." The authors believe that *obtaining an accurate reduction is the first goal to be achieved in the fixation of sacral fractures.*

Displaced sacral fractures that extend through zone II of the sacrum require an *open reduction* and internal fixation. Malreduction of these fractures reduces the diameter of the sacral foramina, with potential injury to the sacral nerve roots. Open reduction affords the ability to precisely reduce the fracture by direct examination of the fracture line across the sacral lamina; additional palpation of the ventral surface of the sacrum ensures that the foramina are not choked by comminuted fragments.

Sacral bars, transiliac plates, and local plate osteosynthesis have been advocated for the internal fixation of sacral fractures. Limited clinical studies and good biomechanical data are described by several authors in the treatment of sacral fractures. In general, these procedures require two posterior approaches to the pelvis; mechanical testing on cadavers indicates that sufficient stability is achieved by these implants.[17,18]

Developed by Letournel and modified with fluoroscopic imaging by Matta, the authors prefer the technique of iliosacral screws, inserted from the iliac wing into the body of $S_1$. The technique of iliosacral screw insertion continues to be refined and modified. Most of these modifications have evolved as a result of the availability of cannulated screw systems. These systems have allowed the percutaneous insertion of iliosacral screws in selected cases.

Duwelius described CT guided fixation of sacral fractures and sacroiliac dislocations. In a series of 13 patients, successful fixation was achieved in all patients, with the late loss of reduction in one patient due to the early removal of an anterior external fixator required by a pin tract infection. General or regional anesthesia was used in the CT suite, with the path of the cannulated screw directed by the CT scan. Most of the patients were positioned in the prone position. Duwelius emphasized that only reducible injuries were selected for this method.[19]

Routt advocates the percutaneous insertion of iliosacral screws in the supine position. In a series of 68 patients, including 35 patients with sacral fractures, union occurred in all sacral fractures with five malunions encountered in the treatment of 27 transforaminal fractures. Importantly, Routt also reported that during this time, an additional 14 patients with transforaminal sacral fractures were treated by open reduction because of bony debris within the foramina.[13] Further series reporting experience with the percutaneous insertion of cannulated screws are expected. The great advantage of percutaneous fixation is avoiding incisions through compromised tissues associated with pelvic fractures. The initial disadvantage appears to be the inability to obtain accurate reductions in all cases.

While cannulated systems can be used, we believe that the tactile sense of using a drill bit and C-arm images allows safer insertion of the screws. During drilling, the AO "push technique" on the drill allows the surgeon to sense that the drill bit remains within bone. The push technique is done in the following manner: by applying intermittent, gentle pushes to the drill, the surgeon feels resistance as the drill strikes against bone; as long as the drill meets resistance, the tip of the drill remains within the sacral bone. The position of the drill is confirmed with cephalad and caudad fluoroscopic images. Once the drill bit is seated in the center of $S_1$, it can be replaced with the guide wire used for cannulated screws. The guide wire is then measured to determine the length of the screw and used to guide the insertion of the screw. Some surgeons may prefer to replace the drill with the guide wire prior to passing the cannulated screws. In one system, a 3.2-mm by 9-inch drill is used. This can be used with the direct reading depth gauge and the appropriate 6.5-mm self-tapping cannulated screw applied directly over the drill. In another, a 2.0-mm drill or guide pin is used. After depth gauge readings, an overdrill must be used to open up the hole in preparation for the shaft of the 7.0-mm cannulated screw. A second check to make sure that the screw is within the bone can be made when the guide wire is inserted. If the drilled tract is within bone, the guide wire should meet resistance and stop. Free penetration of the guide wire indicates that the wire has penetrated outside the sacrum.

The importance of obtaining clear fluoroscopic images during the procedure is essential to performing the procedure. Fluoroscopic images are obtained before prepping and draping. Excessive bowel gas, contrast medium, and obesity prevent accurate imaging of $S_1$ and are therefore absolute contraindications to the use of iliosacral screws.

The screws must be placed in the center of the $S_1$ body. Asnis has shown that the density of the bone into which the screw is placed is the most important factor in pullout strength.[20] Appropriate screw placement by the surgeon markedly increases the quality of the fixation.

In general, screws with 16-mm or short threads are used, both to ensure that the threads cross the fracture line and to avoid placing the thread-shaft junction at the fracture line, thereby placing this stress riser at high mechanic loading. Cannulated screws with threads of 6.5 mm or 7.0 mm (root diameters 4.5 mm or greater) generally do not have a decrease in the root diameter at the thread shaft junction as is found in the solid AO cancellous screws (root diameter 3.0 mm) and, therefore, show no local weakness in this location. They are also of larger shaft and root diameter than their equivalent cancellous screw, making the cannulated screws generally stronger even though they are cannulated (see Chapter 2).

Positioning of the screws is critical. Careful insertion is necessary to avoid penetrating the sacral canal posteriorly, the sacral promontory anteriorly, and the sacral foramina. Frequent fluoroscopic images in both the cephalad and caudal views are mandatory.

Sufficient fixation is usually achieved by the insertion of two iliosacral screws. However, if when the reduction clamp is released the fracture line through the sacral lamina begins to open, a posterior tension band plate is applied. This occasionally occurs when the cephalad part of the sacrum is compressed by the lag screws and causes the caudal portion of the sacrum to gap open. The tension band plate is placed inferior to the posterior inferior iliac spine, across the sacral lamina, and onto the opposite iliac wing. The posterior tension band plate requires a second incision on the opposite side of the pelvis. Depending on the size of the patient, a 12- to 16-hole pelvic reconstruction plate is usually applied. In our experience and based upon the above logic, the posterior tension band plate is used infrequently; however, other clinicians routinely use the plate as a form of supplemental fixation.

## Postoperative Care

The use of an epidural catheter, which is an excellent adjuvant in the control of postoperative pain, is used for 2 to 3 days after surgery. The high incidence of venous thrombosis associated with pelvic fractures mandates that some form of prophylaxis be used; the combination of oral Coumadin and pneumatic compression devices are recommended.

In addition to obtaining anteroposterior, inlet, and outlet roentgenograms, we recommend ordering a postoperative CT scan. The CT scan is the most accurate method to document the position of the iliosacral screws and the quality of the reduction.

Patients are mobilized as other injuries permit. We prefer to keep patients non–weight bearing for 8 to 10 weeks. Recent reports that emphasize loss of reduction underscore the need to protect the fixation until the fracture is united.

## References


1. Scheidegger D, Suter PM. Fracture management and pulmonary care. In: Border JR, Allgower M, Hansen S, Ruedi T, eds. *Blunt Multiple Trauma.* New York: Marcel Dekker, 1990;61–75.
2. Tile M. Pelvic ring fractures. Should they be fixed? *J Bone Joint Surg* 1988;70B:1.
3. Letournel E. Fractures of the pelvis and acetabulum. Symposium, Los Angeles, CA, November, 1992.
4. Bucholz RW. The pathological anatomy of the Malgaigne fracture dislocation of the pelvis. *J Bone Joint Surg* 1981;63A:400–404.
5. Bonin J. Sacral fractures and injuries to the cauda equina. *J Bone Joint Surg* 1945;27A:113.
6. Schmidek H, Schmith D, Kristiansen D. Sacral fractures. *Neurosurgery* 1984;15:735.
7. Sabiston C, Wing P. Sacral fractures: classification and neurological implication. *J Trauma* 1986;26:1113.
8. Denis F, Comfort T. Sacral fractures—an important problem. Retrospective analysis of 230 cases. *Clin Orthop Rel Res* 1985;240:192.
9. Gilland MD, Ward RE, Barton RM, Miller PW, Duke JH. Factors affecting mortality in pelvic fractures. *J Trauma* 1982;22:691–693.
10. Fallon B, Wendt JC, Hawtrey CE. Urological injury and assessment in patients with a fractured pelvis. *J Urol* 1984;131:712–714.
11. Matta J, Saucedo T. Internal fixation of pelvic ring fractures. *Clin Orthop Rel Res* 1989;242:83.
12. Routt ML, Kregor PJ, Simonian PT, Mayo KA. Early results of percutaneous iliosacral screws placed with the patient in the supine position. *J Orthop Trauma* 1995;9:215.
13. Williams P, Warwick R. *Gray's Anatomy.* Edinburgh, New York: Churchill Livingstone 1989.
14. Tornetta P III, Matta J. Long-term follow-up of operatively treated unstable posterior pelvic ring disruptions. OTA National Meeting, Los Angeles, 1994.
15. Semba RT, Yasukawa K, Gustilo RB. Critical analysis of results of 53 Malgaigne fractures of the pelvis. *J Trauma* 1983;23:535–537.
16. Helfet DL. Intraoperative somatosensory evoked potential monitoring during acute pelvic fracture surgery. *J Orthop Trauma* 1995;9:28–34.
17. Albert MJ, Miller ME, MacNaughton M, Hutton WC. Posterior pelvic fixation using a transiliac 4.5 reconstruction plate: a clinical and biomechanical study. *J Orthop Trauma* 1993;7:226–232.
18. Pohleman T, Angst M, Schneider E, Ganz R, Tscherne H. Fixation of transforaminal sacrum fractures: a biomechanical study. *J Orthop Trauma* 1993;7:107–117.
19. Duwelius PJ, Van Allen J, Bray TJ, Nelson D. Computed tomography-guided fixation of unstable posterior pelvic ring disruptions. *J Trauma* 1992;6:420–426.
20. Asnis SE, Ernberg JJ, Bostrom MPG, Wright TM. Bone screw thread design and holding power. Annual Meeting of the American Academy of Orthopaedic Surgeons, February, 1995.

# 10

# The Knee: Tibial Plateau Fracture Reduction Techniques Utilizing Cannulated Screw Fixation

Paul J. Duwelius and David C. Templeman

The objective in treatment of tibial plateau fractures is to obtain a stable, pain-free knee joint with a functional range of motion. Several authors advocate open reduction and internal fixation (ORIF).[1–5] Other authors have reported good results with limited internal fixation in combination with functional bracing or various traction techniques.[6–13] Determining which type of treatment is best depends on a multitude of factors.

Rasmussen's[12] indications for operative treatment are not based on radiographic criteria. His indication for operative treatment is the degree of varus/valgus instability of the knee in complete extension. Lansinger et al.[14] studied 102 patients treated according to Rasmussen's criteria. Ninety percent of patients followed for a 20-year minimum had good to excellent results. Their treatment utilized ligamentotaxis for reduction and stabilization with percutaneous cerclage wire or screw fixation. Duwelius and Connolly[9] have found this technique to be extremely successful in the treatment of tibial plateau fractures. This technique includes meticulous preoperative evaluation, intraoperative radiography and examination of the knee under anesthesia, and precise intraoperative surgical technique. The examination of the knee allows the surgeon to determine the need for operative intervention.

## Structural Anatomy

A fracture of the tibial plateau is an intraarticular fracture of a major weight-bearing joint. This fracture occurs as a result of a combination of lateral bending and vertical thrust. This mechanism of loading and fracture results in depression of the articular surface and shearing off of portions of the metaphysis.

The adult tibial plateau has a 10° slope. The dimensions of the medial and lateral plateau are different. The anatomic differences between the weight-bearing surfaces of the lateral and medial tibial plateaus should be considered when treating these fractures. In cadaver experiments Walker and Erkman[15] demonstrated that almost the entire load borne on the lateral compartment is carried by the lateral meniscus (Figure 10.1). In contrast, load distribution on the medial side is shared equally by the medial meniscus and exposed articular cartilage. The weight-bearing function of the lateral meniscus may explain why functional results after lateral plateau fractures are usually quite good to excellent despite not achieving a perfect roentgenographic appearance. This may also explain the relatively higher frequency of less satisfactory functional results in the bicondylar and medial plateau fracture.

Understanding the association between the cancellous metaphyseal bone, the surrounding collateral ligaments, the central anterior and posterior cruciate ligaments, and the meniscus allows the surgeon to utilize these structures to facilitate reduction of fracture fragments in the treatment of tibial plateau fractures. The ligaments and surrounding soft tissue can be utilized in the treatment of these injuries by applying traction and using ligamentotaxis to assist in the reduction of plateau injuries. The cancellous nature of the metaphyseal region of the tibial plateau is often of low density and often iliac crest bone graft or a tricortical strut is necessary to elevate a central depression-type plateau fracture. Various artificial bone graft substitutes

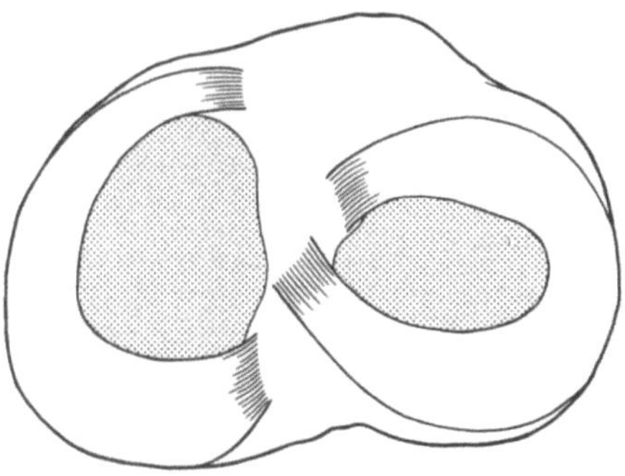


**FIGURE 10.1.** Exposed surface area of the medial and lateral tibial plateaus.

hold some promise, but the greatest limitation of these have been their lack of structural support.[16]

Several authors have reported on the number of associated injuries seen with tibial plateau fractures.[17–19] Browner reported a 56% incidence of associated soft tissue injuries in a series of 30 tibial plateau fractures.[17] The medial collateral ligaments were injured in 20% (6 of 30), the lateral collateral ligaments in 3% (1 in 30), the menisci in 20% (6 in 30), the peroneal nerve in 3% (1 in 30), and the anterior cruciate ligaments in 10% (3 in 30).[17]

Delmarter et al.[18] reported on ligament injuries associated with tibial plateau fractures. Thirty-nine patients with tibial plateau fractures and concomitant ligament injury were evaluated at least one year after injury. Ligamentous injury was determined by stress roentgenograms, plain roentgenograms, operative findings, and Pellegrini-Stieda's ossification. There were 22 isolated medial collateral, eight lateral collateral, one isolated anterior cruciate, and eight combined ligament injuries. All types of tibial plateau fractures were associated with ligamentous injury, although split compression and local compression were most common. This study confirms the view that instability is a major cause of unaccepted results in tibial plateau fractures. Operative repair of medial and lateral collateral ligaments, with appropriate treatment of the bony plateau fracture, may reduce late instability and may improve overall morbidity in these concomitant injuries. Cruciate ligament injury associated with a tibial plateau fracture carries a poor prognosis in their series.

## Clinical Relevance and Preoperative Evaluation

All tibial plateau fractures are clinically evaluated with an examination of the knee in extension, and are determined to be stable or unstable. Unstable fractures have greater than 1 cm of opening to varus or valgus stress testing. If pain precludes an adequate examination, the patient requires examination under anesthesia to document stability in extension. With a stable examination cast bracing is all that is necessary. For fractures that are more complex a molded, hinged cast brace is applied after longitudinal traction. For simple fractures a Bledsoe-type cast brace is used.

Unstable fractures with greater than 1 cm of opening in extension necessitate stabilization. This is best determined with an examination under general anesthesia. This also allows an attempt at reduction utilizing only ligamentotaxis.

An examination of the neurovascular status is mandatory. With suspicion of a knee fracture dislocation, arteriography should be performed. Compartment syndromes are a distinct possibility with these types of fractures.

Routine radiographs include a 105° Moore anteroposterior (AP) view and a lateral view of the knee (Figure 10.2). Fractures that are unstable should have tomography or computed tomography (CT) scan with sagittal and coronal reconstruction. These radiologic studies allow the surgeon a three-dimensional preoperative planning scheme. This will allow accurate placement of screws, plates, or external fixation devices into good bone. Regions that are highly comminuted can be filled with autogenous bone or bone graft substitutes.

If the patient is not going to surgery emergently, or abrasions and skin lesions such as fracture blisters preclude surgery, then the knee can be aspirated and a local anesthetic injected. The leg should then be splinted and evaluated.

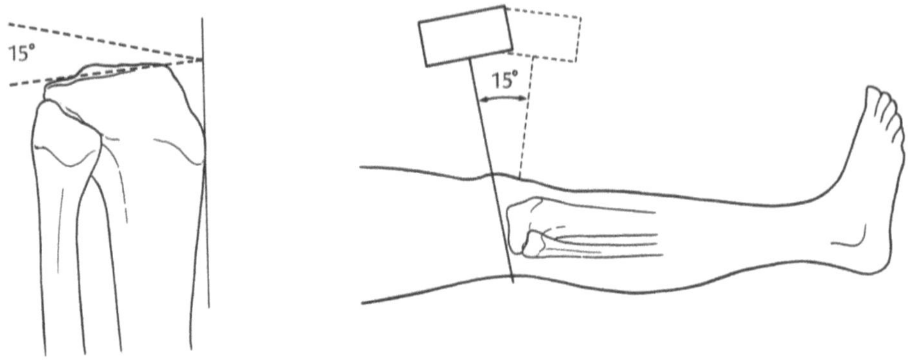


**FIGURE 10.2.** Moore 105° AP view.

## Classification

There are several tibial plateau fracture classifications. The authors feel that no one fracture classification is all encompassing. The Association of Osteosynthesis (AO), Rasmussen, and Hohl classification systems are similar and describe most plateau fractures quite well. The AO classification is described in Figure 10.3. The Schatzker classification describes in more detail the plateau fracture that extends distally into the metaphyseal region of the tibia. This is an ominous fracture pattern and not well described in the AO or Rasmussen classification systems. The Schatzker classification system is illustrated in Figure 10.4. Classification systems are important in evaluating these injuries. These classification systems include the frequently observed patterns and provide guidance for making treatment decisions. In these three classification systems, fractures are divided into minimally displaced (usually less than 3 to 4 mm of depression or displacement) and displaced. Displaced injuries are further subdivided into local compression, split compression, total condylar depression, and split, rim, and bicondylar fractures. Schatzker's classification includes the type six or condylar/metaphyseal/diaphyseal separation. However, the bony classification is insufficient. One must also consider the soft tissue injuries. Open plateau fractures and bumper injuries are usually high-energy injuries. Benirschke et al.[20] reported on immediate fixation of open complex tibial plateau fractures utilizing a standardized treatment protocol. This study emphasized the importance of aggressive soft tissue management, immediate open reduction and fixation after thorough washout, and soft tissue coverage within 5 days.

The authors have found that the AO C3 fracture pattern, regardless of treatment in our series, had the highest complication rate and the poorest outcome.

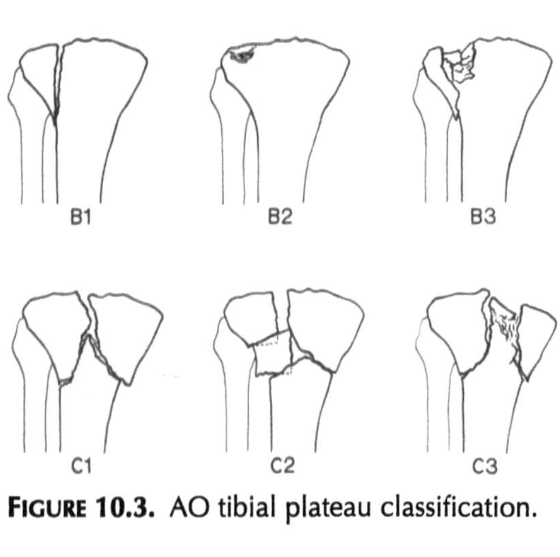


**FIGURE 10.3.** AO tibial plateau classification.

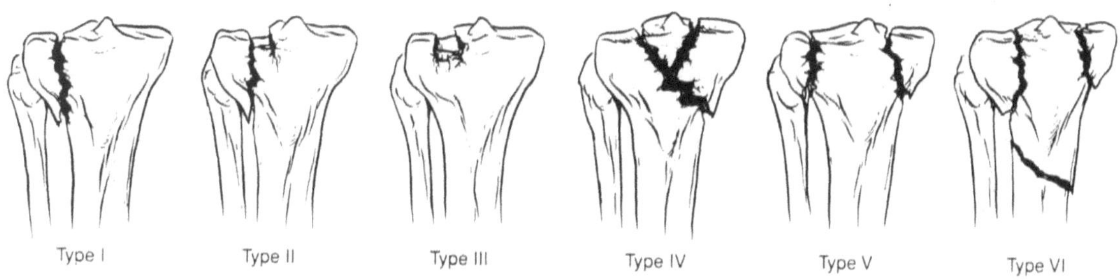


**FIGURE 10.4.** The Schatzker classification of tibial plateau fractures. Type I is a wedge (split) fracture of the lateral tibial plateau. Type II is a split-depression fracture of the lateral plateau. Type III is a pure central-depression fracture of the lateral plateau without an associated split. Type IV is a fracture of the medial tibial plateau, usually involving the entire condyle. Type V is a bicondylar fracture, which typically consists of split fractures of both the medial and lateral plateaus without articular depression. Type VI is a tibial plateau fracture with an associated proximal shaft fracture. (Reprinted with permission from Koval and Helfet.[23])

## Clinical Relevance

The choice between open or closed treatment must be based on examination of the knee in extension. If there is any instability because of malalignment or joint depression, a satisfactory result will require operative treatment. Operative treatment of tibial plateau fractures must take into account the "personality" of the fracture. Personality factors include the patient's age, lifestyle, and the treatment expectations. Hohl and others have stressed the importance of early range of motion of the knee regardless of the treatment selected.

## Specific Indications for Treatment Based on Fracture Classification

### *Type I or Split Fractures*

These most commonly are wedge-type fractures of the lateral tibial plateau in young adults whose good bone quality resists depression. Undisplaced types can be placed in a cast brace immediately with full range of knee motion. If displaced, the majority of these fractures are ideal candidates for percutaneous screw fixation utilizing ligamentotaxis, fluoroscopy, and possibly arthroscopy. Displaced fractures occasionally have a trapped meniscus, which precludes reduction. Arthroscopy or limited open reduction can allow reduction of the fracture (Figure 10.5).

### *Type II or Split Central Depression Fractures*

These fractures in addition to the wedge split have varying amounts of central depression of the lateral plateau (Figure 10.6). The mechanism of injury is similar to the first type. Generally, the quality of the bone is not as good and therefore the weakened bone fails in a compressive load. These fractures commonly occur in older patients with some degree of osteoporosis. If the knee examination is stable in extension, then no treatment is necessary. The lateral meniscus covers the vast majority of the joint surface and the fracture will do well if the joint is moved. Unstable fractures will result in joint incongruity and they need to be addressed by an attempt at closed reduction utilizing ligamentotaxis followed by percutaneous fixation. Usually a limited anterior incision is required, being careful not to undermine any soft tissue or strip any periosteum. The incision should be centered over the split fragment so that maximum visualization of the depressed fragment as well as joint surface can be utilized. The central depressed portion needs to be elevated with a bone tamp and supported by bone graft (Figure 10.7). The fracture can be stabilized with percutaneous screws to avoid further dissection or with a buttress plate and screws if the depressed area is significant or if the lateral wedge is very thin, so as not to allow for screw fixation with washers alone (Figure 10.7).

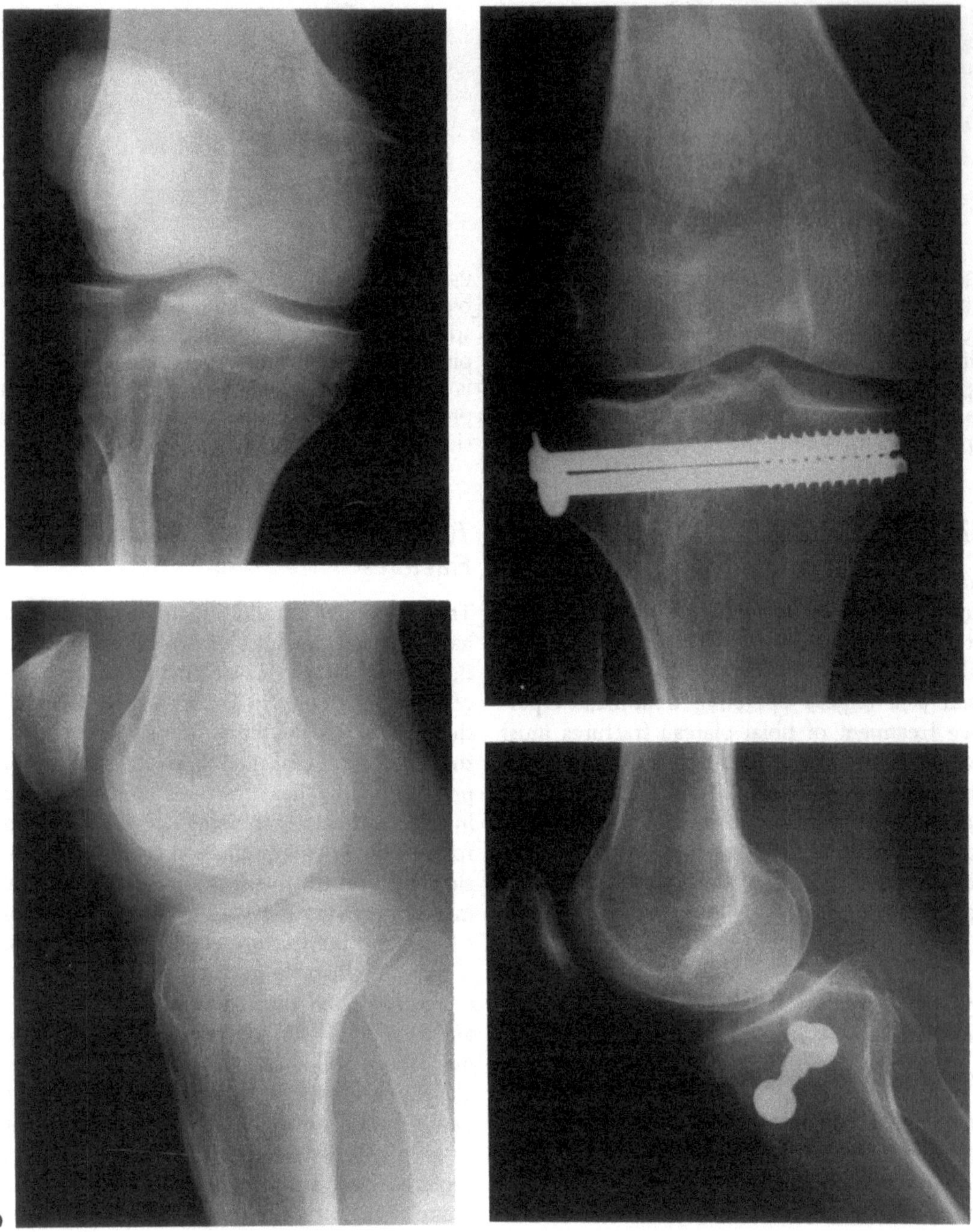

**FIGURE 10.5.** Treatment of simple fractures of the tibial plateau. (a) Anterior-Posterior view of displaced split, central depressed tibial plateau fracture. (b) Lateral view of split-central depressed tibial plateau fracture. (c,d) Post-operative views of split-central depressed tibial plateau view. (d) Lateral view of tibial plateau joint surface post reduction and percutaneous screw fixation.

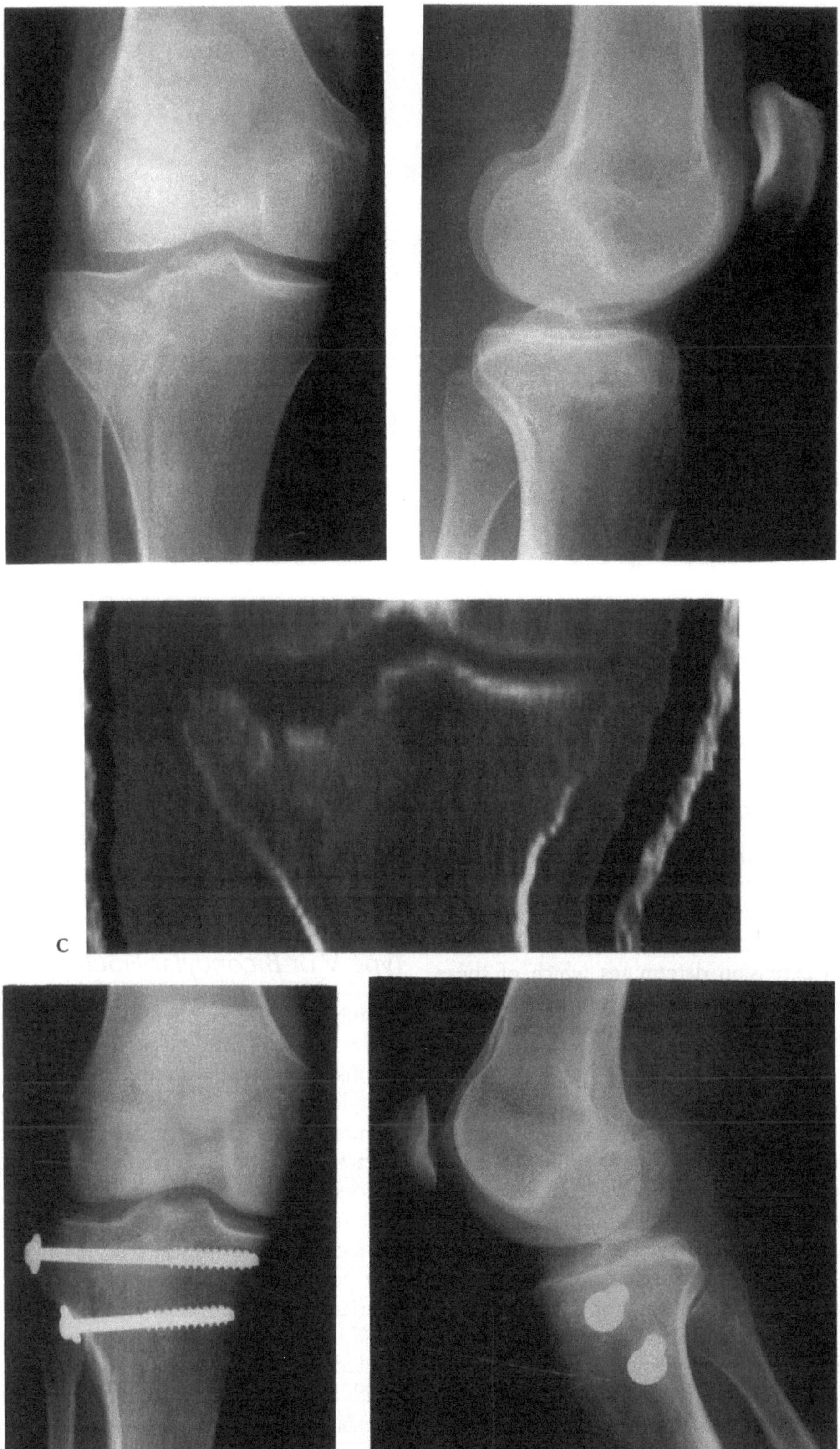

a b c d e

**FIGURE 10.6.** Treatment of split-central depressed tibial plateau fractures. (a,b) AP and LAT views of central depressed lateral plateau view. (c) CT view defining amount of depression. (d,e) Postoperative views of tibial plateau fracture post elevation and iliac crest bone grafting and screw fixation.

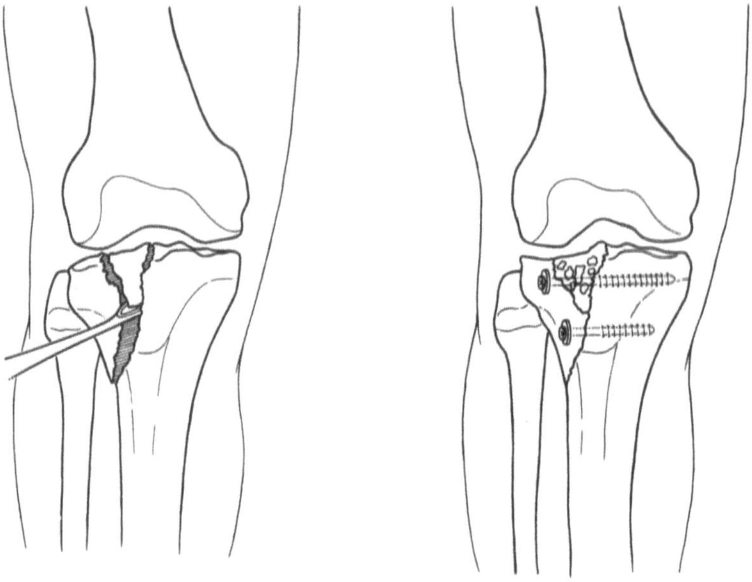

**FIGURE 10.7.** Irreducible fractures or split centrally depressed fractures are elevated through limited arthrotomies or from limited incisions below the plateau and bone graft applied to elevate the fracture. This may also be done under arthroscopic control. Successful treatment with limited internal fixation and bone grafting.

## *Type III or Central Depression Fractures*

A depression of the central portion of the lateral plateau occurs without an associated wedge fracture. Generally, this occurs in older patients with significant osteoporosis. The knee examination in extension determines which of these fractures need surgery. The treatment protocol is the same as for split or split central depression fractures types.

## *Type IV or Medial Plateau Fractures*

These fractures are particularly prone to problems (Figure 10.8). Generally they are associated with younger patients with a higher degree of injury. They almost always are unstable. Fractures of the medial plateau that are nondisplaced are prone to fall into varus, especially with an intact fibula. This fracture pattern needs to be stabilized regardless of examination of the knee. Depending on the fracture pattern, percutaneous screws or plates are indicated to reconstruct the joint surface and prevent subsequent varus deformity. The poor prognosis associated with these injuries is caused by the amount of joint surface that is exposed on the medial plateau compared with the lateral plateau. Also, soft tissue injury may cause knee instability as well as peroneal nerve injury or popliteal artery injury.

## *Type V or Bicondylar Fractures*

Bicondylar fractures have many different types of fracture patterns. Generally these fractures are unstable in extension because of the medial condyle involvement. If traction can align these fractures, many can be treated by cast bracing. Generally for the unstable fracture patterns the authors advocate plating the condyle with the most severe articular involvement with an anterior incision. If the other condyle can be treated with percutaneous screw fixation or some type of triangular external fixator or circular ring frame, less soft tissue dissection is required. Limited fixation of the less-injured condyle avoids the soft tissue dissection and subsequent vascular problems entailed with double plating. If both sides require plate, then small counter-incisions with adequate skin bridges and minimal biologic fixation or use of a small external fixator should be employed. Figure 10.9 illus-

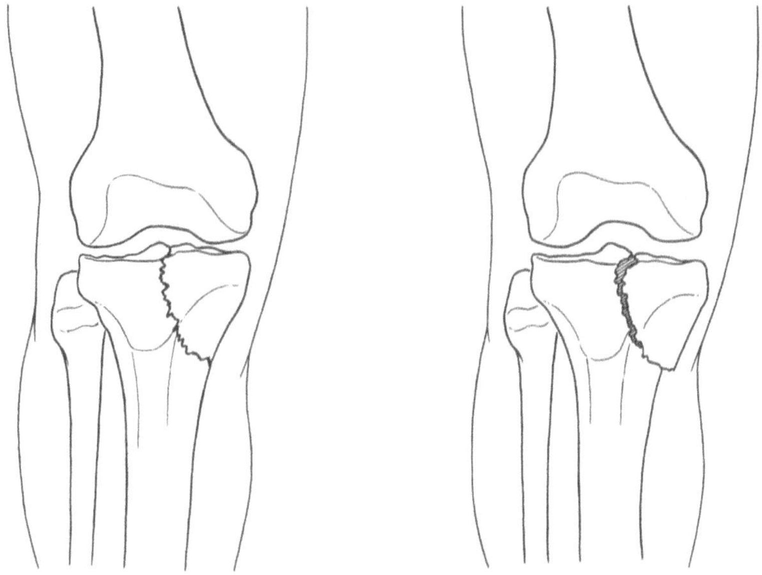

**FIGURE 10.8.** Medial plateau fractures.

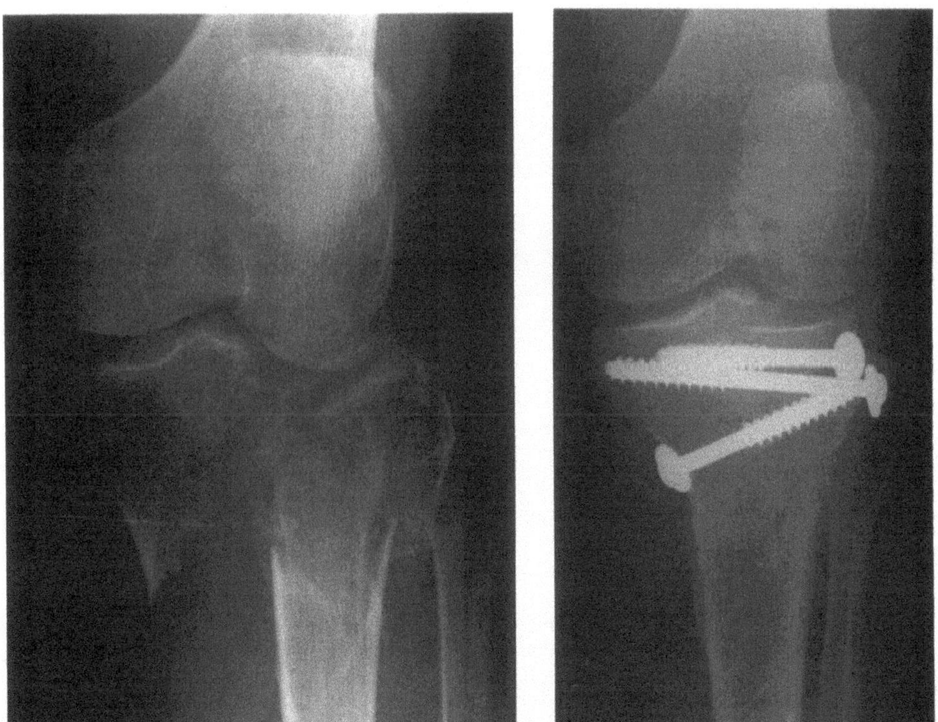

a b

**FIGURE 10.9.** Bicondylar plateau fixation in osteoporotic elderly patient. (a) Severely comminuted bicondylar fracture in elderly osteoporotic patient. (b) Limited internal fixation and plaster cast bracing was performed because of concerns about the quality of bone and the need for excessive soft-tissue stripping ORIF.

trates a case in which limited internal fixation was utilized in a patient with severe osteoporosis. Placement of a midline skin incision is generally preferable in severely injured bicondylar tibial plateau fractures, as this is the approach needed for a subsequent total knee arthroplasty. Many of the type V and VI plateau injuries are associated with significant cartilage injury.

### *Type VI*

The hallmark of the type VI fracture is a fracture line that separates the metaphysis from the diaphysis. These fractures usually are extremely high-energy mechanisms of injury with resultant complex fracture patterns. The resultant separation of the condyles from the metaphyseal-diaphyseal junction makes nearly all of them unstable to examine; therefore, this severe injury almost always requires surgical intervention.

The best surgical approach involves an incision over the fractured condyle with the most involved fracture pattern. If the condyles can be assembled with limited internal fixation to restore condylar widening and joint depression, this is optimal. The shaft component can be restored to the condyles via a triangular or ring external fixator (Figure 10.10). If plates are chosen, then there is no place for external fixation because of the high incidence of infection. If a plate is chosen to reestablish the condyles to the shaft, then percutaneous fixation of the other, less-injured plateau is optimal. Double plating should be used only in instances where a small counterincision is made with limited internal fixation to avoid soft tissue and bone necrosis from the excessive surgical dissection required in placement of double plates. These significant injuries require anatomic reduction, bone grafting, and early mobilization of the knee for best results.

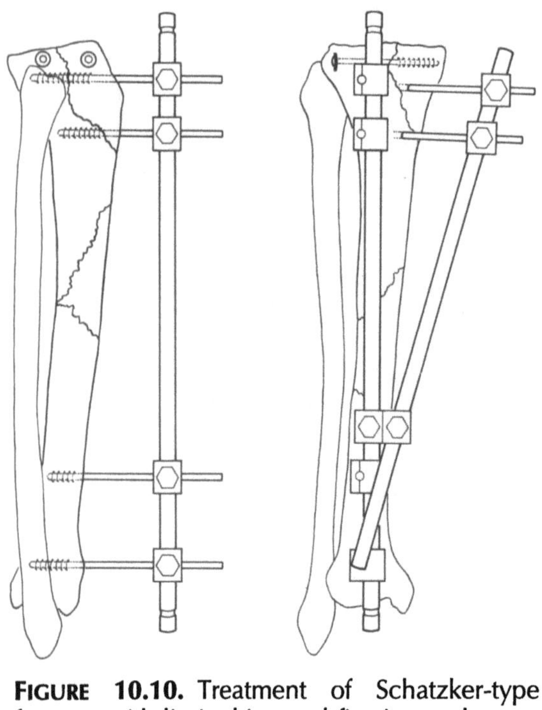

**FIGURE 10.10.** Treatment of Schatzker-type fracture with limited internal fixation and external fixation.

## Treatment Controversy

Tibial plateau fracture treatment is based most importantly on the examination of the knee in extension. The goal of treatment is to restore the fractured knee anatomically and functionally to a condition that is as near normal as possible. Rasmussen[12] revealed that unstable knees with tibial plateau fractures treated surgically and stable knees treated nonsurgically did well. Lansinger et al.[14] support Rasmussen's classic work with 20-year follow-up utilizing these principles based upon the examination of the knee in extension. The authors feel no incisions should be made until an examination of the knee utilizing ligamentotaxis and fluoroscopic evaluation is completed. This gives the surgeon the critical preoperative planning information.

Several previous studies have advocated open reduction and internal fixation with plates and screws. Although good radiographic results sometimes are achieved several report high (25% to 30%), fair, to poor results.[2–4] Others advocate more limited types of internal fixation, possibly in association with ring or external fixation.[9,11,12,14] Whichever treatment is utilized, the surgeon must have established criteria for the surgical indications. The authors feel examination of the knee in extension is the best indicator for surgical intervention. Regardless of which type of treatment is chosen, the knee must be allowed immediate and protected free range of motion postoperatively in a hinged brace. The patient should be doing touchdown weight bearing for 8 to 12 weeks.

# Potential Complications with Internal Fixation

## Problems in Healing

Tibial plateau fractures have a very low incidence of nonunion.

## Open Fracture

Stability in addition to debridement of the open wound with early closure, whether by delayed primary closure, skin grafting, or local or free tissue transfer, and early motion are the best ways to restore function and prevent sepsis.[21] Benirschke et al.'s[20] series illustrates that open reduction and stable internal fixation of the open tibial plateau yields good to excellent results.

## Malunion

This complication is most uncommon when an adequate initial examination has not documented the fracture instability or if documented, adequate internal fixation has not been achieved. This complication is most commonly seen in type IV, V, and VI injuries as the medial plateau component tends to fall into varus. Biologic fixation should not imply inadequate reduction (Figure 10.11).

## Compartmental Syndrome

No chapter on any type of tibial fracture would be complete without mentioning the possibility of a compartmental syndrome. If a compartmental syndrome exists, this fracture must be opened with fasciotomies. Fasciotomies, while saving the muscle from death, create instability of the fracture patterns. Fractures of the tibial plateau associated with compartmental syndromes require fasciotomy and appropriate open reduction and internal fixation to restore fracture stability.

## Multiply Injured Patient

The multiply injured patient at the authors' institution are generally treated regardless of the examination of the knee in extension by some type of percutaneous fixation or ORIF to allow for early mobilization of the patient.

## Neurovascular Injury

Neurologic or vascular injuries are associated most commonly with fracture/dislocations of the knee or medial plateau fractures. The vascular injury should be repaired and the fracture stabilized. If a peroneal nerve injury is documented, postoperatively the knee should be treated in an elevated sling with the knee flexed to decrease traction on the nerve.

Incisions should be carefully planned with adequate skin bridges and good flaps down to bone to avoid iatrogenic vascular injury from excessive soft tissue dissection required. A "perfect" reduction obtained at the expense of the soft tissues usually results in disaster.

## Prominent Hardware

Care should be taken to avoid any protruding hardware especially on the medial aspect of the knee, as this will cause the patient pain especially around the pes anserine bursae and require hardware removal.

# Authors' Preferred Surgical Technique

The key to operative reduction is ligamentotaxis, using longitudinal traction or a femoral distractor (Figure 10.12). The patient is placed in a supine position on a standard operating table. The foot of the table is dropped in order to allow 90° of knee flexion. This position is ideal

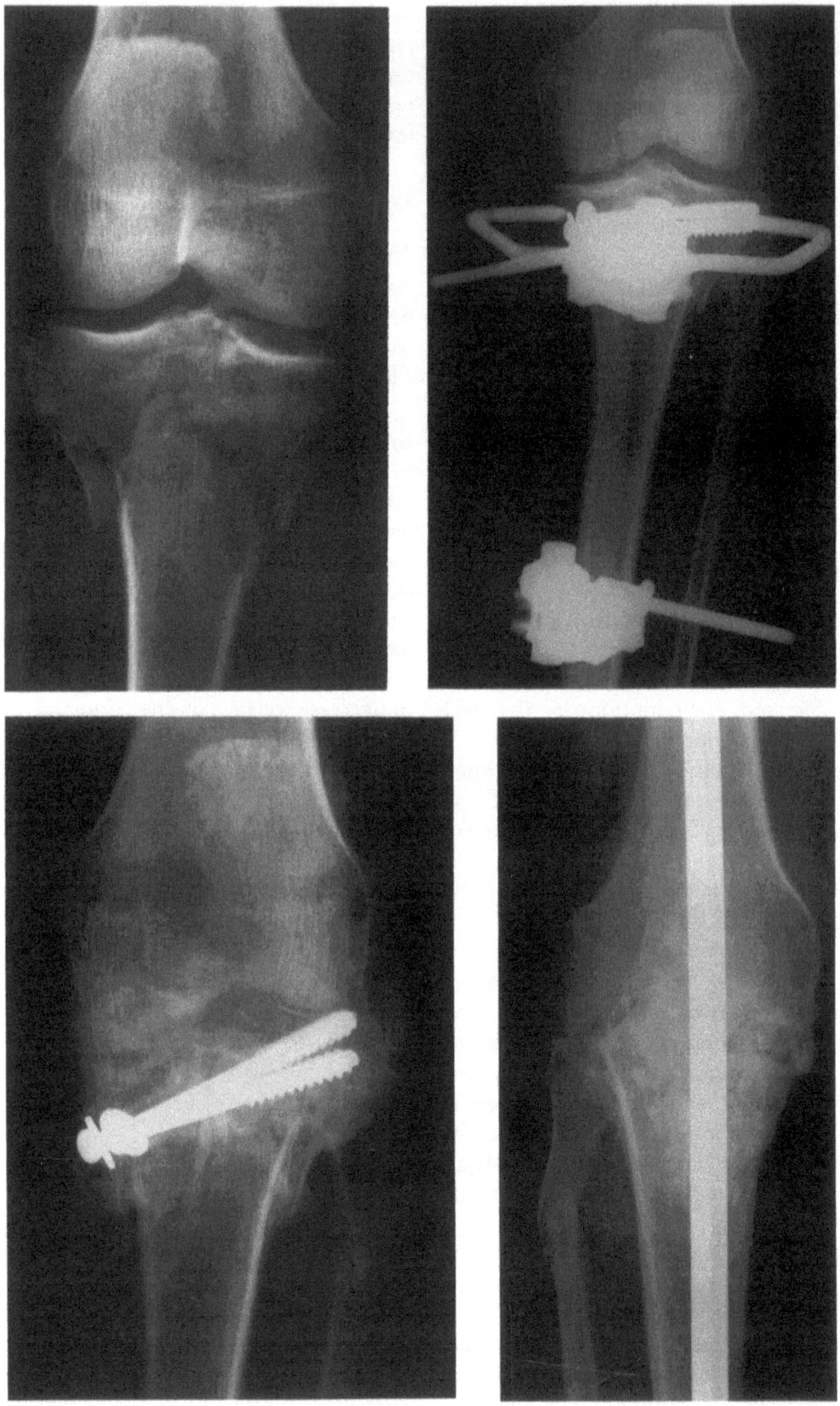

a b c d

**FIGURE 10.11.** Failure of treatment utilizing limited internal fixation and external fixation in open fracture. Arthrotomy required for infection. (a) Open bicondylar tibial plateau fracture. (b) Limited internal fixation plus external fixation was chosen. (c) Subsequent collapse secondary to inadequate fixation. ORIF would have been a better choice. (d) Ultimate fusion required because of infection and malunion.

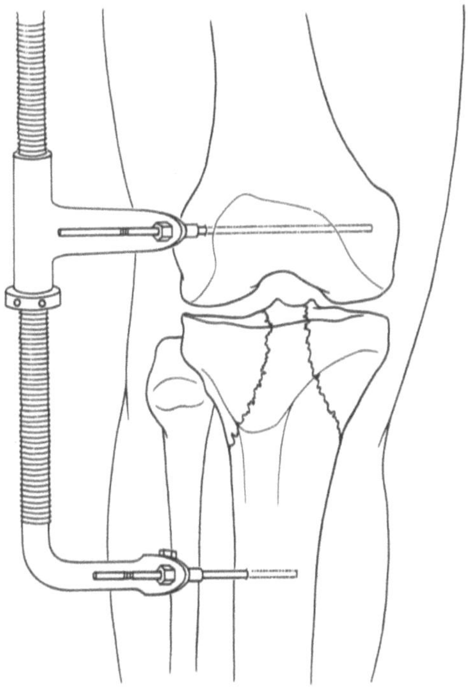

**FIGURE 10.12.** Ligamentotaxis achieved with the distractor.

for open reduction and internal fixation, percutaneous screw fixation, and arthroscopically assisted reduction of the joint. An arthroscopic leg holder is used, allowing the surgeon to apply the forces to the knee required for the reduction (Figure 10.13). Fluoroscopy provides excellent AP and lateral views during the procedure (Figure 10.14). If reduction is satisfactory, then percutaneous screw fixation is utilized. Cannulated stainless steel cancellous screws, 6.5 or 7.0 mm, and washers are used. Multiple screws serve as "one hole plates" and the washer acts as a buttress. Screw size and thread length are selected to allow maximum fracture compression. AO C3 Schatzker IV, V, and VI tibial plateau fracture patterns with extensive metaphyseal comminution require a buttress plate or external fixator.

Most plateau fractures reduce well by ligamentotaxis alone. Fixation with percutaneous screws placed under fluoroscopy maintain the reduction. Preferably, screws are placed parallel, although a more distal screw with a washer used to catch the apex of the fracture may serve as a buttress support.

When ligamentotaxis was unsuccessful in reducing the fracture, because of, for example, trapped meniscus or split central depression bone fragments precluding reduction, then a limited arthrotomy utilizing a parapatellar medial or lateral incision was made for the respective medial or lateral plateau fractures, and stabilization with a buttress plate and/or cannulated screws and iliac crest bone graft is accomplished.

## Equipment

### *System 1*

*Screw thread*: Outer diameter—6.5 mm; pitch—2.5 mm; reverse cutting flutes; self-cutting, self-tapping positive rake tip. *Screw head*: Round head with an internal hexagon. *Drill*: A 230-mm-long 3.2-mm steel drill, which can be used directly with a direct reading 9-inch depth gauge. *Guide pin*: A 230-mm-long 3.2-mm guide pin. *Material*: 22-13-5 stainless steel. *Washers* (optional): 6.5-mm system washers.

### *System 2*

*Screw thread*: Outer diameter—7.0 mm; pitch—2.7 mm. *Screw head*: Round head with an internal hexagon. *Guide pin*: 2.0-mm guide pins with a threaded tip. *Cannulated overdrill*. *Material*: 316 L stainless steel. *Screw tap*: 7.0 mm. *Washers* (optional): 7.0-mm system washers.

The 6.5- and the 7.0-mm cannulated stainless steel screw systems are most familiar to the authors in the reconstruction of the split compression tibial plateau fractures. Preoperative evaluation and planning are essential. In the comminuted split compression fracture with a depressed fragment of articular surface, preoperative tomograms and CT scanning can be most beneficial. Surgical goals are (1) to reconstruct the articular surface, and (2) to stabilize the articular surface in its normal alignment with the tibial shaft. The articular surface is first reassembled, and depressed fragments elevated. This surface is then supported on two guide pins placed the same distance apart as the prox-

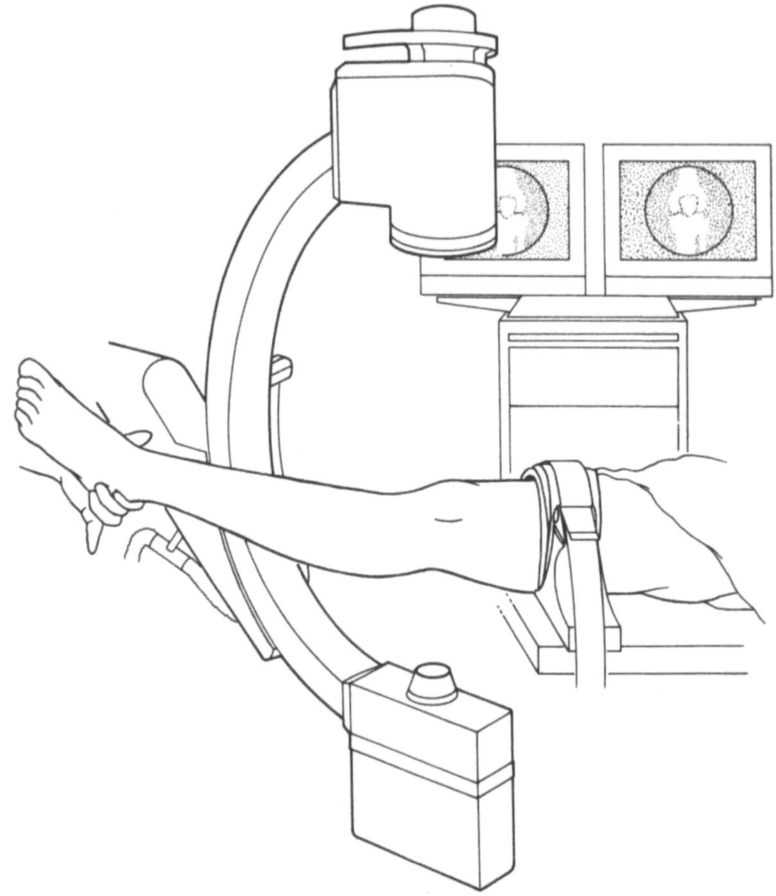

**FIGURE 10.13.** Routine patient position for examination of knee under anesthesia and for percutaneous fixation.

imal two holes in a buttress plate. A bone graft, if needed, is placed below this surface. A buttress plate is bent to conform to the proximal tibia and applied, using two cannulated screws through the proximal holes in the plate.

## Operative Technique for Comminuted Split Compression Fracture of a Lateral Tibial Plateau

1. The patient is placed in a supine position with a sandbag under the ipsilateral hip. The leg is prepped and draped, and exsanguinated with an elastic Esmarch bandage. A well-padded pneumatic tourniquet is inflated about the upper thigh.
2. The anterior compartment muscles are elevated off the lateral tibia, and the fracture exposed. Proximally, the joint is opened to visualize the articular surface. The lateral meniscus may have to be detached anteriorly, but extreme care should be taken to preserve it if not badly torn. At the end of the procedure it should be repaired.
3. Exposure of the depressed fragment is frequently facilitated by retracting the lateral cortical fragment laterally, thus opening the proximal tibia like a book still hinged posteriorly (Figure 10.15).
4. The depressed central articular fracture is then elevated with a periosteal elevator (Figure 10.16). A determination can be made as to the amount of bone loss beneath

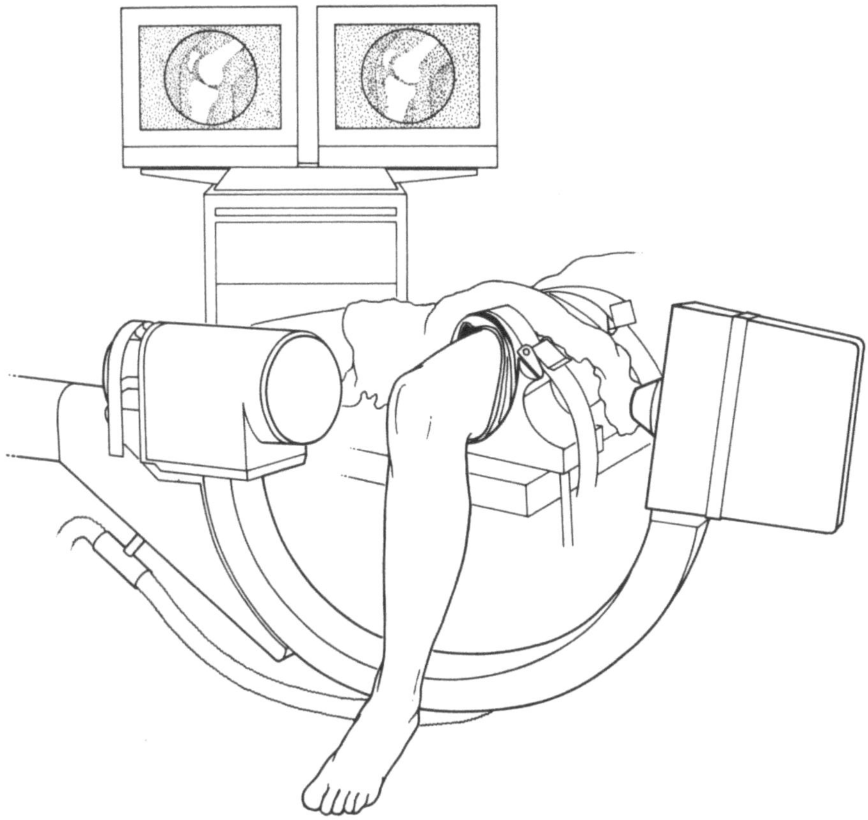

**FIGURE 10.14.** This position allows reduction by ligamentotaxis free access for fluoroscopy, arthroscopy, and for fixation.

the articular and subchondral bone. If necessary, an autogenous iliac crest bone graft is prepared and placed.

5. The hinged lateral fragment is closed. Two 3.2- × 230-mm guide pins are placed approximately 1 cm distal to the joint surface. It is not necessary to predrill the cortex of the tibia at this level. After the first guide is placed, the buttress plate is held with the first guide pin through one of the proximal holes. Using the buttress plate as a template, a second guide pin is placed in the center of the open hole in the buttress plate, then advanced parallel with the original guide pin (Figure 10.17).
6. The guide pins should be passed until their threads engage into the opposite medial tibial cortex. This is confirmed by fluoroscopy.
7. The depth can be read directly off the guide pin or with the depth gauge.
8. The first cannulated screw is placed through the appropriate hole in the buttress plate, advanced over the guide pin, and then driven through the opposite ("far") cortex. *Note*: The self-cutting, self-tapping tip is a major advantage over those cannulated screws that are not self-cutting and self-tapping. Those screws, which require guide pin overreaming and tapping, disengage the guide pin in the far cortex. The threaded guide pin is placed in the far cortex. This then maintains the position of the cannulated screw as it advances itself through the cortex.
9. The second screw is then advanced over its guide pin.
10. Both screws are then tightened with the

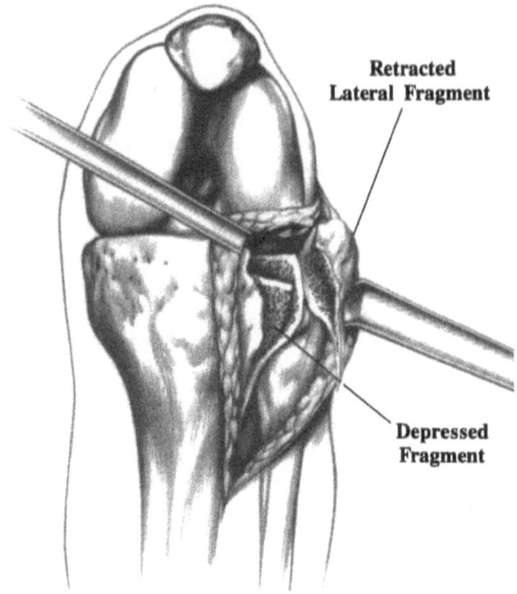


**FIGURE 10.15.** The depressed lateral plateau fragment is often exposed by retracting a lateral cortico-cancellous fragment. (Reprinted with permission from Asnis.[24])

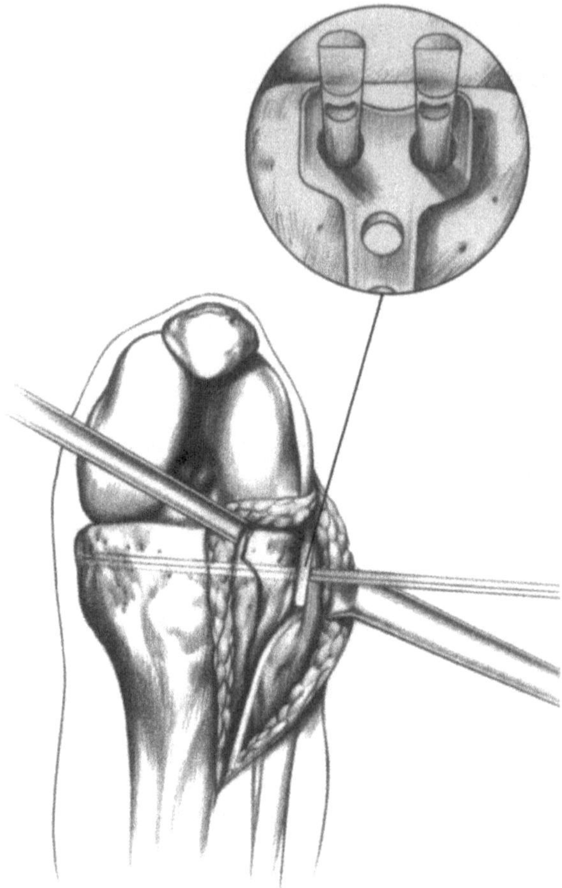

**FIGURE 10.17.** The buttress plate is used as a template for the placement of parallel 3.2 mm guide pins. (Reprinted with permission from Asnis.[24])

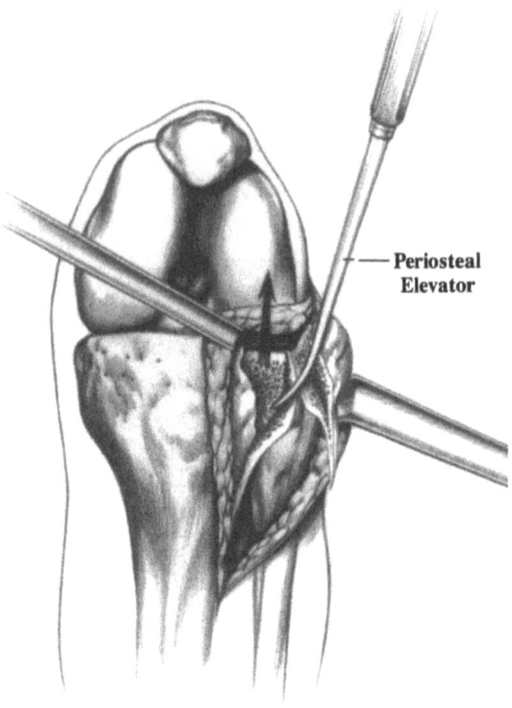


**FIGURE 10.16.** The depressed central articular fracture is elevated with a periosteal elevator. (Reprinted with permission from Asnis.[24])

cannulated screwdriver. If either screw is found to be too long as the fracture compresses, it is replaced with a shorter screw while the second screw holds the fracture compressed. One or two screw threads should pass beyond the medial cortex to provide optimal fixation.

11. The guide pins are removed, and the distal end of the plate is attached to the tibial shaft with cortical screws (Figure 10.18).
12. The lateral meniscus is reattached anteriorly and peripherally. Soft tissues are closed, and a bulky leg dressing and knee immobilizer splint applied.

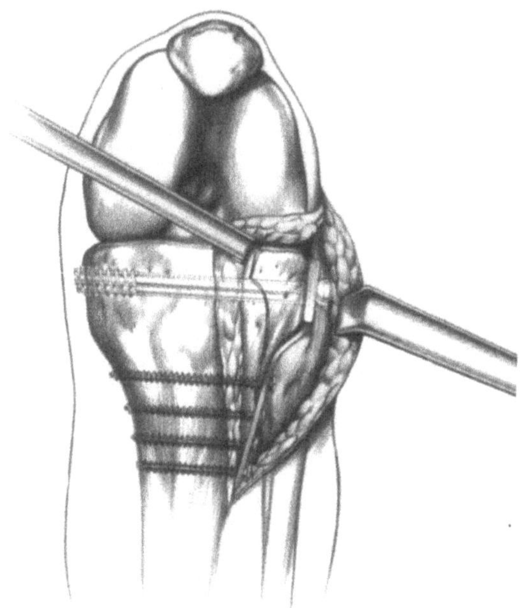

FIGURE 10.18. The 6.5 mm self-tapping cannulated screws are placed over the guide pins. The guide pins are then removed and the distal end of the plate is attached to the tibial shaft with 4.5 mm solid cortical screws. (Reprinted with permission from Asnis.[24])

## Operative Technique for Simple Split Fractures of the Tibial Plateau

When the fractures are slightly separated, yet not depressed, they can often be fixed percutaneously (Figure 10.19).

1. The skin is opened 1 cm distal to the joint line. The first guide pin is then passed through the opposite tibial cortex (Figure 10.20).
2. A second 1-cm incision is then made, and a second guide pin placed. Pin guides can be used to make the guide pins parallel. This is important to allow compression of the fracture. Fluoroscopy confirms the pins' positions.
3. The depth gauge is placed under the guide pin and against the near cortex. Appropriately sized screws are selected.
4. The first screw is then placed through a washer (optional), then over a guide pin, and advanced until compression is applied.

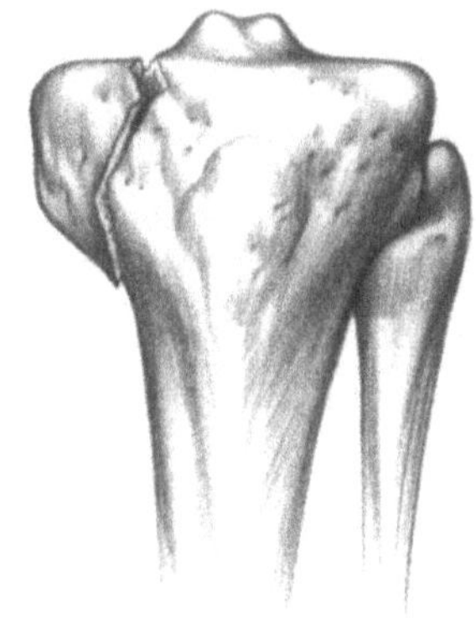

FIGURE 10.19. The slightly separated plateau fractures can usually be fixed percutaneously. (Reprinted with permission from Asnis.[24])

The second screw is similarly placed (Figure 10.21).

5. The guide pins are removed and the skin closed.

Bicondylar fractures required a midline incision or a lateral hockey stick incision. Generally in our series the incision was made on the side of the significant injury. No fracture underwent double plating. Longitudinal midline incisions were used whenever possible to avoid difficulties with total knee replacement or other surgical procedures in the future. When ligamentotaxis failed to reduce the fracture, a drill portal

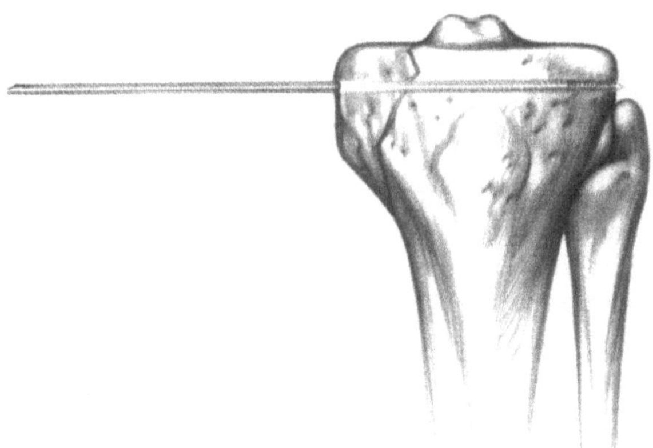

FIGURE 10.20. The 3.2 mm guide pins are placed across the fracture and to the opposite tibial cortex. (Reprinted with permission from Asnis.[24])

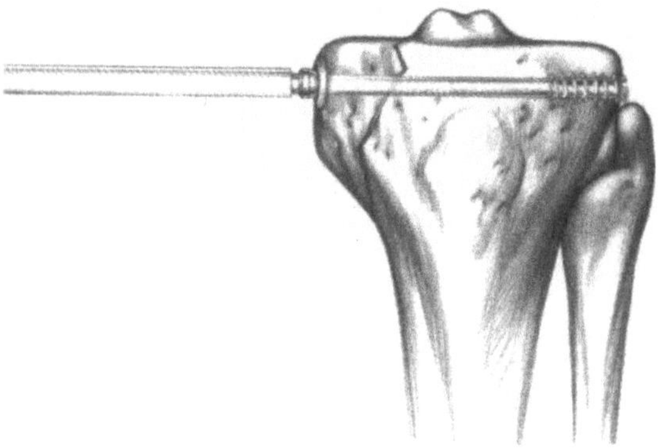

FIGURE 10.21. The 6.5 mm self-tapping cannulated screws are passed over the guide pins and tightened to compress the fracture. (Reprinted with permission from Asnis.[24])

from below was used to allow elevation of depressed fragments with a curette or bone tamp. Autogenous iliac crest bone grafter bone graft substitute is then inserted to support the articular surface (Figure 10.5). Pelvic and acetabular fracture instruments were found to be beneficial in fracture reduction and compression of bony fragments.

All medial plateau or bicondylar fractures with an intact fibula are fixed regardless of examination because of the potential to drift into varus or collapse.[22] Routine fixation is preferred in patients who have concomitant severe lower extremity or pelvic fractures to facilitate mobilization and transfer. Fractures that extend to the tibial diaphysis are stabilized with an external fixator. The plateau fracture is usually stabilized first.

Arthroscopic fixation and joint evaluation have been utilized in the authors' experience. They have been helpful in obtaining and evaluating the reduction. Arthroscopic-assisted reduction as a routine tool in reduction of plateau fractures should be considered experimental at the present time. This study found that simple split or split/decompression-type fractures are amenable to arthroscopic-assisted reduction techniques. However, more complex fracture patterns become more technically challenging, and visualization is more difficult secondary to bleeding. An Esmarch bandage should be used to prevent extravasation of arthroscopic fluid. Time is important during arthroscopy as the irrigation can cause a compartment syndrome. Use of the Esmarch and rapid visualization decrease this problem. Intraarticular injuries such as meniscal tears or ligament reconstruction can be done after fracture healing on an elective basis or acutely via arthroscopy or limited arthrotomy.

## Clinical Results of a Long-Term Follow-Up of Operative Fixation for Tibial Plateau Fractures

Greater than 12 months' follow-up was obtained in 55 out of 75 patients treated between 1988 and 1992, using a prospective tibial plateau protocol with examination of the knee in extension as the determinant of operative stabilization. Thirty-five patients were male and 20 female. The left extremity was injured in 29 patients and the right in 26. Six fractures were open injuries. Three were grade I, two were grade II, and one was grade IIIB injury by Gustilo's classification.[8] The average age was 44 years with a range from 18 to 83 years.

The mechanism of injury was a motor vehicle accident in 19 patients, and a motorcycle accident in seven patients. Pedestrian versus motor vehicle accidents accounted for nine injuries, 11 fractures were due to falls, and miscellaneous injuries occurred in nine cases.

Associated injuries occurred in 49% of the patients. Twenty-four patients sustained multiple fractures ranging from complex pelvic fractures to long bone fractures. Meniscal injuries occurred in four patients. There was one anterior cruciate ligament (ACL) and one medial collateral ligament (MCL) injury. One arterial injury resulted in an above-the-knee amputation. Two nerve contusions occurred. Five patients required prophylactic fasciotomies for elevated compartment pressures.

Eight fractures were noted to be stable and were treated via cast bracing. Thirty-six patients were treated by percutaneous cannulated screws. Five of these were in combination with an external fixator or intramedullary rod. Thirty-one fractures were reduced by ligamentotaxis alone. Two fractures were treated by traction methods due to soft tissue injuries—skin abrasions and fracture blisters that precluded surgery. Ten fractures required supplemental iliac crest bone graft. Eight fractures required open reduction and internal fixation with buttress plates. This treatment method was used in one patient who had a 3-week delay in treatment, and four others were judged by the attending surgeon to have inadequate reduction with limited internal fixation. Two of the eight patients were treated with buttress plating because of marked obesity, which was thought to be a deterrent to successful postoperative bracing.

Fourteen of the patients who had reduction and fixation with cannulated screws also had arthroscopic evaluation at the time of surgery.

Results were assessed using Rasmussen's criteria. A score was assigned to each patient from 0 to 30. The categories used to assess functional outcome were pain, walking capacity, extension, range of motion, and stability.

Fifty-five patients had greater than 12 months' follow-up. Three patients died, and the patient requiring an above-the-knee amputation was excluded. Six patients were from other states and could not be located. Ten additional patients also could not be located; two of these were last seen at a nursing home and eight had no permanent address. All fractures included in this study were healed at the time of follow-up.

Patients with a Rasmussen's score of 20 or greater were considered acceptable results. Twenty-seven fracture results were excellent, 20 good, 10 fair, and none poor. The average score for all patients was 25.9 with a range of 11 to 30. The average score for stable fractures treated with cast bracing was 29. The average score for C3-type fractures was 22.74.

Complications occurred in four patients. Superficial infections occurred in external fixator pin tracts in one case, which were treated with antibiotics and local pin tract care without residual problems. Deep infections occurred in three patient: two were treated with buttress plating required repeat debridement and local wound care, and the third patient was treated with limited internal and external fixation, and subsequently a knee arthrodesis.

There were seven clinical failures according to Rasmussen's criteria. All were AO C3-type fractures. Two were treated by buttress plates with iliac crest bone grafts. Three were treated with limited internal screw fixation and an external fixator. Two of these patients were treated with percutaneous screw fixation alone. The overall failure rate was 13% for the 55 cases in whom adequate follow-up was obtained. The complication rate was 7%. Excellent results were obtained in all patients who had stable knee examinations with no complications. Good/excellent functional results were obtained in all fracture classifications except the AO C3 fracture pattern. The severely comminuted bicondylar fracture pattern had the highest complication rate regardless of treatment type.

Arthroscopic evaluation postreduction in this series and in the previous study reveals the lateral plateau to be consistently well covered by the lateral meniscus, which therefore is the true weight-bearing surface. In contrast, the medial condylar fracture frequently was much more involved. Extensive fracture patterns with split central depression osteochondral defects in the weight-bearing surface medial to the meniscus were much more common than lateral plateau patterns. An intact fibula associated with a medial condylar fracture may also aggravate the problem in the medial compartment by contributing to a varus deformity.[12] Fixation of medial or bicondylar fractures prevents varus deformity. One patient in our series with a medial plateau fracture and intact fibula was treated with a cast brace and developed slight varus (2°).

All seven failures in this study were AO C3 tibial plateau fractures. Percutaneous screw fixation alone or in combination with external fixation may not necessarily lead to a satisfactory result as the failure rate was 30% in this group. The type of treatment was not predictive of results in patients with AO C3 fractures in our study.

In one patient that had an ORIF with an iliac crest bone graft, an anatomic reduction on postoperative x-ray was obtained. He was a clinical failure. The reduction, however, made subsequent total knee arthroplasty (TKA) much easier. The authors recommend in these severely comminuted tibial plateau fractures that the incision should be made midline so that subsequent arthroplasties or arthrodesis can be done without soft tissue complications. This study substantiates the importance of the examination of the knee in extension. All patients with stable knees treated by cast bracing had excellent results. Ligamentotaxis for reduction and percutaneous or limited open reduction and internal fixation is successful in all but AO C3 fractures. Treatment of severely comminuted fractures must be individualized to include soft tissue consideration, bone quality, surgical experience, and overall patient compliance and expectations. Newer reduction clamps assist the surgeon intraoperatively. Arthroscopic evaluation of the reduction is helpful, but in polytrauma situations it is not always practical.

## References


1. Agnew SG, Benirschke SK, Mayo KA, et al. Open reduction internal fixation of complex proximal tibial fractures. *J Orthop Trauma* 1991;5: 236.
2. Blokker CP, Rorabeck CH, Bourne RB. Tibial plateau fractures. An analysis of the results of treatment in 60 patients. *Clin Orthop* 1984;182: 193–199.
3. Rombold C. Depressed fractures of the tibial plateau. Treatment with rigid internal fixation and early mobilization. A preliminary report. *J Bone Joint Surg* 1960;42A:783–797.
4. Schatzker J, McBroom R, Bruce D. The tibial plateau fracture. The Toronto experience 1968–1975. *Clin Orthop* 1979;138:94–104.
5. Tscherne H, Lobenhoffer P. Tibial plateau fractures. Management and expected results. *Clin Orthop* 1993;292:87–100.
6. Apley AG. Fractures of the lateral tibial condyle treated by skeletal traction and early mobilization. A review of sixty cases with specific reference to the long-term results. *J Bone Joint Surg* 1956;38B:699–708.
7. Brown GA, Sprague BL. Cast brace treatment of plateau and bicondylar fractures of the proximal tibia. *Clin Orthop* 1976;119:184–193.
8. Drennan DB, Locher FG, Maylahn DJ. Fractures of the tibial plateau. Treatment by closed reduction and spica cast. *J Bone Joint Surg* 1979;61A: 989–995.
9. Duwelius PJ, Connolly JF. Closed reduction of tibial plateau fractures. A comparison of functional and roentgenographic end result. *Clin Orthop* 1988;230:116–126.
10. Holzach P, Matter P, Minter J. Arthroscopically assisted treatment of lateral tibial plateau fractures in skiers: use of a cannulated reduction system. *J Orthop Trauma* 1994;8:273–281.
11. Koval KJ, Sanders R, Borrelli J, et al. Indirect reduction and percutaneous screw fixation of displaced tibial plateau fractures. *J Orthop Trauma* 1992;6(3):340–346.
12. Rasmussen PS. Tibial condylar fractures. Impairment of knee joint stability as an indication for surgical treatment. *J Bone Joint Surg* 1973;55A: 1331–1350.
13. Scotland T, Wardlaw D. The use of cast-bracing as treatment for fractures of the tibial plateau. *J Bone Joint Surg* 1981;63B:575–578.
14. Lansinger O, Bergman B, Korner L, et al. Tibial condylar fractures. A twenty-year follow-up. *J Bone Joint Surg* 1985;68A:13–19.
15. Walker PS, Erkman MJ. The role of menisci in force transmission across the knee. *Clin Orthop* 1975;109:184–192.
16. Bucholz RW, Carlton A, Holmes R. Interporous hydroxyapatite as a bone graft substitute in tibial plateau fractures. *Clin Orthop* 1989;240:53–62.
17. Bennett WF, Browner B. Tibial plateau fractures: a study of associated soft tissue injuries. *J Orthop Trauma* 1994;8:183–188.
18. Delmarter RB, Hohl M, Hopp E Jr. Ligament injuries associated with tibial plateau fractures. *Clin Orthop* 1990;250:226–233.
19. Vangsness CT Jr, Ghaderi B, Hohl M, et al. Arthroscopy of meniscal injuries with tibial plateau fractures. *J Bone Joint Surg* 1994;76B:488–490.
20. Benirschke SK, Agnew SG, Mayo KA, et al. Immediate internal fixation of open, complex tibial plateau fractures: treatment by a standard protocol. *J Orthop Trauma* 1992;6:78–86.
21. Gustilo RB. Current concepts in management of open fractures. *Instr Course Lect* 1987;36:357–369.
22. Sarmiento A, Kinman PB, Latta LL. Fractures of the proximal tibia and tibial condyles: a clinical and laboratory comparative study. *Clin Orthop* 1979;145:136–145.
23. Koval JK, Helfet DI. Tibial plateau fractures: evaluation and treatment. *J Am Acad Orthop Surg* 1995;3(2):86–93.
24. Asnis SE. The Asnis 2 guided screw system: Howmedica Surgical Techniques. Rutherford, NJ, 1991; 6–8.

# 11

# The Knee: Arthroscopic Surgery with Screw Fixation

Robert E. Schwartz

## Advantages of Cannulated Screws

Cannulated screws and arthroscopic surgery share the common advantage of being minimally invasive to the patient. Just as large dissections are no longer needed for many of the surgical procedures performed with arthroscopy, cannulated screws allow fracture work to be done indirectly with minimal surgical exposure. This results in less surgical morbidity, rapid healing, and a potential for an earlier recovery.

Cannulated screws offer multiple benefits over conventional screws in arthroscopic surgery. First, a cannulated screw travels down a wire "pathway" and can always be retrieved as long as the guide wire remains seated in the bone intended to receive the screw. In comparison, a conventional screw may be lost inside the joint during an arthroscopy, as it can fall off the end of a screwdriver.

Second, conventional screws, if not directed manually exactly down the intended drill path, will miss the far side drill hole and will separate the fragment or fracture intended to be fixed. Achieving correct screw alignment may be more difficult in arthroscopic surgery, as the view provided by the arthroscope is two-dimensional. However, the intraarticular space is three-dimensional. This discrepancy opens the possibility of an error in the third dimension resulting in inaccurate screw insertion. A cannulated screw will follow the guide wire and eliminates insertion alignment errors.

Third, when utilizing a cannulated screw, the final resting place of the screw can be predicted visually and/or radiographically prior to drilling. This allows more accuracy in screw placement and less potential for harm to the repair or fixation site. For example, changing a guide wire position if it is undesirable will have little effect on the repair construct. However, changing a screw once seated can cause a significant problem with poor purchase by the next screw. Guide wires also are important when more than one screw is planned to be used and interference between screws is to be avoided.

Fourth, the guide wire can be used to assist in the manipulation and reduction of a free osteochondral fragment. Once the fragment is aligned, reduced, and held provisionally by a guide wire it can be moved away from its correct position temporarily by pulling the fragment along the guide wire. This allows debridement to be performed on either the fragment or the crater and allows an easy re-reduction prior to internal fixation.

Finally, the cannulation within the screw can serve as a locating device. This is particularly helpful when attempting to remove a previously seated intraarticular cannulated screw. The guide wire is used as a probe to locate the cannulation in the screw head. Once the cannulation is found, the guide wire is pushed into the cannulation. The wire now serves as a guide for the screwdriver to follow to assist in screw removal.

Because of these benefits, cannulated screws are most commonly used with arthroscopy for osteochondritis dissecans (OCD) and tibial plateau fractures. Interference fit fixation in anterior cruciate ligament reconstruction is discussed in Chapter 12.

## Osteochondritis Dissecans

Osteochondritis dissecans presents in a juvenile onset and an adolescent/adult form. The juvenile onset carries with it a better prognosis and can most commonly be treated nonoperatively with limited weight bearing and immobilization.[1] Lesions that are large or involve the weight-bearing areas have been reported to have a worse prognosis with up to 50% of these types of lesions failing conservative treatment.[2,3] Furthermore Twyman[4] has shown radiographic degenerative change in up to 32% in juvenile OCD patients followed long term. The later onset form of the disease is less likely to heal and commonly requires operative intervention.

Many etiologies have been considered for OCD. Direct trauma to the knee in flexion, vascular/ischemic events, and abnormal epiphyseal ossification have all been postulated.[5,6] An excellent review article that covers this area has been written by Clanton and Delee,[7] and cites 97 references.

The arthroscopic appearance of OCD lesions can be divided into the following categories: type I—intact articular surfaces, not mobile; type II—early separation lesion (intact articular cartilage but fragment is mobile); type III—disrupted articular surfaces (flap or window-type lesion); and type IV, crater with loose or fragmented lesion.[8,9]

## Historical Background

Current treatment of OCD still follows Smillie's[10] original treatment recommendations from 1957. He described treating type I lesions by drilling from the intraarticular exposure defined as retrograde drilling. Type II, III, and IV lesions were treated by curettement and debridement to remove fibrous tissue, and fixation was performed with screws or pins. An attempt was made to restore the articular surface geometry by an accurate reduction of the fragment in the displaced lesions. Unfortunately, a second arthrotomy was necessary to remove fixation.

The need for a second surgical procedure was made unnecessary by utilizing bone peg fixation of the lesion as described by Bandi and Allgower[11] and others.[12,13] Internal fixation with buried Kirschner wires in addition to cortical bone peg grafts was reported by Scott and Stevenson[14] in 1971. This procedure also did not require a second arthrotomy to remove the pins except when there was migration of the pins into the joint.

With the advent of arthroscopic surgery, it became possible to address OCD with less morbidity. Ewing and Voto[8] described 72% satisfactory results in 29 patients with excision and retrograde drilling of the lesions arthroscopically. Guhl[9] described arthroscopic treatment of OCD, which involved drilling type I lesions, pinning type II, and curettement and pinning of type III lesions. Type IV lesions were replaced, if possible and arthroscopically bone grafted. Guhl utilized pin fixation inserted through the metaphysis into the lesion defined as an antegrade method of fixation. Lipscomb et al.[15] were the first to describe this method, which allowed for easy removal of the Kirschner wires. The wires that fix the lesion are drilled into the articular surface and out the adjacent metaphyseal cortex. They are left long on the metaphyseal side and remain subcutaneous, so that their removal is easily performed under local anesthesia after healing.

Use of cannulated compression screw fixation for OCD was first described in 1984 by Johnson[16]; 4.0-mm cannulated screws were designed specifically to be used for arthroscopic treatment of OCD. Johnson's technique followed Smillie's[17] principles of debridement of fibrous tissue in the interface of the lesion, freshening of the crater to bleeding bone, and cancellous grafting to fill voids left by the debridement. The procedure mandated non–weight bearing for 2 months and a second arthroscopic surgery for removal of screws. Eighty-four percent satisfactory results were reported.[18]

In 1984, the Herbert screw was reported for intraosseous use in scaphoid fractures.[19] This screw is a unique design as it has no head but instead has a second set of threads (trailing threads) in place of the screw head. Compression is applied to the repair site by using a differential thread pitch in the head and leading thread zone of the screw. The leading thread pitch is greater than the trailing thread pitch. The pitch difference results in the leading threads

**TABLE 11.1.** Small cannulated lag screw mechanical specifications commonly used in arthroscopy, by manufacturer.

| Manufacturer | Thread diameter (mm) | Shaft diameter (mm) | Head diameter (mm) | Guide pin diameter (mm) | Pitch (mm) | Material | Design |
|---|---|---|---|---|---|---|---|
| Ace | 4.0 | 2.8 | 6.35 | 1.6 | 1.8 | Ti 6Al 4V | Conventional |
| Instrument Makar | 4.0 | 2.3 | 6.0 | 0.9 | 2.0 | 316L stainless | Conventional |
| Synthes | 4.0 | 2.4 | 5.0 | 1.25 | 1.75 | 316L stainless | Conventional |
| Zimmer Herbert/Whipple | 3.0 (leading) | 2.5 | 3.9 (trailing) | 1.0 | 1.22 (leading) 1.0 (trailing) | Titanium | Differential pitch |

traveling farther with an insertional revolution than the trailing threads travel. Therefore, compression occurs across the fixation site with insertion.

Herbert screws were described for use in fixation in OCD first by Lange et al.[20] in 1986 and later by Thomson[21] in 1987. Subsequent to those reports, the cannulated Herbert/Whipple bone screw was developed. The Herbert/Whipple screw retained the original leading and trailing thread major diameters of the original Herbert screw, but because of the cannulation the minor diameter increased from 1.75 to 2.5 mm (Table 11.1). The consequences of a larger minor diameter, and therefore a lesser thread depth, is reduced pullout strength.[22]

Shaw[23] demonstrated superiority of a conventional 4.0-mm cancellous lag screw compared with a single Herbert screw in pedilen polyurethane foam simulated scaphoid bones and cadaver bone specimens. Herbert screws were able to generate only 20% of the compressive forces generated by the 4.0-mm cancellous lag screws.

Lange[20] compared the 4.0-mm synthes cancellous lag screw to one and also two Herbert screws in matched vertebral body pullout tests. The 4.0-mm cancellous screw produced a mean pullout strength of 98.4 N (newtons) $\pm$ 4.2 N (mean $\pm$ standard error of the mean). The single Herbert screw pullout strength was 56.5 N $\pm$ 5.8 N. However, two Herbert screws tested together produced a pullout force of 129.2 N $\pm$ 5.0 N.

From these findings, use of more than one Herbert screw is necessary to approach the mechanical performance achieved by a single 4.0-mm cancellous screw. At this time there has not been any direct comparison between cannulated lag screws and cannulated Herbert/Whipple bone screws. One could postulate that the pullout performance of both would be reduced as a direct proportion of the reduced thread depth necessary to accommodate the guide wire pathway through the shaft diameter[24] (see Chapter 2).

Despite the reduced pullout forces and compressive forces achieved by the Herbert screw, not having a head may have an advantage over a 4.0-mm cannulated screw with a head diameter of 5.0 mm. The smaller size of the trailing threads (3.9 mm) theoretically may cause less damage to the articular cartilage during insertion. Another advantage is that Herbert screws are designed to be countersunk into the subchondral bone. This allows them to remain without removal and obviate the need for a later surgical procedure.

## Principles of Surgical Treatment

At this time there does not seem to be a need for internal fixation in type I lesions. The lesions that are symptomatic are uncommon in adults, and are usually seen prior to epiphyseal closure in children. Symptomatic type I OCD lesions can be drilled to a depth of 2.0 cm with non-threaded diamond-point tip 2-mm-diameter depth-marked Kirschner wires, as described by Aglietti et al.[25]

Type II lesions should be drilled the same as a type I lesion. Fixation with a cannulated compression screw should then be performed as described by Johnson.[16,18] If this fixation method results in significant fragment depression, one cannot expect the region involved to participate in physiologically normal load sharing with the surrounding intact articular cartilage. Also a significant depression is most likely to be associated with a large lucent zone in the subchondral bone on radiographs and should be anticipated to need bone grafting.

Retrograde bone grafting[26,27] is an attractive alternative for type II lesions. The subchondral center of the lesion is drilled from the metaphyseal side and packed with bone graft. This procedure is more involved and carries the risk of fracture of the femoral condyle, or conversion to a type III lesion.[17] In addition, internal fixation may be more difficult to achieve as the compression screw does not have as large an intact epiphyseal bony bed to attach to securely.

Transarticular debridement and bone grafting to raise the articular surface[16] and subsequent internal fixation with multiple Herbert/Whipple screws may maintain articular surface geometry better than lag screw techniques alone. Bone grafting offers some resistance to compressive forces that tend to depress the repaired fragment during fixation and physiologic loading. However, Johnson[18] reported that depression of the articular fragment after fixation did not adversely affect the clinical result in his experience.

Type III lesions routinely require bone grafting to reestablish articular contours. After debridement of granulation tissue, there commonly is loss of subchondral bone in the fragment and bed of the lesion. If possible, the lesion should be elevated from the intact cartilage in a fashion that takes into consideration preservation of the articular surface and preservation of any blood supply. Commonly with classic medial condyle lesions there is a soft tissue attachment with synovium at the posterior cruciate ligament. This should be spared. The bed of the lesion is debrided to remove soft tissue and prepared with Steadman picks.™ Low-density cancellous bone graft is harvested from the tibial metaphysis and delivered to the crater as described by Johnson.[16]

Type IV lesions commonly become larger if loose in the joint for any period of time. This is due to articular cartilage overgrowth from the loss of the normal contact inhibition of the cells at the periphery of the lesion and edge of the crater. Principles of debridement of the lesion and bed, cancellous bone grafting to restore articular congruity, and internal fixation also apply to these lesions.

Extremely large lesions often involving posterior femoral condyle locations undergo fragmentation and compression damage due to the high loads experienced by the fragment when there is no surrounding intact articular surface and bone to protect the fragment. In these circumstances fresh osteoarticular allografts[28,29] may be the only reasonable option to repair the defect without resorting to prosthetic replacements.

## Results After Surgical Repair

Type I OCD lesions treated by transarticular drilling show good to excellent result, with 95% healing in preadolescent type I lesions.[25] Type II or III lesions treated with K-wire fixation as reported by Guhl[9] had less than 80% healing. Herbert screw fixation treatment of type II or III lesions were found to have an 88% healing rate in the series reported by Thomson.[21]

Johnson et al.[18] reported 94% early healing of OCD treated by 4.0-mm cannulated screw fixation in a series of 35 knees when evaluated by second-look arthroscopy at 8 weeks postoperative. Two failures were identified early and four failures occurred later, representing an average overall successful healing rate of 83%. It should be noted that 11 of 35 were reoperations in this series.

Convery[28] reported 76% successful results in 90 knees treated with fresh osteochondral allografts for large osteochondral defects of the knee. Garrett[29] reported 94% successful results in patients followed 2 to 9 years after treating lateral condyle OCD lesions with fresh osteochondral allografts.

## Author's Arthroscopic Surgical Technique: 4.0-mm Cannulated Screws

An initial three-portal arthroscopy approach is used. A 5.0-mm outflow cannula is placed superior and medial through the vastus medialis muscle. This cannula should be placed in a more cephalad position than usual so that it can be introduced and remain in the medial gutter. This ensures better flow rates with the knee flexed than when the cannula is in the suprapatellar pouch. When approaching the most common medial femoral condyle OCD lesions, the arthroscope is placed in the midpatella lateral portal to visualize the intercondylar notch and medial compartment. Usually the ligamentum mucosa and a portion of the fat pad must be resected to allow good visualization of the defect with the knee in flexion. This point is most important with the more posterior lesions. The geographic limits of the lesion can usually be defined best by loading the center of the lesion with a large blunt probe or trocar and observing the surface behavior of the surrounding articular cartilage. This is important in type II and III incomplete lesions as the articular involvement is commonly much larger than the radiographic appearance. Once the limits of the lesion are defined, treatment decisions based on size and separation can be made. If the lesion location and periphery cannot be accurately determined, fluoroscopy is used to delineate the lesion.

Type I lesions do not require internal fixation. These lesions if symptomatic require only arthroscopic transarticular drilling through a central articular access drill hole. For each 1.0 $cm^2$ area, a single articular cartilage access channel should be used allowing three to four diverging bone channels to be drilled using a smooth diamond point tip 2.0-mm Kirschner™ wire.[25] The author has found that the best perpendicular access frequently involves resting the wire on the anterior margin of the tibial plateau in the midline, through the patellar tendon, and traversing just cephalad to the anterior horn attachment of the medial meniscus to reach the OCD lesion in the medial femoral condyle. This usually requires that the arthroscope be placed in the midpatella lateral visualization portal. This is to allow freedom of approach for drilling the lesion (Figure 11.1).

Postoperative treatment includes non–weight bearing for 8 weeks and a hinged postoperative knee brace. The brace range of motion limits are adjusted to prevent loading of the repair site for activities of daily living for 6 weeks.

Type II lesions less than or equal to 1.0 $cm^2$ are treated as type I lesions with transarticular drilling with a smooth K-wire as described above. For type II lesions larger than 1.0 $cm^2$ in dimension, this author prefers Herbert/Whipple cannulated screw fixation to stabilize the fragment after drilling. This technique is discussed in the next section.

Type III lesions are elevated partially and debrided. It is advisable, if possible, to save the hinge attachment toward the intercondylar notch, preserving any synovial-derived blood supply. If the hinge attachment cannot be retained, provisional fixation by a 4.0-mm cannulated screw threaded tip guide wire (1.25 mm) is used as Herbert/Whipple screw guide wires (1.0 mm) are too fragile and bend easily. The provisional fixation is inserted obliquely from an ipsilateral portal (Figure 11.2). This is to allow easier visualization of the bony bed when the fragment is withdrawn down the wire away from the crater of the lesion (Figure 11.3). If the fragment is large, two guide wires are used to control rotation. The bony bed must be debrided of fibrous tissue utilizing a small 3.5 mm full radius shaver to remove granulation tissue and freshen the crater of the lesion. An arthroscopic burr must be used carefully as the fragment can be easily damaged (Figure 11.4). Steadman picks™ are very helpful to further prepare the base of the lesion. Alter debridement and preparation, the lesion is replaced anatomically. The decision regarding the need for bone grafting is based on the ability to achieve and restore articular surface geometry.

Cancellous bone is harvested as follows. A 6.5 mm drill hole is placed in the proximal and medial tibial metaphysis 2 to 3 cm below the epiphyseal scar. Cancellous bone from this region has a low enough density that it can be easily shaped and molded in the crater defect and not interfere in obtaining congruence when compression fixation is applied. Through the drill hole a 4.0 mm Instrument Makar Bone Grafter™ is used to harvest and deliver cancellous bone to the fragment bed (Figure 11.5).

Net the fragment is reduced into the crater. Then the guide wire for the cannulated screw should be inserted perpendicular to the articular surface of the lesion. The guide wire should also be centered in the bony lesion if one screw is planned to be used. To insure that the cannulated screw guide wire is centered fluoroscopy in two planes is utilized. If the lesion is large,

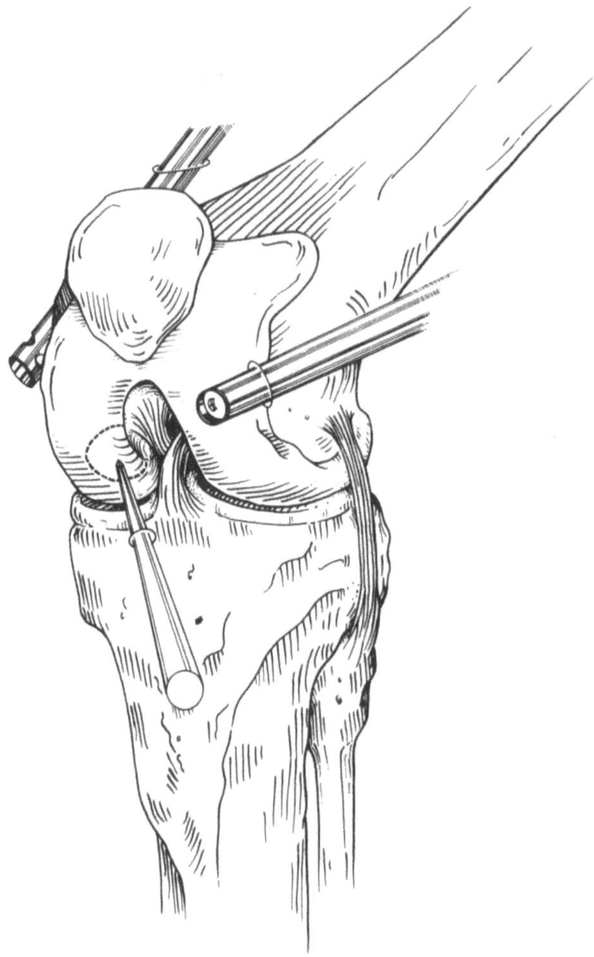

**FIGURE 11.1.** Example of a type I medial femoral condyle osteochondritis dissecans (OCD). Drilling an articular access channel perpendicular to the lesion is depicted utilizing a 2.0-mm smooth diamond-point tip Kirschner wire directed through the patellar tendon.

planning for more than one screw is necessary. If the guide wire must traverse the patellar tendon to meet the above criteria, a longitudinal 1.5-cm incision is made through that area of the tendon to allow atraumatic passage of the guide wire and screw through an 8.0-mm arthroscopic utility cannula. Next the cannulated screw measuring device is passed over the guide wire. This automatically selects a screw 5.0-mm shorter than the guide wire. Maintaining the guide wire within the femoral condyle is very helpful if retrieval of the screw is necessary. Fragment reduction is maintained by applying pressure manually to the utility cannula. The fragment is overdrilled using the 2.7-mm cannulated drill. This lessens the chance of fragmenting the lesion during screw insertion. The 4.0-mm cannulated screw can now be passed over the guide wire and through the 8.0-mm utility cannula. The screw is seated and the next guide wire is inserted if a second screw is planned to be used. Completion of one screw insertion is necessary to prevent bending of the second screw guide wire, as bent guide wires are subject to failure

repair is checked next in two planes with fluoroscopy. The screw must be seated at a subarticular level because prominence of the screw

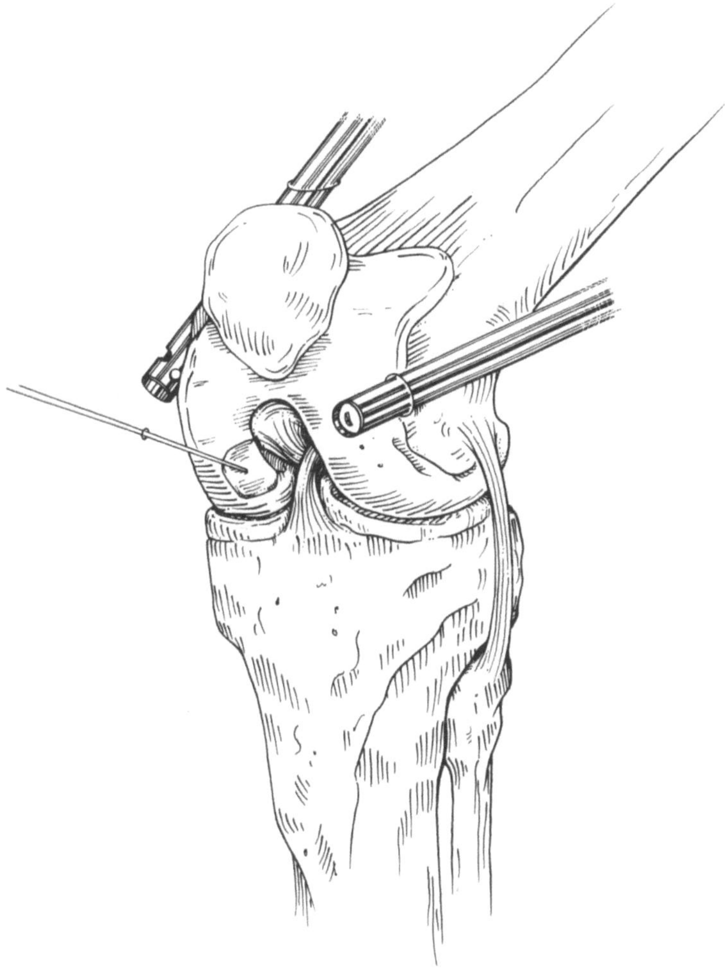

FIGURE 11.2. Use of a threaded-tip, 1.25-mm cannulated screw guide wire as a provisional fixation to assist in later replacement of a type III OCD lesion after crater debridement.

head results in predictable damage to the adjacent corresponding articulating surface.[18] The guide wires and any provisional fixation now can be removed.

Postoperative treatment includes non–weight bearing and restricting range of motion in a brace for 8 weeks. Screws are removed at a second arthroscopy before beginning weight bearing. This allows for accurate assessment of healing.

Type IV lesions present differently from the other lesions because they are free in the joint and most often do not fit correctly in the defect. If the lesion is oversized, the crater and the lesion must be debrided to fit each other anatomically. Debridement of rounding a the crater edge is best accomplished with an arthroscopic ring curette. The fragment is next manipulated into the crater defect and aligned to lie adjacent to one edge of the crater. The periphery of the fragment is fixed temporarily using a 1.25-mm threaded-tip guide wire into the periphery of the crater. This allows one edge of the fragment to be aligned with the crater's corresponding margin and the remaining free edges to remain accessible for debridement. By use of a basket punch the lesion can be reduced in size to fit the crater. Once the fragment is sized correctly it can be rotated around the peripheral guide wire fixation point exposing the bed of the lesion

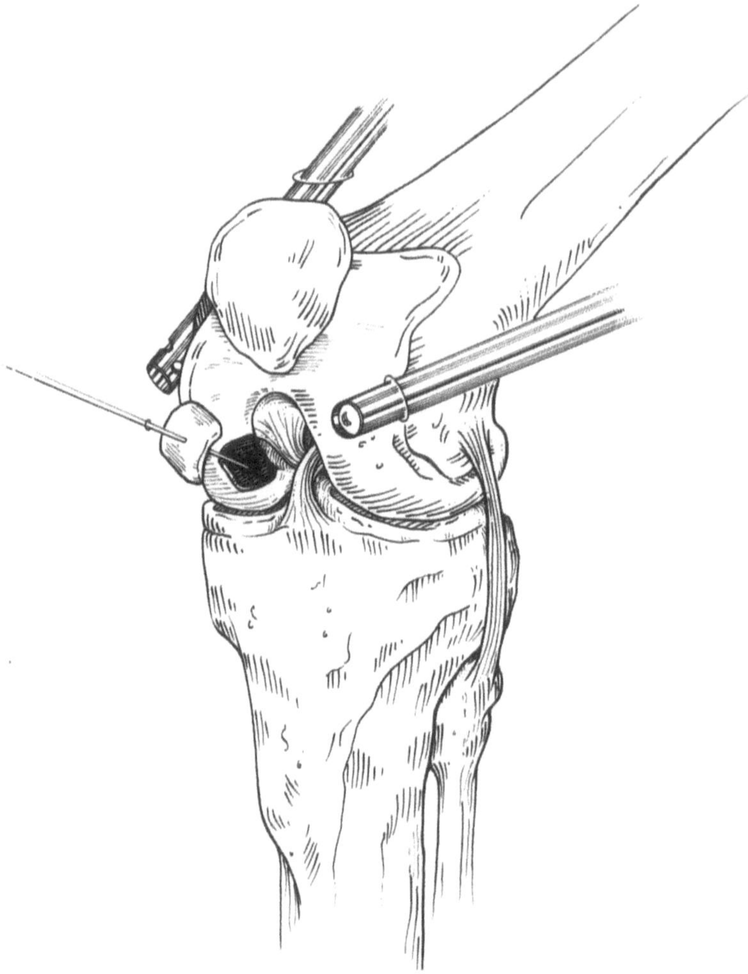

FIGURE 11.3. Displacement of the lesion away form the crater and down the provisional guide wire fixation. This allows access to the crater for debridement and cancellous bone grafting.

for grafting and definitive fixation thereafter. Because of the lesser stability of these lesions, it is best to fix them with multiple screws if size allows.

## Surgical Technique for Type II OCD: Herbert/Whipple Bone Screws

The surgical principles in treatment of OCD are unchanged from those described above when using the Herbert/Whipple cannulated bone screw. The author prefers this device for type II OCD lesions because the articular surface is intact and usually no bone grafting is needed. Successful fixation requires the bone portion of the lesion to be thick enough to support purchase by the trailing threads of the Herbert/Whipple screw. The screws are left in situ and do not require later removal.

The arthroscopic portals are set up as described above. The midpatella medial or lateral portals are very helpful to move the arthroscope from the access pathway necessary for perpendicular approach to the lesion. After anatomic reduction, the OCD cannula and obturator are placed centrally against the fracture fragment.

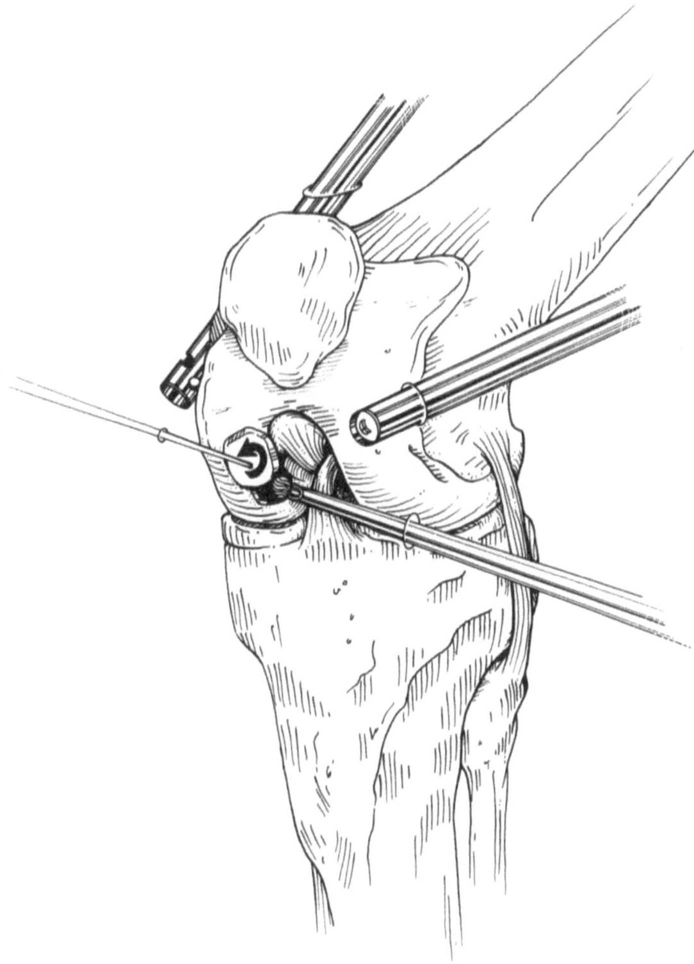

**FIGURE 11.4.** After provisional fixation of an OCD lesion the fragment also may be rotated to allow access to the crater for debridement and cancellous bone grafting.

Pressure on the cannula maintains the fracture reduction (Figure 11.6).

Using the cannulation through obturator, the 1.0-mm guide wire is drilled through the fragment and into the femoral condyle for a depth of at least 25 mm. Radiographic confirmation of the guide wire position and length is necessary. The obturator is removed and the free hand depth gauge replaces it to obtain the proper screw length (Figure 11.7).

The step drill is next set to the chosen screw length and delivered down the cannula. If the desired screw length exceeds the length of the guide wire, the guide wire should be advanced 5.0 mm beyond the desired screw length after replacing the obturator within the cannula. Continued use of the cannula lessens the likelihood of bending the guide wire. The step drill can also damage the guide wire, so drilling should be done only with a sharp drill bit and gentle axial force, taking care to not bend the guide wire (Figure 11.8). If the guide wire is removed inadvertently with drill removal, the obturator should be replaced and another guide wire should be reinserted blunt end first to assist in redirecting the wire into the original channel in the femoral condyle.

The desired screw is mounted onto the modular screwdriver and passed over the guide wire, down the cannula, and inserted into femoral

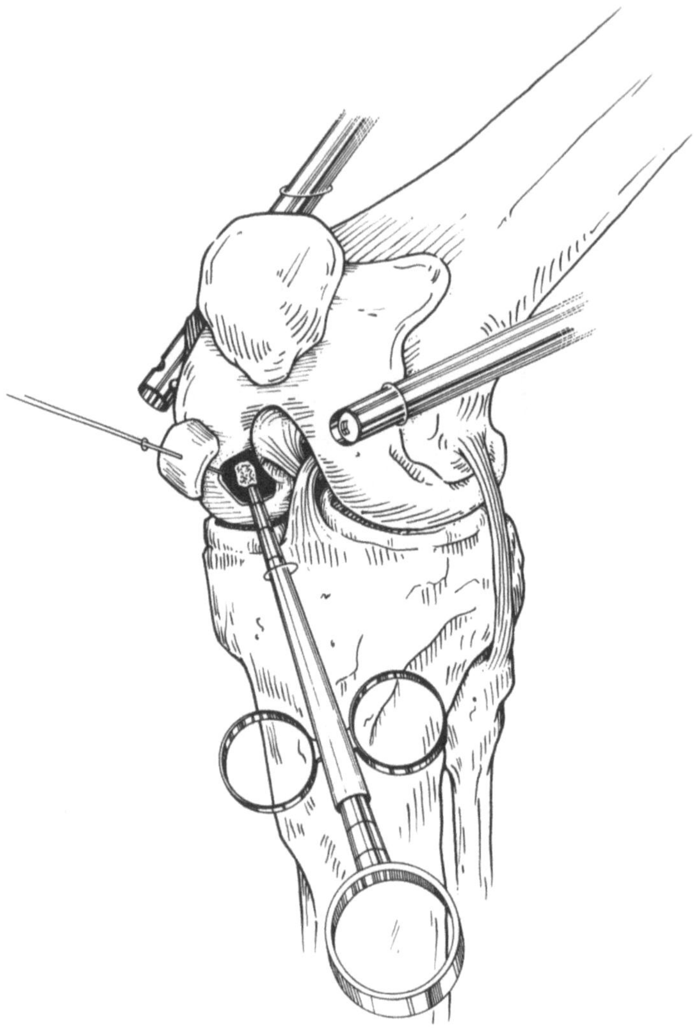

**FIGURE 11.5.** Delivery of low density cancellous bone graft to a type III OCD crater with an Instrument Makar 4.0-mm bone grafter. This elevates the lesion to achieve congruency with the surrounding articular surface.

condyle. The screwdriver has a built-in stop at the end of the cannula. Upon reaching the stop, the screwdriver should continue to be turned to allow the screw to "walk off" the end of the screwdriver and seat the screw into subchondral bone (Figure 11.9). Radiographic confirmation of the screw location and depth is now performed.

A second screw should be considered unless the fragment is smaller than 1.0 cm$^2$. The second screw guide wire must be inserted in such a way that it does not interfere with the first screw (Figure 11.10).

## Arthroscopically Assisted Cannulated Screw Fixation of Lateral Tibial Plateau Fractures

Fixation of tibial plateau fractures utilizing arthroscopic visualization was first reported by Caspari et al.[30] and Jennings[31] in separate reports in 1985. Use of cannulated screws with this technique was mentioned by Jennings. Guanche and Markman[32] described the technical steps to arthroscopic reduction and percutaneous cannulated screw fixation (ARPF) in

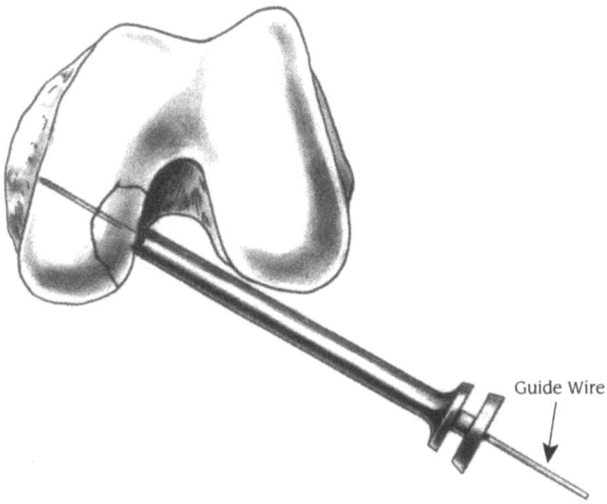


FIGURE 11.6. Herbert/Whipple cannulated screw system technique. The double sleeve OCD cannula is pressed against the lesion's articular surface to assist in perpendicular passage of the 1.0 mm threaded tip guide wire. (Reprinted with permission from Whipple.[37])

Schatzker I, II, and III fractures. Fowble et al.[33] reported the superior results obtainable by arthroscopy and percutaneous cannulated screw fixation when compared with standard open reduction and internal fixation techniques.

## Tibial Plateau Fractures Amenable to Arthroscopic Reduction and Percutaneous Fixation (ARPF)

Prior to treatment of tibial plateau fractures with ARPF, preoperative tomography, or a computed tomography (CT) scan examination is mandatory to identify fracture lines and to plan the location of the hardware. Lateral cortex comminution may preclude utilizing a percutaneous technique requiring a lateral buttress plate to maintain the reduction.

Classification of tibial plateau fractures is covered in Chapter 10. Schatzker I or a split lateral condyle fracture is an ideal fracture for ARPF. The surgical dissection necessary to perform a standard open reduction includes an anterior longitudinal incision, an arthrotomy, and frequently dissection of the lateral meniscus to adequately expose the plateau for reduction. This exposure is avoided with ARPF and fluoroscopically assisted techniques (see Chapter 3).

Schatzker II or a split compression injury of the lateral tibial condyle, also can effectively be evaluated, reduced, and repaired with arthroscopic techniques. The "open-book" dissection necessary to align the depressed area results in

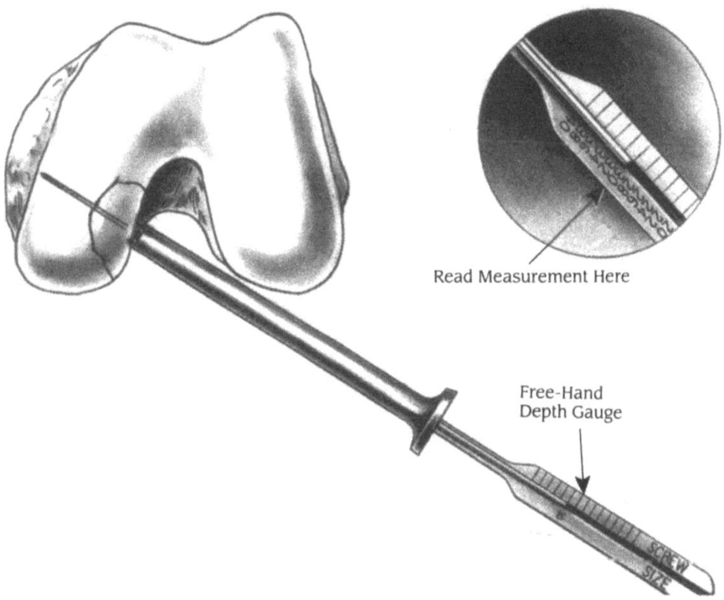


FIGURE 11.7. Herbert/Whipple cannulated screw system technique. Indirect depth gauge reads proposed drill and screw lengths off the tail of the inserted guide wire. (Reprinted with permission from Whipple.[37])

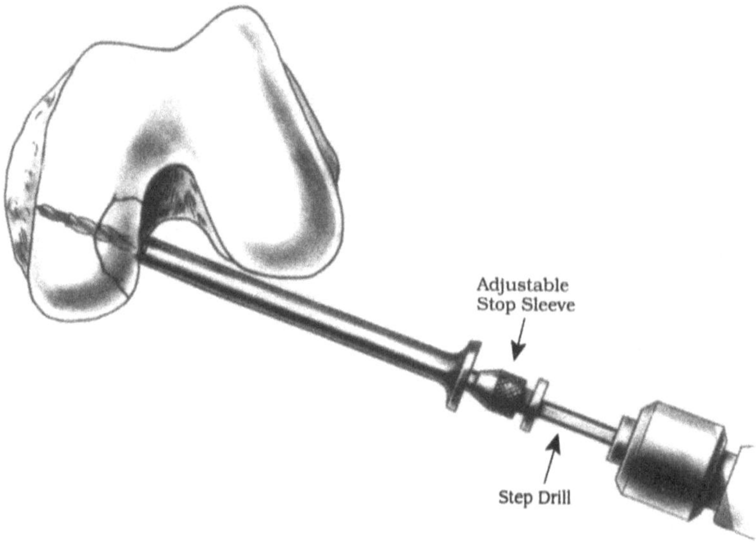


**FIGURE 11.8.** Herbert/Whipple cannulated screw system technique. Step drill passes over guide wire, inside the outer OCD cannula. Depth is controlled by setting the adjustable stop sleeve to correspond to the desired screw length. (Reprinted with permission from Whipple.[37])

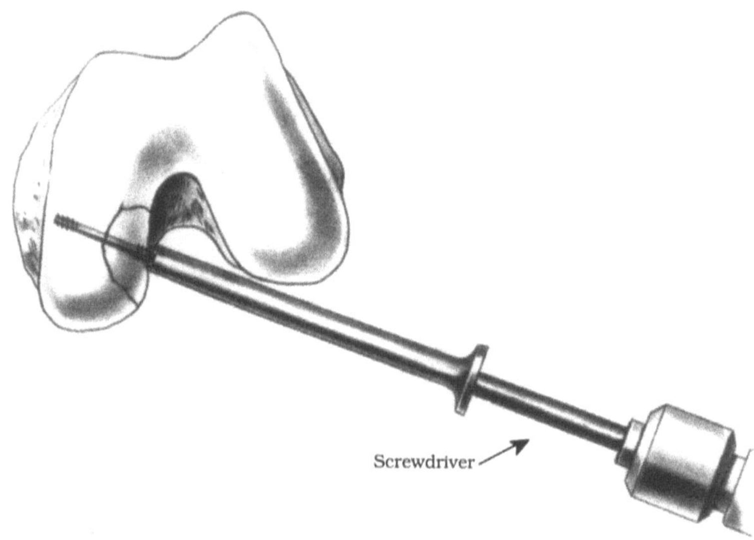


**FIGURE 11.9.** Insertion of Herbert/Whipple screw over the guide wire and through the outer OCD cannula. Once the screwdriver stop reaches the top on the cannula, the cannula is removed and the screw is advanced under direct vision to bury the trailing threads below the articular surface, into the subchondral bone of the fragment. (Reprinted with permission from Whipple.[37])

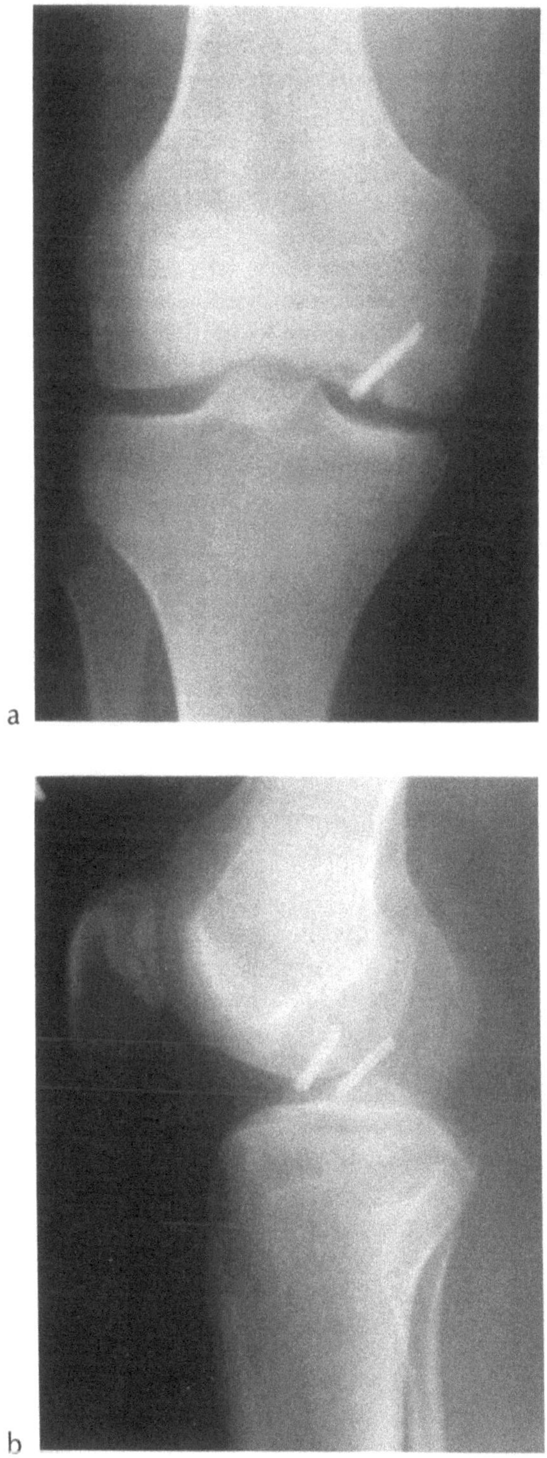

FIGURE 11.10. Anteroposterior (a) and lateral (b) radiographs of a type II OCD lesion after transarticular drilling and internal fixation with Herbert/Whipple bone screws.

significant further displacement of the split portion of the fracture and may contribute to the delayed healing with this approach when compared with ARPF.[32]

Schatzker III or central depressed lateral condyle fractures without a split component are a challenge using open techniques, also because visualization of intraarticular comminution in these fractures is extremely difficult. Arthroscopic visualization of the depressed area is easily accomplished. Creation of a lateral metaphyseal window is needed to gain access and raise the depressed lateral articular fracture fragments. Bone grafting to fill the compressed metaphyseal void created in the reduction process adds to the morbidity in open treatment of this fracture.

Percutaneous fluoroscopic techniques alone of closed reduction and percutaneous screw fixation do not allow investigation of the commonly found intraarticular injuries of the menisci and cruciates reported to accompany these fractures.[34] There is a 25% incidence of peripheral lateral meniscal tears, a 25% incidence of grade III medial collateral ligament tears and a 25% incidence of anterior cruciate ligament tears in Schatzker I, II, and III fractures. For these reasons arthroscopic evaluation of patients with tibial plateau fractures is extremely helpful.

One of the most apparent concerns with ARPF in tibial plateau fractures is egress of saline from the knee through capsular rents created at the time of injury.[35,36] Delays of 3 to 4 days after injury have been proposed to allow healing of capsular rents and to help prevent these occurrences.[35] However, with the advent of pressure-monitored arthroscopy pump systems, it is possible to maintain capsular distension and monitor fluid pressure within the knee. If capsular distension cannot be maintained at the usual intraarticular pressures, loss of intracapsular fluid must be suspected. The surgeon should pay close attention to the calf and thigh circumference in this setting and be prepared to address a compartment syndrome.

## Results of ARPF

Traditional open reduction treatment versus ARPF treatment of split compression and local compression fractures of the lateral tibial plateau were reported by Fowble et al.[33] Their results determined that in 100% of the patients treated by ARPF and fluoroscopic guidance, an anatomic reduction was achieved. In only 55% of the open reduction treatment group was an anatomic reduction achieved. Length of hospital stay was longer as was time to full weight bearing in the open reduction treatment group. Associated soft tissue injuries were comparable. Iliac crest bone graft was used in only 2 of 12 (17%) in the ARPF group and 10 of 11 (91%) of the open reduction group. They concluded that ARPF was superior to traditional open reduction methods.

## Author's Technique for Arthroscopic Reduction and Percutaneous Cannulated Screw Fixation of Lateral Tibial Plateau Fractures

After induction of anesthesia, the knee is examined for stability while visualizing the joint under fluoroscopic imaging. An arthroscopic thigh holder is used as this allows distraction of the lateral compartment while allowing an anteroposterior (AP) orientation to the knee, which assists in using the fluoroscopy equipment. AP positioning allows fluoroscopic confirmation of the reducibility of the lateral plateau with ligamentotaxis. Observation of the medial compartment fluoroscopically allows indirect examination of the medial collateral ligament integrity, which is difficult to assess if the lateral plateau is depressed or unstable. The extremity is exsanguinated and the tourniquet is inflated.

A large (5.0-mm) inflow cannula is placed into the suprapatellar pouch through a superior-medial portal. A standard anteromedial portal is established that is 1.5 cm proximal to the lateral joint line just off the lateral patellar border inferiorly. An anteromedial portal that is also proximal enough to clear the tibial eminence when crossing into the lateral compartment is also created. Intraarticular clots are cleared most rapidly using a 5.5-mm full-radius shaver.

A thorough diagnostic arthroscopy is performed to evaluate for meniscal or concomitant cruciate ligament injury. The author has found the method described by Fowble et al.[33] to be the most effective in localizing the tibial window for elevation of a depressed portion of the tibial plateau. Using an Acufex (Norwood, MA) tibial tunnel guide, a 2.0-mm smooth diamond-point tip guide wire is introduced through the central/inferior metaphyseal fracture line into the center of the depressed area in the lateral plateau (Figure 11.11). Fluoroscopic location is checked to confirm that the tunnel to be drilled will preserve the lateral cortex without splitting the lateral fragment into anterior and posterior fragments, as this makes subsequent percutaneous fixation less reliable. Drilling from the contra-

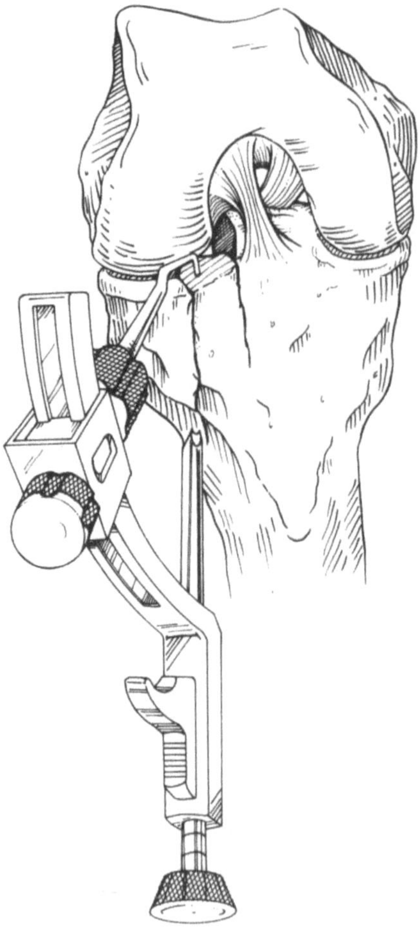

**FIGURE 11.11.** Acufex Multi-Trac tibial-tip guide to locate a 2.0-mm guide wire in the center of the lateral tibial plateau joint depression.

lateral metaphyseal cortex is another option if the split fragment is not large enough to allow an ipsilateral access tunnel.

A 8.0-mm cannulated drill is passed over the guide wire and drilled into the cortex to create a window to allow access to the depressed area of the lateral plateau (Figure 11.12). The opening is created to be as shallow as possible. This retains some of the cancellous bone well below the depressed area, which can be elevated with a bone tamp to act as a graft into the crushed subchondral region. The bone fragments cut from the lateral cortex are collected from the drill recesses to be returned to the tibia as graft material. The guide wire is now removed.

Using a Synthes™ bone tamp introduced through the drilled window, the larger depressed articular surface fracture fragments are elevated while observing the process on the image intensifier. Often the fracture can be overreduced intentionally, and using the lateral condyles as a negative mold the lateral compartment can be loaded carefully to achieve an anatomic alignment, which can be observed on fluoroscopy and confirmed on arthroscopy. If bone graft is required, it is delivered through the cortical window and packed below the subchondral region of the fracture with the bone tamp. The bone tamp is left in position to assist in maintaining the reduction. Proximal reduction of the split component of the fracture is performed by varus positioning using ligamentotaxis. If this maneuver does not achieve reduction, the author uses a 1/4-inch straight osteotome to elevate the split fragment. The osteotome is placed transversely through the cortical window and advanced to the intact posterior cortex medially. Lifting the osteotome moves the split fragment proximally. One or two large tenaculum reduction clamps are used to close the split portion of the fracture.

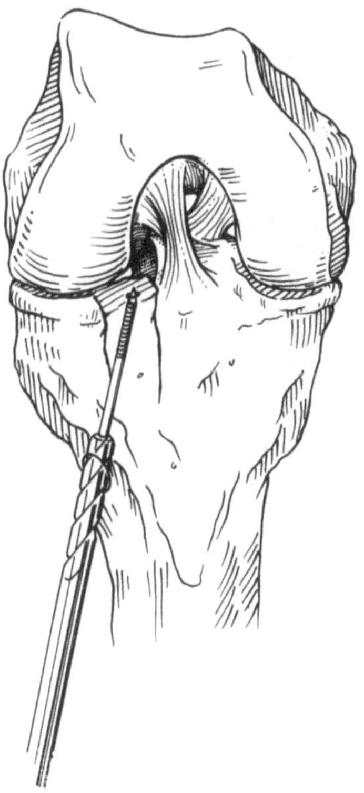

**FIGURE 11.12.** An 8.0-mm cannulated drill bit is used to enter the lateral tibial cortex and create a window to elevate the area of joint depression.

Definitive fixation is performed by using two 6.5-mm Asnis II guided screws as described in Chapter 10. Two 3.2-mm threaded tip guide pins are placed parallel to each other and also parallel to the joint, 10 mm below the articular surface. Pin placement is confirmed with image intensification in two planes. Screw length is determined from measurement off the guide pins, and screws 5 mm shorter than measured are selected to accommodate the compression of the split portion of the fracture. In osteoporotic bone, use of washers is mandatory to assist in fragment compression during seating of the screws. The bone tamp and guide wires are removed and any remaining harvested bone is returned to the tibia. If the split portion of the fracture had also been depressed prior to reduction, a third cannulated screw and washer may be used as a mini-buttress at the most interior aspect of the split fragment to assist in preventing distal migration of the fragment with postoperative mobilization (Figure 11.13).

Postoperative management involves continuous passive motion until flexion beyond 90° is achieved. Non–weight bearing for 8 weeks is necessary to prevent loss of reduction during early healing. A hinged, long-leg postoperative knee brace is used for 12 weeks. At 8 weeks partial weight bearing in the brace is usually

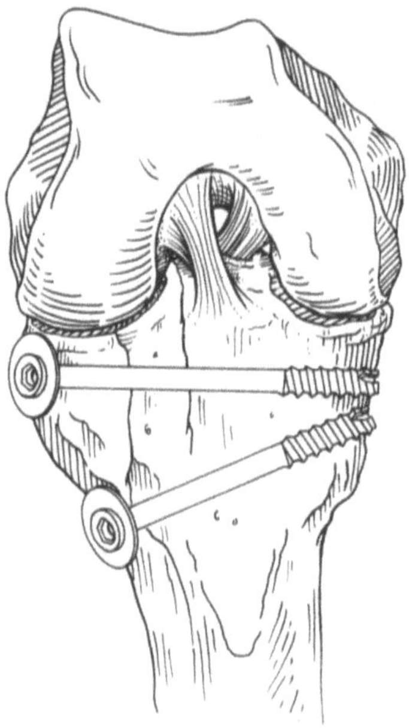

FIGURE 11.13. Split portion of the lateral tibial plateau fracture reduced and supported by a "mini-buttress" cannulated screw. Placement of a 6.5-mm cannulated screw and washer at the inferior aspect of the fracture assists in maintaining reduction of a depressed split fragment.

allowed and advanced to full weight bearing by 12 weeks postoperative.

## References


1. Linden B. Osteochondritis dissecans of the femoral condyles. *J Bone Joint Surg* 1977;59A:769–776.
2. Crawfurd EJ, Emery RJ, Hansel DM. Stable osteochondritis dissecans—does the lesion unite? *J Bone Joint Surg* 1990;72B:320.
3. Cahill BR, Phillips MR, Navarro R. The results of conservative management of juvenile osteochondritis dissecans using joint scintigraphy. A prospective study. *Am J Sports Med* 1989;17(5):601–605.
4. Twyman RS, et al. Osteochondritis dissecans of the knee. A long term study. *J Bone Joint Surg* 1991;73B:461–464.
5. Aichroth P. Osteochondritis dissecans of the knee: a clinical survey. *J Bone Joint Surg* 1971;53B:440–447.
6. Enneking WF. In: Enneking WF, ed. Circulatory diseases of bone. *Clinical Musculoskeletal Pathology*. Gainesville, FL: Storter Printing, 1986;166–168.
7. Clanton H, Delee J. Osteochondritis dissecans: history, pathophysiology and current treatment concepts. *Clin Orthop* 1982;167:50–64.
8. Ewing J, Voto S. Arthroscopic surgical management of osteochondritis dissecans of the knee. *Arthroscopy* 1988;4(1):37–40.
9. Guhl J. Arthroscopic treatment of osteochondritis dissecans; preliminary report. *Orthop Clin North Am* 1979;10:671–683.
10. Smillie I. Treatment of osteochondritis dissecans. *J Bone Joint Surg* 1957:39B:248.
11. Bandi W, Allgower M. Zur Therapie der Osteochondritis dissecans. *Helv Chir Acta* 1959;26:552.
12. Lindholm S, Pylkkanen P, Osterman K. Internal fixation of the fragment of osteochondritis dissecans in the knee by means of bone pins. A preliminary report on several cases. *Acta Chir Scand* 1974;140:626–629.
13. Johnson E, McLeod T. Osteochondral fragments of the distal end of the femur fixed with bone pegs. *J Bone Joint Surg* 1977;59A:677–679.
14. Scott D, Stevenson C. Osteochondritis dissecans of the knee in adults. *Clin Orthop* 1971;76:82–86.
15. Lipscomb P Jr, Lipscomb P Sr, Bryan R. Osteochondritis dissecans of the knee with loose fragments. *J Bone Joint Surg* 1978;60A:235–240.
16. Johnson L. Arthroscopic repair of osteochondritis. In: *Arthroscopy Video Digest*. Okemos, MI: Instrument Makar, August 1984.
17. Smillie I. Osteochondritis dissecans. In: *Injuries of the the Knee Joint*, 4th ed. Edinburgh: E and S Livingstone, 1971:268–330.
18. Johnson L, Utivlugt G, Austin M, et al. Osteochondritis dissecans of the knee: arthroscopic compression screw fixation. *Arthroscopy* 1990; 6(3):179–89.
19. Herbert TJ, Fisher WE. Management of the fractured scaphoid using a new screw. *J Bone Joint Surg* 1984;66B:124–127.
20. Lange R, Engber W, Clancy W. Expanding applications for the Herbert scaphoid screw. *Orthopedics* 1986;8:1393–1397.
21. Thomson N. Osteochondritis dissecans and osteochondral fragments managed by Herbert screw fixation. *Clin Orthop* 1987;224:71–78.
22. Leggon R, Lindsey RW, Doherty BJ, et al. The holding strength of cannulated screws compared with solid core screws in cortical and cancellous bone. *J Orthop Trauma* 1993;7(5):450–457.
23. Shaw J. A biomechanical comparison of scaphoid screws. *J Hand Surg* 1987;12A:347–353.
24. Asnis SE, Ernberg JJ, Bostrom MPG, et al. Cancellous bone screw design and holding power. Scientific exhibit, 62nd Meeting of the American Academy of Orthopedic Surgeons, Orlando, Florida, 1995.
25. Aglietti P, Buzzi R, Bassi P, et al. Arthroscopic drilling in juvenille osteochondritis dissecans of the medial femoral condyle. *Arthroscopy* 1994; 10(3):286–291.

26. Lee C, Mercurio C. Operative treatment of osteochondritis dissecans in situ by retrograde drilling and cancellous bone graft: a preliminary report. *Clin Orthop* 1981;158:129–136.
27. Johnson R, Aaberg T. Use of retrograde bone grafting in the treatment of osseous defects of the lateral condyle of the knee. *Orthopedics* 1987; 10(2):291–297.
28. Convery F, Botte M, Akeson W, et al. Chondral defects of the knee. *Contemp Orthop* 1994;28(2): 100–107.
29. Garrett JC. Fresh osteochondral allografts for treatment of articular defects of the knee in osteochondritis dissecans of the lateral femoral condyle in adults. *Clin Orthop* 1994;303:33–37.
30. Caspari R, Hutton P, Whipple T, et al. The role of arthroscopy in the management of tibial plateau fractures. *Arthroscopy* 1985;1(2):76–82.
31. Jennings J. Arthroscopic management of tibial plateau fractures. *Arthroscopy* 1985;1(3):160–168.
32. Guanche C, Markman A. Arthroscopic management of tibial plateau fractures. *Arthroscopy* 1993; 9(4):467–471.
33. Fowble C, Zimmer J, Schepsis A. The role of arthroscopy in the assessment and treatment of tibial plateau fractures. *Arthroscopy* 1993;9(5): 584–590.
34. Bennett W, Browner B. Tibial plateau fractures: a study of associated soft tissue injuries. *J Orthop Trauma* 1994;8(3):183–188.
35. Noyes FR, Spievack ES. Extraarticular fluid dissection in tissues during arthroscopy. *Am J Sports Med* 1982;10(6):346–351.
36. Peek RD, Haynes DW. Compartment syndrome as a complication of arthroscopy. *Am J Sports Med* 1984;12(6):464–468.
37. Whipple TL. Bone screw system, surgical techniques for fixation of scaphoid and other small bone fractures. In: *Zimmer Surgical Technique.* Warsaw, IN: Zimmer, 1992, 1993.

# 12

# Use of Cannulated Screws in Anterior Cruciate Ligament Reconstruction

Nicholas A. Sgaglione

The management and surgical approach to anterior cruciate ligament (ACL) tears has dramatically evolved over the last 15 years. Advances in basic science, clinical studies of knee ligament pathophysiology, more precise diagnostic skills, and the use of magnetic resonance imaging have contributed to a heightened focus on the ACL. The increased emphasis on fitness and sports participation as well as the greater demand by recreational athletes for return to preinjury knee function have led to an increase in ACL surgery. In the United States, ACL injury rates have been reported to occur at 0.38 per 1,000 per year and it is estimated that over 75,000 ACL reconstructions are performed each year.[1-3] As further attention is directed toward the ACL and the success of ACL surgery becomes more predictable, an increase in these numbers may be seen.

Numerous treatment techniques have been reported and over 20 various reconstructive methods have been published in the literature.[4-20] The current methods used to surgically treat ACL tears have developed in parallel with the advances seen in operative arthroscopy and most practitioners currently utilize arthroscopy as part of the technique of ACL reconstruction.[13,21] Knee arthroscopy aids in the diagnostic evaluation of the entire joint as well as treatment of chondral and meniscal injuries and repair and/or substitution of the torn ACL. ACL reconstruction usually involves replacement of the torn ligament with a biomechanically and functionally suitable ligament graft. Graft selection, placement and fixation may vary depending on clinical preferences. Graft choices include the use of autografts such as the central-third patellar tendon, combinations of semitendinous and gracilis hamstring tendons, or segments of fascia lata.[4,6,8,12,13,17,22] Allograft tissue has also been used in addition to various synthetic ligament devices including stents, scaffolds, and prostheses.[21]

The precise placement of graft tissue is predicated upon the concept of isometry and reproduction of the graft insertion site or footprint. Selection of graft fixation depends upon the graft construct. Fixation options for hamstring tendons or fascia lata grafts include the use of staples, sutures tied around a screw and washer ("suture post"), plate and screw devices, or metallic or plastic buttons.[23-25] Bone-tendon-bone constructs such as central-third (patella) bone tendon (tibia tubercle) bone autografts or allografts that include bone block attachments such as Achilles tendon–calcaneal bone blocks, are more commonly fixed using interference fit screws.[12,26-29] Proponents of the use of patella tendon bone-tendon-bone grafts feel that grafts harvested with bone insertions attached provide immediate optimal stability through the use of interference-fit screws and ultimate fixation by bone-to-bone union.[30-35] Since the introduction of interference-fit screws, several modifications and screw technique advances have developed including the addition of cannulated systems. This chapter details the use of interference-fit screws, specifically cannulated screw designs, used in ACL reconstruction.

## History and Design

Intraarticular reconstruction of the ACL using a patellar tendon bone block technique was described by Jones[36] in 1963 and further modified and popularized by Clancy[9] in 1981 and

Noyes et al.[37] in 1983. Initial fixation techniques included the use of nonabsorbable sutures placed through drill holes in the graft bone block brought out of the bone tunnels and tied over a plastic button or secured with a staple. In 1983, Lambert[38] first reported on the use of a 30-mm-long AO 6.5-mm cancellous screw to produce an "interference" fit. This allowed for a cog-wheel type of fixation whereby the screw engages within the bone tunnel both the bone block and inner side wall of the tunnel. The first report of a fixation screw specifically designed for ACL reconstruction use was in 1987 when Kurosaka et al.[34] introduced and reported on a custom-designed large diameter 9.0-mm self-tapping screw.

The "M. Kurosaka" interference fit screw (DePuy, Warsaw, IN) became available for clinical use in 1987 (Figure 12.1). The original self-tapping screw design was not cannulated and was made of titanium alloy (Ti6AL4V). The original size specifications included 5.5-, 7-, and 9-mm outer diameter screws in lengths of 20 to 40 mm in 5-mm increments. The original tip angle of the screw was 35° (it has recently been changed to 29°) and the minor diameter 4.2 mm (for the 7-mm screw design) and 5.5 mm (for the 9-mm screw design). The thread pitch was 2.25 mm and the screwdriver insertion slot design was a hexagonal broach (2.5 mm wide for the 7-mm and 3.5 mm wide for 9-mm screw).

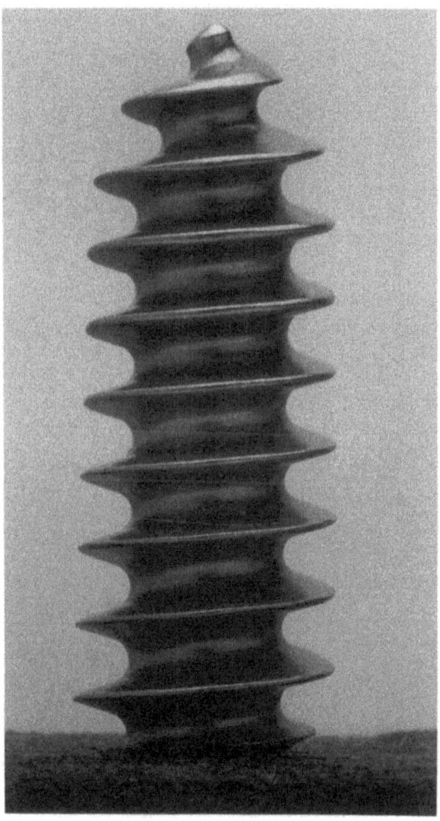

**FIGURE 12.1.** M. Kurosaka interference screw. (Photograph used with permission from DePuy, Inc., Warsaw, IN.)

As demand for ACL surgery increased and in particular use of the patellar tendon bone-tendon-bone graft became more popular, interference screw fixation options rapidly evolved. Numerous commercial equipment companies expanded upon existing technologies and provided for innovative design modifications. In 1989, the first cannulated screw design was introduced (Concept; Linvatec, Largo, FL) with a spiral tip titanium alloy screw design available in 5.75-, 7-, 8-, and 9-mm outer diameter screws of 20- to 40-mm lengths (in 5-mm increments). The minor diameters were 3.9, 4.8, 5.2 and 5.6 mm for the 5.75-, 7-, 8-, and 9-mm screws respectively. The larger screws (7, 8, and 9 mm) all had a 1.67-mm screw cannulation and were used in conjunction with a 1.5-mm diameter nitinol nickel alloy or stainless steel cannulated guide wire.

Design modifications included sharper starting threads and blunted body threads for ease of insertion and less potential for graft injury. The endoscopic transtibial modifications of the original arthroscopic-assisted technique, which was introduced in 1989 by Rosenberg, heightened the concern that the graft could be injured by intraarticular retrograde (distal to proximal from the arthroscopic portal toward the femoral tunnel) insertion of the femoral interference screw.[16,39,40] Several design modifications followed to address this issue. Screw polishing using a tumbler finish was marketed in 1992 to further reduce the chance that the screw could injure the graft when placing it endoscopically into the femoral tunnel (Cannu-Flex Silk; Acufex Microsurgical, Mansfield, MA). Rounded head femoral screws were also developed to increase the safeness of endoscopic insertion (Guardsman; Linvatec, Largo, FL, and Arthrex Inc.,

Naples, FL). Sheathed screw systems have also been introduced to allow for intraarticular advancement and delivery of the femoral screw toward the femoral tunnel in a plastic cannula (Arthrex Inc., Naples, FL) (Figure 12.2). The spiral tip design of the screw was modified in 1992 with the introduction of a double helix insertion tip, which would presumably facilitate more precise insertion (Figure 12.3) (Propel; Linvatec, Largo, FL).

Cannulated interference screw systems have become more commonly used and most designs now incorporate cannulation since it affords more precise screw placement. The initial problems reported with cannulation use including breakage and wire incarceration, have been reduced by improvements in the guide wires.[41] Wire diameters have been enlarged in some designs to 1.5 mm (Cannu-Flex Silk 1.5; Acufex, Mansfield, MA) and 2.0 mm (Arthrex Inc., Naples, FL).

Most recently, attention has been turned to the use of bioabsorbable implants.[37,42–46] This technology has begun to be applied toward interference-fit screws. A bioabsorbable design was released in 1994 (Bioscrew; Linvatec, Largo, FL) which is made of a homopolymer derived from poly-L-lactide, a synthetic polyester associated with delayed absorption (up to 2 years). The screw is available cannulated in 7-, 8-, and 9-mm diameters and 20- to 30-mm lengths (in 5-mm increments). The driver hexagonal broach has been replaced by a tri-lobed broach design. A bioabsorbable screw composed of lactic acid and glycolic acid has also been developed, and is available in the United States after being clinically studied in Europe (Biodegradable Screw; Instrument Makar, Okemos, MI). Further specifications of commercially available interference screws are listed in Table 12.1.

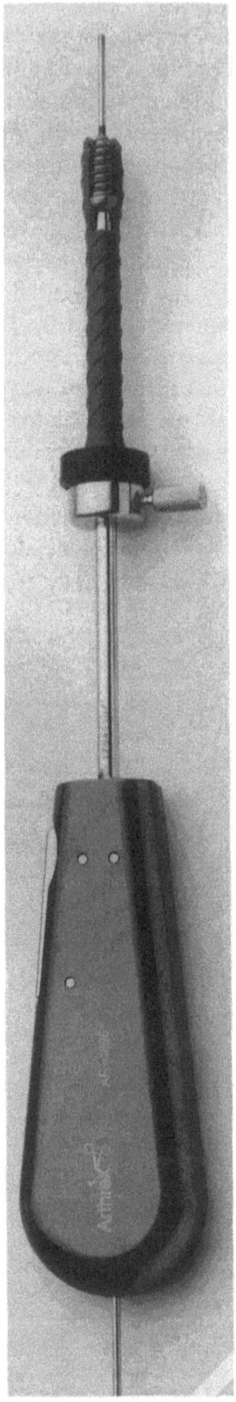

FIGURE 12.2. Arthrex sheathed cannulated screw. (Photograph courtesy of Arthrex Inc., Naples, FL.)

## Advantages of Cannulated Interference Screws

Cannulated interference screw systems provide multiple advantages over the initially introduced first-generation noncannulated systems. Endoscopic placement of the femoral interference

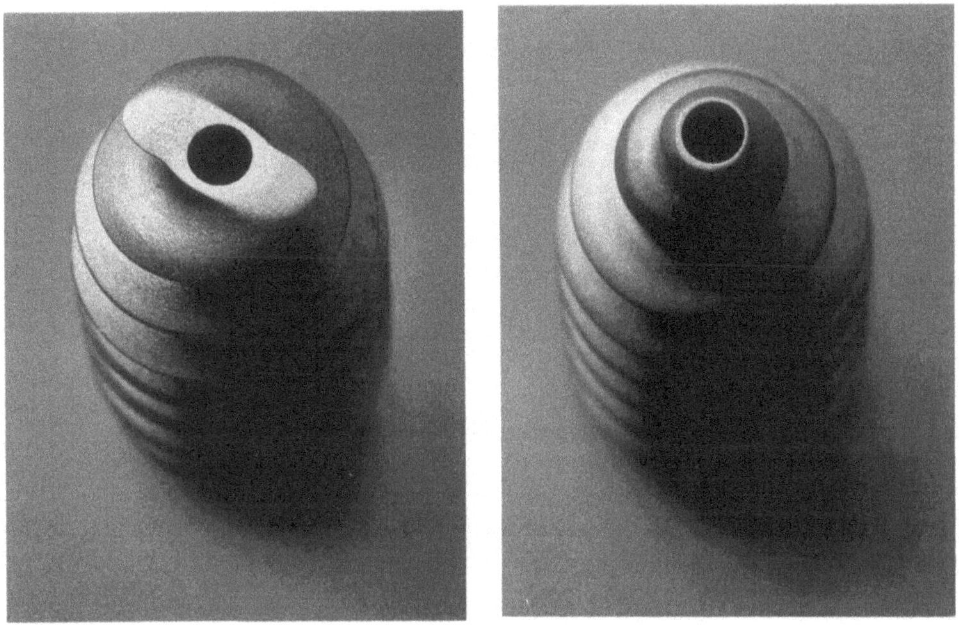
a b

FIGURE 12.3. (a) A double-helix thread permits the screw to engage bone evenly on both sides, limiting veering associated with (b) single-helix designs. (Photograph courtesy of Linvatec, Inc., Largo, FL.)

screw is particularly facilitated by the use of cannulated interference screw systems. The cannulation wire can reduce the potential for screw divergence or convergence at the time of insertion by reproducible guiding of the screw into the specifically desired position.[47] Avoidance of divergence ensures optimum contact between the screw and bone block, which contributes to higher pullout strengths.[41,48] Avoidance of convergence reduces the chance that the bone block can be overly compressed by the screw, thereby leading to block disruption or fracture. The use of cannulated interference-fit screws also reduces the chance of graft translocation, which can occur when the screw is being inserted and the bone block then spins (usually in a clockwise manner) leading to an altered position placement of the screw. This can lead to graft tendon injury or laceration of the graft itself usually at the bone-tendon junction. Another advantage to the use of the cannulated screw systems is that at the time of screw insertion, either through one of the arthroscopic portal incisions (usually the inferomedial joint line portal) or through the central-third patellar tendon harvest site defect, the guide wire serves as a track to facilitate smooth screw passage through the soft tissues. This is particularly helpful when passing the screw through the tendon defect, since the infrapatellar fat pad tends to catch the screw. The guide wire also eliminates the possibility that the screw can become dislodged from its driver and then become loose in the joint. Finally, more precise depth can be gauged using a cannulated guide wire. Several commercially available cannulated systems have calibrated markings on the tip of the guide wire that allow for more exact assessment of the depth of insertion, thereby reducing the chance for an abnormal graft–screw length relationship.

## Biomechanics

Fixation is critical to the success of ACL reconstruction and numerous studies reveal that most failures of the graft construct do so at the weak link, which is the point of graft attachment.[29,34,49–53] The patella tendon bone-tendon-

**TABLE 12.1.** Specifications of commercially available interference screws.

| Company | Trademark name | Release | Material[1] | Type[2] | Sizes[3] | Minor diameter[4] | Thread pitch[4] | Guide wire diameter[4] | Guide wire material[4,5] | Driver broach |
|---|---|---|---|---|---|---|---|---|---|---|
| Acufex Microsurgical, Mansfield, MA | Interference | 1989 | Ti | NC | 5.5 × 20–30 | – | 2.75 | – | – | – |
| | | | | | 7 × 20–30 | 3.5 | 2.75 | – | – | 2.3 |
| | | | | | 9 × 20–30 | 5.5 | 2.75 | – | – | 3.4 |
| | Cannu-Flex | 1990 | Ti | C | 7 × 20–30 | 4.14 | 2.75 | 1 | N | 2.3 |
| | | | | | 9 × 20–30 | 5.5 | 2.75 | 1 | N | 3.4 |
| | Cannu-Flex Silk | 1992 | Ti | C | 7 × 20–30 | 4.14 | 2.75 | 1 | N | 2.7 |
| | | | | | 8 × 20–30 | – | 2.75 | 1 | N | – |
| | | | | | 9 × 20–30 | 5.0 | 2.75 | 1 | N | 3.4 |
| | Cannu-Flex Silk 1.5 | 1995 | Ti | C | 7 × 20–30 | 5.0 | 2.75 | 1.5 | N | 3.4 |
| | | | | | 8 × 20–30 | – | 2.75 | 1.5 | N | – |
| | | | | | 9 × 20–30 | 6.95 | 2.75 | 1.5 | N | 3.4 |
| Arthrex Inc., Naples, FL | Nonsheathed | 1993 | Ti | C/NC | 6 × 20–40 | 4.2 | 2.0 | 1.5 | N | 2.5 |
| | Sheathed | 1993 | Ti | C/NC | 7 × 20–40 | 5.1 | 2.1 | 2.0 | N | 3.5 |
| | | | | | 8 × 20–40 | 5.5 | 2.3 | 2.0 | N | 3.5 |
| | T-Screw | 1993 | Ti | C/NC | 9 × 20–40 | 6.0 | 2.5 | 2.0 | N | 3.5 |
| | | | | | 10 × 20–40 | 6.6 | 2.7 | 2.0 | N | 3.5 |
| DePuy, Inc., Warsaw, IN | M. Kurosaka | 1987 | Ti | NC | 5.5 × 25–30 | – | – | – | – | 2.5 |
| | | | | | 7 × 20–40 | 4.2 | 2.25 | – | – | 2.5 |
| | | | | | 9 × 20–40 | 5.5 | 2.25 | – | – | 3.5 |
| | M. Kurosaka cannulated | 1989 | Ti | C | 7 × 20–40 | 4.2 | 2.25 | 1.14 | SS/N | 2.5 |
| | | | | | 9 × 20–40 | 5.5 | 2.25 | 1.57 | SS/N | 3.5 |
| | Advantage | 1993 | Ti | C/NC | 7 × 15–40 | 5.0 | 2.25 | 1.57 | SS/N | 3.5 |
| | | | | | 9 × 15–40 | 5.8 | 2.25 | 2.28 | SS/N | 4.0 |
| Instrument Makar, Okemos, MI | Perfixation | 1993 | SS | NC | 6,7,8,9 × 25 | – | 1.25 | – | – | Threaded reversible |
| | Biodegradable | 1995 | LA + GA | NC | 9 × 25 | – | – | – | – | |
| Linvatec, Inc., Largo, FL | Conical tip interference screw | 1988 | Ti | NC | 6.5 × 20–40 | – | – | – | – | 2.5 |
| | | | | | 9 × 20–40 | – | – | – | – | 3.5 |
| | Cannulated interference screw | 1989 | Ti | C | 5.7 × 20–30 | 3.9 | 2.3 | < 1 | N | 2.5 |
| | | | | | 7 × 20–40 | 4.8 | 2.5 | 1.5 | SS/N | 3.5 |
| | | | | | 8 × 20–40 | 5.2 | 2.5 | 1.5 | SS/N | 3.5 |
| | | | | | 9 × 20–40 | 5.6 | 2.5 | 1.5 | SS/N | 3.5 |
| | Propel | 1993 | Ti | C | 7 × 20–30 | 4.8 | 5 | 1.5 | SS/N | 3.5 |
| | | | | | 8 × 20–30 | 5.2 | 5 | 1.5 | SS/N | 3.5 |
| | | | | | 9 × 20–30 | 3.5 | 5 | 1.5 | SS/N | 3.5 |
| | Guardsman femoral interference screw | 1993 | Ti | C | 7 × 20–30 | 4.8 | 5 | 1.5 | SS/N | 3.5 |
| | | | | | 8 × 20–30 | 5.2 | 5 | 1.5 | SS/N | 3.5 |
| | | | | | 9 × 20–30 | 5.6 | 5 | 1.5 | SS/N | 3.5 |
| | Bioscrew | 1994 | PL | C | 7 × 20–30 | 4.8 | 2.5 | 1 | SS/N | Trilobe |
| | | | | | 8 × 20–30 | 5.3 | 2.5 | 1 | SS/N | |
| | | | | | 9 × 20–30 | 5.6 | 2.5 | 1 | SS/N | |

[1] Ti, titanium alloy Ti6A14V; LA + GA, lactic acid + glycolic acid; PL, poly-L-lactide; SS, stainless steel.
[2] C, cannulated; NC, noncannulated.
[3] Diameter by lengths (mm); length in 5-mm increments.
[4] Minor diameter (mm); thread pitch (mm); guide wire diameter (mm); driver broach (mm).
[5] N, nitinol; Ss, stainless steel.

bone autograft strengths have been reported to have ultimate load to failure values of 2,000 to 3,000 newtons (N), whereas most time-zero fixation strengths have been reported to be 50 to 1000 N.[34] Furthermore, during the early postoperative period the newly implanted graft may be mechanically vulnerable since revascularization has been shown to reduce the strength of the graft.[54,55] Therefore, the need to obtain the most optimal initial fixation strength at the point of graft attachment is important.

The use of an intraarticular bone-tendon-bone graft construct secured at the time of surgery with interference fit screws has many mechanical and biologic advantages. Early secure fixation ensures maintenance of the intraoperatively preset graft tension, contributes to the loading of the graft itself, and anchors the graft allowing earlier weight bearing, motion, and return to functional activities. Biologically, ligament graft bone-block to bone-tunnel healing has been shown to occur in 6 to 8 weeks, which appears to be sooner than animal model studies of tendon graft healing in bone tunnels.[4,31,56] Mechanical studies of fixation methods have shown that the comparative pullout strengths of interference-fit screws used with ligament bone blocks are superior. Kurosaka compared patellar tendon cadaveric grafts fixed to the femur and tibia with staples versus using no. 5 nonabsorbable sutures tied over a plastic button versus using a 6.5-mm AO cancellous screw to achieve interference fit with the bone block.[34] Analysis of load-deformation curves revealed the interference screw constructs were associated with significantly higher values in terms of linear load, stiffness, and maximum tensile strength than either the suture/button or staple fixation methods. In that same study, data indicated that use of a 9.0-mm diameter interference-fit screw custom designed for use in fixing ligament graft bone blocks in tibial/femoral tunnels demonstrated statistically significantly increased stiffness, linear load, and maximum tensile strength compared with the 6.5-mm AO cancellous screw. The 9.0-mm Kurosaka screws provided more than twice the pullout strength of the 6.5-mm cancellous screws used as interference-fit screws. The Kurosaka screw was associated with a 436.5 N linear load compared with 160.9 N for the 6.5-mm cancellous screw, and stiffness was noted to be 57.9 N/mm for the Kurasaka screw compared with 36.2 N/mm for the 6.5-mm cancellous screw. Similar findings were reported in a porcine model by Paschal et al.,[51] who found that interference screw fixation was stronger than postfixation (sutures tied over a cancellous screw and washer). Using 9-mm diameter Kurasaka screws (DePuy, Warsaw, IN) and 10-mm bone blocks, the mean ultimate loads were higher (535 N) compared with postfixation (309.1 N) using no. 5 nonabsorbable sutures tied around a 6.5-mm AO cancellous screw.

Matthews and coworkers[33] reported in 1993 on fixation strengths of patellar tendon-bone grafts using several different fixation methods. Force-displacement curves were generated and the mode of failure was studied. They found that the interference-fit screw fixation constructs afforded fixation strengths equal to or even stronger than the graft itself. Failure during testing was observed to occur by ligament rupture and bone plug pullout in most cases. One interesting finding was that when the interference screw path adjacent to the graft bone block diverged, which occurred in three cases, then reduced fixation strength was noted. The use of a cannulated interference screw system using a guide wire for direction to reduce the chance that divergence can occur is cited by the study.

Recent data reported by Steiner et al.[57] assessed graft fixation techniques and compared biomechanical testing variables including maximum load, stiffness, displacement at yield load, and mechanism of failure. The ACL reconstructions using patellar tendon grafts had a strength of $423 \pm 125$ N and a stiffness of $46 \pm 24$ N/mm. The study found that ACL reconstructions using patellar tendon grafts and interference screws have a closer to normal ACL stiffness than reconstructions using hamstring grafts.

## Factors Affecting Screw Fixation Biomechanics

The strength of the interference-fit screw construct is dependent on the quality of the specific bone, the degree to which compression is achieved in the bone tunnel including insertion torque, the design and size of the particular screw, its relationship with the bone block including level of insertion, and the direction and magnitude of forces acting upon the ligament graft.[30,53,58–63] In addition the effect of the bone block shape has also been shown to affect mechanical strength.[64] Interference fixation has been shown to be affected by bone density, particularly as it relates to age.[26,53] This has been studied in animal and cadaveric models. Reznik et al.[61] observed that a lower pullout strength was associated with studies in human cadavers with a mean age of 58.6 years compared with those specimens with a mean age of 20.3 years. Similar findings were identified by other authors.[26,30,62]

## Insertion Torque

The influence of insertion torque as well as screw diameter has been studied by Kohn and Rose,[28] who analyzed the comparative effectiveness of 20-mm-long interference-fit screws of 7- and 9-mm diameters. Maximum insertion torque was also recorded and it was shown that when the insertion torque exceeded 250 N/cm, bone block stability was noted. Insertion torque was reported on by Brown et al.,[62] who analyzed the failure strength of interference screw fixation. The group coined the phrase "interference," defined as the screw diameter (outer thread diameter) minus the gap or maximum bone-block tunnel gap distance. Interference would essentially be equivalent to the screw thread engagement in the bone and was evaluated to be a predictor of failure load with an optimal interference or optimal screw size for a given bone-block tunnel gap size.

## Gap Size

The concept of gap size was originally reported by Reznik and Daniel.[61,65] In the laboratory, they found that gap size (which is the measured gap between the bone tunnel and bone block) can affect screw pullout strength and is related to screw insertion torque. In their healthy porcine bone model, the pullout load was noted to be more optimal and the screw insertion torque

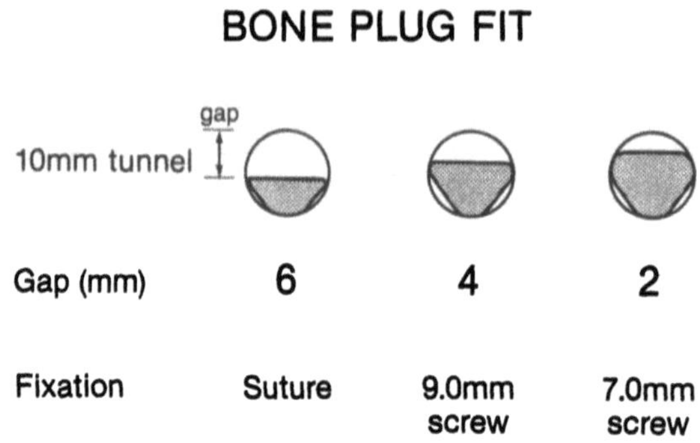


FIGURE 12.4. Gap size. (Photograph used with permission from Alan Reznik, M.D.)

higher when the gap between the bone block and tunnel was less than 4 mm. Reznik concluded that when the gap size was greater than 4 mm, then a 9.0-mm-diameter screw rather than a 7.0-mm should be utilized (Figure 12.4). Attention to the actual construct gap size was recommended using rod-like gap gauges of increasing diameter (1 to 6 mm) to clinically determine whether a 7- or 9-mm screw should be used. Clearly, both bone block and tunnel geometry can affect gap size.

## Bone Block Geometry

Regarding the effect of geometry on bone block fit and strength, Shapiro et al.[64] found that circular bone plugs were 19.9% stronger than trapezoidal matched plugs with greater pullout strengths and decreased stress concentration effects on the patellar harvest site. They recommend a new technique of harvesting circular patellar bone blocks.

## Screw Design

Screw design, specifically screw size, can affect biomechanical stability and has been reported by Brown et al.[60] in human cadaveric studies. The effect of screw thread length, screw diameter, and screw core size on the fixation strength of the patellar tendon graft constructs was evaluated. The authors found that when comparing 5.5- and 7-mm diameter screws, there was a highly significant increase in pullout force for the 7-mm compared to the 5-mm screw. It was also noted that the effect of screw diameter was not the same for each screw length. For the 20-mm-long screws, the pullout force increased 120%, when 7-mm screws rather than 5-mm were inserted. However, for longer (25-mm) screws, the pullout increased only 21% when the diameter was increased from 5.5 to 7 mm. When the 7-mm screws were (endoscopically and retrograde) inserted compared with 9-mm screws (which were inserted using an antegrade "rear entry" method), no significant difference in pullout strength could be found. A similar result was noted by Hulstyn et al.,[63] who also noted superior biomechanical properties in bovine bone associated with using 7- and 9-mm diameter screws compared with 5.5-mm screws but with no real difference between the 7- and 9-mm diameter for both the tibia and the femur. It is important to point out that the gap was limited to 2 to 4 mm for all specimens. Hulstyn et al. also studied screw length and found that for a 10-mm bone block, a 20-mm-long screw can be exchanged for the 30-mm length without compromising stability.

Brown et al.[60] also studied the screw core diameters, comparing standard (3.5-mm core) versus increased core diameter (4.42-mm core) in 5.5- and 7-mm overall diameter screws. No significant difference was noted in pullout force or insertion torque between the standard and increased core screws.

The length of the interference screw used during reconstruction is more likely to be determined by the bone block more than anything else; however, the question of what screw and bone block length is optimal has been addressed by Fulkerson et al.[41,47] They reported that equivalent pullout strength could be expected for bone blocks as short as 10 mm long compared to blocks 20 mm long in porcine and human cadaveric models. However, for blocks 5 mm long a marked weakening of the fixation strength was noted with significant decrease in pullout.

## Tunnel Site

Screw size selection is also dependent on whether the tibial or femoral side is being approached. In contrast to C. Brown's[60] work, Kohn and Rose[28] found that the 7-mm screws are not recommended for the tibial side tunnel and that the tibial fixation was predictably weaker using a 7- versus 9-mm screw. Presumably the tibial tunnel bone wall consists of substantially more cancellous bone than the corresponding femoral side, which could affect pullout.

# Pitfalls Associated with Interference Screw Fixation

Several pitfalls exist in the use of interference screws and have been described by Bach[66] as graft–screw length mismatch, tunnel-graft-screw mismatch, tunnel-screw divergence, graft advancements, graft fracture or transection, graft translocation, and suture laceration.

## Graft–Screw Length Mismatch

Graft–screw length mismatch can occur when the interference-fit screw length is too long or inserted too far and intraarticular penetration occurs. With advancement of the screw beyond the bone graft the screw may ultimately lie in contact with the tendinous portion of the graft resulting in graft abrasion and damage. If an oversized screw is left proud and not inserted to its full length, then its prominence can result in overlying soft tissue inflammation (Figure 12.5). Franco et al.[67] studied and reported on postoperative radiographs, which they found could be misleading with regard to the exact location of the tibial interference screw. They advised careful measurement of the tibial tunnel and bone block lengths prior to selecting the appropriate screw length.

## Tunnel-Graft-Screw Mismatch

Tunnel-graft-screw mismatch can occur when an inappropriately sized tunnel is drilled relative to the size of the graft bone block. This has been described in further detail by Reznik et al.[61] in their study of gap sizing. Difficulty can then arise with insertion of the interference screw causing damage to the bone block or advance-

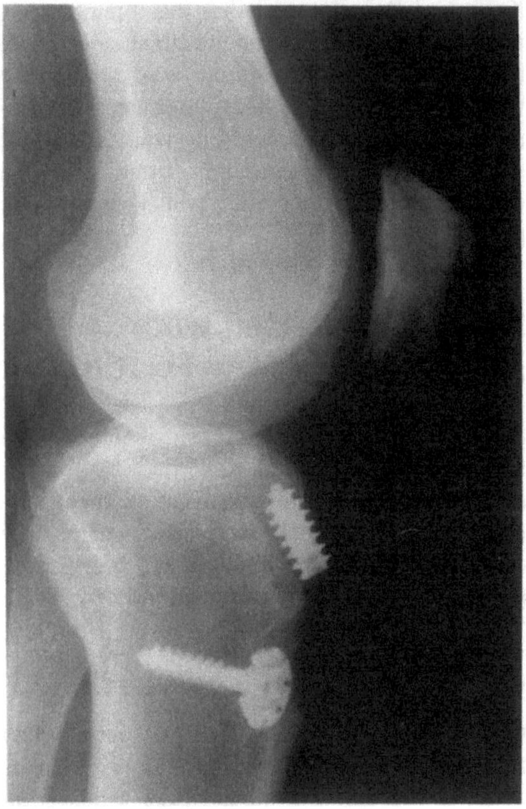

FIGURE 12.5. Radiograph of graft-screw length mismatch. The tibial screw is too superficial and is not engaging the bone block.

ment of the graft. Screw divergence also tends to occur more easily if the gap size is smaller and a larger screw is used as "gap size assessment," thereby making it more difficult to initiate the self-tapping screw, which can diverge.

## Divergence

Screw divergence has been reported on by numerous authors including Pierz et al.,[68] Fulkerson et al.,[47] Jomha et al.,[48] Lemos et al.,[69] and Fanelli et al.[70] A divergent interference screw pathway is defined by the position of the screw relative to a guide wire placed laterally in the tunnel along the length of the bone plug (Figure 12.6a). Attention to divergence has been heightened by the increasing popularity of the endoscopic technique of femoral interference screw placement. Use of a cannulated screw design can theoretically reduce divergence (Figure 6b). Intraarticular insertion of the femoral screw can be technically difficult and can be associated with graft advancement (pushing and countersinking of the bone block by the interference screw ahead of the screw instead of parallel) and graft translocation (spinning of the bone block around the screw). In addition, divergence or especially convergence of the interference screw can contribute to graft injury including bone block fracture, tendon transection, and leader suture laceration.[39,40,71,72] A clinical radiographic analysis of interference screw placement revealed that divergence significantly occurs.[69] Furthermore, the study revealed that anteroposterior and lateral screw angles measured on the postoperative radiographs were significantly different depending on whether the femoral screws were placed endoscopically (retrograde, from distal to proximal) or open (via an antegrade—from proximal to distal—technique using exposure of the distal femur through a lateral femoral incision). In the endoscopic group, 36% were noted to have divergent screws with only one screw measured to diverge > 15° compared with no divergence noted in the open group.

The clinical significance of divergence was questioned by Fanelli et al.,[70] who retrospectively reviewed 97 patients who underwent endoscopic ACL reconstruction. In that study, radiographic analysis revealed that despite attempted parallel placement of the femoral interference screw (using a cannulation wire) 46% of 48 patients had divergence between the bone plug and the tunnel. Of the 46%, the divergence was in the medial/lateral plane in 7 patients with a mean angle of 20.3°, and in 5 patients the divergence was in the anterior/posterior plane with a mean angle of 20.6°. A second group of patients in which no attempt to achieve parallel screw placement was made (screw placement through inferomedial portal) was noted to have a higher incidence of divergence as measured on postoperative radiographics with 84% being divergent (49% on the anterior/posterior views and 71% on the lateral views). Fanelli et al. reported on the clinical out-

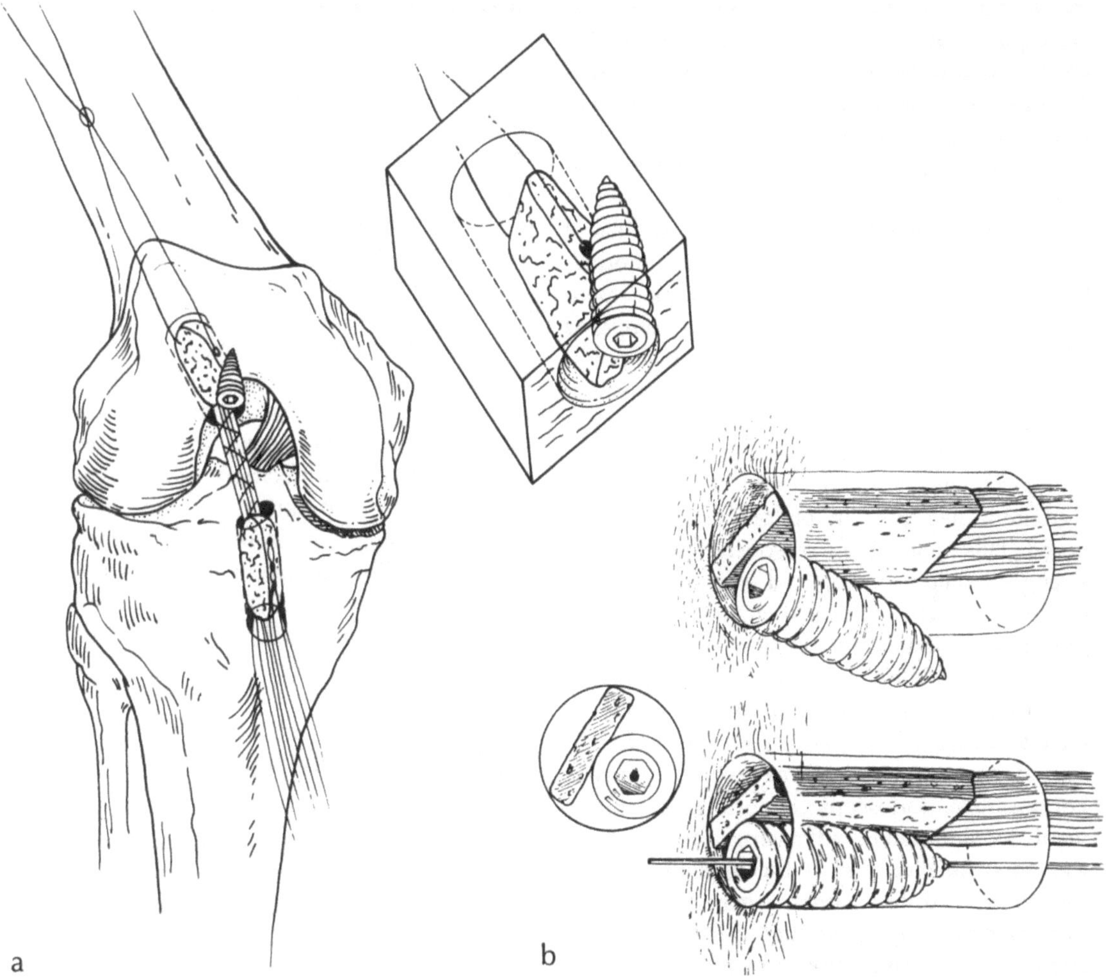


**FIGURE 12.6.** (a) Divergence of femoral interference screw and bone block. (b) Divergence and cannulated screw design. The cannulated screw theoretically should prevent divergence of the screw and the bone plug. (Reprinted with permission from Matthews, L. et al.[33])

come of these patients with a 1-year minimum follow-up (maximum of 2.5 years) and found that despite the high incidence of divergence, no perioperative sequelae or clinical failure could be demonstrated. These clinical results are important to consider since several authors have demonstrated in the laboratory in animal and cadaveric bone models that divergence can significantly reduce the pullout strength of the interference screw–bone block construct.

Jomha et al.[48] found in the porcine animal model that there was a significant weakening of fixation for screw angles measuring > 20° of divergence with respect to the bone plug. The effect on pullout strength was studied in four model groups in which the interference screw and bone block divergence angles were 0°, 10°, 10° versus 20°, and 20° versus 30°. The most significant difference was between 0° and 30° with a mean pullout strength noted to be 607 N for 0° and 10° and 497 N for 20° and 30°. Jomha et al. concluded that divergent screw placement (from parallel with respect to the bone plug) could affect fixation mechanical properties. These results are corroborated by a study by Fulkerson et al.[47] in the bovine knee model that found that when interference screws were placed at 15° and 30° of divergence, 15° gave little dropoff in holding strength, whereas 30° of divergence resulted in a 77% reduction in screw holding strength.

Fulkerson and coworkers[41] have further reported on the effects of divergence interference screws on linear load to failure in simulated ACL reconstructions in porcine knee models. Endoscopic (retrograde) tibial screw placement (tibial articular side-entry point) was compared to rear-entry (tibial cortical side-entry point) placements. The endoscopic screw placement was associated with a higher holding strength than the rear-entry method. In addition, at divergence angles greater than 30°, statistically significant decreases in pullout strength were noted. Fulkerson et al. reasoned that holding strength would be maximized when more of the interference screw threads engaged both the graft bone block and the tunnel wall. They point out that in addition to the angle of divergence, the actual tracking direction of the screw in relation to the forces that act on the graft (retrograde versus antegrade) may also play a role. For example, endoscopic femoral screw placement would require advancing the screw in the opposite direction of the applied load on the graft, and this contact may actually be more mechanically stable than if the loads were applied in the same direction as the screw is advanced.[47,68]

## Guide Wire Pitfalls

Pitfalls that are specific to cannulated wire systems include complications related to screw guidewire use. In five human cadaveric knees, a 1.1-mm-diameter stainless steel guide wire for a 7-mm interference screw was studied.[41] Intentional divergence was then achieved with the screws placed off the parallel plane of bone block and tunnel. Radiographics were obtained and revealed bending of the wire in all cases. This study points out that divergence can lead to guide wire bending, incarceration, or even breakage. When the experiment was repeated with rigid guide wires, intended divergence was not as easy to achieve.

## Screw Depth Placement

The effect of interference screw depth placement has recently been studied.[73] Three levels of graft fixation on the tibia were evaluated to see if the actual level to which the screw is inserted has any affect on knee stability. Ishibashi et al.[73] measured anteroposterior tibial translation under robotic loading conditions. They compared placement of the tibial screw proximally (just distal to the ACL insertion site on the tibial plateau) with central block and screw position in the tibial tunnel and distal fixation, just outside and distal to the tibial tunnel (for the distal group an interference screw was not used). Presumably the distal fixation model would be analogous to extratunnel fixation constructs such as stapling a bone block in a trough just distal to the tibial tunnel or using a suture post. The study found significant differences for the proximal fixation model, which resulted in the most stable knee.

# Author's Preferred Technique

The technique of arthroscopic ACL reconstruction using a central-third patellar tendon graft has evolved from open methods and utilizes arthroscopy to approach graft tunnel, preparation, placement, and fixation. In general, the following steps make up the author's preferred technique and surgical approach to ACL reconstruction using cannulated interference screw fixation.

## Setup

After anesthesia is administered the patient is positioned supine and a well-padded tourniquet is applied to the affected thigh as proximally as possible. (The tourniquet is infrequently used; however, it is advised that it be applied and be available for inflation if needed.) A lateral post (Telos; Fallston, MD) is affixed to the operating table at the level of the distal junction of the tourniquet cuff and lateral to the affected limb, leaving approximately a four-finger-breadth distance between the patient's lateral thigh and the inner surface of the post. The lateral post provides the surgeon with a point of leverage allowing opening of the medial compartment via valgus stress application. (Other surgeons may prefer a leg holder.)

## Examination Under Anesthesia (EUA)

Both the affected knee and the contralateral presumed "normal" control knee are then examined under anesthesia to assess the extent and degree of patholaxity. Instability testing is performed in all planes and rotary instability is graded. The extent and degree to which the surgeon can accurately document patholaxity on EUA determines whether the patellar-tendon autograft is procured prior to arthroscopic examination of the knee. If the surgeon has any doubt as to whether the EUA of the affected knee confirms the preoperative diagnosis of ACL deficiency, then diagnostic arthroscopy should be performed prior to harvesting of the ligament graft.

## Graft Harvesting

After prepping and draping of the knee, the proposed incision and peripatellar graft harvest sites are infiltrated with an injection of local anesthetic with epinephrine or sterile arthroscopic irrigation fluid injected with 1 cc of 1:1000 epinephrine in 3,000 cc of 0.9% normal saline. An intraarticular injection of the fluid with epinephrine is also given. If the graft is harvested first (preferred technique if corroborated by EUA), then two types of incisions may be utilized. To accomplish an endoscopic single anterior approach to the ACL reconstruction (retrograde placement of the femoral interference screw), the incision (or incisions) are limited to the anterior aspect of the knee. For two-incision arthroscopic approaches, in addition to the anterior incision a lateral incision over the lateral femoral condyle is also approached to allow antegrade placement of the femoral interference screw.

The endoscopic modification of the arthroscopic-assisted ACL reconstruction technique can be performed via two types of anterior knee incisions. One method is to use a single longitudinal midline incision extending from the inferior pole of the patella and curving slightly distally and medially to the tibial tubercle. The alternative endoscopic incision technique uses two mini-transverse (2 to 3 cm) incisions placed at the inferior pole of the patella and just medial to the tibial tubercle overlying the proposed tibial drill tunnel site (Figure 12.7). The proposed advantages of the mini-transverse incisions include cosmesis, less dissection, presumably less postoperative pain, and less chance for localized cutaneous nerve injury. After incising the skin, the patellar tendon is identified and the patellar tendon paratendon is carefully incised and retracted, allowing for later repair. The central-third patellar tendon is identified, measured, and marked out with methylene blue. The patellar bone block is procured first after clearing the prepatellar bursal tissue and fascia. An electrocautery facilitates marking out of the proposed bone cut sites.

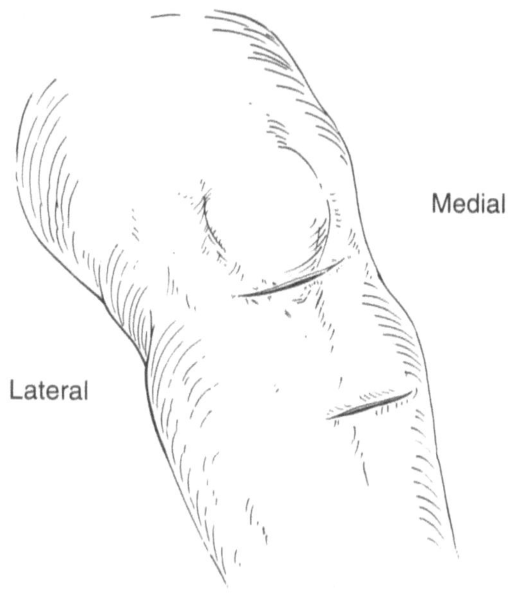


**FIGURE 12.7.** Endoscopic skin incisions.

## Graft preparation

A 1.0-cm oscillating saw is then used to cut the patellar bone block, which is generally harvested as 20 mm long, 10 mm wide, and 8 mm deep. A trapezoidal rather than square shaped bone block is preferable to reduce the chance of inducing a stress riser at the patellar harvest site, which could predispose to fracture. One oblique drill hole is placed in the patellar bone block using a $\frac{3}{32}$-inch drill bit and a no. 5 nonabsorbable braided polyester suture (Mersilene, Ethicon; Somerville, NJ) is passed through the block (which will be used as the proximal femoral bone block). A graft template is then used to outline and sharply cut the central third of the patella tendon taking care not to diverge (which can result in transection of the remaining tendon) or converge (which can result in transection of the graft). The underlying fat pad is left intact.

The tibial tubercle bone block is then approached and a similarly sized block is harvested, only instead of a 20-mm-long block a 25-mm block is procured. The tibial block is similarly drilled but three drill holes are spaced out passing three no. 5 nonabsorbable sutures (the tibial tubercle bone block is used on the tibial side). The free graft is then further cleared and debrided of all fat and adventitia and then tubed using a running 2-0 absorbable suture. The femoral bone block–tendon junction is marked with methylene blue to facilitate later arthroscopic visualization of the graft as it is seated in the femoral tunnel. The bone blocks are carefully chamfered to produce a rounded bullet-shaped configuration and to allow easy passage through appropriately diameter-graft sizing tubes (9-, 10-, and 11-mm diameter). The overall graft length is measured to assess whether the graft–tunnel length relationships will result in graft-tunnel mismatch (the result of a graft that after femoral fixation is achieved ends up proud on the tibial side with protrusion of the tibial bone block, which can limit placement of an interference fit screw in the tibial tunnel. The graft is then protected and stored on the back operative table in a towel moistened with antibiotic-impregnated saline.

## Patellar Donor Site Grafting

Cancellous bone is obtained with a curved curette from the proximal tibial metaphyseal bone through the tibial tubercle bone-block harvest site. The bone is then transferred and packed into the patellar defect to restore continuity of bone stock and presumably reduce the potential for patellar fracture and localized pain.

## Arthroscopy Examination

Arthroscopic examination is commenced through an inferolateral portal placed at the level of the joint line and a saline pump inflow is used on the scope sheath. Instrumentation is passed through a corresponding inferomedial portal. The joint line portals can both be made through the retinaculum to avoid further skin portal incisions, and this can be facilitated with an 18-gauge spinal needle, particularly if using the dual mini-transverse incision technique. A third superomedial or superolateral portal may sometimes be necessary for outflow. A complete diagnostic examination of the joint is performed after lavage (especially if hemarthrosis exists). Operative debridement and articular surface and meniscal tissue surgery is then undertaken. If meniscal repair is to be performed, sutures are passed at this time but may be tied down after the ACL reconstruction is completed.

## Notchplasty

Soft tissue and bony debridement of the notch is then performed. Any remaining ACL stump tissue is removed, allowing better definition of the preferred tibial and femoral drill sites as well as the location of the intact posterior cruciate ligament (PCL) position. Intercondylar notch stenosis and the potential for graft impingement are corrected. Landmarks include the most superior and posterior margin of the medial wall of the lateral femoral condyle (the "over-the-top" position), the "12 o'clock" midline position of the notch, the PCL insertion on the lateral wall of the medial femoral condyle, the intercondylar eminences or tibial spines, and the anterior horn of the lateral meniscus.

## Selection of Tunnel Drill Sites

Selection of the tibial and femoral tunnel sites is extremely important, and many studies have addressed the concept of isometric placement of the ACL graft. The key points are that the graft attachment sites should provide the graft with a passage free of bony impingement, with optimal tension and appropriate load distribution through a full arc of motion. Several commercial isometer devices are available and their use can be invaluable depending on the individual surgeon's preference. The author, however, prefers reliance on clearly defined landmarks and reproducible selection of bone tunnel positions.

## Tibial Tunnel

Both the endoscopic technique (using a transtibial tunnel to drill the femoral tunnel) from distal to proximal in a retrograde fashion and the arthroscopic-assisted technique (approaching the femoral tunnel via a transiliotibial band incision overlying the condyle and antegrade drilling of the femoral tunnel) start with selection and drilling of the tibial tunnel. The tibial ACL insertion site, the central region just anterior to the intercondylar eminence approximately 7 mm anterior to the PCL bulk, and the posterior margin of the anterior horn of the lateral meniscus all serve as tibial tunnel landmarks. A posterocentral site is preferable taking into account the vector direction toward the proposed femoral tunnel site and its relationship with the anterosuperior, medial, and lateral walls of the intercondylar notch.

A nonthreaded $\frac{3}{32}$-inch-diameter trochar-tipped smooth Steinmann guide pin is used to drill the tibial tunnel using a commercially available drill guide. The angle of the tibial tunnel in relation to the longitudinal tibial axis can be adjusted accordingly, depending on the length of the graft (if graft-tunnel mismatch is anticipated, a longer tibial tunnel may be preferable and therefore use of a more widely angled tunnel position).[74–76] The drill guide pin entrance site is approximately at the level of the tibial tubercle and 1 to 2 cm medial to it. The guide pin is passed up into the joint under arthroscopic visualization through the inferolateral joint line portal and its position is carefully checked. It is helpful to advance the guide wire toward the possible femoral drill tunnel site to allow assessment of potential notch impingement and the direction of the graft position. If the position is unsatisfactory, then the guide wire is redrilled. If the position is optimal, then a 10-mm cannulated reamer is used to drill over the guide wire, which is brought back and "capped" with a curette to protect inadvertent injury to the surrounding tissues. In most cases, the tibial tunnel is drilled to accept a 10-mm-diameter graft and a 10-mm tunnel is drilled. The intraarticular edges of the tunnel are chamfered, especially the posterior margins, to reduce graft abrasion. After the tunnel is drilled, all bony debris should be lavaged out of the joint and fluid extravasation can be reduced by using a commercially available covered cannula.

## Femoral Tunnel

If an arthroscopic-assisted technique is used, the lateral transiliotibial band approach is made and a femoral drill guide selected to guide the positioning of the femoral tunnel. Drilling of the guide pin is then performed in an antegrade manner under arthroscopic visualization through the inferolateral joint line portal.

If an endoscopic transtibial technique is used, then a 2.4-mm-diameter guide pin is passed retrograde up the tibial tunnel through the joint and into the notch toward the femoral tunnel site. A position 3 to 5 mm from the "over-the-top" margin is selected. It is important to clearly define the bony margins since soft tissue can obstruct visualization of the femoral tunnel site location. Knee flexion of at least 90° facilitates guide pin passage and commercially available transtibial femoral drill guides can be helpful. The coronal plane positioning of the tunnel in the notch is approximately at 1:00 to 1:30 on the face of a clock for a left knee and 10:30 to 11:00 for a right knee. Another helpful landmark can be that the guide pin should cross and be directly anterior the bulk of the intact PCL.

The femoral guide pin must be of sufficient length to be able to advance it in a retrograde fashion into the femur and out the anterior thigh. The 2.4-mm-diameter extra-long guide pin with suture eye (Arthrex Inc., Naples, FL) is preferred, since it allows guide pin drilling, reamer drilling of the femoral tunnel over the guide pin, and graft passage all in sequence, thereby reducing surgical time. The guide pin is drilled retrograde up through the femoral tunnel site and out the anterior femoral cortex, through the anterior thigh musculature and out the skin in one pass. The guide pin must be with the knee securely positioned in flexion and then precisely captured upon visualization of its exit over the anterior thigh (prepping and draping of the thigh as well as positioning of a cuff tourniquet must allow for ease of access to the pin exit site). After the drill pin is passed, its relationship at the femoral tunnel is carefully assessed. The drill pin is then reamed with an appropriately sized reamer, usually 10 mm in diameter. The potential for the tunnel to be too posterior (posterior cortical breakout or disruption) or too anterior should be constantly monitored and avoided. If posterior disruption does occur, then the endoscopic technique can be converted to the arthroscopic-assisted technique with the use of a lateral femoral condylar incision. If the tunnel is too anterior, then this is far more significant and a new tunnel may need to be drilled. In general, after reaming of the femoral tunnel, a 2- and 3-mm posterior cortical wall of bone is usually optimal. It is imperative to assess the femoral tunnel prior to continuing the procedure. After satisfactory position is assured, the tunnel's edges are gently chamfered and all bony debris thoroughly lavaged out of the joint.

## Graft Passage

The graft is passed using the nonabsorbable leader suture in a retrograde manner through the tibial tunnel using the endoscopic technique. Graft passage using the arthroscopic-assisted technique is dependent on the individual surgeon's preference whether the graft is passed distal to proximal or proximal to distal. Commercially available passers or looped 20-gauge stainless steel wire can facilitate the smooth passage of the graft. Placement and use of no. 5 nonabsorbable leader sutures is advised to allow for the incorporation of the sutures in a suture-post method of fixation if it is so desired. Positioning of the femoral bone block under direct arthroscopic visualization can be performed with an arthroscopic probe, although the author has found a small Freer elevator to be helpful.

## Femoral Tunnel Keying

Endoscopic femoral bone block fixation is accomplished first. Keying the junction of the bone block and tunnel marks out and provides a starting point for placement of the interference screw guide wire and the femoral side interference-fit screw. Positioning of the tendinous-insertion side to the femoral bone block (in general, the bone block is harvested from the patella) posteriorly tends to slightly posteriorize the femoral graft insertion site, but more importantly places the tendinous portion of the graft further away from the screw insertion site. The guide wire insertion site is then usually placed at the anterior junction of the femoral bone block, which is the preferred placement site for the interference screw.

## Femoral Screw Placement

After positioning the femoral bone block, a guide wire is passed through the central-third patellar tendon defect harvest site, through the infrapatellar fat pad and into the keyhole at the junction of the bone block and tunnel wall under direct arthroscopic visualization. (The inferomedial joint line portal or accessory medial portal can also be used.) It is important that the knee be flexed to at least 90° or more during the endoscopic femoral screw placement. The cannulated interference screw (using a $7 \times 20$ mm) is then passed over the guide wire and seated with the cannulated screwdriver. The screw is advanced over the guide wire and the bone block fixed into place. Care is taken not to have the screw advance or translocate the bone block upon insertion. To avoid guide wire incarceration fatigue or even breakage, the guide wire is slowly backed out as the screw becomes approximately halfway seated. The final screw insertion is carried out without the guide wire. Upon final fixation of the femoral block the graft is inspected and tension is manually applied to ensure a stable construct and secure screw purchase. Palpation of the construct should always be performed with an arthroscopic probe.

## Tibial Screw Placement

The graft may be twisted 90° upon itself at this point (to increase strength) and tensioned with the knee brought close to full extension.[77] It is important to ensure that the tibial bone block is freely mobile and not hung up in its tunnel, since appropriate graft tensioning cannot be accomplished. The tibial bone block is then positioned to avoid suture laceration upon insertion of the tibial screw. A cannulated screw system facilitates this and, as on the femoral side, reduces the incidence of divergence, convergence, block disruption, injury, or translocation. With tension applied at all times on the tibial block, using the bone block sutures, the tibial screw is passed over its guide wire and inserted into position.

## Final Inspection

Upon completion of graft fixation, the graft is once again arthroscopically inspected for position, ensuring that there is no notch impingement and that appropriate tension is palpable in the graft fiber bulk. Patholaxity tests are repeated and documentation of elimination of the preoperatively noted instability should be confirmed. In addition, the knee should be taken through a full range of motion. All meniscal repair sutures would at this time be tied and secured and the joint is irrigated and lavaged of any possible remaining debris.

## Closure

The closure begins by loosely approximating the central-third patellar tendon defect with a continuous 2-0 absorbable suture. It is advisable to place a drain usually adjacent to the tibial tunnel block since occasionally postoperative oozing can occur and result in a hematoma. The drain is removed in 12 to 24 hours. Upon completion of the skin incisional closure, a postoperative intraarticular injection of morphine and bupivacaine with epinephrine can, along with Ketorolac tromethamine (Toradol; Syntex, Palo Alto, CA) reduce early postoperative discomfort. A bulky cotton dressing is applied that allows full motion and the knee is then placed in a hinged postoperative brace. Cryotherapy and continuous passive motion (0–90°) are encouraged immediately beginning in the recovery room. The patients are usually discharged within 24 hours on crutches, advising partial weight bearing as tolerated. An outpatient rehabilitative program is begun the following day.

# Summary

Significant advances in the surgical approach to ACL reconstruction have resulted in a reproducible and in general successful technique to help restore the function of this ligamentous stabilizer. The evolution of ACL reconstruction surgery has proceeded toward methods associated with less perioperative morbidity through the use of limited-incision arthroscopic-assisted techniques. The central-third patellar tendon bone-tendon-bone autograft is currently favored by many surgeons, since it is associated with optimal mechanical and biologic properties and because it can be securely fixed using interference-fit screw fixation.

Multiple biomechanical and clinical studies have supported the use of interference screws for graft fixation, and numerous improvements in the design and delivery of these screws have been seen since they were first introduced in 1988. The use of cannulated interference screw systems has significantly contributed to the technique by affording a more precise and reproducible method of achieving secure screw fixation with greater ease of use.

The potential pitfalls of perioperative loss of fixation, divergence, graft translocation, and graft injury may all be reduced and avoided through the appropriate use of cannulated fixation systems. Technical attention to gap sizing, graft-tunnel mismatch, and screw insertion with guide wire retrieval may all further contribute to less potentially associated morbidity. A specific endoscopic-ACL reconstruction technique preferred and used by the authors with clinical success was described.

## References


1. Miyasaka K, Daniel D, Stone M, et al. The incidence of knee ligament injuries in the general population. *Am J Knee Surg* 1991;4:3–8.
2. Fu F. Personal communication, 1993.
3. Daniel DM, Stone ML, Dobson BE, et al. Fate of the ACL-injured patient. A prospective outcome study. *Am J Sports Med* 1994;22(5):632–643.
4. Baker C, Graham J. Intraarticular ACL reconstruction using the patellar tendon: arthroscopic technique. *Orthopedics* 1993;16(4):437–441.
5. Bach B. Arthroscopy-assisted patellar tendon substitution for anterior cruciate ligament insufficiency. *Am J Knee Surg* 1989;2(1):3–20.
6. Bach RB, Jones GT, Sweet FA, et al. Arthroscopy-assisted anterior cruciate ligament reconstruction using patellar tendon substitution. *Am J Sports Med* 1994;22(6):758–767.
7. Beck C, Paulos L, Rosenberg T. Anterior cruciate ligament reconstruction with the endoscopic technique. *Oper Tech Orthop* 1992;2:86–98.
8. Buss D, Warren R, Wickiewicz T, et al. Arthroscopically assisted reconstruction of the anterior cruciate ligament using autogenous patellar ligament grafts. Results after twenty-four months. *J Bone Joint Surg* 1993;75A:1346–1357.
9. Clancy W. ACL reconstruction using one-third of the patellar ligament augmented by extraarticular tendon transfers. *J Bone Joint Surg* 1981;64A:352–359.
10. Garfinkel M, Miller L, Antich T. The "one-incision" (endoscopic) technique versus the "two-incision" technique of anterior cruciate ligament reconstruction. A preliminary report. Presented at the 24th Annual EOA Meeting, Orlando, FL, October 1993.
11. Harner C, Marks P, Fu F, et al. Anterior cruciate ligament reconstruction: endoscopic versus two-incision technique. *Arthroscopy* 1994;10(5):502–512.
12. Jackson D, Jennings L. Arthroscopically-assisted reconstruction of the anterior cruciate ligament using a patellar tendon bone autograft. *Clin Sports Med* 1988;7:785–800.
13. Johnson R. Current concepts review: the treatment of injuries of the ACL. *J Bone Joint Surg* 1992;74A:140–151.
14. Lambert KL, Cunningham RR. Anatomic substitution of the ruptured ACL using a vascularized patellar tendon graft with interference fix fixation. In: Feagin JA Jr, ed. *The Cruciate Ligaments. Diagnosis and Treatment of Ligamentous Injuries about the Knee.* New York: Churchill Livingstone, 1988, 401–408.
15. Jones KG. Reconstruction of the anterior cruciate ligament. A technique using the central one-third of the patellar ligament. *J Bone Joint Surg* 1970; 52A:1302.
16. Rosenberg T, Paulos L, Abbott P. Arthroscopic cruciate repair and reconstruction: an overview and description of technique. In: Feagin JA, ed. *The Cruciate Ligaments.* New York: Churchill Livingstone, 1988;409–423.
17. Sgaglione N, Warren R, Wickiewicz T, et al. Primary repair with ST augmentation of acute ACL injuries. *Am J Sports Med* 1990;18:45–57.
18. Shelbourne KD, Rettig AC, et al. Miniarthrotomy versus arthroscopic-assisted anterior cruciate ligament reconstruction with autogenous patellar tendon graft. *Arthroscopy* 1993;9(1):72–75.
19. Malek M, DeLuca J, et al. Outpatient anterior cruciate ligament surgery: review of safety, practicality and economy. *Arthroscopy* 1992;8(3):404–405.
20. Odensten M, Gillquist J. Functional anatomy of the anterior cruciate ligament and a rationale for reconstruction. *J Bone Joint Surg* 1985;67A:257–262.
21. Bessette G. The anterior cruciate ligament. *Orthopedics* 1990;13:551–561.
22. Larson RL, Taillon M. Anterior cruciate ligament insufficiency: principles of treatment. *J Am Acad Orthop Surg* 1994;2:26–35.
23. Acker JH, Drez D. Angulation of fixation screw in knee ligament procedures. *Orthopedics* 1989; 12(6):823–826.
24. Amis AA. The strength of artificial ligament anchorages. A comparative experimental study. *J Bone Joint Surg* 1988;70B:397–403.
25. Straight CB, France EP, Paulos LE, et. al. Soft tissue fixation to bone. A biomechanical analysis of spiked washers. *Am J Sports Med* 1994;22(3): 339–343.
26. Butler DL. Evaluation of fixation methods in cruciate ligament replacement. *Instr Course Lect* 1987; 36:173–178.
27. James P. Stable fixation of bone-tendon-bone grafts in ACL reconstruction. *Am J Knee Surg* 1989;2(2):71–75.
28. Kohn D, Rose C. Primary stability of interference screw fixation. *Am J Sports Med* 1994;22(3):334–338.
29. Cerullo G, Puddu G. Arthroscopic placement of the interference screw for anterior cruciate ligament reconstruction. *Arthroscopy* 1993;9(6): 712–713.
30. Noyes FR, Butler DL, Grood ES, et al. Biomechanical analysis of human ligament grafts used in knee ligament repairs and reconstruction. *J Bone Joint Surg* 1984;66A:344–352.
31. Bosch U, Kasperczyk W. Healing of the patellar tendon autograft after posterior cruciate ligament reconstruction. *Am J Sports Med* 1992;20(5):558–566.
32. Arnoczky SP, Torzilli PA, Warren RF, et al. Bio-

logic fixation of ligament prostheses and augmentations. An evaluation of bone ingrowth in the dog. *Am J Sports Med* 1988;16(2):106–112.
33. Matthews LS, Lawrence SJ, Yahiro MA, Sinclair MR. Fixation strengths of patellar tendon-bone grafts. *Arthroscopy* 1993;9(1):76–81.
34. Kurosaka M, Yoshiya S, Andrish JT. A biomechanical comparison of different surgical techniques of graft fixation in anterior cruciate ligament reconstruction. *Am J Sports Med* 1987;15(3):225–229.
35. Grana WA, Egle DM, Mahnken R, et al. An analysis of autograft fixation after anterior cruciate ligament reconstruction in a rabbit model. *Am J Sports Med* 1994;22(3):344–351.
36. Jones KG. Reconstruction of the anterior cruciate ligament. A technique using the central one-third of the patellar ligament. *J Bone Joint Surg* 1963;45A:925.
37. Noyes FR, Butler DL, Paulos LE, et al. Intra-articular cruciate ligament reconstruction. Perspectives on graft strength, vascularization and immediate motion after replacement. *Clin Orthop* 1983;172:71–77.
38. Lambert KL. Vascularized patellar tendon graft with rigid internal fixation for anterior cruciate ligament insufficiency. *Clin Orthop* 1983;172:85–89.
39. Godbout B, Tearse D. Endoscopic-assisted anterior cruciate ligament reconstruction with autogenous patellar tendon graft: technical recent advances to improve technique. Presented at the 59th Annual AAOS Meeting, Washington, DC, February 1992.
40. Meade T, Dickson T. Technical pitfalls of single incision arthroscopic-assisted ACL reconstruction. *Am J Arthroscopy* 1992;2(2):15–19.
41. Fulkerson J, Hosick WB, Malkani A, et al. Potential problems in Kurosaka screw fixation of bone-tendon-bone graft transplants. Presented at the 60th Annual AAOS-AOSSM Specialty Day Meeting, San Francisco, CA, February 1993.
42. Bostman OM. Foreign-body reaction to fracture fixation implants of biodegradeable synthetic polymers. *J Bone Joint Surg* 1990;73B:592.
43. Bostman OM. Current concepts review: absorbable implants for the fixation of fractures. *J Bone Joint Surg* 1991;73A:148–153.
44. Bucholz RW. Prospective study of bioabsorbable screw fixation of ankle fractures. *J Orthop Trauma* 1992;6:505.
45. Bucholz RW, Henry W, Henley B. Fixation with bioabsorbable screws for the treatment of fractures of the ankle. *J Bone Joint Surg* 1994;76A:319–324.
46. Pihlajmaki H, Bostman O, Hirvensalo E, et al. Absorbable pins of self-reinforced poly L-lactic acid for fixation of fractures and osteotomies. *J Bone Joint Surg* 1992;74B:883–857.
47. Fulkerson J, Hosick W, Cautilli R, et al. Fine points in Kurosaka screw fixation of bone-tendon-bone graft transplants. Presented at the AAOS Sports Medicine Course, Steamboat Springs, CO, 1994.
48. Jomha NM, Raso VJ, Leung P. Effect of varying angles on the pullout strength of interference screw fixation. *Arthroscopy* 1993;9(5):580–583.
49. Burks R, Daniel D, Losse G. The effect of continuous passive motion on anterior cruciate ligament reconstruction stability. *Am J Sports Med* 1984;12(4):323–327.
50. Robertson DB, Daniel DM, Biden E. Soft tissue fixation to bone. *Am J Sports Med* 1986;14(5):398–403.
51. Paschal SO, Seemann MD, Ashman RB, et al. Interference fixation versus post-fixation of bone-patellar tendon-bone grafts for anterior cruciate ligament reconstruction. A biomechanical comparative study in porcine knees. *Clin Orthop* 1994;300:281–287.
52. Good L, Tarlow SD, Odensten M, et al. Load tolerance, security, and failure modes of fixation devices for synthetic knee ligaments. *Clin Orthop Rel Res* 1990;253:190–196.
53. Ivey M, Li F. Tensile strength of soft tissue fixations about the knee. *Am J Knee Surg* 1991;4(1):18–23.
54. Clancy W, Narechania R, Rosenberg T, et al. Anterior and posterior cruciate ligament reconstruction in Rhesus monkeys. *J Bone Joint Surg* 1981;63A:1270–1283.
55. McFarland E. The biology of anterior cruciate ligament reconstructions. *Orthopedics* 1993;16:403–410.
56. Rodeo S, Arnoczky S, Torzilli P, et al. Tendon healing in a bone tunnel. *J Bone Joint Surg* 1993;75A:1795–1803.
57. Steiner ME, Hecker AT, Brown CH, et al. Anterior cruciate ligament graft fixation. Comparison of hamstring and patellar tendon grafts. *Am J Sports Med* 1994;22(2):240–247.
58. Fithian D, Daniel D, Casanave A. Fixation in knee ligament repair and reconstruction. *Oper. Tech. in Orthop* 1992;2:63–70.
59. DeCoster TA, Heetderks DB, Downey DJ, et al. Optimizing bone screw pullout force. *J Orthop Trauma* 1990;4:169–174.
60. Brown CH, Hecker AT, Hipp JA, et al. The biomechanics of interference screw fixation of patellar tendon anterior cruciate ligament grafts. *Am J Sports Med* 1993;21(6):880–886.
61. Reznik AM, Davis JL, Daniel DM. Optimizing interference fixation for cruciate ligament reconstruction. *Trans Orthop Res Soc* 1992;15:519.
62. Brown G, Pena F, Grontredt T, et al. Failure strength of interference screw fixation in bovine, young human, elderly human cadaver knees: influence of insertion torque, tunnel-bone block gap and interference. *Acta Orthop Scand* 1994; submitted.

63. Hulstyn M, Fadale P, Abate J, et al. Biomechanical evaluation of interference screw fixation in a bovine patellar bone-tendon-bone autograft complex for anterior cruciate ligament reconstruction. *Arthroscopy* 1993;9(2):417–424.
64. Shapiro J, Cohn B, Jackson D, et al. The biomechanical effects of geometric configuration of bone-tendon-bone autografts in anterior cruciate ligament reconstruction. *Arthroscopy* 1992;8(4): 453–458.
65. Reznik A, Daniel D. ACL graft placement, tension, and fixation. *Surg Rounds Orthop* 1990;Sept: 21–24.
66. Bach BR. Potential pitfalls of Kurosaka screw interference fixation for ACL surgery. *Am J Knee Surg* 1989;2(2):76–82.
67. Franco MG, Bach BR, Bush-Joseph CC. Intraarticular placement of Kurosaka interference screws. *Arthroscopy* 1994;10(4):412–417.
68. Pierz K, Baltz M, Fulkerson J. Effect of Kurosaka screw divergence on the holding strength of bone-tendon-bone grafts. *Am J Sports Med* 1995; 23(3):332–335.
69. Lemos MJ, Albert J, Simon T, et al. Radiographic analysis of femoral interference screw placement during ACL reconstruction: endoscopic versus open technique. *Arthroscopy* 1993;9(2):154–158.
70. Fanelli GC, Desai BM, Cummings PD, et al. Divergent alignment of the femoral interference screw in single incision endoscopic reconstruction of the anterior cruciate ligament. *Contemp Orthop* 1994;28(1):21–25.
71. Doerr AL, Cohn BT, Ruoff MJ, et al. A complication of interference screw fixation in anterior cruciate ligament reconstruction. *Orthop Rev* 1990; 19(11):997–1000.
72. Matthews LS, Soffer SR. Pitfalls in the use of interference screws for anterior cruciate ligament reconstruction: a brief report. *Arthroscopy* 1989;5: 225–226.
73. Ishibashi Y, Rudy T, Kim H, et al. The effect of the ACL graft fixation level on knee stability. Presented at the 14th Annual Meeting of the Arthroscopy Association of North America, San Francisco, CA, May 6, 1995.
74. Kenna B, Simon T, Jackson D, et al. Endoscopic ACL reconstruction: a technical note on tunnel length for interference fixation. *Arthroscopy* 1993; 9(2):228–30.
75. Miller R, Dandy D. Graft length for anterior cruciate reconstruction. *J Bone Joint Surg* 1991;73B: 920–921.
76. Shaffer B, Gow W, Tibone J. Graft-tunnel mismatch in ACL reconstruction: a new technique of intraarticular measurement and modified graft harvesting. *Arthroscopy* 1993;9(6):633–646.
77. Cooper D, Deng X, Burstein A, et al. The strength of the central third patellar tendon graft. *Am J Sports Med* 1993;21(6):818–824.

# 13
# Ankle Fractures

Stanley E. Asnis and Mathias P.G. Bostrom

Ankle fractures form part of the spectrum of ankle injuries, which range from simple low-energy closed ankle sprains to high-energy open fractures and dislocations of the tibiotalar joint. The ankle joint is an intrinsically unstable complex hinge joint that depends on both bony and ligamentous anatomy for stability. Although there are no clear boundaries to the ankle, by convention injuries of the ankle are defined as those involving the supramalleolar region of the tibia and fibula, including the soft tissues that support the tibiotalar joint. It is a joint that requires precise structural integrity for proper function. Accordingly when it is injured, it requires anatomic restoration for a satisfactory outcome regardless of whether operative or nonoperative techniques are employed.[1]

## Structural Anatomy

The bony anatomy of the ankle joint is complex with functional articulations not only between the tibiotalar joint but also between the fibulotalar joint and the tibiofibular joint. The tibia and fibula are structurally aligned to form a partially constrained mortise as first described by Maisonneuve in the 19th century.[2] Within this mortise sits the wedge-shaped talus, which is slightly wider anteriorly than posteriorly.[3] This bony anatomy allows for dorsiflexion and plantar flexion of the ankle, with pronation, supination, eversion, external rotation, and internal rotation occurring at the subtalar joints. Stability is achieved by four groups of bony and ligamentous structures[4]:

*Medial*: Medial malleolus
- Medial collateral ligament
  - Superficial deltoid ligament
  - Deep deltoid ligament

*Lateral*: Lateral malleolus
- Lateral collateral ligament complex
  - Anterior talofibular ligament
  - Posterior talofibular ligament
  - Calcaneofibular ligament

*Anterior*: Anterior tibiofibular ligament

*Posterior*: Posterior tibiofibular ligament
- Posterior malleolus

In addition to the anterior and posterior tibiofibular ligaments, the fibula and tibia anatomy is maintained by the transverse tibiofibular ligament and the more proximally by the interosseous ligament (Figure 13.1).

While no muscles cross the ankle joint, numerous tendons cross the ankle joint: posteriorly the Achilles and plantaris tendons; medially the tibialis posterior, flexor digitorum longus, and flexor hallucis longus; anteriorly the tibialis anterior, extensor digitorum longus, extensor hallucis longus, and peroneus tertius; and laterally the peroneus longus and brevis (Figure 13.2).

## Clinical Relevance

The bony and ligamentous structures are vital to maintaining the integrity of the joint and to maintaining the talus within the mortise. The importance of maintaining full congruity of the joint is emphasized by the fact that a 1-mm shift laterally of the talus reduces the contact area of the tibiotalar joint by 42%.[5] With further lateral displacement of the talus the contact area was progressively reduced but then rate of change for each increment of shift was less marked. The clinical significance of this con-

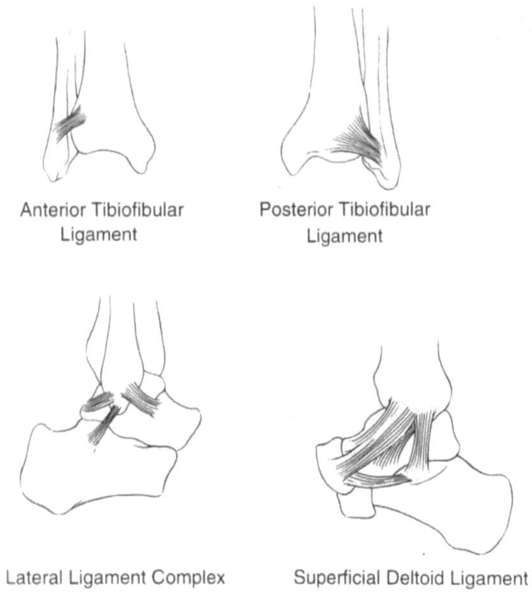


**FIGURE 13.1.** Bony and ligamentous anatomy of the lateral and medial ankle.

tact loss is still not fully understood; however, many surgeons believe that this will predispose the ankle to later degenerative arthritis. The stability of the ankle joint is dependent upon the anterior, posterior, lateral, and medial complexes. If only one group is lost, stability will be maintained, but as further groups are lost the stability of the ankle joint becomes further compromised regardless of the pattern of injury sustained. Thus if there is complete disruption of the medial structures with displacement of the lateral complex there is gross instability. Similarly if all four groups are lost the ankle will be completely unstable.

In addition to the importance of the bony and ligamentous anatomy for proper joint function, care must also be taken in preserving the soft tissue envelope surrounding the ankle joint, since only tendons and skin and no muscles make up this envelope. The significance of this is that wounds may be difficult to heal and the surgical incision must be well planned to avoid skin compromise. In general the skin on the lateral and medial sides of the ankle is very thin and must be treated with special care during any manipulation or intervention involving the ankle. If two incisions are used the skin bridge separating the incisions should be maximized to avoid wound problems.

# Neurovascular Anatomy

There are two major neurovascular bundles that cross the ankle joint. The anterior neurovascular bundle consisting of the deep peroneal nerve and the dorsalis pedis artery cross the ankle joint beneath the extensor retinaculum between the tibialis anterior and the extensor hallucis longus tendons. The posterior bundle consisting of the posterior tibial artery and tibial nerve crosses posterior to the medial malleolus between the tendons of the flexor digitorum longus and the flexor hallicus longus. Three other nerves cross the joint: (1) the saphenous nerve, which passes anterior to the medial malleolus and runs along the saphenous vein; (2) the superficial peroneal nerve, which lies just lateral to the anterior midline; and (3) the sural nerve, which lies posterior the fibula along with the short saphenous vein (Figure 13.3).

## Clinical Relevance

Avoidance of injury to tendons, nerves, or vessels during surgery is essential for proper motor function and sensation of the foot and to avoid vascular compromise and painful neuroma formation. Care must be taken with incisions about the ankle to avoid and/or protect these tendons and neurovascular structures. During open procedures these structures are under direct visualization. When performing percutaneous techniques these structures are not visualized. The specific areas of concern are the anterior ankle, posteromedial ankle, and the area just posterior to the distal fibula. The first two areas contain a complex of tendons, vessels, and nerves, whereas the third contains the peroneal tendons. The remaining ankle circumference can be utilized more safely, with some care reserved for the saphenous nerve and vessel anteromedially and the sural nerve laterally (Figure 13.3).

When approaching the ankle, proper technique dictates that after making the initial skin incision, the subcutaneous tissues should be bluntly spread with a hemostat and retracted. A

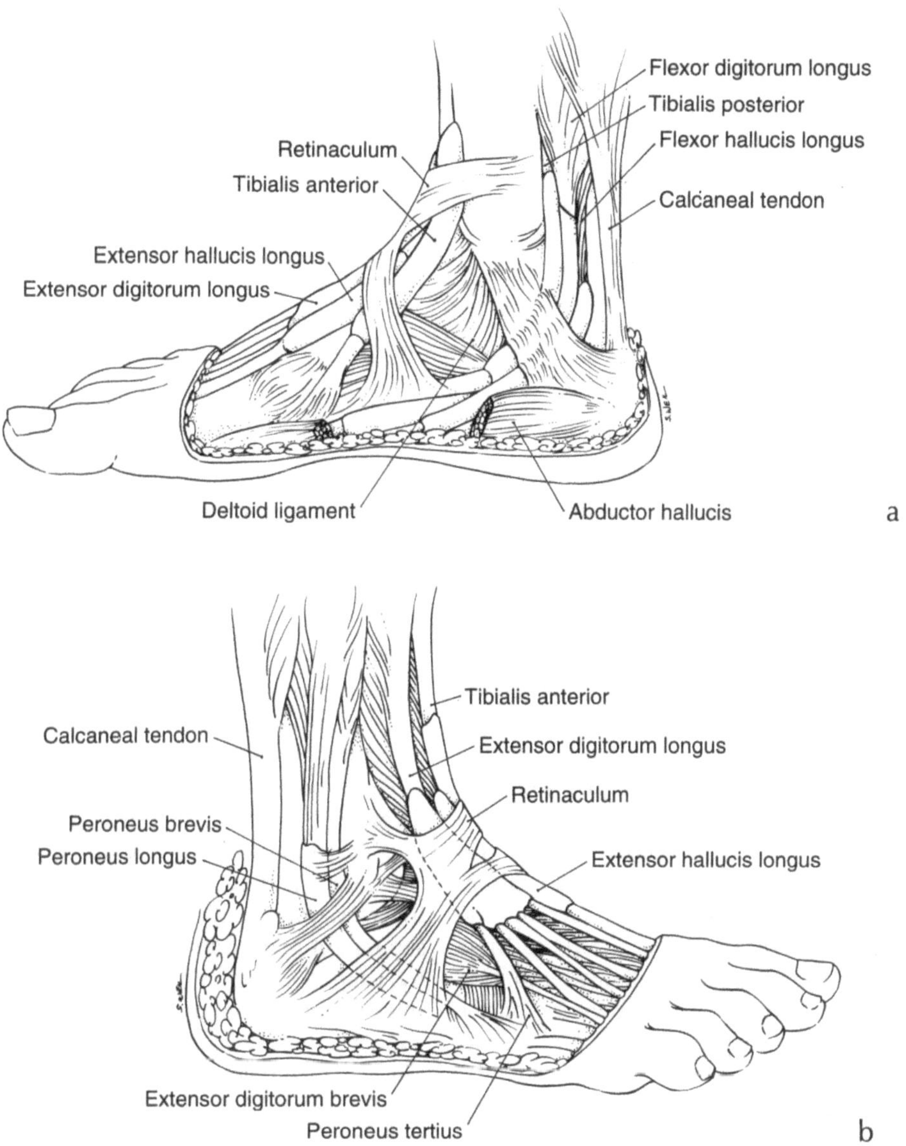


**FIGURE 13.2.** Soft tissue anatomy of the ankle joint. (a) medial view and (b) lateral view.

cylindrical tissue protector is placed onto the bone prior to drilling or guide pin placement. A self-tapping cannulated screw system with a positive rake cutting tip is advantageous (see Chapter 2). At the time of initial screw placement over the guide pin, the screw is initially turned counterclockwise so that it is blunt and does not grab or cut soft tissues. After the screw tip has been advanced past the soft tissues and down to the bone's cortex, the direction is reversed into a clockwise direction allowing for the positive rake cutting flutes to cut and tap the bone with advancement of the screw.

# Classification

Since Henderson[6] in 1932 proposed his ankle fracture classification system consisting of uni-, bi-, and trimalleolar fractures, there have been numerous more-involved classification schemes proposed. Lauge-Hansen proposed what is prob-

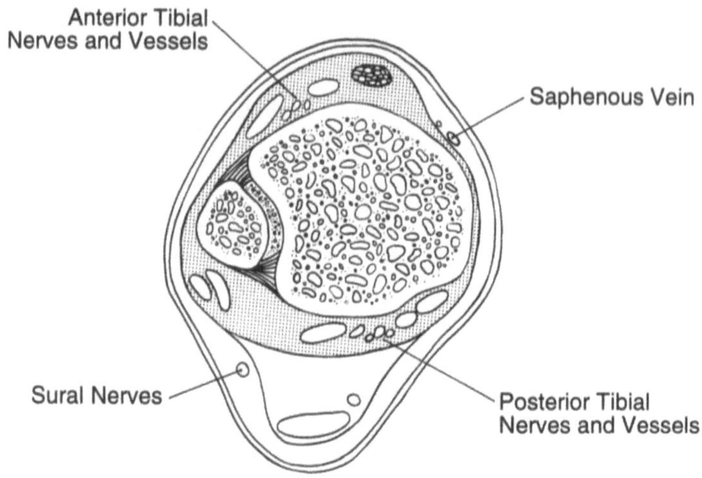


**FIGURE 13.3.** Cross section just proximal to ankle joint indicating location of major neurovascular structures.

ably the most comprehensive scheme in 1950 based on clinical, radiographic, and experimental observations.[7] Specifically he proposed a system of fracture classification that is based on the position of the foot at time of injury followed by the direction of the deforming force on the foot. There are four main subdivisions of this system: (1) supination-adduction, (2) supination-external rotation, (3) pronation-abduction, and (4) pronation-external rotation. Each of these injury patterns can then be subdivided into various stages, depending on the severity of the injury. Thus each group is composed of a spectrum of injuries depending on the severity. While comprehensive, this system is cumbersome and of limited clinical usefulness.

Weber and Danis separately proposed a system that classified the injury dependent on the location of the fibula fracture, with higher fibula fractures indicating more extensive damage to the tibiofibular ligaments with concomitant increase in mortise instability.[8,9] A type A injury is a fibular fracture below the tibial plafond and corresponds to the Lauge-Hansen supination-adduction injury pattern. With this injury the tibiotalar joint is stable and rarely requires internal fixation. Type B injuries are oblique spiral fractures of the fibula caused by external rotation. This injury is equivalent to the supination-external injuries of Lauge-Hansen. Weber proposed a type C injury pattern with the fibula fracture above the syndesmosis, which may be either a pronation-external rotation injury or a pronation-abduction injury.

Tile[10] proposed a system depending on the deforming force on the ankle at time of injury. A type I injury consists of an adduction-inversion injury pattern causing a lateral injury below the syndesmosis. The injury pattern matches the supination-adduction injury pattern proposed by Lauge-Hansen and the Weber type A injuries. A type II injury is an external rotation-abduction injury pattern producing an injury to the lateral complex at or above the syndesmosis. This type of injury corresponds to the supination-external rotation, pronation-abduction, and pronation-external rotation injuries seen in the Lauge-Hansen system and the type B and C injuries of the Weber system Tile further classified these injuries as being stable or unstable depending on the stability of the ankle mortise with stable injuries being defined as those that cannot be displaced by physiologic forces.

## Clinical Relevance

To be useful, a classification system must help in the management of the fracture and allow comparison of treatment results. While all the classification systems described above are useful in understanding the injury sustained, the clinician is most concerned about how to best manage the injury. Thus, which classification scheme one uses is not as important as understanding how to reduce the fracture and understanding which injury patterns are unstable and will require operative intervention to achieve stability and restore the congruity of the joint.

# Management

Since Pott[11] first stressed the importance of anatomic reduction of ankle fractures in the late 18th century, restoring joint stability and congruity remain essential in the treatment of ankle fractures. Ideally, the goals of treatment are to obtain anatomic reduction, maintain this reduction, and recover prefracture function with a mobile painless ankle. The choice of operative versus nonoperative treatment depends on many factors including the expectations of the patient, the general medical condition of the patient, the weight of the patient, bone quality, skin swelling and condition, the patient's other injuries, and the expertise and equipment of the surgical team. If a closed reduction and immobilization will result in a congruous stable joint, then nonoperative management is indicated. If stable anatomic restoration is not achievable by closed techniques, then operative intervention is usually indicated.

# Operative Techniques

The operative techniques to be described are outlined by anatomic region. These fractures may be solitary or in the different combinations as described by Lauge-Hansen or Weber and Danis. It is important to plan the operative procedure from good anteroposterior, lateral, and mortise radiographs. If needed, a radiograph of the entire tibia and fibula including the knee may also be indicated. A contralateral mortise view may be of value. On occasion a computed tomography (CT) scan can be very helpful in planning the fixation of the comminuted distal tibia. The entire injury pattern should be analyzed so as to adequately plan the incision(s) and type of internal fixation necessary.

Evaluation of the entire patient is also essential prior to operative intervention. Surgery should be carried out as soon after injury as the condition of the patient and soft tissues allow. This is ideally within 6 to 8 hours or before any true swelling or fracture blisters develop.[9] If delay cannot be avoided, then the ankle should be gently reduced, immobilized, and elevated to prevent further soft tissue injury and to decrease swelling. Occasionally skeletal traction or external fixation is indicated.

Ankle procedures are frequently performed with the patient in the supine position with a sandbag under the affected buttock. With a large posterior malleolar fragment, a prone or lateral position is often advantageous. For open procedures, a tourniquet is highly recommended.

In the treatment of ankle fractures cannulated screw techniques are commonly mixed with standard AO-ASIF techniques, i.e., fixation of the fibula with an AO interfragmentary screw and a one-third tubular plate, and the medial and posterior malleoli with cannulated screws.

## Advantages of Cannulated Screws

The use of cannulated screws in the treatment of ankle fractures is not intended to replace standard AO/ASIF procedures of open fracture fixation but rather to supplement these techniques. There are several advantages of using cannulated screws in ankle fracture fixation:

1. Ankle fractures are very accessible to fluoroscopic use. Fluoroscopic controlled guide pin placement can improve accuracy of positioning the screw.
   a. The guide pin can be used as a handle for reducing the fracture fragment.
   b. The guide pin can be repositioned with minimal host bone disturbance as compared with repositioning an already-placed screw.
   c. Guide pins can allow temporary fixation of one element of a complex fracture while another is being fixed.
   d. Guide pins used for temporary fixation can be positioned in the ideal position in

the fracture fragment and left in place for the final screw placement. Temporary wire fixation in solid screw techniques can get in the way of the solid screw need for final fixation.

   e. The guide pin can be used to establish the ideal screw's length prior to screw placement.

2. Percutaneous or very limited exposures can be utilized. This is advantageous compared with the wide exposures often needed to access the posterior malleolus.
3. Guide pins can be passed entirely through the bone and allowed to exit the opposite side of the leg (i.e., the treatment of posterior malleolar fractures). The final cannulated screw can then be passed over the guide pin from either direction depending on the fracture configuration.
4. Parallel placement of screws if desired is facilitated with the use of jigs and guide pins.

## Authors' Preferred Equipment

*Drill* (optional): A 2.0-mm by 150-mm steel drill, which can be used with a direct reading depth gauge. *Guide pin*: A 2.0-mm by 150-mm guide pin with a threaded tip and tapered root diameter (see Chapter 2). *Screw head*: Round head with an internal 3.5-mm hexagon. *Screw thread (cancellous type)*: Outer diameter—5.0 mm; reverse cutting flutes; self-cutting, self-tapping positive rake tip. *Cortical type*: Outer diameter: 4.5 mm fully threaded. *Material*: 316 LVM stainless steel. *Washers*: 5.0-mm system washers. *System accessory equipment*: A 20- to 70-mm depth gauge, 2.0-mm pin guide, soft tissue protection sleeve, and cannulated overdrill. (This reams over the guide pin to the diameter of the root of the screw thread or the shaft of the lag screw and not to the outer diameter of the screw thread. This is a smaller hole than a glide hole used to obtain a lag effect with a fully threaded screw.) Occasionally smaller cannulated screws are utilized; however, the authors prefer the 4.5- to 5.0-mm sizes for holding power and the ability to use a 2.0-mm guide pin for preliminary placement and fixation. Smaller guide pins have the disadvantage of increased flexibility.

# Lateral Malleolar Fractures

## Indications

Since the fibula is often considered the key to stability of the ankle, most displaced fractures of the distal fibula require operative reduction and fixation.[9] Although rigid fixation with an interfragmentary compression screw and a neutralization or compression plate gives excellent fixation, in the elderly rodding techniques have also been shown to be very effective even though there is less inherent stability. Pritchett studied 50 patients over 65 years of age randomized in two 25-patient groups.[12] One group was treated with Rush rods and the other with AO plates. Eighty-eight percent of patients treated with intramedullary rods had good or fair result compared with 76% undergoing plate and screw fixation. Full weight bearing was possible 6 weeks earlier with Rush rods than with AO plates, and there was less morbidity in the intramedullary rodded group. The authors have had a similar experience and agree with more limited fixation than AO plating in selected cases.

Nondisplaced avulsion fractures of the fibula (supination-adduction/Weber type A) may not require operative repair, but displaced unstable avulsion injuries generally require reduction and fixation. This is especially true if there is an associated medial complex injury and/or an osteochondral fracture of the tibia or talus.

Similarly, in stable nondisplaced eversion-abduction-type injuries nonoperative treatment is indicated. If the stability of the ankle remains uncertain, then examination under anesthesia is indicated. In unstable injuries even if an adequate reduction is achieved by closed means, the ankle must be placed in internal rotation with a high incidence of redisplacement due to the lack of a stable medial buttress. Therefore, most eversion-abduction (Weber B and C) injuries require operative reduction and fixation.

Fractures of the proximal fibula associated with ankle injuries (Maisonneuve-type) usually do not require internal fixation but may need a syndesmotic screw for adequate stabilization depending on the other associated injuries to the ankle.

## An Approach Specific to Percutaneous and Limited Open Reductions

The fibula is readily accessible to percutaneous and limited exposures. The area posterior to the lateral malleolus is avoided to prevent interference with the peroneal tendons. If necessary, the fracture can be reduced open with a small incision and a separate incision or distal extension of the first incision used for screw or rod entry. With an intramedullary screw or rod, the long proximal wound extension often needed for plating is eliminated. In plating, the proximal portion of such an incision must be made carefully to avoid the superficial peroneal nerve as it crosses the fibula, since injury to this nerve may cause a painful neuroma.

## Techniques

Transverse or short oblique fractures at the level of the top of the talar dome or below (Weber A and B) are fixed with a cannulated screw or Rush rod, either of which may or may not also utilize a tension band wire (Figure 13.4). The Weber C fracture is treated either with a Rush rod or AO plate technique depending on the stability of the associated fractures of the ankle and the fixation necessary to maintain adequate length of the fibula (Figure 13.5).

The key in the limited fixation of the fibula is in obtaining anatomic alignment of the fibula and fracture, then determining where the internal fixation device should enter. In the lateral malleolar fracture, the proximal fibula is usually held fixed to the distal tibia by its ligamentous attachments. Since the fixation device will pass up into the intramedullary canal of the proximal fibula, the distal fragment alignment is determined by where the fixation lies within it. Once the fracture is reduced, the critical entrance point in the fibula tip must be determined. If too anterior an entrance point is chosen, the lateral malleolus may displace posteriorly as the intramedullary devise aligns itself in the proximal fibula; if too posterior a site is chosen, the lateral malleolus may displace anteriorly. Likewise the site must be satisfactory in the medial-lateral direction. Too lateral an entry site may displace the lateral malleolus medially and tend to close the ankle mortise. Because of the increased width at the end of the fibula the entrance site for a screw may be slightly lateral and the screw directed slightly medially across the fracture. Since the Rush rods are much longer they are committed completely by the direction of the proximal fibula. A slightly lateral entrance site can be selected by prebending the distal end of the rod 10° to 15°. Once the surgeon is aware of the importance of this positioning and can determine the entrance site satisfactorily, the procedure is usually simple.

The fibula is reduced if necessary and a determination made as to the entrance site in the tip of the lateral malleolus. If an open reduction is performed, the entrance site is determined by direct visualization. If closed, the site is chosen with the aid of the fluoroscope and a small incision made over the appropriate site at the end of the lateral malleolus. A 2.0-mm guide pin is placed through the fibular cortex, across the fracture, and into the proximal fibula. The position of the guide pin is confirmed by fluoroscopy. The depth gauge is used to determine screw length. The cannulated overdrill is then used to open the fibula cortex and widen the channel in the distal fragment only. This allows easier cutting by the self-cutting screw and puts less torque and strain on the distal fibula when the screw is passed. The 5.0-mm self-cutting, self-tapping screw is then passed over the guide pin and passed retrograde across the fracture. If desired, a 20-gauge wire or no. 5 braided Dacron suture is then passed through a transverse drill hole proximal to the fracture site and placed in a figure-eight shape around the screw head.

For more proximal and oblique fractures (Weber C), the authors utilize a small or more commonly medium Rush rod. Again the entry site is of major importance. The length of rod selected will go well up into the medullary canal of the fibula. The entry site is opened with the appropriate Rush awl. The rod is then directed across the fracture and up the proximal fibula. The bevel at the leading end of the rod is used to direct the rod until it has passed the fracture site. It is oriented such that the point of the bevel is always kept toward the center of the

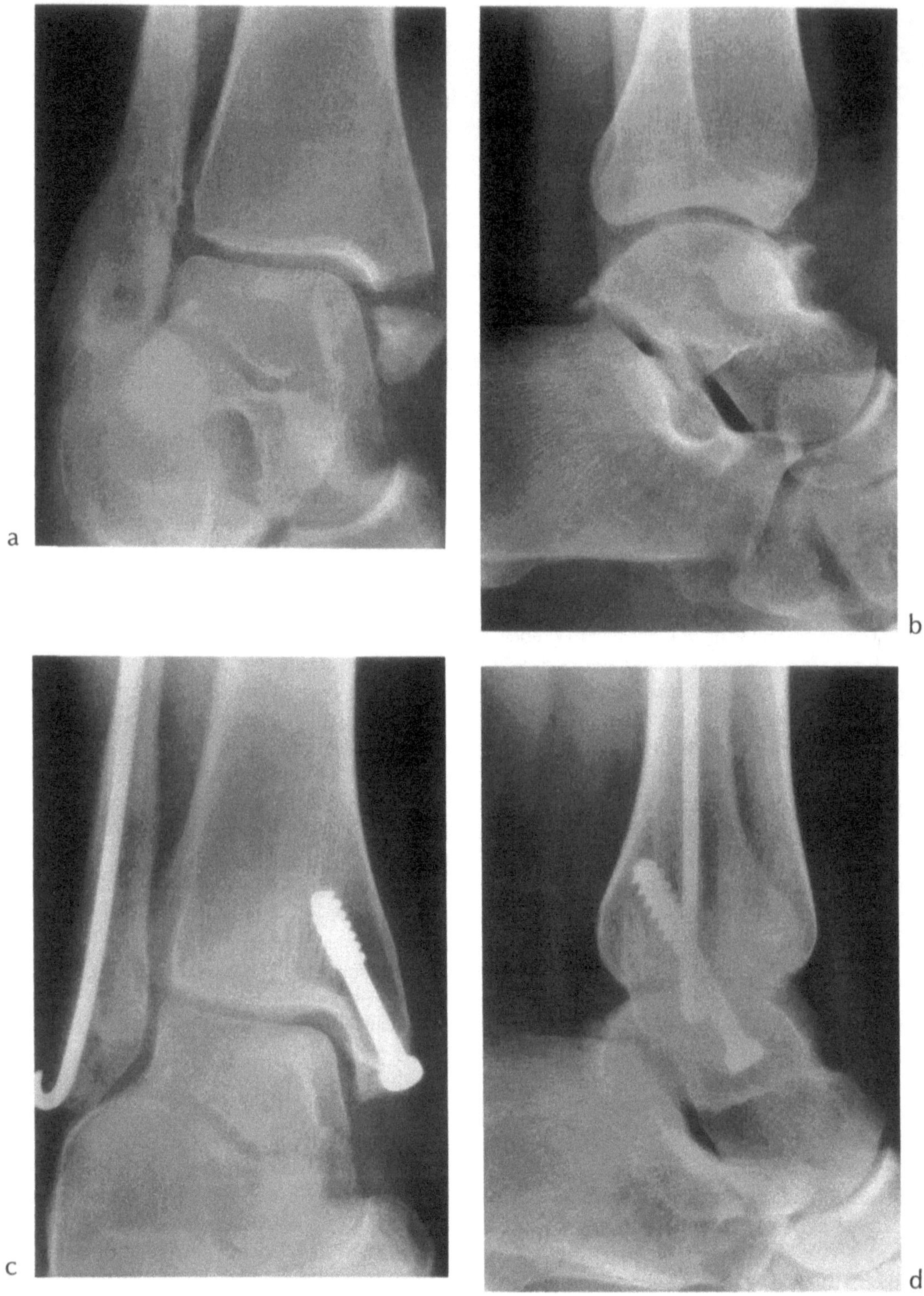


**FIGURE 13.4.** (a) The mortise and (b) lateral radiographs demonstrate transverse lateral malleolar and medial malleolar fractures. The post-fixation (c) mortise and (d) lateral views demonstrate the fibula fixed percutaneously with a Rush rod and the medial malleolus fixed percutaneously with a cannulated 5.0-mm partially threaded cancellous screw.

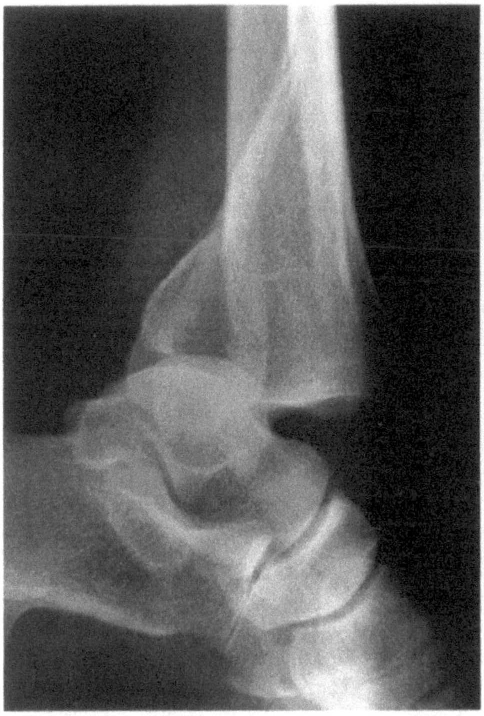

a

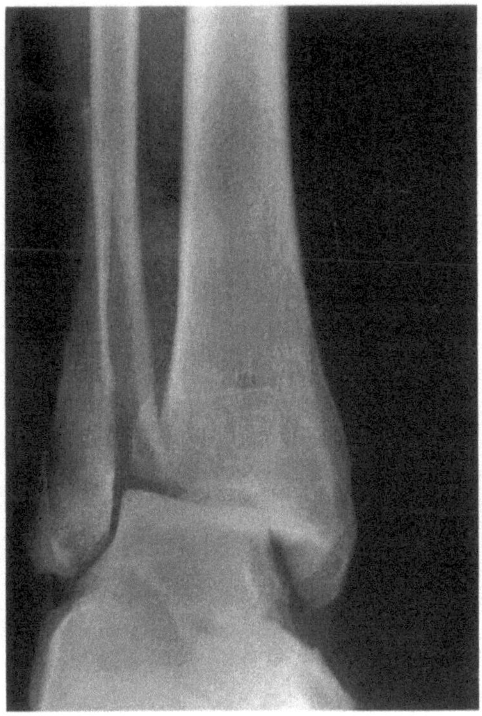

b

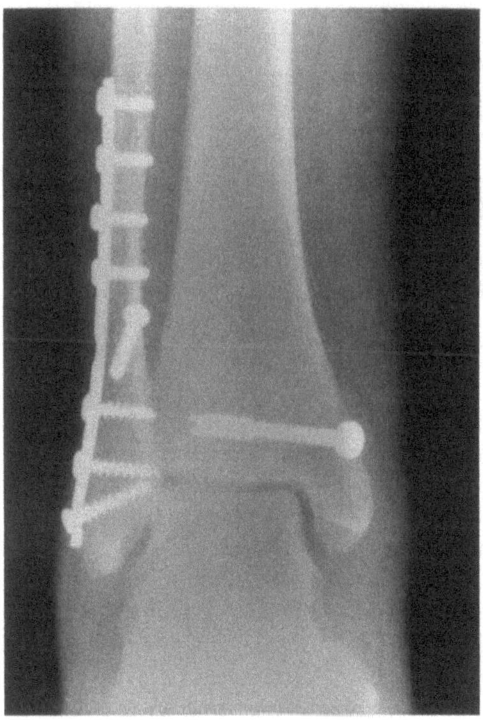

c

**FIGURE 13.5.** (a) The lateral and (b) mortise radiographs demonstrate a trimalleolar fracture dislocation of the ankle. (c) The oblique lateral malleolar fracture was fixed with a one-third semitubular plate. The posterior malleolar fragment was secured with a cannulated 5.0-mm partially threaded cancellous screw.

medullary canal. Prior to placement the Rush rods are prebent approximately 10° at their distal end to flare slightly away from the ankle joint and the talus. This conforms well to the shape of the distal fibula. A figure-eight tension band wire or suture can be utilized if necessary in the Weber B fractures or in a cerclage fashion in the oblique Weber C fractures.

### Clinical Relevance

The determination of the fixation method used for the lateral malleolus is dependent on the combination of injuries to the ankle. If the medial and posterior complexes are stable or can be stability fixed, limited procedures with cannulated screws or Rush rods and wires are preferred. These procedures require less dissection and appear to heal rapidly. The key is the reduction of the fibula in its proper position in relation to the tibia. AO/ASIF plating techniques are used in the more comminuted fibula fractures or the pylon fracture where rigid rotational and axial stability are required.[13] After the ankle fractures are fully healed the authors prefer to remove the fixation devices in the younger patients. Removal of a cannulated screw or Rush rod from the fibula is a simple procedure. The authors feel that the healed fibula that has had a Rush rod or cannulated screw removed may be stronger than that which has had a plate removed.

## Medial Malleolar Fractures

### Indications

Eversion-abduction injuries to the ankle often result in either deltoid ligament injuries or avulsion injuries to the medial malleolus. Substantial controversy surrounds the need for operative intervention with these injuries. If the mortise can be reduced with an intact medial malleolus or small distal avulsion and an anatomic position of the fibula, then operative intervention on the medial side is not always indicated. However, if the mortise remains widened or the fibula or medial malleolus cannot be reduced, then the medial ankle should be explored to remove any interposed tissue such as periosteum, the deltoid ligament, or the posterior tibial tendon. In these cases, the medial and/or lateral malleolar fractures are reduced and fixed.

Supination-adduction injuries resulting in a medial injury usually cause a vertical fracture of the medial malleolus and may be associated with either a crush injury to the medial articular surface of the tibia or talus.[14] This fracture may include the posteromedial tibia. This injury pattern requires internal fixation occasionally with bone grafting.[11,13]

### Incisions

Medial malleolar avulsion fractures are approached using a standard anteromedial approach that may be extended proximally. The skin flap of such an incision is based posteromedially and derives its blood supply from the adjacent posterior tibial artery. When utilizing this incision, care must be taken to protect the saphenous nerve and vein anteriorly. Although the saphenous vein can be sacrificed if necessary, avoidance of the adjacent saphenous nerve is essential. If the fracture is associated with a large posteromedial fragment, then a posteromedial approach may be preferred.

### Techniques

Vertical fractures of the medial malleolus require fixation with cancellous screws. These are usually placed perpendicular to the fracture plane if the size of the fragment permits. Due to the vertical shear forces on the fragment, a buttress plate may be necessary. If there is comminution or impaction of the tibial surface, precise reconstruction of the articular surface should be attempted with supplementary bone graft as necessary.

The large fragment of the vertical fracture, which includes the medial malleolus and either the medial or posteromedial tibia, can be readily reduced. The fracture can be windowed open anteriorly (hinged posteriorly) to examine the joint. The joint can be irrigated and intra-articular debris removed. The proximal fracture line usually does not require full visualization. The fracture is then reduced and held with two

2.0-mm guide pins placed parallel to each other and perpendicular to the fracture. The guide pins are spaced to be in the desired position of the screws. The pins must be placed proximal enough to assure that the screw will not enter the ankle joint. When the desired pin position is confirmed by fluoroscopy, measurements are taken with the direct reading depth gauge for screw length. The tibial cortex is optionally opened with the cannulated overdrill. The overdrill enlarges the hole to the size of the root diameter of the thread or the diameter of the shaft of the screw, not the outer diameter of the thread. This is not the same as a glide hole used to make a fully threaded cortical screw lag. If a washer is not to be used, the cortex is countersunk slightly with the cannulated countersink. The first 5.0-mm cancellous screw is then passed over the guide pin across the fracture and into the tibia. Likewise, the same steps are followed for the second screw over the second guide pin. If desired, washers may be utilized.

The very common oblique medial malleolar fracture is very amenable to screw fixation (Figure 13.4 and 13.6). The authors feel that one well-placed cancellous screw will give excellent fixation of the medial malleolus. The fracture must first be evaluated in regard to the size and integrity of the medially malleolar fragment. If comminuted or very small, then the wire and tension band construct should be used. Most medial malleolar fragments will readily accept a 5.0-mm cannulated cancellous screw. The larger medial malleolar fragments will often accept a 6.5-mm cannulated cancellous lag screw. The fracture is first exposed with an anterior medial approach as just described. The fracture is reduced with a fracture reduction forceps. A 2.0-mm guide wire is placed in the middle of the fragment, then directed through the midportion of the fracture and into the tibia. When using this configuration, the screw threads need only engage 2 to 4 cm beyond the fracture and not to the lateral tibial cortex unless the

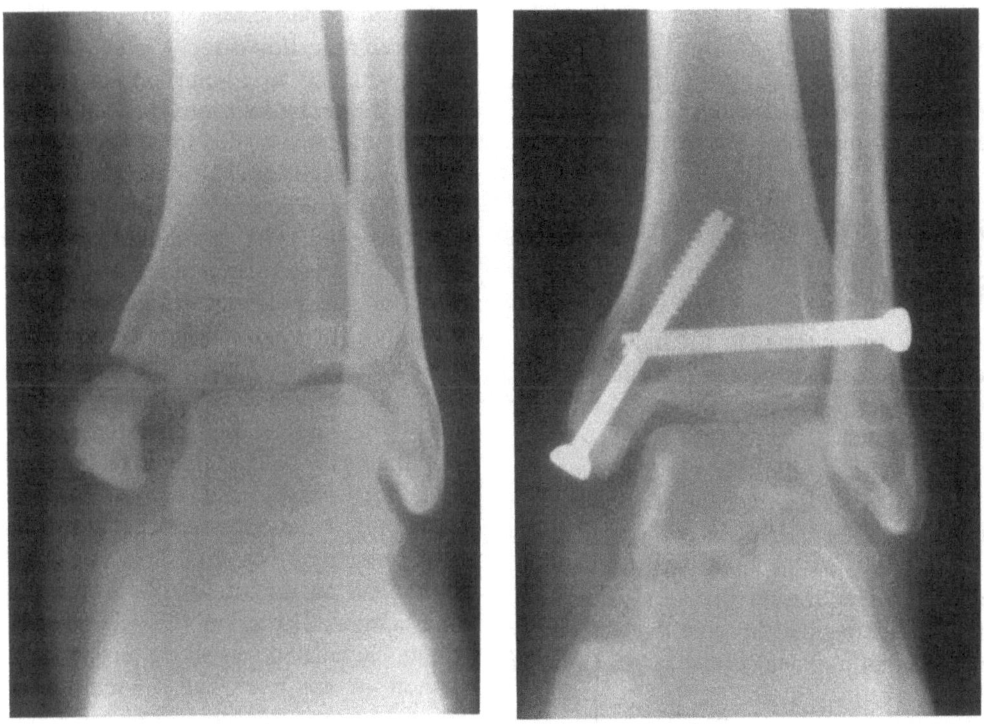

a b

**FIGURE 13.6.** (a) A displaced medial malleolar fracture is shown with a syndesmotic injury. (b) The medial malleolar fracture was fixed with a cannulated 5.0-mm partially threaded cancellous screw and the syndesmosis was fixed with a cannulated 4.5-mm fully threaded cortical screw.

bone is osteoporotic. The position of the guide wire is confirmed with fluoroscopy or radiographs. The direct reading depth gauge is used to determine the screw length. The medial malleolar fragment is reamed with the cannulated overdrill to the size of the shaft of the screw. The overdrill is passed completely through the fragment, across the fracture, and approximately 5 mm into the tibia. This enlarges the hole in the bone fragment to the size of the smooth shaft of the 5.0-mm screw and will decrease the strain on this fragment when the screw threads pass. The selected 5.0-mm self-cutting and self-tapping screw is then threaded through the fragment and across the fracture into the tibia while the fracture is supported by the bone reduction forceps. The fragment may rotate slightly as the screw thread passes, but can very easily be anatomically realigned when the fragment rests on the smooth shaft of the lag screw. The fragment is firmly compressed into anatomic position as compression is applied. The authors have found that the compression of one 5.0- or 6.5-mm cannulated screw applies adequate rotational control without the need of an additional second screw. With this technique there is less chance of fracturing the medially malleolar fragment.

# Posterior Malleolar Fractures

## Indications

Controversy continues as to the indications for operative treatment of posterior malleolar fractures, with open reduction indicated with fragments greater than 25% to 35% of the articular surface or if the fracture is displaced greater than 2 mm.[13–16] Additional indications include continued posterior talar dislocation or subluxation, incongruity of the tibial articular surface, the need for stabilization of the syndesmosis, and those fractures that involve the tibiofibular groove where a fragment prevents reduction of the fibula.

## Incisions

Using standard AO/ASIF techniques, patients with large posterolateral fragments should be approached via a posterolateral approach, just as patients with large posteromedial fragments should be approached via a posteromedial approach. This usually requires a large incision for full exposure and visualization. If cannulated screws are utilized and indirect reduction techniques are successful, percutaneous screw placement may eliminate the need for these more extensive incisions that may compromise wound healing.

## Techniques

Generally as the fibula is reduced many posterior malleolar fragments are pulled into anatomic position, with dorsiflexion of the ankle assisting in the reduction by ligamentotaxis. If the large posterior malleolar fracture is nondisplaced or reduces with closed means, then percutaneous fixation is indicated (Figures 13.5 and 13.7). If the posterior malleolar fracture is mildly displaced, then reduction may be possible by manipulation of the fragment using the guide pins as handles. If a reduction of the fragment and articular surface is not obtainable, then a full open reduction is required.

Two small 5- to 10-mm incisions are made. One is placed just lateral to the Achilles tendon and the other just medial to it. These are placed at a level approximately 10 mm proximal to the posterior lip of the ankle joint as determined by fluoroscopy. The first guide pin is passed through the posterolateral incision down to the cortex of the posterior malleolus. It is then driven into the fragment. The second guide pin is likewise passed through the posteromedial incision. Care is taken with this pin to stay toward the middle of the posterior tibia and avoid the flexor hallicus longus tendon and posterior tibial artery and nerve. The surgeon should review the cross-sectional anatomy prior to the procedure. The sizes of screws to be used will depend on the size of the posterior malleolar fragment. The authors prefer to use 6.5- or 5.0-mm cannulated cancellous screws or a combination of the two. The 6.5-mm cannulated screws are used over the 3.2-mm guide pins and the 5.0-mm screws over the 2.0-mm guide pins. The 3.2-mm guide wire for the 6.5-mm screw serves as a stiffer handle to maneuver the fragment. After the fracture is reduced with the guide pins, they are driven across the fracture

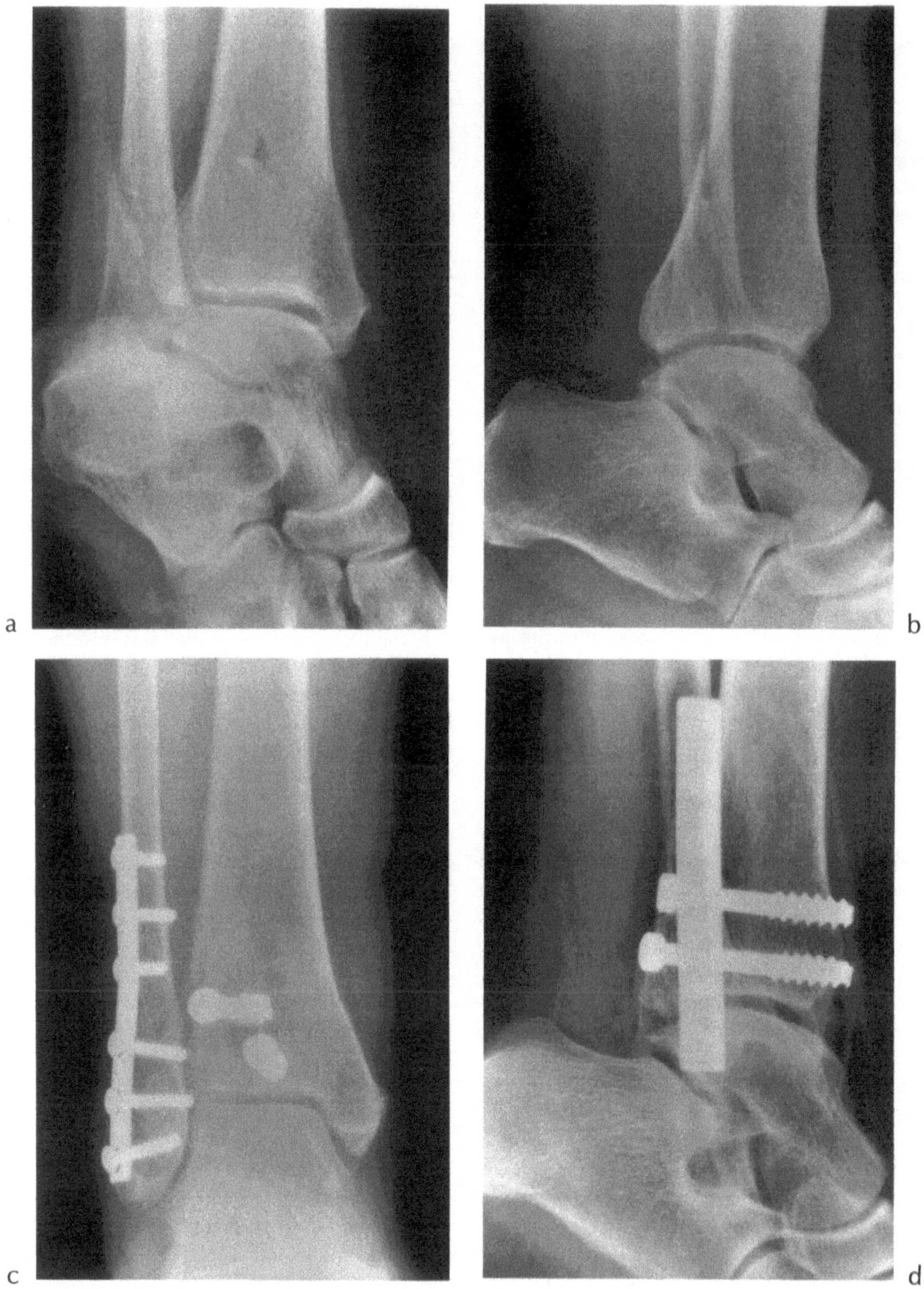

FIGURE 13.7. (a) The mortise radiograph demonstrates an oblique fibular fracture (b) while the lateral radiograph shows a large posterior malleolar fracture. (c) The fibular fracture was fixed with a one-third semitubular plate and (d) the posterior malleolus was fixed with two cannulated 5.0-mm partially threaded cancellous screws placed by a percutaneous technique.

and into the distal tibia. The position is confirmed by fluoroscopy. The depth gauge is then used to determine the proper screw length. The first screw is then slowly advanced over the guide pin turning the screw in a counterclockwise direction. This allows the screw to pass through the soft tissue as a blunt object. This is continued until the cortex of the posterior malleolus is firmly met; the direction of the screw is then reversed and the positive raked cutting flutes start advancing into the bone. The second screw is similarly passed and both screws tightened to compress the fracture.

On occasion, with a large fragment, the surgeon may prefer to place the screw from anterior to posterior. This is permitted only if the posterior fragment is large enough to allow the entire screw thread to pass the fracture and be contained in the posterior malleolus or posterior tibial fragment (and allow lag). The same procedure is followed except the guide pin is carefully advanced through the anterior tibial cortex. A cut down is then made over the pin anteriorly and the screw can be passed retrograde over the guide pin, leaving the head of the screw at the anterior tibial cortex.

# Anterior Malleolus

While the anterior malleolus is rarely fractured in isolation, it may be fractured in association with either medial or lateral injuries. This is especially true of the avulsion fracture of the anterior tibiofibular ligament from the tibial tubercle of Tillaux-Chaput. If the fragment is large enough, then it may warrant fixation via either the lateral or medial wounds. It may also be fixed more easily via the limited exposure techniques using cannulated screws. The techniques and approaches for accomplishing this would be similar to fixing posterior malleolar fractures via either anteromedial or anterolateral stab incisions.

# Syndesmosis

After the reduction and fixation of medial, lateral, posterior, and anterior complexes, the syndesmosis should be examined. If there continues to be widening of the tibiofibular joint, then fixation of the syndesmosis is recommended.[15,17] The most common recommendations for operative fixation include syndesmotic rupture associated with the following: medial ligamentous injury, talar shift without fracture of the fibula (tibiofibular diastasis), Maisonneuve fracture, and the continued evidence of syndesmotic instability after fixation of the fibula and any avulsion fractures.

## Technique

Fixation of the syndesmosis is recommended with one 4.5-mm cannulated fully threaded cortical screw placed through the fibula and the lateral cortex and trabecular bone of the tibia, i.e., three cortices. In that the fibula shaft lies posterolateral above the level of the tibiotalar joint, the screws should be directed from posterolateral to anteromedial. The ankle should be held in neutral to slight dorsiflexion to bring the wider anterior portion of the talus into the mortise. This avoids overtightening the mortise and the permanent loss of dorsiflexion. The level of the screw should be at the level of the tibiofibular ligaments or 1 to 2 cm proximal to the joint.

The level of the screw is first selected with the aid of the fluoroscope, and a free guide wire is placed as a marker on the surface of the leg. A 1-cm incision is made over the palpated cortex of the fibula. Soft tissues are retracted with a hemostat. The ankle is placed in neutral to slight dorsiflexion. Since a fully threaded screw is to be used, the distance between the fibula and the tibia will remain set as the final screw threads into the tibia. A 2.0 × 150 mm Gray bone drill is used rather than the same length guide pin. This will allow easier and more controlled passage through the hard cortical bone of the fibula. The drill is directed anteromedially. The drill is placed in a cylindrical soft tissue protector and passed through both cortices of the fibula and the lateral cortex of the tibia short of the medial cortex. Position is confirmed with fluoroscopy. The direct reading depth gauge is used and screw length determined. The lateral fibular cortex may optionally be reamed with the overdrill. The 4.5-mm fully threaded self-cutting self-tapping screw of appropriate length is then passed over the drill. The screw is advanced until its head comes in contact with the lateral cortex of the fibula. The patient should be non–weight bearing for 6 to 8 weeks after insertion. Surgeons suggest syndesmotic screw removal at 3 months after repair (Figure 13.6).

# Complications of Internal Fixation

Despite generally satisfactory results with open reduction internal fixation techniques, complications do occur.

## Neurovascular Injuries and Compartmental Syndrome

Despite the proximity of major neurovascular bundles about the ankle, the frequency of neurovascular injury is rare.[18] Compartmental syndrome of the foot is also a rare complication of ankle fractures, but may occur especially when there has been direct vascular compromise as seen with fracture dislocations. As always with compartmental syndromes, early recognition and treatment avoids the long-term sequelae of this syndrome.

## Nonunion and Malunion

Nonunions after ankle fractures are relatively rare but if they occur they are usually associated with the medial malleolar fractures that were not fixed at the time of injury.[19,20] In these situations union can be achieved with open reduction and internal fixation but may be difficult due to resorption at the fracture site, remodeling at the fracture edges, and osteoporosis. Bone grafting is often necessary. Nonunions of the lateral and posterior malleoli are less common.

Malunions of the fibula, especially with inadequately reduced external rotation injuries, occur more frequently, resulting in incongruity of the articular surface and instability of the mortise.[21,22] If not corrected early by fibular osteotomy and lengthening, they can lead to persistent symptoms, degenerative arthritis, and loss of function of the joint. Medial malleolar malunions also occur with less frequency and are usually asymptomatic.

## Wound Problems and Infection

The infection rate associated with internal fixation of closed fractures is less than 2%, and marginal wound necrosis has been reported to be as high as 3% with even higher rates reported with complex fractures of the distal tibia and ankle.[15,21–23] Multiple techniques can be employed to minimize the incidence of wound problems and infections including careful handling of the soft tissues, minimizing tourniquet time, gentle retraction, avoiding implants that are too large, appropriate wound drainage, wound closure without tension, and avoiding restrictive dressings. Since trauma to the soft tissues is minimized with percutaneous techniques, wound problems and infections should be less.

## Postoperative Arthritis and Reflex Sympathetic Dystrophy

The incidence of degenerative arthritis following ankle fractures is directly related to the adequacy of the reduction. Specifically if the anatomic reduction is achieved, then the incidence of arthritis is about 10%.[21,24–26] If, however, the reduction is inadequate, then the incidence is 85%. Osteochondral fractures and the more severe injury patterns also have increased rates of degenerative arthritis, even when adequate reduction has been achieved. This increased rate may be related to damage to the articular surface at the time of injury.

Reflex sympathetic dystrophy has been associated with all types of ankle injuries regardless of severity or whether operative or nonoperative techniques were utilized. Prompt restoration of the anatomy and early return to function may decrease the incidence. Prolonged immobilization should be avoided.

# Conclusion

The use of cannulated screws in the treatment of ankle fractures supplements the use of more established techniques. They provide internal fixation while minimizing the soft tissue dissection, and therefore help achieve the ultimate goal of restoration of the ankle mortise while allowing for early motion and satisfactory functional results.

## References


1. Hughes JL. The medial malleolus in ankle fractures. *Orthop Clin North Am* 1980;11:649–660.
2. Maisonneuve JG. Recherches sur la fracture du perone. *Arch Gen Med* 1840;7:165–187.
3. Inman VT. *The Joints of the Ankle.* Baltimore: William & Wilkins, 1976.
4. Pankovich AM, Shivaram MS. Anatomical basis of variability in injuries of the medial malleolus and the deltoid ligament I. Anatomic studies. *Acta Orthop Scand* 1979;50:217–223.
5. Ramsey PL, Hamilton W. Changes in the tibiotalar area of contact caused by lateral talar shift. *J Bone Joint Surg* 1976;58A:356–357.
6. Henderson MS. Trimalleolar fracture of the ankle. *Surg Clin North Am* 1932;12:867–872.
7. Lauge-Hansen N. Fractures of the ankle. Analytic historic survey as the basis of new experimental, roentgenologic, and clinical investigation. *Arch Surg* 1948;56:259–317.
8. Brunner CF, Weber BG. *Special Techniques in Internal Fixation*, New York: Springer-Verlag, 1982.
9. Muller ME, Allgower M, Schneider R, et al. *Manual of Internal Fixation.* Techniques recommended by the AO-ASIF Group. Berlin: Springer-Verlag, 1991.
10. Tile M. Fractures of the ankle. In Schatzker J, Tile M (eds). *The Rationale of Operative Fracture Care.* New York: Springer-Verlag, 1987;371–405.
11. Pott P. *Some Few General Remarks on Fractures and Dislocations.* London: Hawes, Clark, and Collins, 1768.
12. Pritchett JW. Rush rods versus plate osteosynthesis for unstable ankle fractures in the elderly. *Ortho Rev* 1993;16:691–696.
13. Wilson JC. Fractures and dislocations of the ankle. In: Rockwood CA, Green DP (eds). *Fractures in Adults*, Philadelphia: J.B. Lippincott, 1984; 1665–1701.
14. Berndt AL, Harty M. Transchondral fractures (osteochondritis dissecans) of the talus. *J Bone Joint Surg* 1959;41A:988–1020.
15. McDaniel WJ, Wilson FC. Trimalleolar fractures of the ankle. An end result study. *Clin Orthop* 1977;122:37–45.
16. McLaughlin HL, Ryder CT. Open reduction and internal fixation for fractures of the tibia and ankle. *Surg Clin North Am* 1949;29:1523–1534.
17. Mast JW, Teipner WA. A reproducible approach to the internal fixation of adult ankle fractures: rationale, technique, and early results. *Orthop Clin North Am* 1980;11:661–679.
18. Tipton WW, D'Ambrosia RD. Vascular impairment as a result of fracture-dislocation of the ankle. *J Trauma* 1975;15:524.
19. Morrey BF, Wiedman GP. Complications and long-term results of ankle arthrodesis following trauma. *J Bone Joint Surg* 1980;62A:10–17.
20. Brighton CT, Black J, Friedenberg ZB, et al. A multicenter study of the treatment of non-union with constant direct current. *J Bone Joint Surg* 1981;63A:2–13.
21. Brodie IA, Denham RA. The treatment of unstable ankle fractures. *J Bone Joint Surg* 1974;56B: 256–262.
22. Offierski CM, Graham JD, Hall JH, et al. Late revision of fibular malunion in ankle fractures. *Clin Orthop* 1982;171:145–149.
23. Lindsjo U. Operative treatment of ankle fractures. *Acta Orthop Scand Suppl* 1981;52:1–131.
24. Meyers ML, Kumler KW. A.S.I.F. Technique and ankle fractures. *Clin Orthop* 1980;150:211–216.
25. Mitchell WG, Shaftan GW, Sclafani JJ. Mandatory open reduction: its role in displaced ankle fractures. *J Trauma* 1979;19:602–615.
26. Klossner O. Late results of operative and nonoperative treatment of severe ankle fractures. *Acta Chir Scand Suppl* 1962;293:1–93.
27. Harrington KD. Degenerative arthritis of the ankle secondary of longstanding lateral ligament instability. *J Bone Joint Surg* 1979;61A:354–361.

# 14

# Composite Fixation for Juxtaarticular Fractures

Lon S. Weiner and Eric C. Mirsky

Composite fixation has emerged as an important modality in the primary treatment of certain juxtaarticular fractures, especially those of the tibia. Composite (or hybrid) fixation refers to the utilization of internal fixation, generally consisting of cannulated screws confined to the metaphysis and articular surface, with an external fixator applied as a neutralization device.

This treatment modality is particularly applicable to fractures of the proximal tibia (including bicondylar tibial plateau fractures with metaphyseal-diaphyseal dissociation) and those of the distal tibia (pilon fractures). Several recent reports have found a high percentage of good and excellent results employing composite fixation for the operative treatment of these fracture patterns.[1–4] The important principles of this treatment include the restoration of normal joint anatomy, stable fracture fixation without compromising soft tissues, and early motion.

In the application of hybrid fixation, cannulated, interfragmentary lag screws are used to obtain stable, anatomic fixation of metaphyseal and intraarticular fragments. The external fixator is then applied, and serves to neutralize shear, bending, and torsional forces. Consequently, the metaphyseal lag screws provide stable and anatomic internal fixation and the external fixator provides for neutralization.

This chapter presents the rationale for the use of composite fixation for the operative management of juxtaarticular tibia fractures, particularly the use of cannulated screws, describes the technique for application, and discusses early reports of outcomes and complications of its practice.

## Historical Background

Juxtaarticular fractures of the tibia are often the result of high-energy trauma and are frequently associated with other injuries. Historically, these injuries have posed difficult treatment problems for the orthopaedic surgeon with limited options, yielding significant complication rates and a high incidence of unsatisfactory results.[1,2,5–15]

The treatment options for tibial plateau and pilon fractures are in many ways similar. These include open reduction and internal fixation with varying degrees and types of internal fixation, external fixation alone or in combination with limited internal fixation, or closed treatment.[1,5,6,16–27]

The closed treatment options include casting, cast braces, and traction. Casting has been largely unsuccessful, since it prevents knee and ankle motion, which is known to promote healing of articular defects, and is generally inadequate to hold those fractures prone to shortening. Skeletal traction allows for limited early joint motion as well as access to open wounds for dressing changes. However, it does not provide for anatomic articular reduction and subjects the patient to a prolonged period of bed rest, with its attendant complications.

The primary benefit of operative treatment is the maintenance of function and longevity of the knee and/or ankle joint secondary to the restoration of normal anatomy. However, traditional open reduction and plating has resulted in a high incidence of soft tissue complications, including skin slough, wound dehiscence, and infection, ultimately leaving many patients with an unacceptable morbidity and clinical result.[2,6,13–15,28–30]

Classic techniques of open reduction and internal fixation of pilon fractures, as developed by Ruedi and Allgower, provide superior results in the treatment of those injuries sustained after less severe, low-energy trauma.[31–37] Ruedi and Allgower[36] reviewed 84 intraarticular fractures of the distal tibia treated by open reduction and internal fixation. In 78 fractures, at an average follow-up of 50.3 months, they reported 74% good and excellent results. However, they did not classify the fractures based on the severity of displacement and comminution on the initial radiographs. Therefore, it is not known how the severity of the injury affected either the early or long-term results. Ruedi and Allgower concluded that anatomic reconstruction of the articular surface was necessary for a good functional outcome. Failure to achieve stable anatomic reduction often leads to compromised results. They recommended a treatment sequence of fibular reconstruction, restoration of articular surface, bone grafting of defects, and the use of an anterior or medial neutralization plate.

The results of treatment for more severe, high-energy fractures have been less promising. Ovadia and Beals[33] found that the most important variables influencing the clinical results following a pilon fracture were the fracture type, the method of treatment, and the quality of reduction. They reviewed 142 tibial plafond fractures treated by a variety of orthopaedic surgeons and methods over a 19-year period in a large metropolitan area. Their articular fractures were classified as type I, nondisplaced; type II, minimally displaced; type III, displaced with several large fragments; type IV, displaced with multiple fragments and a large metaphyseal defect; and type V, displaced with severe comminution. All 21 type I fractures had excellent or good final clinical results, regardless of the method of treatment. In contrast, only 4 of 18 patients (22%) with a type V fracture had good or excellent clinical results. They concluded that the fracture type was the most important factor accounting for their 35% unacceptable results in severe fractures.

Teeny et al.[14] reviewed the clinical results of 58 patients with 60 tibial plafond fractures treated by open reduction and internal fixation using principles of the Arbeitsgemeinschaft für Osteosynthesefrogen/Association for the Study of Internal Fixation (AO/ASIF) group over a 5-year period. They found that the Ruedi fracture classification correlated closely with overall clinical results. In this study, 18 of 30 patients (60%) with a Ruedi type III fracture had a poor clinical result. They concluded that the fracture severity, combined with the inability to achieve an anatomic reduction, were the variables significantly contributing to a poor result.

Analysis of severe proximal tibia fractures is more difficult. Most large series include all tibial plateau fractures. Agnew et al.[38] noted that only 592 Schatzker V and VI fractures have been reported in the English-language literature since 1956, and of those only 140 were treated by definitive internal fixation. In Schatzker et al.'s[39] own series of 219 fractures, only eight were types V or VI and treated with open reduction and internal fixation (ORIF). Several recent reports have focused specifically on comminuted and bicondylar fractures and have emphasized the soft tissue problems associated with internal fixation. Agnew et al. studied 46 complex tibia fractures, 14 of which were open tibial plateau fractures. Using ORIF, they had good functional results with a low complication rate. Within this group, however, diverse treatment methods were used to accommodate variable fracture patterns. These included double plating, lateral plating with a medial external fixator, and antiglide techniques. The goal was stable fixation without compromising soft tissues. Christensen et al.[8] reported on composite fixation using a medial external fixator in order to avoid soft tissue stripping and the need for multiple plates. Fernandez[40] described a specialized surgical approach; however, the series is small and the surgical approach is extensive.

Historically, results for juxtaarticular tibia fractures have generally correlated with the amount of comminution of the articular surface, with severely comminuted fractures portending a worse prognosis.[5,7,27] Waddell et al.[27] reported that adequacy of reduction of a tibial plateau fracture is a crucial factor in obtaining a satisfactory result. They reviewed 95 patients with tibial plateau fractures, and found this to be true regardless of the type of fracture treated.

Blokker et al.[5] confirmed this finding in their analysis of the results of treatment in 60 patients. Regardless of whether these fractures were treated by closed methods or by ORIF, the single most important factor in predicting outcome following a tibial plateau fracture was the adequacy of the initial reduction. The method of achieving the reduction was not as critical of a factor.

The concept of limited open reduction in combination with external fixation for pilon fractures is not new and was in fact introduced by Scheck[41] in 1965. He first identified, reduced, and fixed "key" fracture fragments, emphasizing minimal soft tissue stripping. He then applied a dual pin external fixator from the calcaneus to the proximal tibia to maintain metaphyseal-diaphyseal alignment. Scheck applied this technique to five cases of comminuted tibial plafond fractures, four of which were open, and reported satisfactory results in all five cases.

Bosse et al.[42] reported a small series with satisfactory results, as did other authors. They prospectively studied 20 patients treated with combined techniques of minimal internal fixation and external fixation for unstable tibial diaphyseal fractures. At a minimum follow-up of 2 years, all fractures healed.

Spiegel and Vanderschilden,[43] however, achieved less-promising results with limited internal fixation in the tibial diaphysis. They employed minimal internal and external fixation together for a select series of open tibial fractures in an attempt to maximize the advantages and minimize the disadvantages of each full system used separately. They used interfragmentary cortical screws for internal fixation and a "half-frame" external fixator. In this case, the external fixator acts as an "external neutralization plate" to protect the minimal internal fixation. They reported a significant complication rate, which included further bone devascularization, loosening and breakage of implants, pin tract infections, osteomyelitis, and pathologic fractures through pinholes that can lead to nonunion. These findings have led to techniques combining the concepts of anatomic reduction, stable fixation, and early rehabilitation, with limited soft tissue dissection and limiting the size of the implant used.

# Classification

Traditional classification systems such as the Schatzker classification for tibial plateau fractures and the Ruedi system for pilon fractures have been important because of their ease of application and their contribution to treatment principles for these injuries.

In the system of Schatzker et al.,[39] fractures are classified topographically as lateral condylar, medial condylar, or bicondylar. The lateral condylar fractures are classified morphologically as split, depressed, or a combination of the two. Types I, II, and III involve the lateral condyle only. Type I is a split fracture, type II is a depression fracture, and type III is a split and depression fracture. Type IV is a medial condyle fracture, type V is a bicondylar fracture, and type VI is a bicondylar fracture with metaphyseal-diaphyseal dissociation (Figure 14.1). This classification system has the advantage of being simple and anatomic. However, it does not address fracture severity and diversity, energy of injury, treatment, or the entire gamut of injury.

The pilon fracture is, by definition, a combination of an ankle and distal tibial metaphyseal fracture, usually with intraarticular comminution. The Ruedi classification[35] is the most widely accepted system for pilon fractures. This system is based on the degree of comminution and displacement and makes a crucial distinction between nondisplaced, low-energy injuries and severely comminuted and impacted fractures. Type I consists of a cleavage fracture of the distal tibia without displacement of the articular surface. A type II fracture consists of significant fracture and displacement of the articular surface but without significant comminution of either the joint surface or the overlying metaphysis. A type III fracture denotes impaction and comminution of the distal tibial cartilage and metaphysis. This classification is simple and addresses injury severity by making the distinction between low-energy injuries and severely comminuted and impacted fractures. However, it

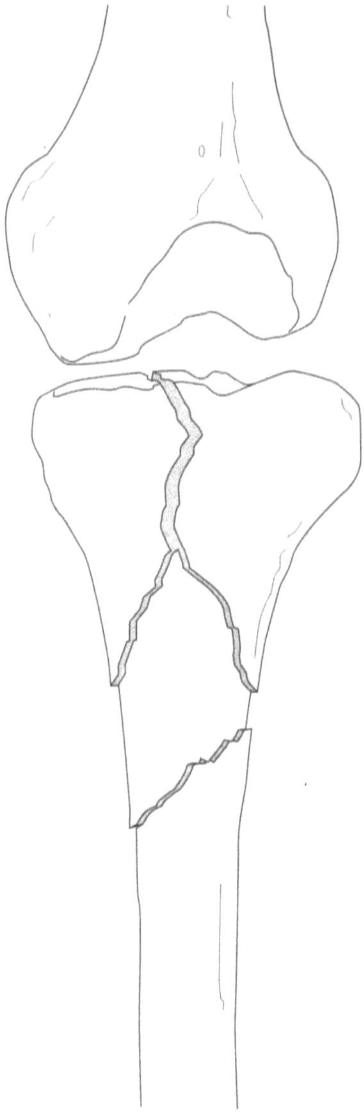

FIGURE 14.1. A type VI tibial plateau fracture (a bicondylar fracture with metaphyseal-diaphyseal dissociation) as classified by Schatzker and McBroom.

is incomplete in assessing the true variety of potential injuries and treatment options.

These classification systems, despite their historical importance and perspective, tend to be insufficient in predicting outcome and delineating treatment. Presently, the updated AO classification[44] is the most appropriate. It divides juxtaarticular fractures of the tibia into type A (extraarticular), type B (partial articular), and type C (complete articular).

Tibial plateau fractures are represented by types B and C (Figure 14.1). A B1 fracture is a pure split fracture and corresponds to a Schatzker I fracture. B2 fractures are pure depressions (Schatzker II), and the B3 subgroup represents a split-depression fracture (Schatzker III). The type C fractures are similar to the Schatzker V and VI groups.

The AO classification similarly divides distal tibia fractures into types A, B, and C. The pilon fractures are represented by the type C fractures. Type C fractures of the proximal or distal tibia are as follows: C1 fractures have simple articular and metaphyseal fracture patterns; C2 fractures are those pilon fractures with simple articular and complex metaphyseal fracture patterns; and in C3 fractures both the joint and the metaphysis are comminuted. The A3 fractures, which are extraarticular fractures with significant metaphyseal comminution, should be considered in the spectrum of pilon and severe proximal tibia fractures because they are high-energy injuries, close to the joint, and have associated metaphyseal-diaphyseal dissociation.

## Preoperative Planning

Careful preoperative planning is an important component of the successful operative management of complex juxtaarticular fractures.[44] Imaging studies should include plain radiographs of both the injured and normal extremities and computed tomography (CT) scans. Because of normal variation, radiographs of the opposite side serve as a template for preoperative planning. Tomograms are effective to evaluate joint depression. A preoperative CT scan is used to evaluate the fracture pattern of the metaphyseal area, which includes the joint surface. This helps to plan the incision(s) to be used. The CT scan should be done in the transverse plane and may be supplemented with multiplanar or three-dimensional reconstructed images.

## Treatment

The key to successful treatment is to obtain stable, anatomic fixation without compromising the soft tissues. The main steps of the procedure

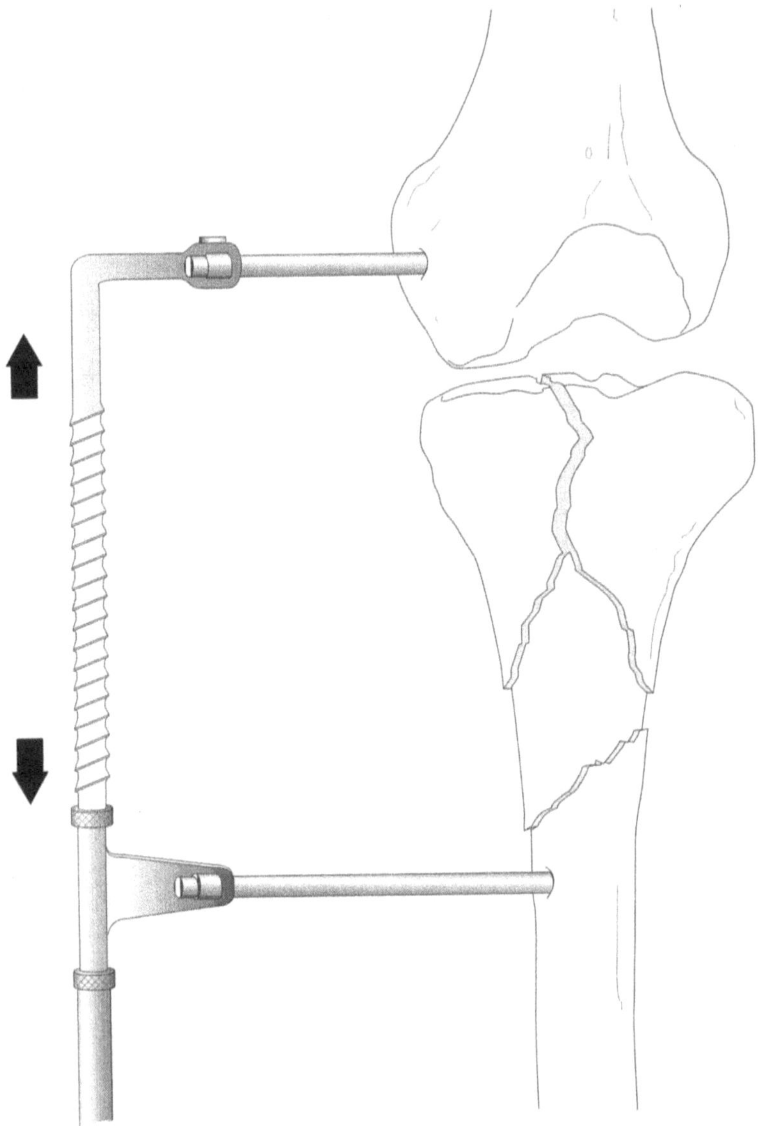

FIGURE 14.2. The application of a femoral distractor to a type VI (Schatzker and McBroom) tibial plateau fracture. The distractor is applied initially to give the surgeon an idea of what reduction can be achieved with ligamentotaxis.

are as follows: (1) distraction of the extremity via a spanning external fixator (femoral-tibial distraction for proximal tibia fractures; tibial-calcaneal distraction for pilon fractures); (2) reduction and stabilization of the joint surface and metaphysis; and (3) revision of the external fixator with reduction and neutralization of the metaphyseal-diaphyseal dissociation.

A femoral distractor or semicircular external fixator can be applied initially as a joint distractor (Figure 14.2). This will give the surgeon an idea of what reduction can be achieved with ligamentotaxis.

Major fragments of the joint and metaphysis are identified so that lag screw fixation can be employed. Fractures of the joint can be thought of as nondisplaced, displaced simple, and displaced comminuted. Percutaneous treatment is employed for fractures with nondisplaced articular components or cases whose joint reduces anatomically after closed reduction. Those fractures with intraarticular displacement are treated by arthrotomy, open reduction and internal fixation, and if necessary, bone grafting. An indirect reduction of the metaphyseal-diaphyseal dissociation is then performed with the external fixator. The goal is anatomic reconstruction of the metaphysis and articular surface with cannulated screws and neutralization of the metaphyseal-diaphyseal extension with the external fixator.

Reconstruction of the metaphysis provides one site of fixation for the external fixator. Minor adjustments may subsequently be made in any plane to correct malalignment. The construct provides immediate stability so that early range of motion is possible postoperatively.

Reproducible fracture patterns are evident in the majority of juxtaarticular tibia fractures despite the fact that these fractures are generally displaced and comminuted. Consequently, the external fixator may be applied in the same manner for each case.

The patient is positioned supine on an image intensifier–compatible table with the extremity draped free.

# Advantages of Cannulated Screws

1. The knee and ankle are very accessible to fluoroscopic placement of guide pins followed by cannulated screws.
2. Jigs may be used to facilitate the placement with parallel guide pins.
3. Open reduction can be performed through the incision that best exposes the joint and fracture fragments. Frequently, this incision is not in the best location for the placement of the fixations screws. Soft tissue dissection is then limited by placing the guide wires and subsequent cannulated screws through separate stab wounds.
4. The joint can be visualized through the primary incision, and guide pins placed through stab wounds can be used as handles in the fracture fragment to reduce the fracture and anatomically restore the joint surface.
5. Guide pins can be used for preliminary fixation. The position of these pins is usually the same as that desired for the cannulated screws.
6. Guide pins offer a means to directly determine the ideal screw length prior to their placement.

# Authors' Preferred Equipment

## Large Cannulated Screws

### System 1

*Screw thread:* Outer diameter—6.5 mm; pitch—2.5 mm; reverse cutting flutes; self-cutting, self-tapping positive rake tip. *Drill:* 3.2-mm steel drill that can be used directly with a direct reading depth gauge. *Guide pin:* 3.2-mm with a threaded tip and tapered root diameter. *Screw head:* Round head with a 4.8-mm internal hexagon. *Material:* 22-13-5 stainless steel. *System accessory equipment:* Washers, depth gauge, pin guide, soft tissue protection sleeve, cannulated overdrill.

### System 2

*Screw thread:* Outer diameter—6.5 mm; pitch—1.9 mm; reverse cutting flutes; self-cutting, self-tapping tip. *Drill:* A 3.2-mm steel drill. *Guide pin:* 3.2-mm with a threaded tip. *Screw head:* Round head with an internal hexagon. *Material:* Titanium alloy. *System accessory equipment:* Washers, depth gauge, pin guide, soft tissue protection sleeve.

## Small Cannulated Screws

### System I

*Screw thread:* Outer diameter—5.0 mm; pitch—1.6 mm; everse cutting flutes; self-cutting, self-tapping positive rake tip. *Screw shaft:* Smooth, 3.5 mm. *Guide pin:* 2.0-mm with a threaded tip and tapered root diameter. *Screw head:* Round head with an internal 3.5-mm hexagon. *Material:* 316 LVM stainless steel. *System accessory equipment:* Washers, depth gauge, 2.0-mm pin guide, soft tissue protection sleeve, cannulated overdrill.

## System 2

*Screw thread:* Outer diameter—4.5 mm; pitch—1.0 mm; self-cutting, self-tapping positive rake tip. *Screw shaft:* Fully threaded 3.5-mm root diameter. *Guide pin:* 2.0-mm with a threaded tip and tapered root diameter. *Screw head:* Round head with an internal 3.5-mm hexagon. *Material:* 316 LVM stainless steel. *System accessory equipment:* Washers, depth gauge, 2.0-mm pin guide, soft tissue protection sleeve, cannulated overdrill.

# Fixation of Proximal Tibia Fractures

Proximal tibia fractures with intraarticular displacement require exposure of the tibial plateau to perform an open reduction. The arthrotomy should be made directly over the fracture line anteriorly to keep periosteal stripping to a minimum. This is usually performed through an anterolateral incision, which extends from the superior pole of the patellar to the tibial tubercle. However, depending upon the fracture pattern, an anteromedial incision may be required. The meniscus is incised between tag sutures and retracted with the tibial condyle, exposing the intraarticular portion of the fracture.[11] Open reduction of the plateau fracture is then performed (Figure 14.3). The 3.2-mm guide wires can be placed through stab wounds away from thc primary incision at the direction most opportune for the final fixation screws. With the guide pins in the fracture fragment, the fragment can be manipulated into an anatomic position while viewing the articular surface through the arthrotomy. If more than one guide pin is to be used in a single fragment, they are usually placed parallel to each other and to the joint surface. Parallel guide pin jigs and fluoroscopy are very useful for this positioning. After the fracture is reduced and the articular surface restored, the 3.2-mm guide pins are advanced across the fracture and into the host bone. Bone graft is used if there is severe comminution or metaphyseal impaction. Fixation is achieved with self-cutting, self-tapping 6.5-mm cannulated screws inserted over the provisional 3.2-mm guide pins.

In simple fractures involving the plateau, the two main fragments include the medial and lateral tibial condyles. More complex patterns can have coronal splits of the medial condyle[38] or posterior condyle fractures. Fractures of the posteromedial condyle often require a secondary incision for reduction.[45] After identification and reduction of major fragments, the articular surface and metaphysis are rebuilt using guide pins and Kirschner wires. The 3.2-mm guide pins are used with the 6.5-mm cannulated screws, while 2.0-mm guide pins are used with the 4.5- and 5.0-mm screws. The direct reading depth gauge is used to measure the ideal screw length. The length of the screw is usually just to, or alternatively one thread length through, the opposite cortex. After depth gauge measurement, a slightly shorter screw is selected if any significant lag of the fracture is expected. Definitive fixation is performed with self-cutting, self-tapping cannulated lag screws (Figure 14.4). The size of the screw is determined by the size of the fracture fragment to be fixed. Minimum requirements for fixation usually include two screws placed in the coronal plane (mediolateral direction), and two screws in the sagittal plane (antereroposterior direction) to secure the tubercle. Washers are occasionally used to buttress the fracture. The appropriate washer is placed around the neck of the cannulated screws prior to the screw's passage over the guide pin. Other fixation may be added or deleted, depending on the fracture configuration.

# Fixation of Distal Tibia (Pilon) Fractures

In the operative treatment of pilon fractures, the restoration of the length of the extremity is a critical step. A distractor placed from the tibia to the calcaneus is valuable. Fractures of the fibula are plated through a standard lateral approach. Segmental fibula fractures or those with marked tibial shortening may require indirect reduction and initial application of a distractor.

The ankle joint and distal tibia are approached through an anteromedial incision placed along the medial border of the tibialis anterior tendon.

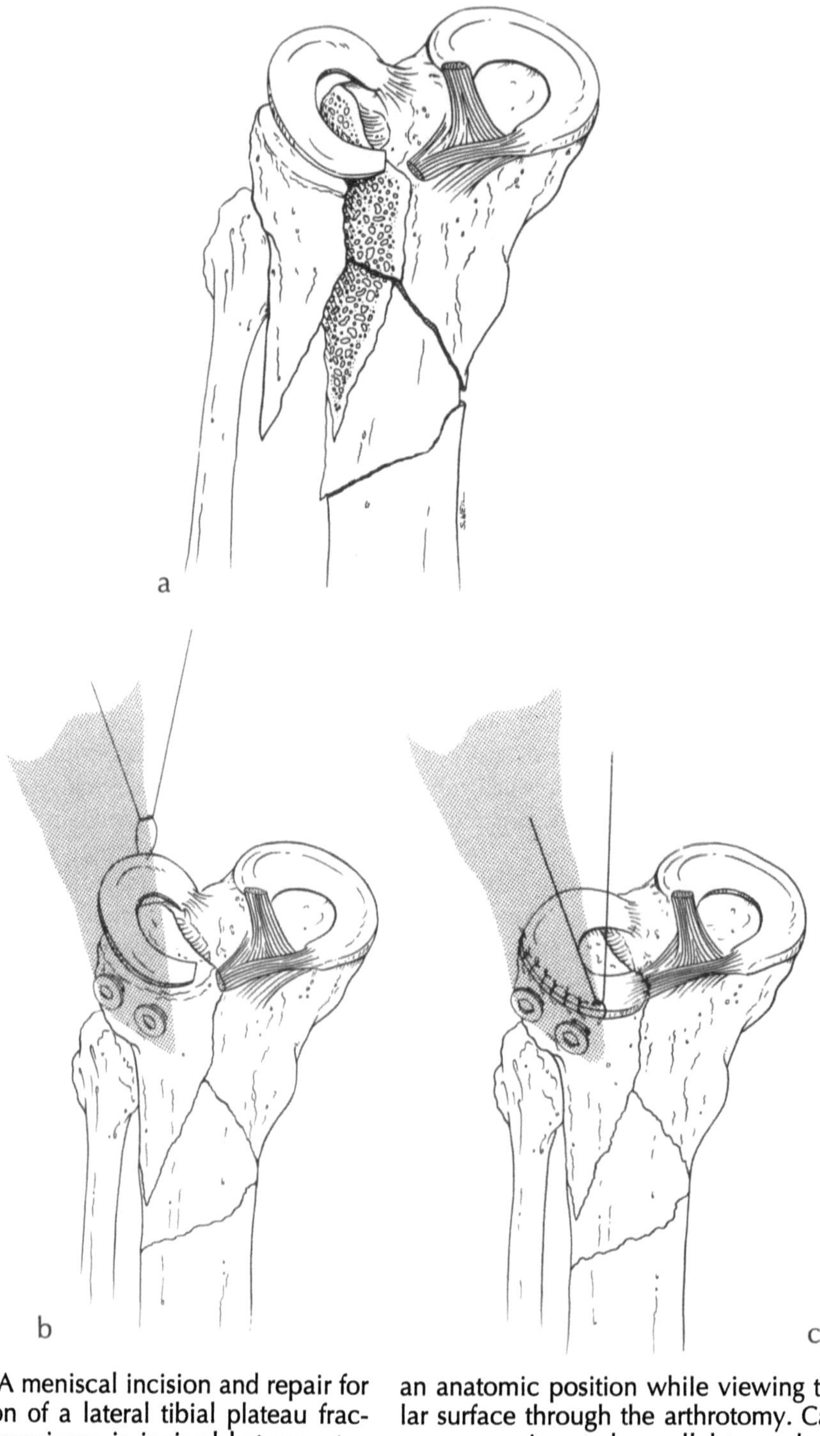

a

b

c

**FIGURE 14.3.** A meniscal incision and repair for open reduction of a lateral tibial plateau fracture. (a) The meniscus is incised between tag sutures and retracted with the tibial condyle, exposing the intraarticular portion of the fracture. (b) With guide pins in the fracture fragment, the fragment can be manipulated into an anatomic position while viewing the articular surface through the arthrotomy. Cannulated screws are inserted, parallel to each other and to the joint surface, over the provisional guide pins for definitive fixation. (c) An open meniscal repair is then performed with the tag sutures.

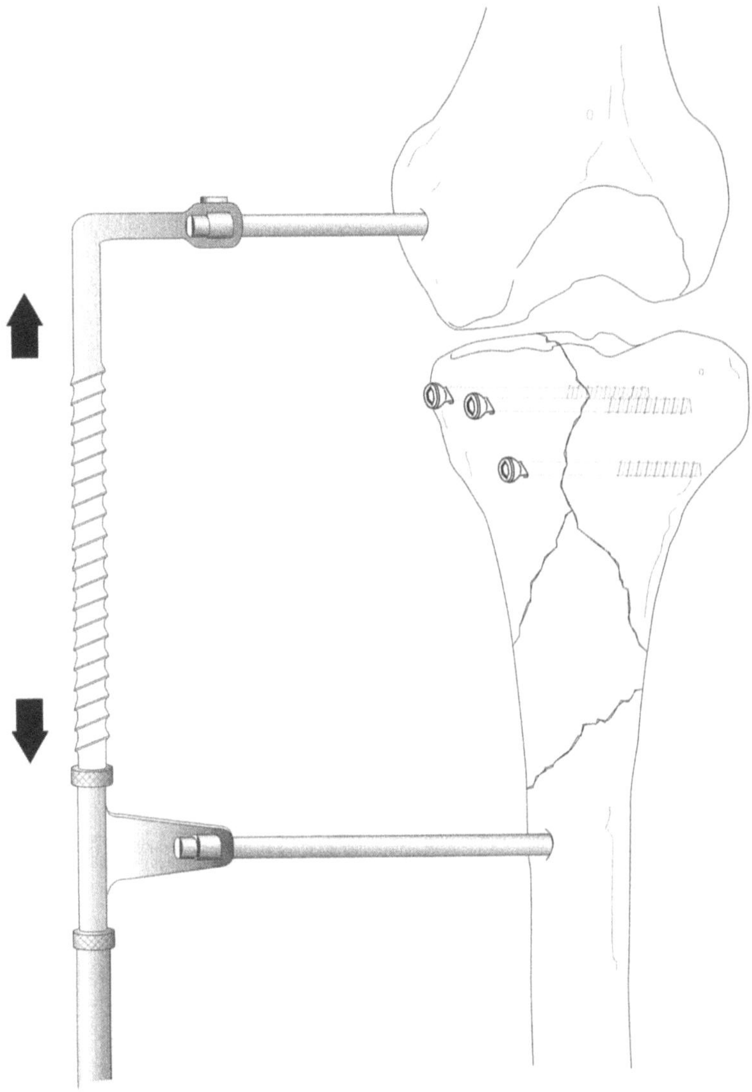

**FIGURE 14.4.** A type VI tibial plateau fracture (Schatzker and McBroom) with a femoral distractor still in place following definitive fixation of the condyles with self-cutting, self-tapping cannulated lag screws.

Provisional fixation of the metaphyseal shell and tibial plafond is accomplished with 3.2- or 2.0-mm guide pins. The major fragments to be fixed include the medial malleolus, and anterolateral and posterior fragments. The size and configuration of the fracture fragments vary, and a CT scan again provides valuable information. The guide pins are replaced by the respective self-cutting, self-tapping 5.0- or 6.5-mm cannulated screws following radiographic confirmation of an acceptable articular reduction. Autologous bone graft is done primarily for metaphyseal defects. Delayed primary or secondary bone grafting of the metaphyseal-diaphyseal junction should be performed if little healing is seen at 6 weeks.

## Application of the External Fixator

The final operative step requires neutralization of the metaphysis to the diaphysis by application of an external fixator.

A proximal tibial ring is used for comminuted or depressed tibial plateau fractures. An adequate construct for a proximal tibial ring includes three tensioned wires, or preferably two wires and a half pin. The initial 1.8-mm wire is inserted from posterolateral to anteromedial approximately 1 cm below the articular surface. The fibular head is used as a landmark. The wire can penetrate the head of the fibula if desired or enter superior and anterior to avoid the peroneal nerve. The wire should be inserted using image intensification. The 2/3 medium-sized ring is connected to the wire with a wire tension assembly and centered on the extremity. The second wire is inserted from posteromedial to anterolateral using the wire assembly and ring as a template. The wires are then tensioned to 100 kg. A half pin or third wire can be added either at this time or after provisional reduction.

The distal tibial ring is used for complex distal tibia and pilon fractures. Depending on fracture configuration, two wires parallel to the articular surface often provide enough fixation. However, three wires or two wires and a half pin are preferable. The initial wire begins posterolaterally in the fibula 5 to 10 mm above the articular surface and exits anteromedially from the distal tibia, medial to the tendon of the tibialis anterior muscle. The wire is connected to the ring with a tension-anchor assembly. The second wire begins in the posterior aspect of the medial malleolus, anterior to the posterior tibialis tendon and exits anterolaterally from the distal tibia. The ring is centered on the leg and the wires are tensioned to 100 kg. A third transverse wire or anterior half pin can be added, depending on the fracture pattern.

The diaphyseal ring is essentially identical for proximal and distal tibia fractures and is assembled using a biplanar half-pin configuration. The diaphyseal ring should be the same size as the metaphyseal ring (Figure 14.5).

The hybrid fixator is then assembled using the proximal tibial ring and diaphyseal ring for tibial plateau fractures, or alternatively using the distal tibial ring and diaphyseal ring for pilon fractures. After application of the hybrid external fixator, reduction of the metaphysis to the diaphysis is performed and visualized with fluoroscopy. Anatomic alignment must be achieved, which includes varus-valgus, translational, anteroposterior, and rotational factors. Three appropriately sized connecting rods stabilize the system. A third wire or half pin in the metaphyseal ring may be added for increased stability at the fracture site if there is gross motion (Figures 14.6, 14.7, and 14.8).

Use of the semicircular external fixator as a neutralization device has the advantages of triaxial reduction capabilities and ease of application. The construct provides immediate fracture stability so that early mobilization of the patient and range of motion at the knee and ankle joints is possible. Fixation across the joint is indicated with some open fractures for primary wound care, or for severely comminuted fractures for which joint fixation is difficult.

## Postoperative Care

Pin care is performed twice a day with half-strength hydrogen peroxide solution. Patients are kept non–weight bearing for 3 months postoperatively for intraarticular fractures. The fixator must be maintained until complete healing can be demonstrated clinically and radiographically, with callus at the metaphyseal-diaphyseal junction. This usually requires a minimum of 8 weeks postoperatively, with an average of about 12 weeks. Braces are often used for 4 to 8 weeks after the frames are removed.

Continuous passive motion (CPM) is generally begun on the first postoperative day for all juxtaarticular tibial fractures. Those patients with pilon fractures should be splinted at night, with active and passive motion during the day.

## Complications

Juxtaarticular tibia fractures are, in general, severe injuries, and many potential complications of treatment exist. These may be consid-

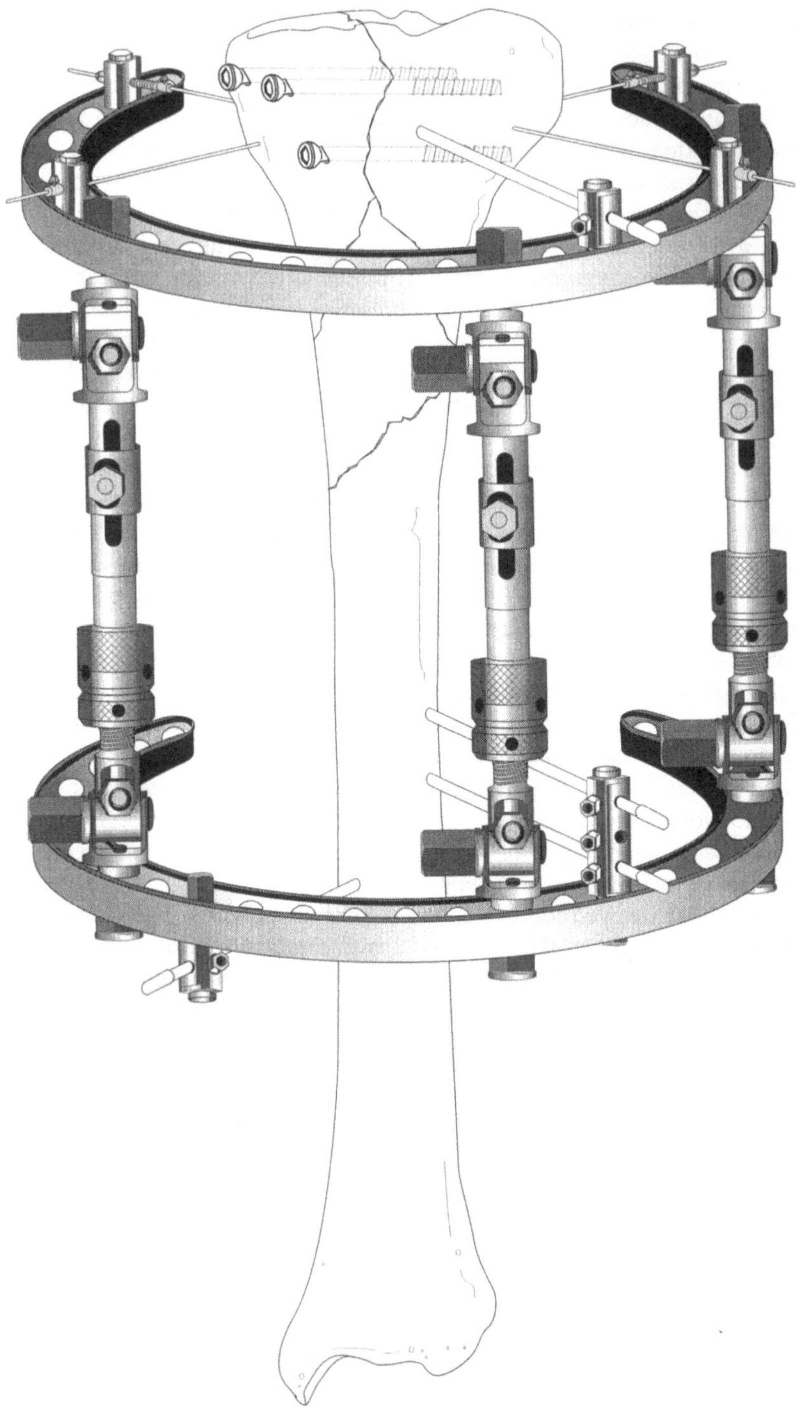

**FIGURE 14.5.** A type VI tibial plateau fracture (Schatzker and McBroom) following definitive fixation of the condyles with self-cutting, self-tapping cannulated lag screws and application of a semicircular, hybrid external fixator with three connecting rods. The diaphyseal ring is assembled using a biplanar half-pin configuration. The metaphyseal and diaphyseal rings should be the same size.

ered to be either technical (intraoperative), acute, or late postoperative complications.

Intraoperative complications such as malreduction of the articular surface, hardware malpositioning, and inadequate internal fixation, are surgeon-dependent and can be kept to a minimum. Malreduction of the articular surface may lead to early arthrosis due to malalignment, rotation, or shortening. This complication may be avoided by careful preoperative templating and scrutiny of the CT scan, and by thorough intraoperative radiographic evaluation. Hardware malpositioning usually results from joint penetration by screws. This must be recognized intraoperatively and adjusted to avoid late arthrosis. Inadequate internal fixation is usually secondary to comminution and bone loss. Metaphyseal comminution can be augmented by bone grafting.

The most problematic complications include infections and soft tissue loss. This is more of a concern in the management of pilon fractures than in those of the proximal tibia, and has been reported to range in incidence up to 36%.[28] Skin slough and wound infection may require secondary procedures for soft tissue coverage.

Meticulous soft tissue handling may help reduce the incidence of soft tissue problems. Leone et al.[28] suggest that delayed wound closure or primary or delayed split-thickness skin graft may help avoid these potential complications. If primary closure with Allgower-Donati sutures is not possible without undue tension on the skin, then wounds should not be closed primarily. Tornetta et al.[46] reported no skin sloughs following the treatment of 26 pilon fractures with combined internal and external fixation. In this series, all surgical incisions were closed primarily without the need for skin grafting.

Pin tract infections are a problematic complication of external fixation. Superficial pin tract infections generally resolve after oral antibiotics and local care. Deep infections of pin sites often require removal or relocation of pins or wires, debridement, and intravenous antibiotics.[46] Tornetta et al.[46] reported one superficial infection treated with antibiotics, and three pin tract infections in three patients, which were treated by antibiotics alone in two and pin removal in one.

Deep infections can occur and have included septic joints or deep wound infections.[4,46] Weiner et al.[4] reported two knee infections, both in cases in which wires were placed in subchondral bone close to the joint space. These are believed to develop secondary to bacterial contamination of an intracapsular wire in the presence of hemarthrosis. Tornetta et al.[46] reported one ankle infection at 6 weeks, which was treated with removal of lag screws and external fixator and intravenous antibiotics.

Late postoperative complications include malunion, nonunion, and degenerative joint disease. McFerran et al.[47] reported malunion rates for pilon fractures as high as 42% and nonunions as high as 18%. Tornetta et al.[46] reported one 10° varus malunion in 26 pilon fractures.

Malunions of tibial plateau fractures have been reported in several series depending on the type of treatment.[1,4,5,7,9,10] Weiner et al.[4] reported two malunions in 50 severe proximal tibia fractures (4%) treated with combined internal and hybrid external fixation, both due to inadequate intraoperative reduction. However, nonunions have been reported rarely for these fractures.

Another potential postoperative complication using composite fixation is nonunion or malunion of the metaphyseal-diaphyseal junction. Fractures with shortening, marked comminution, and compromised vascularity to the fracture site are at risk for nonunion. This complication may be avoided to a large extent by early bone grafting.

Posttraumatic arthritis and avascular necrosis are additional late postoperative complications. They also appear to be related to both the severity of the initial injury and the ability to achieve a stable, anatomic reduction with minimal dissection. Some authors have reported their incidence to be as high as 54%.[4,5,7,10,32,33,37,39,47]

## Results

There are several recent reports documenting a high percentage of good and excellent outcomes following the use of composite fixation

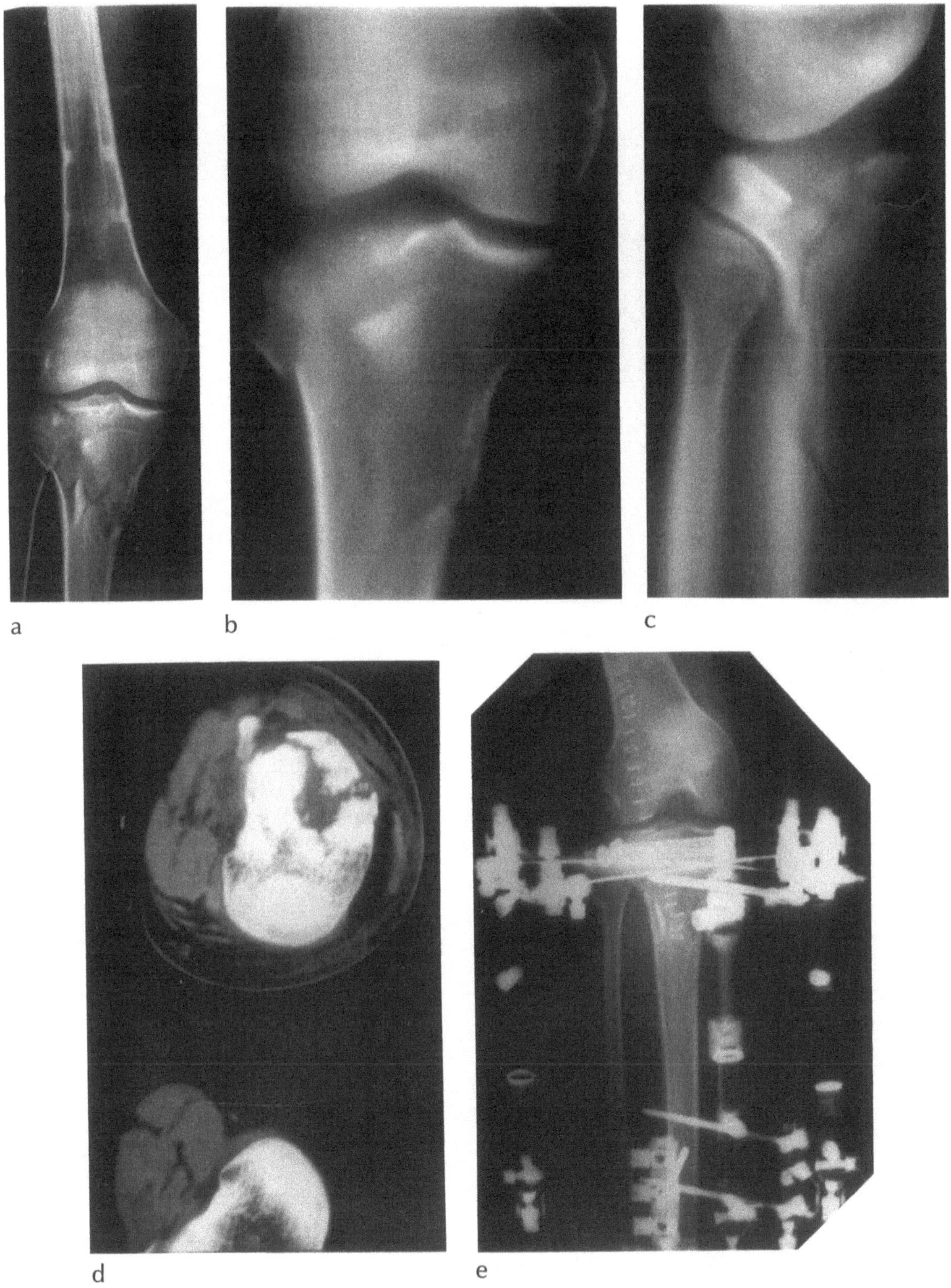

**FIGURE 14.6.** A type VI (Schatzker and McBroom) tibial plateau fracture treated with limited internal fixation and hybrid external fixation. (a) Preoperative anteroposterior radiograph demonstrating a bicondylar fracture with metaphyseal-diaphyseal dissociation. (b and c) Preoperative tomograms in the anteroposterior and lateral planes demonstrate several large articular fragments. (d) Preoperative axial CT scan again demonstrates the articular fragments. (e) Immediate postoperative anteroposterior radiograph following articular reduction and fixation with self-cutting, self-tapping 6.5-mm cannulated lag screws and neutralization with a hybrid semicircular external fixator, employing three connecting rods.

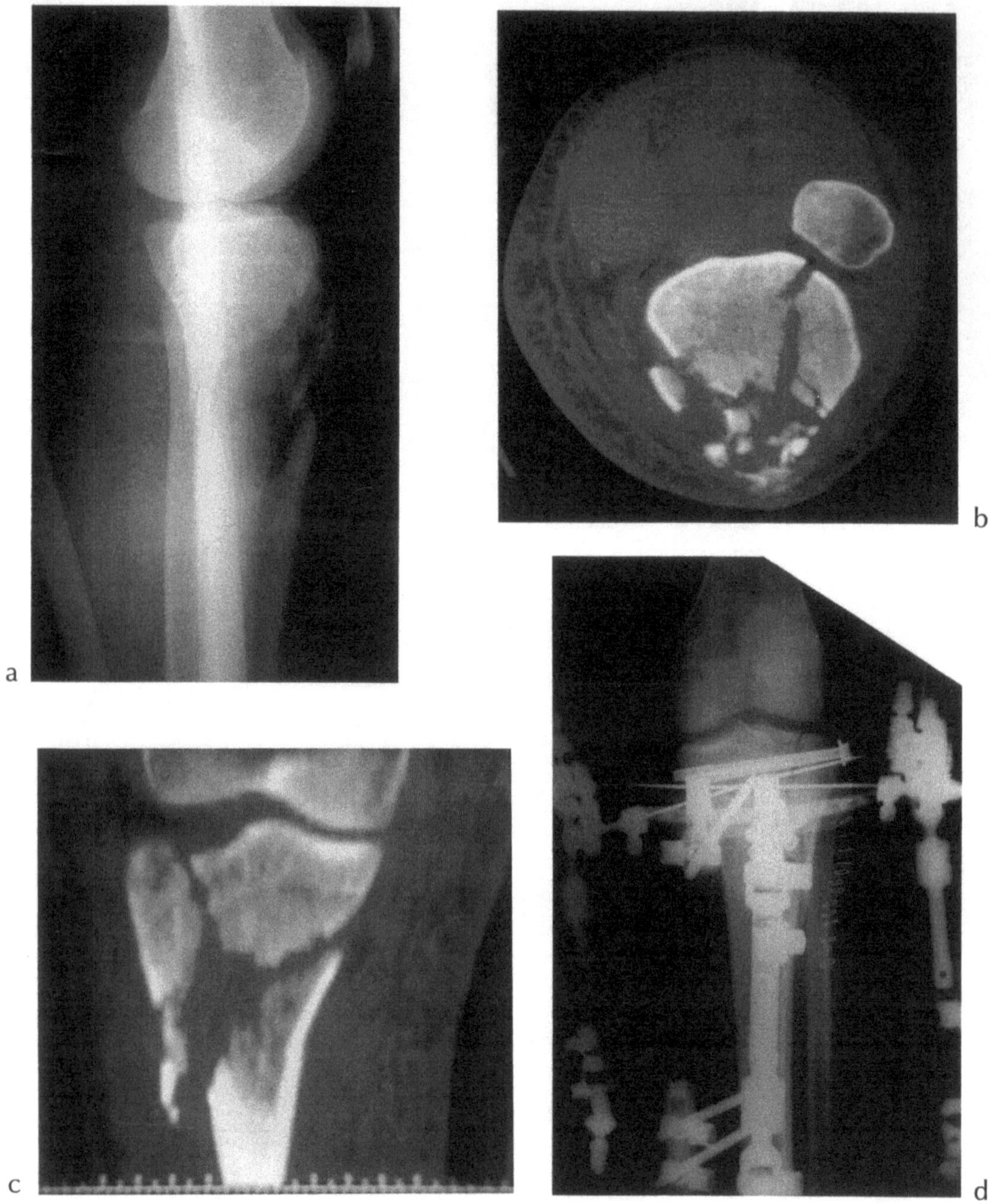

**FIGURE 14.7.** A type VI (Schatzker and McBroom) tibial plateau fracture treated with composite fixation. (a) Preoperative lateral radiograph demonstrating a bicondylar fracture with extensive comminution and metaphyseal-diaphyseal dissociation. (b and c) CT scan in the axial and coronal planes demonstrate extensive comminution of the articular surface and metaphyseal-diaphyseal dissociation. (d) Postoperative anteroposterior radiograph following open reduction and limited internal fixation of the articular surface with self-cutting, self-tapping cannulated 6.5-mm lag screws and reduction and neutralization of the metaphyseal-diaphyseal dissociation with a hybrid semicircular external fixator with three connecting rods.

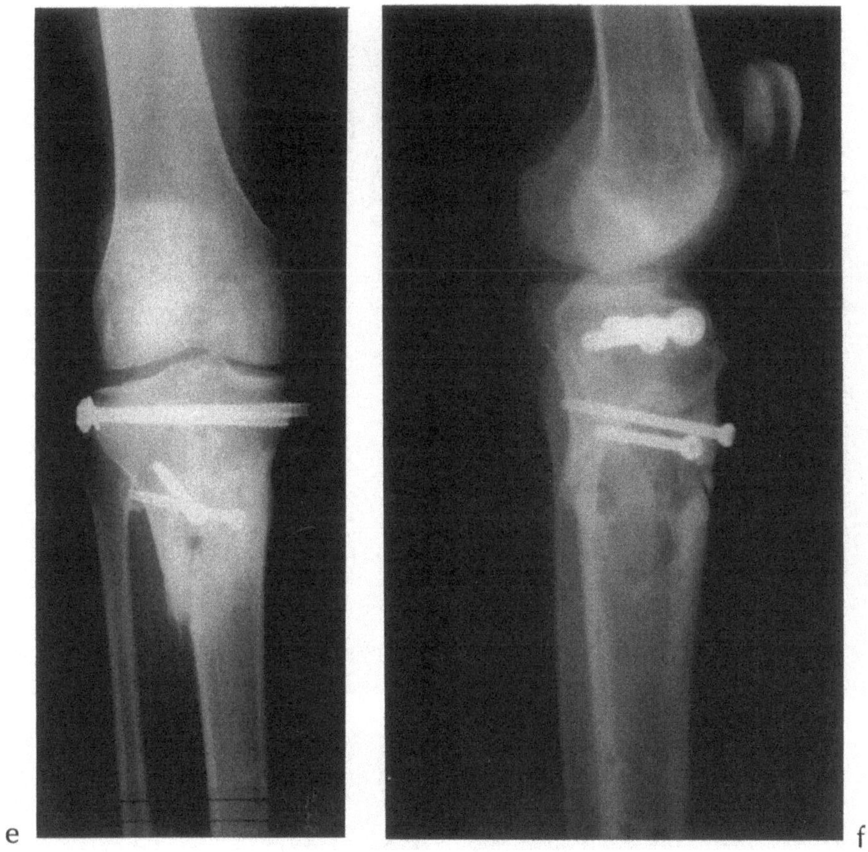

FIGURE 14.7 (e and f) Anteroposterior and lateral radiographs taken 3 months postoperatively, after the external fixator was removed. The articular surface and major fragments are well reduced. There is some bridging callus at the fracture site.

for juxtaarticular tibia fractures.[3,4,46,48] Tornetta et al.[46] reported 81% overall good or excellent results in 26 patients who were followed for 8 to 36 months following treatment of severe tibial plafond fractures with composite fixation. Moreover, 69% of patients in their series with Ruedi type III injuries and 70.5% of those with intraarticular fractures had excellent or good results. They concluded that this method reduces the amount of soft tissue dissection and especially periosteal stripping necessary for fixation with larger plates while yielding comparable results. This technique offers a low complication rate while providing stable fixation and allowing for early motion.

Mills[3] reported on five patients with oblique fractures of the tibia treated with combined interfragmentary lag screw fixation and external fixation. All fractures in this series healed without complications. He concluded that this method represents mechanically lag screw fixation with a neutralization plate and biologically is minimally traumatic to bone or soft tissue. These fractures healed by primary bony union in spite of crush injury, devascularization, or local infection.

Weiner et al.[4] reported on 50 severe fractures of the proximal tibia that were treated with limited internal fixation combined with external fixation. In this series, all fractures healed, at an average of 12 weeks. There were two nonunions, which required bone graft. Average Hospital for Special Surgery (HSS) knee score was 90 (68–100). Overall, they reported 82% good or excellent anatomic results. They concluded that this treatment modality is an

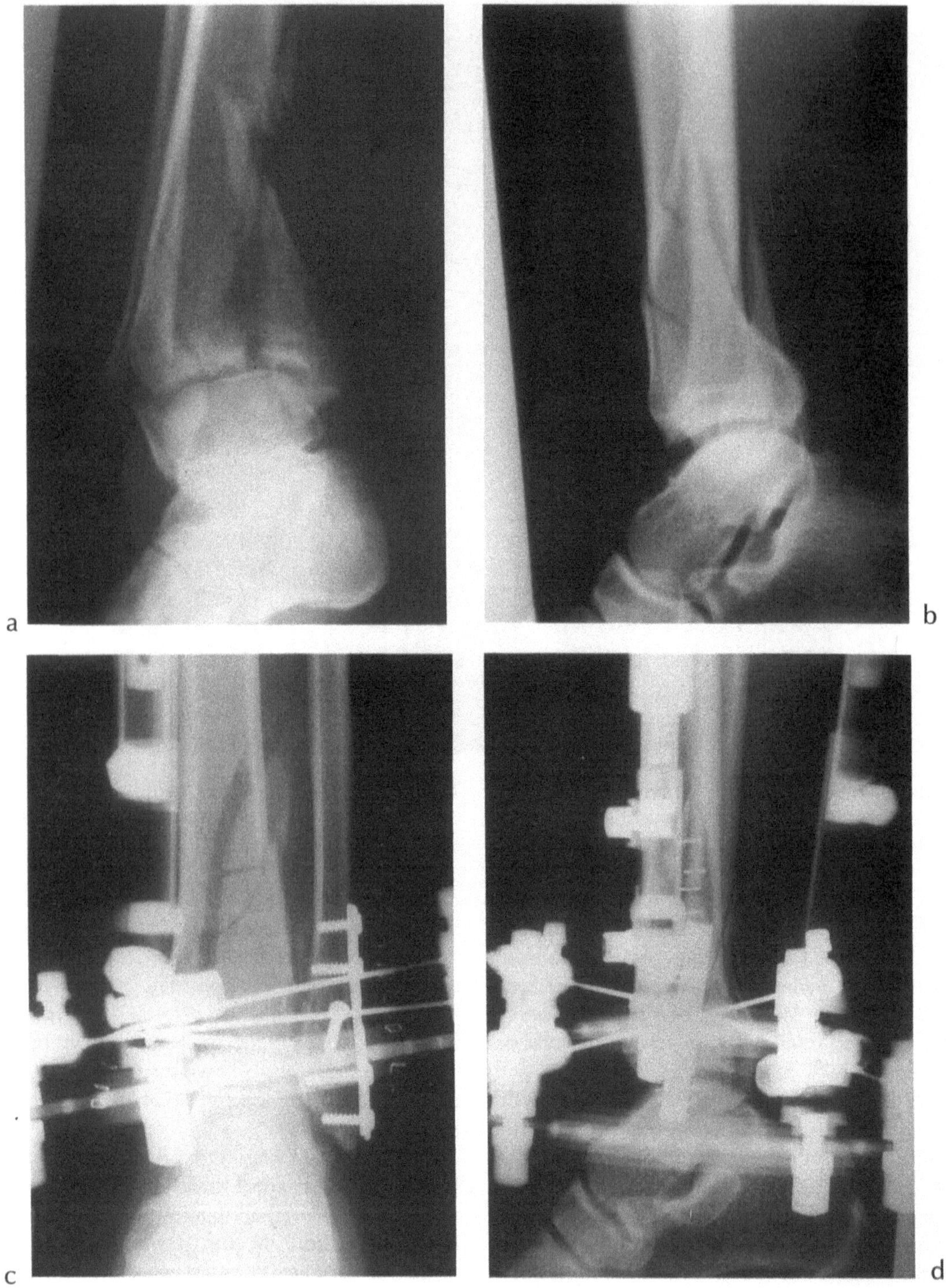

**FIGURE 14.8.** (a) Anteroposterior and (b) lateral views of a pilon fracture with simple joint pattern, complex metaphyseal pattern (A0-C2). (c, d) It was treated with limited internal fixation and hybrid external fixation requiring minimal exposure and fixation of joint surface.

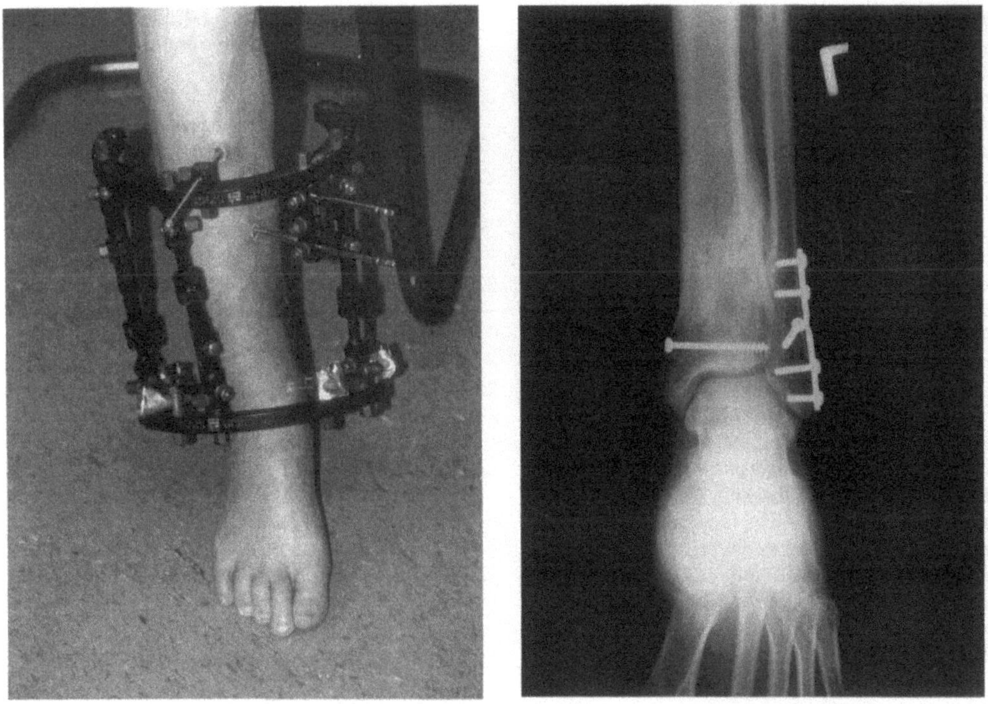

e f

**FIGURE 14.8** (e) Clinical appearance during treatment. (f) Radiographic appearance after treatment. (Reprinted with permission from Karas EH and Weiner LS: Displaced pilon fractures: An update. *Orthop Clinic North Am* 1994;25:651–63.)

excellent alternative for severe proximal tibia fractures, allowing the surgeon to achieve a high rate of union and good clinical outcome with little jeopardy to the soft tissue structures. In general, results correlate with the amount of proximal comminution of the articular surface, with severely comminuted fractures portending a worse prognosis.

Saleh et al.[48] treated 12 patients with comminuted pilon fractures using limited open reduction and interfragmentary fixation of the major articular fragments combined with an articulated external fixator to maintain diaphyseal alignment, neutralize joint movement, and encourage early motion. Only one of the patients in this study had a poor functional result.

## Conclusion

As techniques of biologic fixation and external fixation are refined, they are playing an increasingly important role in the management of severe juxtaarticular tibia fractures. Accordingly, composite fixation, emphasizing biologic principles, has been shown to increase healing rates and to decrease infections without compromising stable fixation. Preliminary studies with composite fixation have yielded excellent functional results with minimal soft tissue and bony complications. Composite fixation provides the patient with a markedly displaced, comminuted, or open juxtaarticular tibial fracture the best chance of a good clinical result with minimal risks, and is therefore an excellent treatment for these complex injuries.

## References


1. Bach AW, Hansen ST. Plates versus external fixation in severe open tibial shaft fractures. *Clin Orthop* 1989;241:89–94.
2. Bone L, Stegeman P, McNamara K, et al. External fixation of severely comminuted and open tibial pilon fractures. *Clin Orthop* 1993;292:101–107.
3. Mills RM. Minimal internal and external fixation in oblique lower extremity fractures: a report of five cases and description of technique. *J Orthop Trauma* 1988;2:250–256.
4. Weiner LS, Kelley M, Yang E, et al. The use of combination internal fixation and hybrid external fixation in severe proximal tibia fractures. *J Orthop Trauma* 1995;9:244–250.
5. Blokker CP, Rorabeck CH, Bourne RB. Tibial plateau fractures and analysis of treatment in 60 patients. *Clin Orthop* 1984;182:193–198.
6. Bone L, Stegemann P, McNamara K, et al. The use of external fixation in severe fractures about the ankle. *Orthop Trans* 1990;14:265.
7. Burri C, Bartzke G, Coldeeway J, et al. Fracture of the tibial plateau. *Clin Orthop* 1979;138:84–93.
8. Christensen K, Powell J, Bucholz R. Early results of a new technique for treatment of high grade tibial plateau fractures. *J Orthop Trauma* 1990; 4:226.
9. King GJW, Schatzker J. Nonunion of a complex tibial plateau fracture. *J Orthop Trauma* 1991; 5:209–212.
10. Lansinger O, Bergman B, Courner L, et al. Tibial condylar fractures: a 20 year follow-up. *J Bone Joint Surg* 1986;68A:13–18.
11. Perry CR, Evans G. New surgical approach to fractures of the lateral tibial plateau. *J Bone Joint Surg* 1984;66A:1236–1240.
12. Rasmussen P. Tibial condylar fractures, impairment of knee joint stability as an indicator for surgical treatment. *J Bone Joint Surg* 1973;55A: 1331–1350.
13. Shelton M, Jones R, Shelton Y. Pilon fractures—a new classification and treatment. *Orthop Trans* 1959;13:762.
14. Teeny SM, Wiss DA. Open reduction and internal fixation of tibial plafond fractures. *Clin Orthop* 1993;202:108–117.
15. Trafton PG, Bray TJ, Simpson LA. Fractures and soft tissue injuries of the ankle. In: Browner BD, Jupiter JB, Levine, AM, et al., eds. *Skeletal Trauma*, vol 2. Philadelphia: WB Saunders, 1992; 1931–1941.
16. Allgower M, Muller ME, Willenegger H. *Technik der Operativen. Frakturbehandlung.* New York: Springer-Verlag, 1963.
17. Apley AG. Fractures of the tibial plateau. *Orthop Clin North Am* 1979;10:61–74.
18. Bone LB. Fractures of the tibial plafond: the pilon fractures. *Orthop Clin North Am* 1987;18:95–104.
19. Burwell HN, Charnley AD. The treatment of displaced fractures of the ankle by rigid internal fixation and early joint movement. *J Bone Joint Surg* 1965;47B:634–660.
20. DeCoster TA, Nepola JV. Cast brace treatment of proximal tibial fractures: ten year follow-up study. *Clin Orthop* 1988;231:196–204.
21. Drennan DB, Locher FG, Maylahn D. Fractures of the tibial plateau: treatment by closed reduction and spica cast. *J Bone Joint Surg* 1975;61A:989–995.
22. Duwelius PJ, Connolly JF. Closed reduction of tibial plateau fractures: a comparison of functional and radiographic results. *Clin Orthop* 1988;230: 116–125.
23. Maale G, Seligson D. Fractures through the distal weight-bearing surface of the tibia. *Orthopedics* 1980;3:517–521.
24. Mast J, Spiegel P. Complex ankle fractures. In: Meyers, MH, ed. *The Multiply Injured Patient with Complex Fractures.* Philadelphia: Lea & Febiger, 1984.
25. Moore TM, Pazkis MJ, Harvey JP. Tibial plateau fractures: definition, demographics, treatment rationale and long term results of closed traction management or operative reduction. *J Trauma* 1987;1:97–119.
26. Ries M, Meinhard B. Medial external fixation with lateral plate internal fixation in metaphyseal tibia fractures. *Clin Orthop* 1990;256:215–223.
27. Waddell AP, Johnston DWC, Neidre A. Fractures of the tibial plateau: a review of 95 patients and comparison of treatment methods. *J Trauma* 1981;21:376–381.
28. Leone V, Ruland R, Meinhard, B. The management of soft tissue in pilon fractures. *Clin Orthop* 1993;292:315–320.
29. Pierce RO, Heinrich JH. Comminuted intraarticular fractures of the distal tibia. *J Trauma* 1979;19:828–832.
30. Young MJ, Barrack RL. Complications of internal fixation of tibial plateau fractures. *Orthop Rev* 1994;23:149–154.
31. Bourne RB. Pylon fractures of the distal tibia. *Clin Orthop* 1989;240:42–46.
32. Kellam JF, Wadell JP. Fractures of the distal tibial metaphysis with intra-articular extension: the distal tibial explosion fracture. *J Trauma* 1979;19: 593–600.
33. Ovadia DN, Beals RK. Fractures of the tibial plafond. *J Bone Joint Surg* 1986;68A:543–551.
34. Ruedi T, Allgower M. The operative treatment of intra-articular fractures of the lower end of the tibia. *Clin Orthop* 1979;138:105–110.
35. Ruedi T, Allgower M. Fractures of the lower end of the tibia into the ankle joint. *Injury* 1969;1:92–99.
36. Ruedi T, Allgower M. Fractures of the lower end of the tibia into the ankle joint: results of nine years after open reduction and internal fixation. *Injury* 1973;5:130–134.

37. Teeny S, Wiss D, Hathaway R, et al. Tibial plafond fractures: errors, complications, and pitfalls in operative treatment. *Orthop Trans* 1990;14:265.
38. Agnew SG, Benirschke SK, Mayo KA, et al. Open reduction and internal fixation of complex tibial plateau fractures. *J Orthop Trauma* 1991;5: 236.
39. Schatzker J, McBroom R, Bruce D. Tibial plateau fractures: the Toronto experience 1968–1975. *Clin Orthop* 1979;138:94–104.
40. Fernandez DL. Anterior approach to the knee with osteotomy of the tibial tubercle for bicondylar tibial plateau fractures. *J Bone Joint Surg* 1988;70A:208–219.
41. Scheck M. Treatment of comminuted distal tibial fractures by combined dual-pin fixation and limited open reduction. *J Bone Joint Surg* 1965; 47A:1537–1553.
42. Bosse MJ, Staeheli JW, Reinert CM. Treatment of unstable tibial diaphyseal fractures with minimal internal and external fixation. *J Orthop Trauma* 1989;3:223–231.
43. Spiegel PG, Vanderschilden J. Minimal internal and external fixation treatment of open tibial fractures. *Clin Orthop* 1983;178:96–102.
44. Mast J, Ganz R, Jacob R. *Planning and Reduction Technique in Fracture Surgery.* Berlin: Springer-Verlag, 1989.
45. Georgiadis GM. Combined anterior and posterior approaches for complex tibial plateau fractures. *J Bone Joint Surg* 1994;76B:285–289.
46. Tornetta P, Weiner L, Bergman M, et al. Pilon fractures: treatment with combined internal and external fixation. *J Orthop Trauma* 1993;7:489–496.
47. McFerran M, Smith S, Boulas HJ, et al. Complications encountered in the treatment of pilon fractures. *J Orthop Trauma* 1992;6:195–200.
48. Saleh M, Shanahan G, Fern ED. Intra-articular fractures of the distal tibia: surgical management by limited internal fixation and articulated distraction. *Injury* 1993;24:37–40.

# 15
# Ankle Arthrodesis

Arthur K. Walling and Brian J. Padrta

While joint replacement has flourished in the majority of joints, its disappointing results in the ankle have contributed to the continued popularity of arthrodesis as a dependable and acceptable method of treatment for disorders of the ankle. Arthrodesis of the ankle has become the most frequently performed fusion procedure of major joints. It is most commonly performed for traumatic arthritis, but it is also an effective and reliable treatment for patients with inflammatory arthridities, instability, or failed arthroplasty (Figures 15.1 and 15.2).

## External Verses Internal Fixation

Charnley[1] initially popularized the use of external fixation to provide compression at the site of fusion. More recent fixateurs, such as the Calandruccio frame, have used triangular configurations in an attempt to improve stability.[2,3] Despite these improvements, biomechanical studies comparing external fixation to internal fixation show superior stability with internal fixation.[4] Moeckel et al.[5] compared the clinical results between internal and external fixation methods for arthrodesis in a group of 68 ankles. Those ankles treated with internal fixation had a union rate of 95% compared with 78% for those treated with external fixation. External fixation is also associated with higher incidences of infection (secondary to pin tracts) and overall complication rates.[6] From the patient viewpoint, external fixation is bulky, requires daily pin care, and thus remains unpopular. Because of these factors, use of external fixation is best reserved for septic situations, and internal fixation has become the most widely accepted method of achieving stability and compression at the fusion site.

Methods of obtaining compression arthrodesis with internal fixation are varied. Studies comparing the use of plates vs. screws for obtaining internal fixation have shown that double-T plating does provide a more rigid construct, but has the disadvantage of requiring more soft tissue stripping and may jeopardize vascularity to the talus and tibia.[7] We also feel that it is more difficult to achieve compression across the fusion site when using only plate fixation. Because of this, we continue to prefer the use of transarticular cancellous screws to obtain compression arthrodesis.

Multiple configurations for screw placement exist, and debate regarding the number of screws needed for fixation and their positioning continues. Most authors use at least two screws to obtain fixation and prefer proximal to distal positioning.[8] Mann et al.[9] describes a technique from distal to proximal with the insertion point beginning in the lateral talus and proceeding upward across the ankle joint into the tibia. Friedman et al.[10] tested paired cadaver ankles and found that two 6.5-mm crossed cancellous screws placed from proximal to distal were superior to parallel screws in resisting torsional stress. A University of Washington study felt strongly that three screws are necessary for fixation and that the crucial screw is one placed from the posterior malleolus of the tibia into the neck and head of the talus.[11] Biomechanically, the three-screw configuration is more rigid but may not affect clinical outcome when compared with the use of two screws in uncomplicated cases[12] (Figure 15.3).

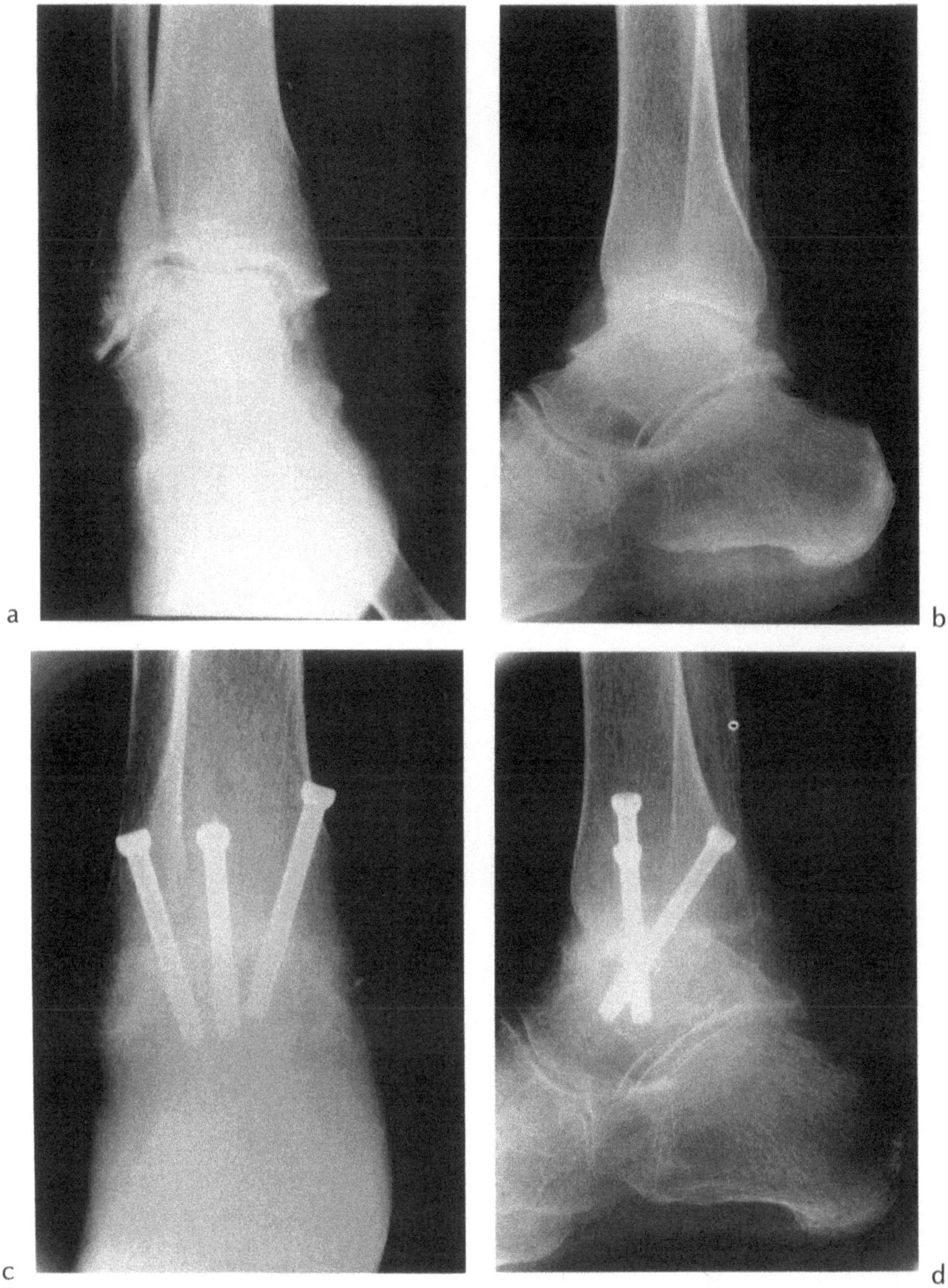
a b c d

**FIGURE 15.1.** (a and b) Preoperative AP and lateral radiographs of a 79-year old man with progressive pain and crepitance of the right ankle. (c and d) Postoperative AP and lateral radiographs illustrating the correct positioning of the posterior-anterior screw when utilizing the three-screw fusion technique.

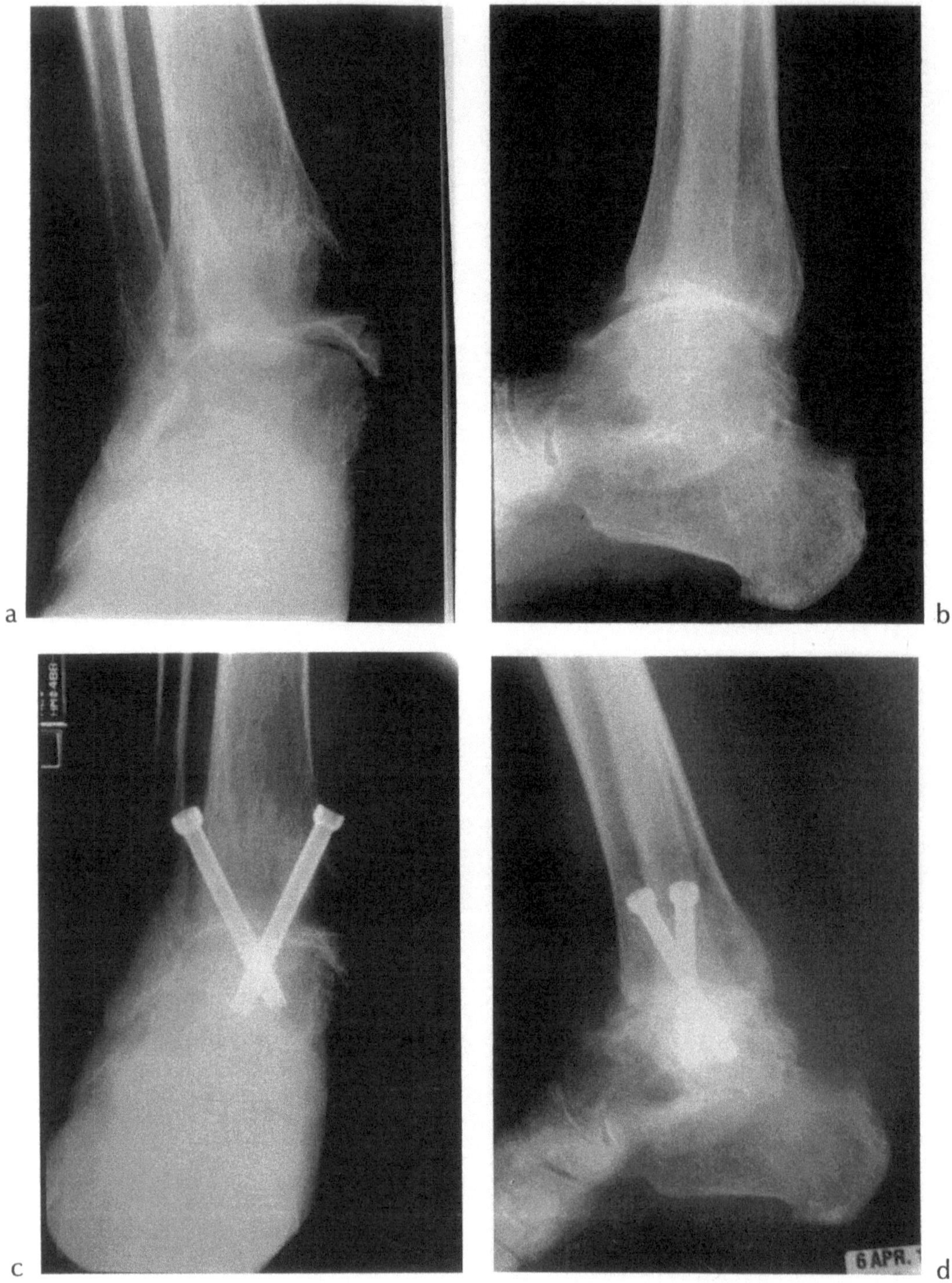


**FIGURE 15.2.** (a and b) Preoperative AP and lateral radiographs demonstrate lateral articular loss secondary to progressive talar tilt in a patient with valgus malalignment. (c and d) Postoperative radiographs of healed fusion, which show correction of the malalignment utilizing the two-screw technique.

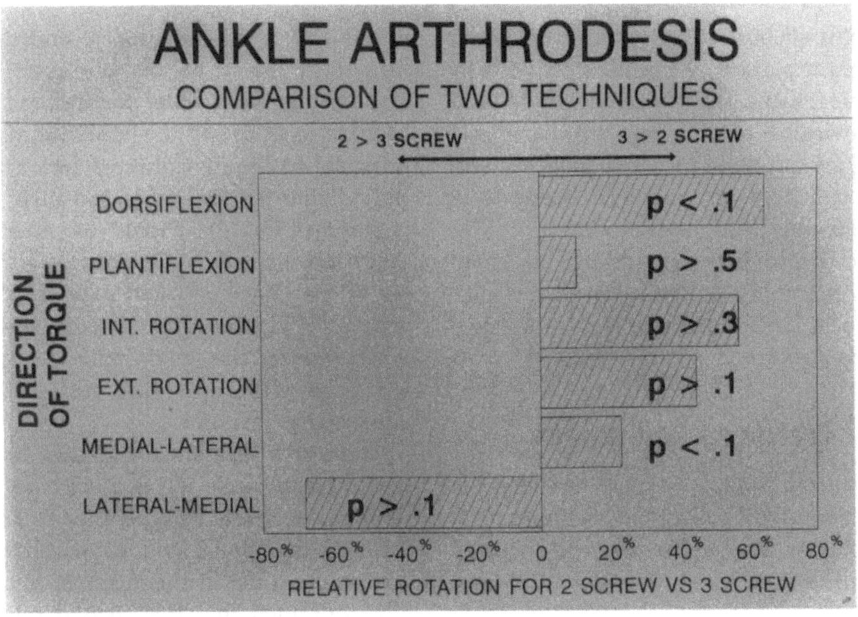


**FIGURE 15.3.** Biomechanical testing of two screws (medial/lateral) vs. three screws (posteroanterior, medial, and lateral) showed greater resistance to rotation in five of six planes with the three-screw technique. This was not statistically significant and may be clinically irrelevant if postoperative immobilization is employed.

# Operative Technique

Multiple techniques and surgical approaches have been described to achieve arthrodesis. We prefer an anterior approach in most instances and utilize a lateral approach when it is necessary to remove internal fixation or when significant anterior displacement of the talus and foot in the ankle mortise exists, as can occur following pilon fractures. When determining which technique to utilize the surgeon must consider the underlying disorder, degree of deformity, bone stock, and patient demands.

The goal of the arthrodesis is to position the ankle in a neutral flexion-extension position with approximately 5° of valgus. It is equally important to position the foot along the weight-bearing line of the tibia, or slightly posterior, so that the overall length of the foot is decreased in relationship to the tibia. This shortens the lever arm and is believed to improve gait dynamics postfusion. External rotation should be approximately 5° to 10° and is best judged by comparison to the opposite ankle. The emphasis should be on rigid internal fixation, minimal bony resection, and meticulous soft tissue handling.

Cannulated cancellous screws are a practical method of achieving rigid internal fixation with compression across the arthrodesis site.[12] Placement of the guide pins under direct vision enables accurate assessment of eventual screw positions. The use of fluoroscopy further confirms screw placement and length. The pins themselves assist in maintaining the arthrodesis in the correct position prior to screw placement. In addition, the ability to place the screws percutaneously leaves soft tissue intact, thereby preserving vascularity. Cannulated screws are invaluable if using an arthroscopic technique for fusion.

## Advantages of Cannulated Screws

1. The ankle is readily accessible to fluoroscopic placement of guide pins.
2. The guide pins can provisionally hold the arthrodesis in position and readily be repositioned if necessary prior to definitive screw placement.

3. Guide pins can be used retrograde from within the articular surface of the tibia through the tibial metaphysis, then later antegrade, after foot provisional positioning, into the talus.
4. Guide pins can be used percutaneously with the aid of fluoroscopy and arthroscopy to do a percutaneous arthrodesis.
5. The use of provisional guide pin placement minimizes soft tissue dissection in the ankle where very little soft tissue covers much of the bony structure.

## Authors' Preferred Equipment

Large cannulated screws: Partially threaded 6.5-mm titanium screws. *Guide pin,* 3.2 mm.
Small cannulated screws: Partially threaded 4.5-mm stainless steel screws. *Guide pin,* 2.0 mm.

## Anterior Approach

The patient is positioned supine on a fluoroscopic-compatible operating room table with a "bump" under the ipsilateral hip. The iliac crest is prepared for bone graft harvest. A tourniquet is used throughout the procedure to control bleeding and enhance visualization. The anterior approach utilizes the interval between the tibialis anterior and extensor hallucis longus tendons. The neurovascular bundle is carefully identified and retracted laterally. The periosteum of the tibia and capsule of the ankle joint are incised in line with the skin incision. The full extent of the ankle joint can then be exposed by subperiosteal and subcapsular dissection. The articular surfaces of the ankle joint are denuded of cartilage with an osteotome, being careful to avoid excessive bony resection. A lamina spreader, pituitary rongeur, and powered osteotome are very helpful in ensuring complete cartilage excision from all surfaces. In addition, the tibiotalar surfaces and the medial-lateral gutters should be fully denuded. Any varus-valgus malalignment is corrected prior to fixation (Figure 15.2). Once the desired position for arthrodesis has been obtained, the placement of the screws can commence.

If utilizing the three-screw technique (Figure 15.1), the most important screw is the posterior to anterior screw. The foot is maximally plantar flexed and a 3.2-mm double-ended guide pin (this may have to be pre-made) is placed through the distal tibial plafond and drilled retrograde so as to exit the posterior malleolus just proximal to the metaphyseal flare and lateral to the Achilles tendon. When the ankle is correctly positioned this pin should be situated so that when advanced it will eventually enter the center of the talar body and extend into the neck and head. Fluoroscopic control is very helpful when placing this guide pin. The guide pin is left flush with the tibial surface and is not advanced at this time.

Through a separate lateral stab incision a second 3.2-mm guide pin is placed just above the tibial metaphyseal flare anterior to the fibula (or through the fibula) and advanced to, but not across, the joint. In this manner, it can be visually confirmed that this second guide pin will exit the tibia in a position to enter the lateral talar body. A third 3.2-mm guide pin is placed through a medial stab incision in the same manner and its exit point from the plafond and its expected entrance point into the talus visually confirmed. By not advancing the pins, their positions can be verified to maximize later cannulated screw purchase.

Iliac crest bone graft is placed into the fusion site to improve contact between any areas of incongruity that remain after denuding and contouring the tibial and talar surfaces. The foot is now carefully returned to the original position selected for arthrodesis. This should be neutral plantar flexion and dorsiflexion with neutral to slight valgus angulation. The talus should be translated slightly posterior within the mortise. The guide pins are then advanced into the talus in the order in which they were initially placed to maintain the position for arthrodesis.

We prefer the use of stout (3.2-mm) guide pins that will hold the position of arthrodesis. Fluoroscopy is used to confirm arthrodesis position and guide pin locations. In the lateral view, the lateral guide pin should be anterior in the talus and the medial should be more posterior in its talar position. The guide pins are then measured with the direct reading depth gauge and the appropriate cannulated 6.5-mm self-tapping cancellous screws selected. The posteroanterior screw is placed first, followed by the lateral and

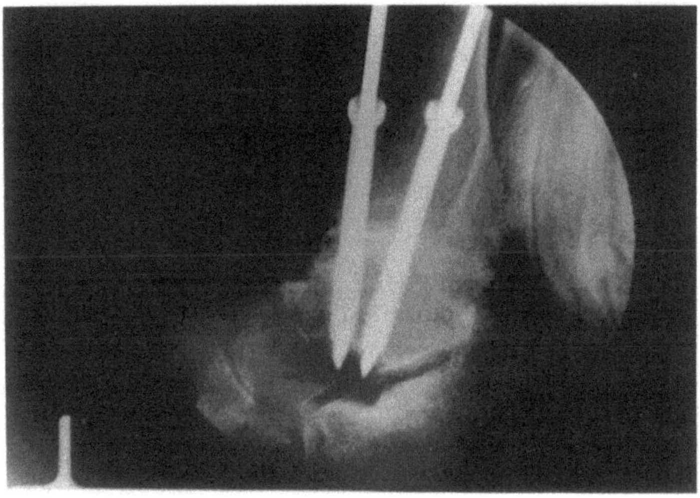

**FIGURE 15.4.** Intraoperative fluoroscopy demonstrating final screw position prior to guide pin removal.

then medial screws. Additional bone graft is placed into a trough created in front of the ankle in a strain-relieving manner.[11] Final anteroposterior and lateral radiographs are obtained to ensure proper position and that the subtalar joint has not been penetrated (Figure 15.4).

The incisions are closed in layers over suction drainage. A well-padded posterior and U-shaped splint is applied. This is changed to a short leg cast at the time of suture removal. Partial weight bearing is allowed and progressed as radiographic evidence of union allows. Most patients are full weight bearing at 8 weeks and can be converted to a removable brace, which is worn only for weight bearing to a total of 12 to 16 weeks depending upon clinical evidence of fusion.

Uncomplicated situations with little or no malalignment may require only two 6.5-mm screws (medial-lateral) for satisfactory stabilization. When in doubt, the small additional time that it requires to place the anteroposterior screw is far less consequential than the risk of nonunion.

## Lateral Approach

The lateral, or transfibular, approach is primarily used when anterior displacement of the talus in the ankle mortise exists, such as occurs following pilon fractures, and to remove previous internal fixation devices. This approach also can be utilized to expose the subtalar joint to perform pantalar arthrodeses. It may be coupled with a medial incision.

The distal fibula is exposed through a straight lateral incision. A 4- to 5-cm segment of fibula is removed exposing the ankle mortise. The talar and tibial surfaces of the ankle are denuded and any angulatory deformity corrected. Once the optimum position for fusion has been obtained the 3.2-mm guide pins are inserted. Under direct vision the same positioning of guide pins and self-tapping 6.5-mm cannulated screws, as was described for the anterior approach, is possible.

The removed section of distal fibula is then prepared for reinsertion. The lateral surfaces of the tibia and talus are denuded to bleeding bone, as is the opposing surface of the removed fibula. The distal fibular section is then secured to the tibia and talus with two additional lag screws placed through the fibula and into the corresponding tibia and talus.[11] This may be performed with 2.0-mm guide wires to give provisional fixation. The position is confirmed by fluoroscopy. The direct reading depth gauge is read and the 4.5-mm partially threaded self-tapping cancellous screws are passed over the guide wires. Bone graft is utilized as with the anterior approach. It is extremely important to restore the lateral integrity by replacing the fibula. We have recently treated three cases where the fibula was either not replaced or insecurely fixed that resulted in valgus malunions. The postoperative regimen is the same for both approaches.

## Arthroscopic Approach

Our experience with arthroscopic-assisted ankle arthrodesis is still being assessed. Our general impression has been that while it is certainly viable, clear-cut advantages to open techniques remain to be seen. There is no question that the arthroscopic technique is best utilized in those patients whom have little or no deformity that requires correction.[13] Differences between open and arthroscopic methods in regard to postoperative pain, time to union, and nonunion rates still need to be assessed.

Our technique has utilized only two portals, anteromedial and anterolateral. A Zimmer ankle distractor is also used to improve visualization. A standard 4-mm, 30° arthroscope with a continuous pressure infusion irrigation setup is satisfactory in most cases. A 4.5-mm resector/shaver is used for the initial debridement, with more aggressive burs utilized as needed. It is important to debride all surfaces including the medial and lateral recesses. Ring curettes and pituitary rongeurs are very helpful in achieving complete debridement.

Once debridement is complete, the 3.2-mm guide pins are introduced percutaneously and their exits from the tibial plafond are visualized arthroscopically. Either two pins (medial and lateral) or three pins (posteroanterior, medial, and lateral) may be utilized. It is much more difficult to place the posteroanterior guide pin arthroscopically as it cannot be placed in an inside-out fashion as in the open technique. After placement of the guide pins, the foot is positioned and the guide pins advanced into the talus. Their positions and the position of the foot in relationship to the tibia is confirmed by fluoroscopy. The appropriate-length screws are determined with the direct reading depth gauge and then advanced over the guide pins and rechecked fluoroscopically. Routine closure and immobilization are utilized as in the open techniques.

# Patient Review

In November 1993 we reported on our results in 42 patients (42 arthrodeses) utilizing the two- or three-screw internal compression technique and anterior approach. These were all performed for traumatic or inflammatory arthritis. Men outnumbered women 3 : 1. All patients went on to successful union using the criterion of trabeculization across at least 50% of the joint in both the anteroposterior (AP) and lateral x-ray views and the patient could bear full weight on the ankle. The average time to union was 14 weeks.[12]

## Difficult Ankle Arthrodeses

Several factors have been identified by multiple authors that may predispose patients to nonunion.[11,12,14] These include, but are not limited to, smoking, neurotrophic joints, talar osteonecrosis, pyarthroses, and extended hindfoot fusions. In our own series, utilizing the conventional compression screw arthrodesis technique, two of three patients with diabetic Charcot changes of the ankle went on to nonunion, and two of four patients treated for compensatory arthritis following previous subtalar arthrodesis developed nonunions. It is important to recognize that these conditions require additional considerations and methods of fixation.

# Conclusion

While ankle arthrodesis remains the operation of choice for most patients with chronic painful conditions of the ankle, it is important to remember that it is a salvage operation. If reconstructive alternatives exist, they should at least be considered prior to fusion.[15] We feel that if arthrodesis is necessary, utilization of internal screw fixation for fusion is a reliable procedure. In most instances, it is well suited to the use of cannulated screws. No matter which surgical approach is utilized, the primary goal, in addition to union, is to obtain functional positioning of the foot. Patient satisfaction is highly dependent upon this. Unfortunately, no matter how good the union rates and initial patient satisfaction, gradual compensatory changes are inevitable in the subtalar and midfoot joints, and we should continue to search for a "better" procedure.

## References


1. Charnley J. Compression arthrodesis of the ankle and shoulder. *J Bone Joint Surg* 1951;33B:180.
2. Hagen RJ. Ankle arthrodesis—problems and pitfalls. *Clin Orthop* 1986;202:152.
3. Malarkey RF, Binski JC. Ankle arthrodesis with the Calandruccio frame and bimalleolar onlay graft. *Clin Orthop* 1991;268:44–48.
4. Scranton PE, Fu FH, Brown TD. Ankle arthrodesis—a comparative clinical and biomechanical evaluation. *Clin Orthop* 1980;151:234–243.
5. Moeckel BH, Patterson BM, Inglis AE, Sculo TP. Ankle arthrodesis: a comparison of internal and external fixation. *Clin Orthop* 1991;268:78.
6. Cracchiolo A, Cimino WR, Lian G. Arthrodesis of the ankle in patients who have rheumatoid arthritis. *J Bone Joint Surg* 1992;74A:903–908.
7. Dohm MP, Benjamin JB, Harrison J, Szivek JA. A biomechanical evaluation of three forms of internal fixation used in ankle arthrodesis. *Foot Ankle* 1994;15:297–300.
8. Mauerer RC, Cimino WR, Cox CV, Satow GK. Transarticular cross-screw fixation: a technique of ankle arthrodesis. *Clin Orthop* 1991;268:56.
9. Mann RA, Van Manen JW, Wapner K, Martin J. Ankle fusion. *Clin Orthop* 1991;268:49.
10. Friedman RL, Glisson RR, Nunley JA. A biomechanical comparative analysis of two techniques for tibiotalar arthrodesis. *Foot Ankle* 1994; 15:301–305.
11. Holt ES, Hansen ST, Mayo KA, Sangeorzan BJ. Ankle arthrodesis using internal screw fixation. *Clin Orthop* 1991;268:21.
12. Walling AK, Dennis J, Latta L. Tibio-talar arthrodesis using two 6.5mm titanium screws. Presented at the Florida Orthopaedic Society, Palm Beach, FL, 1993.
13. Myerson MS, Quill G. Ankle arthrodesis: a comparison of an arthroscopic and an open method of treatment. *Clin Orthop* 1991;268:84.
14. Scranton PE Jr. An overview of ankle arthrodesis. *Clin Orthop* 1991;268:96.
15. Marti RK. Malunited ankle fractures—the late results of reconstruction. *J Bone Joint Surg* 1990; 72B:4.

# 16
# The Foot

Charles N. Cornell

Until recently, interest in operative management of fractures of the foot and use of internal fixation for reconstruction and arthrodesis has been minimal. But over the past two decades advances in fracture surgery have conclusively documented that lower extremity function is better when normal anatomy is restored and prolonged casting is avoided following injury. In view of the realization that the lower extremity cannot function without a sound foot, there has been an explosive increase in interest in applying principles of internal fixation to the foot.[1] As with open reduction and internal fixation (ORIF) elsewhere, the four goals of internal fixation in the foot are (1) restoration of normal anatomy with rapid union, (2) preservation of blood supply to the operative area, (3) achievement of stable internal fixation that meets the biomechanical demands of the foot, and (4) mobilization and functional weight bearing as early as possible.

Not all fractures in the foot require internal fixation to heal with satisfactory results. In addition, in the foot full range of motion (ROM) is not essential for all joints, especially the midtarsal and tarsometatarsal joints as well as the IP joints of the toes. Nonetheless, displaced intra-articular fractures require near anatomic reduction. The subtalar, transtarsal, and metatarsophalangeal joints require almost full ROM to restore normal foot function. In addition, the intricate interrelationships of the joints of the foot require proper alignment for proper function. In this sense, even when joints stiffen or become arthrodesed precise anatomic alignment is needed to preserve maximal overall function.[2] It is in these instances that ORIF can be vitally important.

## Clinical Relevance

Due to the intricate soft tissue and skeletal anatomy of the foot, ORIF is extremely challenging. Surgical exposures must be carefully planned to avoid unnecessary injury to neurovascular structures. In addition, exposures should be minimized to avoid excessive devascularization of the small and poorly vascularized bones of the foot. A large portion of the bony surfaces of the foot is subcutaneous or of very limited soft tissue coverage. The individual bones are small. Too short a screw may not give maximum potential fixation and holding power, whereas too large a screw may have its threaded tip extend into the joint or the adjacent bone. Small implants are needed, and the screw heads should be small to allow countersinking below articular cartilage surfaces. Due to the peculiar geometrics encountered especially when transfixing the metatarsals, special insertion techniques are needed. For all these reasons cannulated screws provide many advantages in the foot. In this chapter the indications and techniques for internal fixation in the foot are reviewed with special emphasis on the use of cannulated screws.

## Advantages of Cannulated Screws

The use of cannulated screws in the treatment of foot fractures can supplement the standard AO/ASIF procedures. There are several advantages of using cannulated screws in foot fracture fixation:

1. The foot is very accessible to fluoroscopy and fluoroscopic placement of guide pins.
2. The incision can be placed to obtain optimum exposure for the reduction of the fracture or dislocation; the guide pins can then be placed either through this wound or percutaneously through new puncture wounds if the orientation of the ideal screw requires a different direction. This minimizes the exposure and soft tissue dissection.
3. The guide pin can be used as a handle for reducing the fracture fragment.
4. Guide pins provide preliminary fixation and can be placed in the most opportune location for fixation, which is usually the site for the final screw.
5. The guide pin can be repositioned in these small bones with minimal bone loss, thus maintaining host bone integrity for final screw fixation.
6. The guide pin can be used to establish the ideal screw's length prior to screw placement.

Several basic rules of technique must be observed when cannulated screw fixation is applied to the foot. If a fracture is reduced and held with a guide pin, additional provisional fixation often is added before overdrilling the guide pin to minimize the loss of reduction. Pointed reduction forceps or additional K-wire fixation will prevent this. When overdrilling a terminally threaded guide pin, especially for smaller cannulated screws, care must be taken to follow the path of the pin and not bend, bind, or cut the guide wire. Reaming should be stopped before the terminally threaded portion or else the guide pin will be extracted by the drill. When screws are used to transfix a joint that has been dislocated and open-reduced, fully threaded screws provide maintenance of reduction but avoid compression of the joint and possible cartilage necrosis. In fixation of the talus and arthrodesis of the subtalar joint, a 6.5- to 7.0-mm cannulated screw should be used. Fixation of the midtarsal bone fractures can be performed with 3.5-mm cannulated screws, but whenever possible 4.5- or 5.0-mm screws should be used to provide sufficient strength to avoid screw breakage, especially when performing arthrodesis or correcting posttraumatic deformity.

# Factors to Consider in Cannulated Screw Fixation

The surgeon should consider several design criteria in determining the system of cannulated screw to be used. Titanium screws are advantageous if computed tomography (CT) or magnetic resonance imaging (MRI) is to be used in the postoperative period. Stainless steel screws are readily used in conjunction with the stainless steel fixation plates used so often in trauma fixation systems.

The size of the guide wire is determined by the cannulation of the intended cannulated screw to be used. This does vary between different available systems. A larger diameter guide wire has the advantage over the smaller wire in being stiffer with less chance of bending or deviation. The larger guide wires also offer better provisional fixation. A tapered root thread has increased strength over a fixed root thread and less chance of threaded tip breakage or incarceration within the screw's cannula (see Chapter 2). Smooth Kirschner wires or drill bits can be used as guide pins in circumstances where a threaded tip is not necessary. Pretapping decreases the screw's holding power, giving self-cutting and self-tapping screws an advantage. If a tap is to be used, only the near cortex is tapped.

The holding power of the screw is proportional to the outer diameter of the screw's thread, while the strength of the screw is proportional to the root diameter of the thread adjusted for the size of the cannulation and the metal used (see Chapter 2). These factors should be considered in relation to the goals of fixation, i.e., to maintain position and/or to provide strength. A surgeon should become familiar with the specifics of his preferred cannulated screw system but may utilize other systems when clinically indicated.

# Author's Preferred Equipment

## Large Cannulated Screws

*Screw thread:* Cancellous; outer diameter—7.0 mm; pitch—2.75 mm; not self-cutting. *Screw shaft:* 4.5 mm. *Thread length:* 16 or 32 mm. *Guide pin:* 2.0 mm with a threaded tip. *Screw head:* Round head with an internal 3.5-mm hexagon. *Material:* 316 LVM stainless steel. *System accessory equipment:* Washers, depth gauge, pin guide, soft tissue protection sleeve, cannulated overdrill.

### *Alternate Systems*

#### System 1

*Screw thread:* Outer diameter—6.5 mm; pitch—2.5 mm; reverse cutting flutes; self-cutting, self-tapping positive rake tip. *Drill:* A 3.2-mm steel drill, which can be used directly with a direct reading depth gauge. *Guide pin:* 3.2 mm with a threaded tip and tapered root diameter. *Screw head:* Round head with a 4.8-mm internal hexagon. *Material:* 22-13-5 stainless steel. *System accessory equipment:* Washers, depth gauge, pin guide, soft tissue protection sleeve, cannulated overdrill.

#### System 2

*Screw thread:* Outer diameter—6.5 mm; pitch—1.9 mm; reverse cutting flutes; self-cutting, self-tapping tip. *Drill:* A 3.2-mm steel drill. *Guide pin:* 3.2 mm with a threaded tip. *Screw head:* Round head with an internal hexagon. *Material:* Titanium alloy. *System accessory equipment:* Washers, depth gauge, pin guide, soft tissue protection sleeve.

## Small Cannulated Screws

### *System 1*

*Screw thread:* Cancellous; outer diameter—4.5 mm; pitch—1.75 mm; not self-cutting. *Screw shaft:* 3.1 mm. *Guide pin:* 1.6-mm with a threaded tip. *Screw head:* Round head with an internal 3.5-mm hexagon. *Material:* 316 LVM stainless steel. *System accessory equipment:* Washers, depth gauge, pin guide, soft tissue protection sleeve, cannulated overdrill.

### *System 2*

*Screw thread:* Cancellous; outer diameter—3.5 mm; pitch 1.25 mm; not self-cutting. *Screw shaft:* 2.5 mm. *Guide pin:* 1.25 mm with a threaded tip. *Screw head:* Round head with an internal 2.5-mm hexagon. *Material:* 316 LVM stainless steel. *System accessory equipment:* Washers, depth gauge, pin guide, soft tissue protection sleeve, cannulated overdrill.

### *Alternate Systems*

#### System 1

*Screw thread:* Outer diameter—5.0 mm; pitch 1.6 mm; reverse cutting flutes; self-cutting, self-tapping positive rake tip. *Screw shaft:* Smooth 3.5 mm. *Guide pin:* 2.0 mm with a threaded tip and tapered root diameter. *Screw head:* Round head with an internal 3.5-mm hexagon. *Material:* 316 LVM stainless steel. *System accessory equipment:* Washers, depth gauge, 2.0-mm pin guide, soft tissue protection sleeve, cannulated overdrill.

#### System 2

*Screw thread:* Outer diameter—4.5 mm; pitch—1.0 mm; self-cutting, self-tapping positive rake tip. *Screw shaft:* A fully threaded 3.5-mm root diameter. *Guide pin:* 2.0 mm with a threaded tip and tapered root diameter. *Screw head:* Round head with an internal 3.5-mm hexagon. *Material:* 316 LVM stainless steel. *System accessory equipment:* Washers, depth gauge, 2.0-mm pin guide, soft tissue protection sleeve, cannulated overdrill.

# Technique

The techniques described in this chapter utilize the author's preferred equipment but also can be performed with other systems as suggested as alternates.

## Fractures of the Talus[3]

Talar fracture patterns vary according to the mechanism of injury. Talar neck fractures usually occur following high-energy mechanisms and result from acute hyperdorsiflexion of the foot. The fracture occurs when the neck of the talus is forced across the anterior lip of the tibia. Fractures of the head of the talus follow indirect medial or lateral displacements of the forefoot. Fractures of the body occur following vertical loading of the plantarly flexed foot. Compression fractures of the facets occur with vertical loading of an inverted or everted foot and often accompany subtalar dislocations.

Two anatomic factors are responsible for the relatively poor prognosis following talar fracture. Sixty percent of the surface of the talus is covered by articular cartilage. The various articular facets form important articulations with the rest of the foot. The talonavicular joint is the cornerstone of midfoot motion. The talar dome provides ankle motion, and the three subtalar facets are needed for eversion and inversion of the foot. Because there are no muscle or tendon attachments, the talus has a limited blood supply. Displaced fractures in the talar neck or body can significantly disrupt the talar articulations and threaten the blood supply to the talus. Exact anatomic reduction of such fractures is needed to preserve joint function. In addition, it is believed that compression of talar fragments by lag screw fixation may permit early revascularization and limit the degree of avascular necrosis (AVN) that occurs.[4]

## Fractures of the Talar Neck

Fractures of the talar neck are classified into four types using the modified Hawkins classification.[5,6] This classification predicts the risk of avascular necrosis based upon the degree of fracture displacement:

Type I: The talar neck is undisplaced. Risk of AVN is less than 10%.

Type II: There is slight displacement of the neck fracture. The risk of AVN is approximately 40%.

Type III: There is complete displacement of the body from both the ankle and subtalar joints, with the chance of AVN approaching 90%.

Type IV: This was added by Canale and Kelly.[6] This category includes subluxation of the head and dislocation or extrusion of the body. This risk of AVN is 100%.

Conditions that favor healing and diminish the risk of AVN are anatomic reduction and compression of the fracture fragments as soon after injury as possible. Lag screws provide this compression and are recommended over K-wire fixation for these fractures.[4]

Hawkins type I fractures can be treated by closed reduction, which involves gentle plantar flexion, and distraction followed by inversion and dorsiflexion, which compresses the fracture site.[1] Posterior to anterior fixation can then be accomplished. A Kirschner wire or 2.0-mm guide pin is placed for preliminary stabilization and then replaced by a countersunk cannulated 7.0-mm short-threaded (16-mm) screw for definitive fixation. Two similarly placed parallel screws may also be used. The talus has very dense bone and the guide pin should be overdrilled to 4.5 mm in the proximal fragment. This hole is overdrilled to the size of the screw's shaft not the outer diameter of the screw thread (7.0 mm). A fracture firmly fixed in this fashion may be treated with early range of motion with little chance of displacement. (Optionally, 6.5-mm titanium screws or 6.5-mm 22-13-5 stainless steel screws are available, which accommodate larger 3.2-mm guide pins.)

For displaced type II, III, and IV fractures ORIF is needed. Exposure of the fracture is gained through combined medial and lateral incisions (Figure 16.1). Although a direct ante-

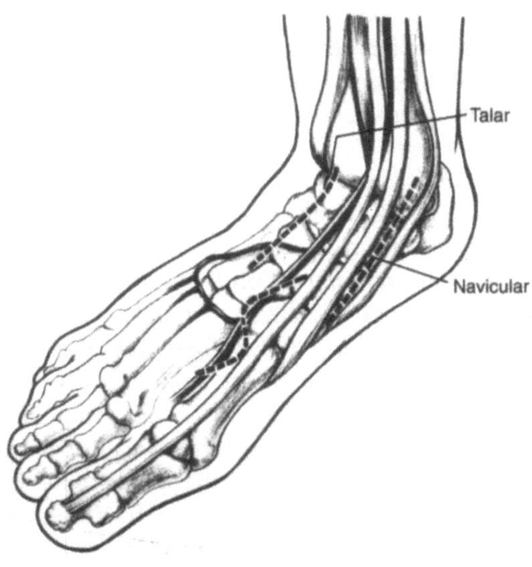


**FIGURE 16.1.** Incisions used to gain access to the talus for reduction and fixation of displaced fractures. (Reprinted with permission from Sangeorzan.[3])

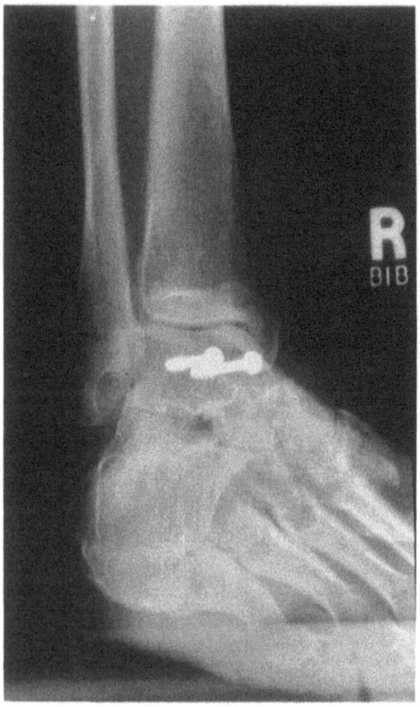

a

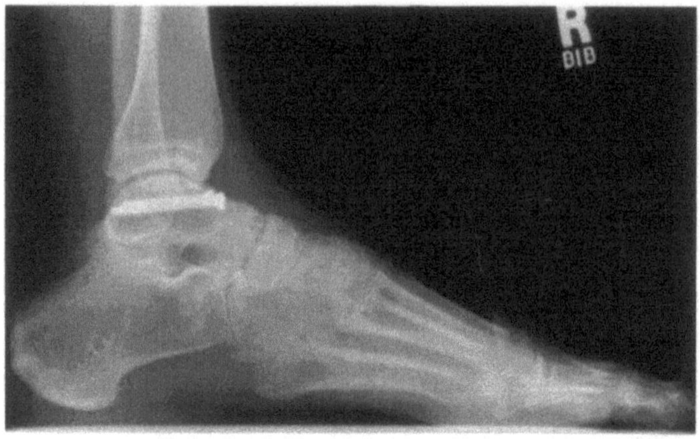

b

**FIGURE 16.2.** (a) An anteroposterior view of the fixation of a talar neck fracture with 4.5-mm cannulated screws placed from anterior to posterior. (b) The lateral radiograph showing anterior to posterior screw placements.

rior incision provides excellent exposure, it risks damage to any remaining blood supply along the dorsal talar neck. The medial incision runs between the anterior and posterior tibial tendons and can be extended so that a medial malleolar osteotomy can be performed if needed. Provisional fixation is provided with parallel or crossed 1.6-mm guide pins, then replaced with 4.5-mm countersunk cannulated screws for fixation (Figure 16.2). Postoperatively, talar fractures are managed with partial weight bearing and active ROM exercises. These fractures are usually united in 8 weeks. Fractures of the body of the talus and impaction fractures of the talar facets are best visualized through the medial malleolar approach. When possible posterior to anterior fixation is used for fixation of the talar body using parallel 3.5- or 4.5-mm cannulated screws (Figure 16.3). A separate small posterior incision is used to place the guide pins followed by the screws. Impaction fractures usually require disimpaction of joint fragments, bone grafting to fill subchondral defects, and fixation with small screws or Kirschner wires (Figure 16.4). Fractures of the head of the talus are exposed through any of the incisions mentioned. Fixation is achieved using countersunk 3.5-mm cannulated screws (Figure 16.2).

## Fractures of the Calcaneus

Calcaneal fractures are usually caused by axial loading injuries. Avulsion fractures can result from indirect force. For example, the Achilles tendon can avulse the dorsal portion of the tuberosity at its insertion site. Seventy-five percent of calcaneal fractures are intraarticular involving the subtalar joint. Currently, CT scanning is essential in the evaluation of calcaneal fracture patterns allowing adequate preoperative planning for ORIF.[7]

Several distinctive components characterize calcaneal fractures.[1,8] The medial sustentacular fragment, which is triangularly shaped on the semicoronal CT scan, may vary in size but remains in its normal position held by the interosseous ligament. The posterior facet is impacted and rotated as much as 30° to 60° anteriorly. A long posterior portion of the calcaneal tuber may remain attached to the facet creating the tongue-type fracture pattern. The lateral wall is

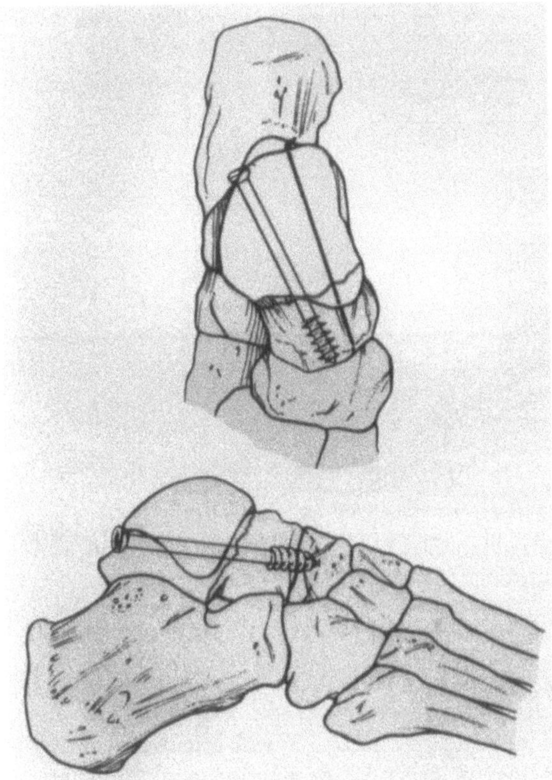

FIGURE 16.3. The technique of posterior to anterior fixation of talar neck fracture. (Reprinted with permission from Hansen.[1])

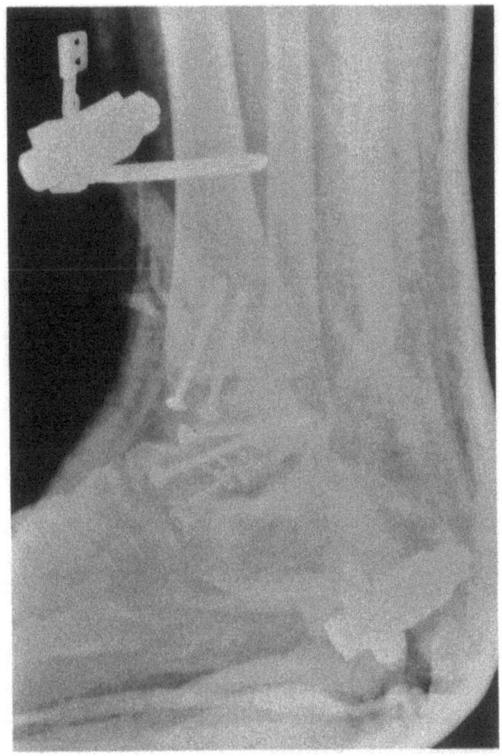

FIGURE 16.4. A radiograph of a technique used for repair of an impaction fracture of the subtalar facets. A medial malleolar osteotomy approach was used for exposure: 3.5-mm screws stabilized a Hawkins type I talar neck fracture. The facet was disimpacted and stabilized with a 1.6-mm K-wire. The defect was bone grafted and the construct neutralized.

usually significantly widened and the anterior process may be shortened and flexed with disruption of the dense cortical bone beneath the sinus tarsi, which form the angle of Gissane.

Open reduction internal fixation is becoming increasingly accepted as the best treatment for the displaced calcaneal fracture. The lateral approach using the Seattle incision is now the approach of choice. The techniques of fixation is well described in the reports by Benirschke.[9,10] The steps involved in restoration and fixation of calcaneal anatomy involves complete exposure of the lateral aspect from the tuber to the calcaneocuboid joint by reflection of the full-thickness lateral flap (Figure 16.5). The subtalar joint is identified and the sustentacular fragment is visualized. The anterior process is reduced to the sustentactular fragment and held with Kirschner wires. The anatomic relationship between the tuberosity and medial wall is restored using a Schanz pin inserted into the tuberosity for distraction and correction of the varus deformity. Preliminary fixation with K-wires maintains the reduction. The joint surface of the posterior facet is then elevated and precisely reduced to the sustentacular fragment and fixed with 3.5-mm cortical lag screws. The lateral wall is then reduced and the entire construct stabilized with reconstruction plates. A combination of an H-plate and 2.7- or 3.5-mm reconstruction plate is popular, but specially designed plates are also available. Cannulated screws may be useful in fixation of the posterior facet fragment. A 1.25-mm guide pin can be used to reduce the anterior process to the sustentaculum; then the 3.5-mm cannulated lag screws can adequately replace

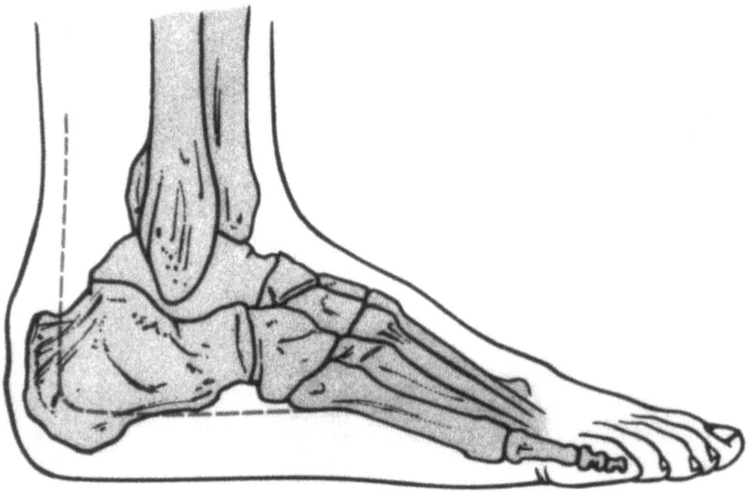

**FIGURE 16.5.** The incision used for exposure of the calcaneous needed for open reduction and internal fixation. (Reprinted with permission from Hansen.[1])

the 3.5-mm cortical lag screws recommended in the Seattle technique. The restoration of the posterior facet to the sustentaculum is key. The sustentaculum is usually composed of dense cancellous bone amenable to a fixation screw; however, it represents a small target. Reduction is performed and held with Kirschner wires and a 1.2-mm guide wire in the position of the desired screw. Confirmation is performed by fluoroscopy or conventional radiographs. A depth gauge measurement predicts the ideal screw length. The optional cannulated screw is then placed and compression applied as desired.

In spite of careful management, both operatively and nonoperatively treated calcaneal fractures are frequently complicated by the development of subtalar arthritis. Reconstruction of the malunited calcaneus reiterates the principles of open reduction and internal fixation. That is, in addition to preservation of the subtalar joint, overall goals include restoration of calcaneal anatomy including height, width, and length, with re-creation of Bohler's and Gissane's angles. In cases of malunion with posttraumatic arthritis, simple fusion of the subtalar joint relieves arthritic pain but fails to achieve the above-stated goals. Subtalar distraction bone block fusion as described by Carr et al.[11] addresses the late complications of os calcis fractures more completely. This procedure is indicated for patients with a painful, deformed calcaneus with loss of heel height, lateral impingement, and tibiotalar neck impingement due to loss of the talar declination angle.[11] A primary subtalar fusion can be considered for patients with arthritis but little deformity. Subtalar bone block fusion is performed with the patient in the contralateral decubitus position. A posterolateral Gallie-type approach or Seattle incision are utilized for exposure of the subtalar joint. Distraction is applied using a medially placed femoral distractor or large laminar spreaders. The subtalar joint is denuded of cartilage, and heel varus or valgus deformity corrected by mobilization of the heel. Correction of the talocalcaneal angle to 25° to 40° can be confirmed by intraoperative x-ray. The subtalar joint gap is measured and a tricortical iliac crest bone autograft is harvested. The graft is triangular in shape to help create talar declination. The graft is placed in the subtalar joint aiming for a heel position of neutral to slight valgus, and distraction is released. Provisional fixation is provided with two 2.0-mm parallel guide pins in the desired location of the screws. Compression arthrodesis is achieved using two 7.0-mm cannulated screws. The guide pins and cannulated screws are inserted under fluoroscopic control through stab wounds in the heel. The screws are aimed proximally to securely fix the talus to the calcaneus with the interposed graft. Cannulated screws are particularly helpful in this case, permitting adjustment of screw length and positioning with minimal trauma to the plantar soft tissues (Figure 16.6). The incisions are closed with the usual attention to the soft tissues. Postoperatively cast immobilization is used for 12 weeks, the final 6 weeks in a walking cast. Carr et al.[11] calls for use of fully threaded cancellous screws in these cases to avoid loss of correction that might occur with compression screws. I have used lag screw fixation with great success. Carr et al. and I have employed this technique with excellent early and late results. For minimal subtalar deformity, compression arthrodesis without bone block using cannulated lag screws inserted in this axial fashion is also extremely effective.

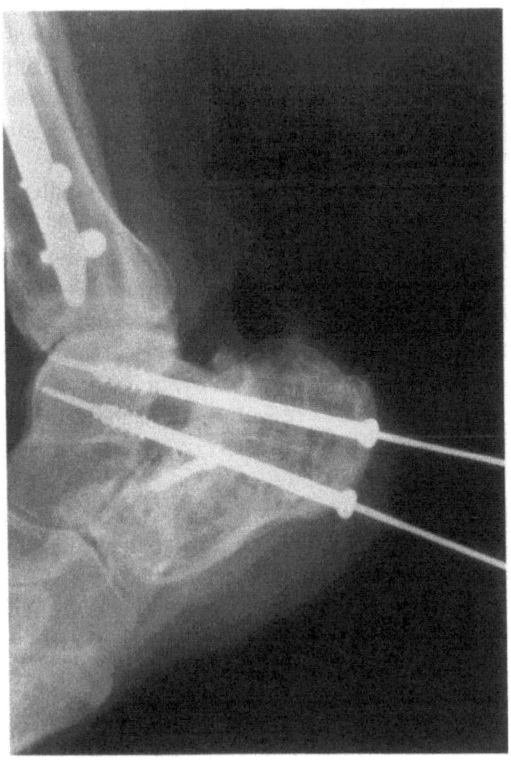

**FIGURE 16.6.** The technique of subtalar bone block fusion; 7.0-mm cannulated screws are inserted through the heel and are aimed into the body of the talus.

## Tarsal Navicular Fractures

The tarsal navicular or scaphoid is the keystone of the medial arch. It articulates with the crucial talonavicular joint proximally and with each of the three cuneiforms distally. The talonavicular joint has significant mobility but the naviculocuneiform articulations are relatively immobile. The posterior tibial tendon inserts upon the navicular medially.

Navicular fractures are usually caused by axial loading directed through the metatarsals along a plantar-flexed foot. The exact fracture pattern depends upon the position of the foot at the time of injury. Avulsion fractures, tuberosity fractures, and dorsal lip fractures result from indirect injury. Navicular fractures are classified according to three categories[12,13]:

Type I: Fractures of the tuberosity, which generally represent avulsion by the posterior tibia tendon.
Type II: Dorsal lip fractures, which generally result from Chopart sprains or subluxations.
Type III: Fractures of the body caused by high-energy axial loading of the foot. These injuries have the worst prognosis and are associated with significant instability of the midtarsal joints (Figure 16.7).

Displaced fractures of the navicular and dorsal lip fractures require ORIF.[3,12] The primary incision is often made dorsally to provide ample exposure of the fracture. A second medial incision can be made over the tuberosity and is helpful in manipulative reduction and placement of lag screws. A medial distractor or laminar spreader can help achieve indirect reduction and improves visualization of the talonavicular and naviculocuneiform joints. In many instances reduction of these joints is necessary, and transfixation with a 2.0-mm K-wire necessary to maintain the joint position. Cancellous bone grafting should be used to fill voids or defects. Cannulated screw fixation is extremely helpful since exposure is limited. Cannulated 3.5-mm lag screws over 1.25-mm guide wires provide excellent fixation of the scaphoid fragment. If K-wire stabilization of the talonavicular joint

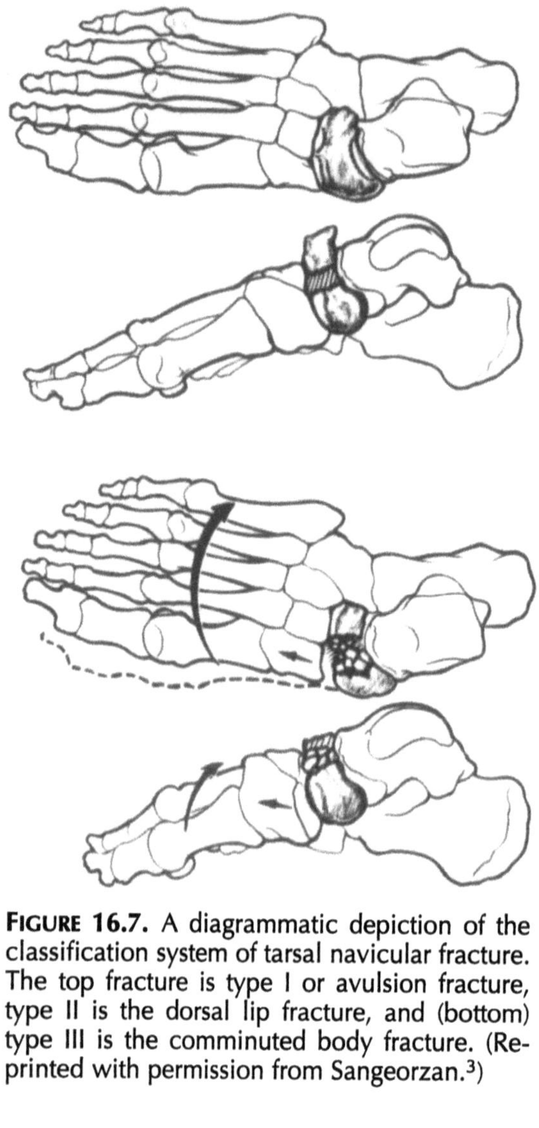

FIGURE 16.7. A diagrammatic depiction of the classification system of tarsal navicular fracture. The top fracture is type I or avulsion fracture, type II is the dorsal lip fracture, and (bottom) type III is the comminuted body fracture. (Reprinted with permission from Sangeorzan.[3])

is necessary, the pin is usually removed after 4 weeks. Cast immobilization without weight bearing is encouraged for 6 weeks. Following this, ambulation in a supportive shoe is recommended.

## Tarsometatarsal (Lisfranc) Fracture Dislocations

The intertarsal and tarsometatarsal joints are very stable and immobile and are disrupted only by high-energy injuries. Isolated injuries may often occur during sports by indirect mechanisms such as a runner catching a foot in a hole. In general, Lisfranc dislocations are part of a larger constellation of multiple trauma. In this setting, the mechanism is often direct crushing violence with severe associated soft tissue injury.

Most tarsometatarsal fracture dislocations are visible on plain radiographs but may be subtle. Stress views can be helpful in delineating the true magnitude of injury and resulting instability. A high degree of suspicion should be aroused in a markedly painful and swollen forefoot in spite of relatively normal plain radiographs.

Prognosis following Lisfranc fracture dislocations appears to be most directly correlated with the accuracy of reduction and maintenance of reduction during the healing period. Poor results develop from posttraumatic deformity and arthritis. The most common posttraumatic deformity resulting from this injury is the planovalgus forefoot, which is painful and impossible to fit into shoes.[14] ORIF of these injuries is therefore advocated. Fears of posttraumatic stiffness caused by transfixation in these joints are not warranted because stiffness in this area is not clinically significant as long as normal anatomy is restored.

The technique of internal fixation[15] calls for exposure of the injured joints through two dorsal incisions. The first is within the first web space, and the second, if needed, is placed between the bases of the third and fourth metatarsals. Cannulated screws are a significant advantage because they allow a more limited exposure. Direct reduction is achieved and maintained using the 1.6- or 1.25-mm guide pins for the cannulated screws. Fixation is provided by 4.5- or 3.5-mm fully threaded transfixation screws. The first metatarsal is usually fixed first. Proper reduction implies re-creation of the normal varus position of the first metatarsal. The base of the second is then reduced and held with an axial screw. The medial screws are generally 4.5-mm thread diameter, with 3.5-mm diameter reserved for the third metatarsals. The fourth and fifth joints often reduce adequately with fixation of the medial joints, but a percutaneous cannulated screw inserted through the base of the fifth metatarsal into the cuboid may be needed (Figure 16.8). One technical

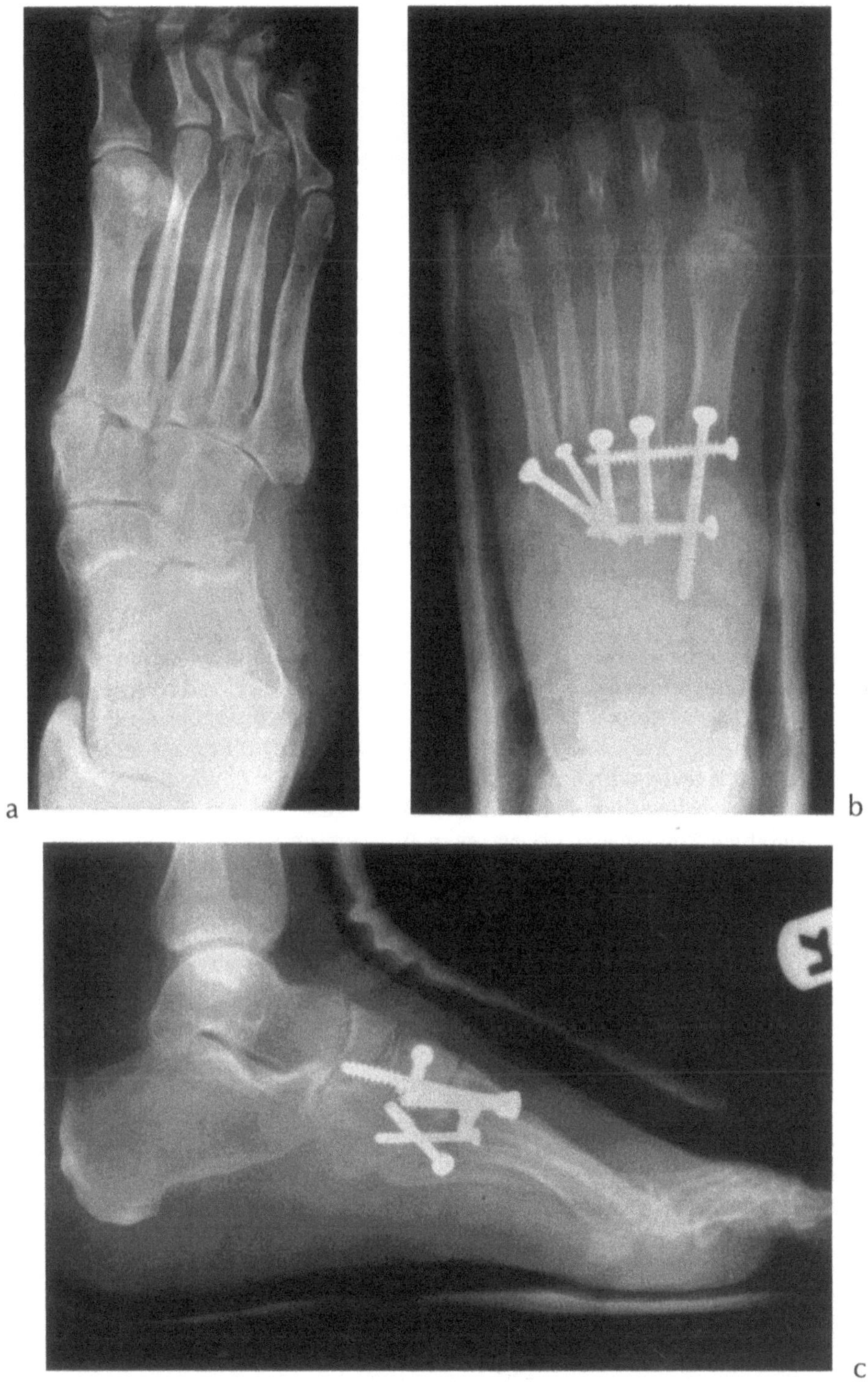


**FIGURE 16.8.** (a) A radiograph of a chronic Lisfranc dislocation following reduction and fusion; (b,c) 4.5-mm cannulated screws are used. The entire medial column was unstable requiring the navicular cuneiform fusion in addition to the tarsometatarsal fusions.

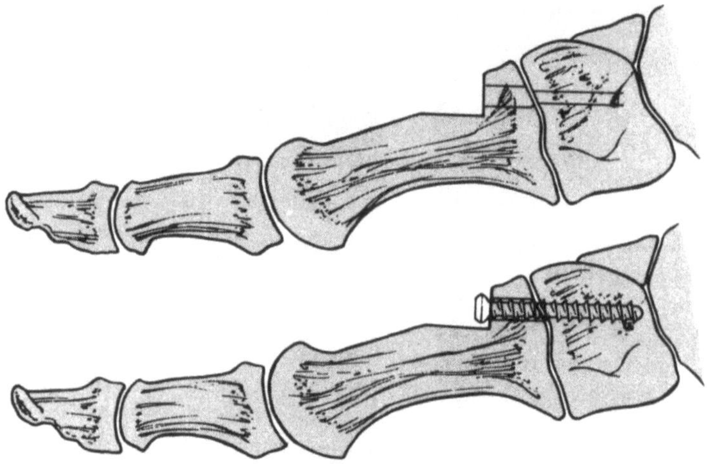

**FIGURE 16.9.** The technique of notching the metatarsal shaft for proper placement of the transfixation screws. (Reprinted with permission from Hansen.[1])

consideration that must be applied for insertion of these screws has been pointed out by Hansen and his coworkers. The metatarsal bases should be notched appropriately 1 cm away from the joint. The notch can be made with a bur or rongeur. The distal cortex below the drill hole must be debrided and then countersunk to accommodate the head of the screw as it is tightened. The cannulated countersink can be used in this step. This notch prevents upward levering of the head of the screw, which can crack the base of the metatarsal. It also permits sufficient countersinking of the screw head to keep it from being in a prominent subcutaneous position (Figure 16.9).

Following fixation of this injury a well-padded short leg cast is applied and limited weight bearing is begun (20 to 30 pounds) as soon as pain and swelling permits. Casting is needed for 8 weeks. Transfixation screws should be removed 3 months postoperative. Vigorous physiotherapy to strengthen foot and calf muscles and to maximize joint range of motion is begun.

In cases of neglected Lisfranc injuries, severe, painful, posttraumatic arthrosis can develop. This is best handled by arthrodesis of the tarsometatarsal joints. The technique of arthrodesis is similar to fixation of the acute injury but requires denuding of cartilage surfaces, correction of deformity, and fixation using large compression lag screws. Generally, 4.5-mm or larger screws up to 7.0 mm are recommended (5.0- or 6.5-mm screws of another system are as good). Breakage of 3.5-mm screws is not uncommon. Bone grafting can favorably improve the chances of securing a stable fusion.[14]

There are multiple other situations where internal fixation using cannulated screws can be of significant advantage. For example, Jones fracture of the fifth metatarsal, notorious for poor healing, can be stabilized with percutaneous placement of a 4.5-mm cannulated lag screw. Interphalangeal fusion of the great toe is often needed for correction of claw toe deformity. A longitudinally oriented cannulated compression screw placed percutaneously through the end of the toe is an excellent technique for this purpose. These are only a few examples of how cannulated screws can be creatively applied for internal fixation in the foot.

## References

1. Hansen ST. Foot injuries. In: Browner D, ed. *Skeletal trauma*, vol 2. Philadelphia: WB Saunders, 1992;1959–1991.
2. Mann R. Biomechanics of the foot and ankle. In:

Mann R, ed. *Surgery of the Foot and Ankle.* St. Louis: Mosby, 1993;3–45.
3. Sangeorzan BJ. Foot and ankle joint. In: Hansen ST, Swiontkowski MF, eds. *Orthopedic Trauma Protocols.* New York: Raven Press, 1993;350–353.
4. Mayo KA. Fractures of the talus: principles of management and techniques of treatment. *Tech Orthop* 1987;2:42–54.
5. Hawkins LG. Fractures of the neck of the talus. *J Bone Joint Surg* 1970;52A:991–1002.
6. Canale ST, Kelly FB. Fractures of the neck of the talus. Long-term evaluation of seventy-one cases. *J Bone Joint Surg* 1978;60A:143–156.
7. Koval KJ, Sanders R. The radiographic evaluation of calcaneal fractures. *Clin Orthop* 1993;290:41–46.
8. Carr JB. Mechanism and pathoanatomy of the intra-articular calcaneal fracture. *Clin Orthop* 1993; 290:36–40.
9. Benirschke SK. Results of operative treatment of os calcis fractures. Paper Presented at AAOS, New Orleans, Feb. 8–12, 1990.
10. Carr JB, Hansen ST, Benirschke SK. Surgical treatement of foot and ankle trauma. Use of indirect reduction techniques. *Foot Ankle* 1989;9:176.
11. Carr JB, Hansen ST, Benirschke SK. Subtalar distraction bone block fusion for late complications of os calcis fractures. *Foot Ankle* 1989;9:81–86.
12. Sangeorzan BJ, Benirschke SK, Mosca V, Mayo KA, Hansen ST. Displaced intraarticular fractures of the tarsal navicular. *J Bone Joint Surg* 1989;71A:1504–1510.
13. Eichenholtz SN, Levine DB. Fractures of the tarsal navicular. *Clin Orthop* 1964;34:142–157.
14. Sangeorzan BJ, Verth RG, Hansen ST. Salvage of Lisfranc's tarsometatarsal joint by arthrodesis. *Foot Ankle* 1990;10:193–200.
15. Arntz CT, Verth RG, Hansen ST. Fractures and fracture dislocations of the tarsometatarsal joint. *J Bone Joint Surg* 1988;70A:173–181.

# 17
# The Spine

Robert A. McGuire, Jr.

## Cannulated Screws in the Spine

During the last decade, the use of cannulated screws in the treatment of spinal disorders has become fairly commonplace. This technique allows direct stabilization of cervical fractures and also facilitates the placement of screws into the thoracic and lumbar vertebral body using the transpedicular approach. The chapter addresses the anatomy, biomechanics, techniques, and potential complications associated with the utilization of cannulated screws in the spine.

## Cervical Spine

The upper cervical spinal anatomy is unique in that both significant rotation as well as flexion and extension at the C-1–C-2 articulation are allowed.[1] Approximately 50% of axial rotation occurs at this segment, and owing to the orientation of the C-1–C-2 facet complex, adequate mechanical stability is not provided in the event of a fracture of the dens, transverse ligament rupture, or burst of the C-1 ring. The use of cannulated screws in the cervical spine permits direct repair of the dens fractures while retaining cervical motion[2,3] or posterior transarticular fixation of C-1–C-2 when transverse ligament rupture or unstable Jefferson's fractures render the segment unstable.[4,5]

## Anterior Fixation of the Odontoid

Anatomically, the dens lends itself to direct repair of the fracture, restoring stability while maintaining motion. The majority of fractures at this level occur at the junction of the dens and the body of C-2, or obliquely into the body of C-2.[6] Blood supply to this watershed area is precarious, with little cancellous bone present. Therefore, displacement of this fracture is associated with a high rate of nonunion when treated nonoperatively.[7]

Biomechanical testing in vitro following internal fixation of this fracture with screws has demonstrated that stability is one half that of the unfractured odontoid.[8] The use of two screws versus a single screw has not been shown to enhance the stability of the construct,[8,9] and in certain anatomic specimens the size of the odontoid precludes the safe use of more than one screw.[10]

Odontoid fractures are classified using the Anderson and D'Alonzo criteria. A type I fracture is described as an oblique fracture through the apex of the dens and probably represents an avulsion of the alar ligaments. This fracture is rare and, when detected, atlanto-occipital dislocation must be considered. Type II fractures occur at the junction of the dens with the body of the axis that is below the level of the transverse ligament. This fracture is the most common as well as the most controversial regarding treatment. The rate of nonunion has been reported to range from 10% to 67% with nonoperative treatment. Several predictors of nonunion of this fracture have been described. These are an initial displacement of greater than 5 mm, posterior displacement, angular displacement of greater than 10°, age greater than 60 years at the time of injury, smoking, and delayed diagnosis. Type III fractures extend in an oblique manner caudally from the base of the dens to the anterior body of the axis. A 13% rate of nonunion with nonoperative treatment has been reported with this fracture.

Jefferson's fractures occur as a result of an axial load to the head, with the resulting force being transferred through the wedge-shaped lateral masses of C-1, resulting in a break of the ring and lateral displacement of the condyles. If the C-1 lateral masses are subluxed greater than 7 mm in relation to the lateral masses of C-2, then the transverse ligament is considered to be compromised with resulting potential instability of this segment.

Indications for direct stabilization include the type II or shallow type III displaced odontoid fracture; the type II fracture with an intact transverse ligament and posterior C-1 arch fracture, which would preclude initial posterior wiring procedure and prolonged halo immobilization to allow healing of C-1 prior to operative stabilization; and those patients who wish to retain the C-1–C-2 mobility.

Contraindications to this procedure include the unstable Jefferson's fracture in addition to the dens fracture, those dens fractures with oblique configurations that prevent adequate stability when compressed following internal fixation, and fractures resulting from a pathologic process.[2]

# Anatomy

The dens is slightly conical in nature and thickest at its base. Before age 7, the transverse synchondrosis, which joins the dens to the body may be mistaken for a type III fracture. In the adult, the dens extends cephalad an average of 15 mm from the body of the second vertebra. Men tend to have odontoids with greater dimensions than women; however, the size has not been shown to correlate with specimen height or weight.

# Technique

## Anterior Fixation of the Odontoid

### *Author's Preferred Equipment*

*Guide pin:* 1.25 mm by 150 mm with a threaded tip. *Screw head:* Round head with an internal 3.5-mm hexagon. *Screw thread:* Cancellous type; outer diameter—4.0 mm. *Material:* 316 LVM stainless steel or titanium. *System accessory equipment:* 4.0-mm system washers, soft tissue protection sleeve, 4.0-mm system cannulated tap, direct reading depth gauge, drill (optional)—2.7 mm.

Prior to the start of the operation, the patient must be positioned appropriately to facilitate fluoroscopic evaluation of the spinal anatomy, which is essential for safe placement of the screws (Figure 17.1). Gardner-Wells tongs can be utilized with the head placed in a padded horseshoe, but a radiolucent three-point head positioning device is superior. The radiolucent

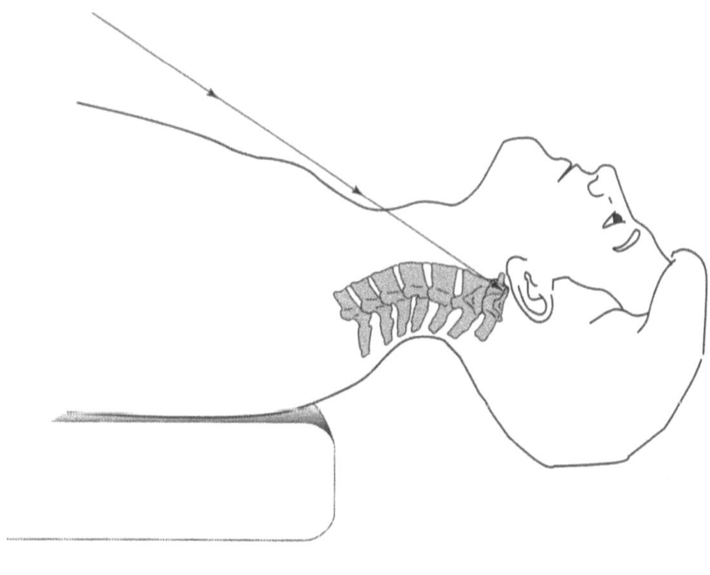

**FIGURE 17.1.** The patient is positioned supine with the shoulders at the end of the bed and the head in a holding device. The fracture is reduced and the proposed line of screw placement is visualized fluoroscopically. There must be no impingement of the guide wire on the sternum.

holding device allows visualization of the C-1–C-2 complex in both the anteroposterior (AP) and lateral planes. The fluoroscope is placed in such a manner to allow visualization in both the true lateral and true AP planes. We have found the use of two fixed units to be superior to a single unit, which must be sequentially rotated from the lateral to AP plane during the procedure. The fracture must be reduced and be able to be fluoroscopically visualized in both planes before the surgical procedure is initiated. When the fracture has been reduced, a trial placement of a guide pin is performed by laying the guide pin along the neck with radiographic monitoring in the lateral plane. The plane of the guide pin must not impinge on the sternum and still allow direct placement from the anterior margin of the C2-3 interspace and the tip of the odontoid. If this unrestricted pathway cannot be attained, then the head must be either flexed or extended so as to facilitate this angle.

When acceptable reduction and visualization have been accomplished, the neck is surgically prepped and draped. If the surgeon is right-handed, a right-sided anteromedial approach to the vertebra may be more comfortable, and the left-handed surgeon would probably use a left-sided approach. The incision is made at the C-6 level and soft tissue dissection continued between the alar and visceral fascia. When the anterior border of the spine is encountered, blunt dissection is continued cephalad until the anterior caudal lip of C-2 is palpated. Soft tissue retractors are placed to prevent inadvertent nerve, vessel, esophageal, or tracheal injury. Guide pins (1.2 mm) may then be placed (Figure 17.2a).

The decision as to whether to place one or two screws must be made prior to the start of the procedure. If two screws will be placed, then the insertion point is selected lateral to the midline and checked fluoroscopically. Using a drill sleeve for additional soft tissue protection, the guide pin is advanced in a lateral to medial direction penetrating the cortex of the tip of the odontoid. Guide pin placement is monitored radiographically in both the AP and lateral planes.

If one screw will be placed, then the initial starting point is the midline of C-2 and directed in the same sagittal plane as with two screws. A second guide pin may be placed to function as an anti-rotation device and then removed after screw placement.

When the guide pins have been correctly positioned, the screw length is determined by direct measurement from the guide pin and the near cortex is tapped (Figure 17.2b). The cancellous bone is not tapped. A 4.0-mm cancellous cannulated (either 316 stainless steel or titanium) screw is inserted and monitored radiographically to assure that the guide pin does not migrate in a cephalad direction as the screw is advanced (Figure 17.2c). Care must be taken during the selection of screw length to prevent crossing of the fracture line with the threaded portion of the screw, which could lead to distraction of the fracture and subsequent nonunion (Figure 17.2d).

Postoperative management includes the use of a hard collar for 6 to 8 weeks as healing progresses, and routine radiographic evaluation. When healing is evident, weaning from the collar is accomplished and exercises designed to return a normal range of motion are instituted.

## Results

Bohler[3] reported a series of 15 patients in whom a 100% arthrodesis was achieved. Montesano et al.[11] treated 14 patients with odontoid screws. The rate of union was 86% (12/14), with six of six fractures that were treated with a single screw achieving a solid arthrodesis and six of eight fractures utilizing two screws attaining solid union. In the report of Etter et al.,[2] 23 patients had a union rate of 87% (20/23) and a complication rate of 17.4%, with one death occurring after successful stabilization. The majority of complications occurred early in the series and were attributable to the learning curve of the procedure.

## Conclusion

Anterior fixation of odontoid fractures provides excellent stability to facilitate fracture union while maintaining normal C-1–C-2 motion. The technique is demanding and requires meticulous attention to detail from positioning to surgical technique, in order to minimize the risks of both intraoperative and postoperative complications.

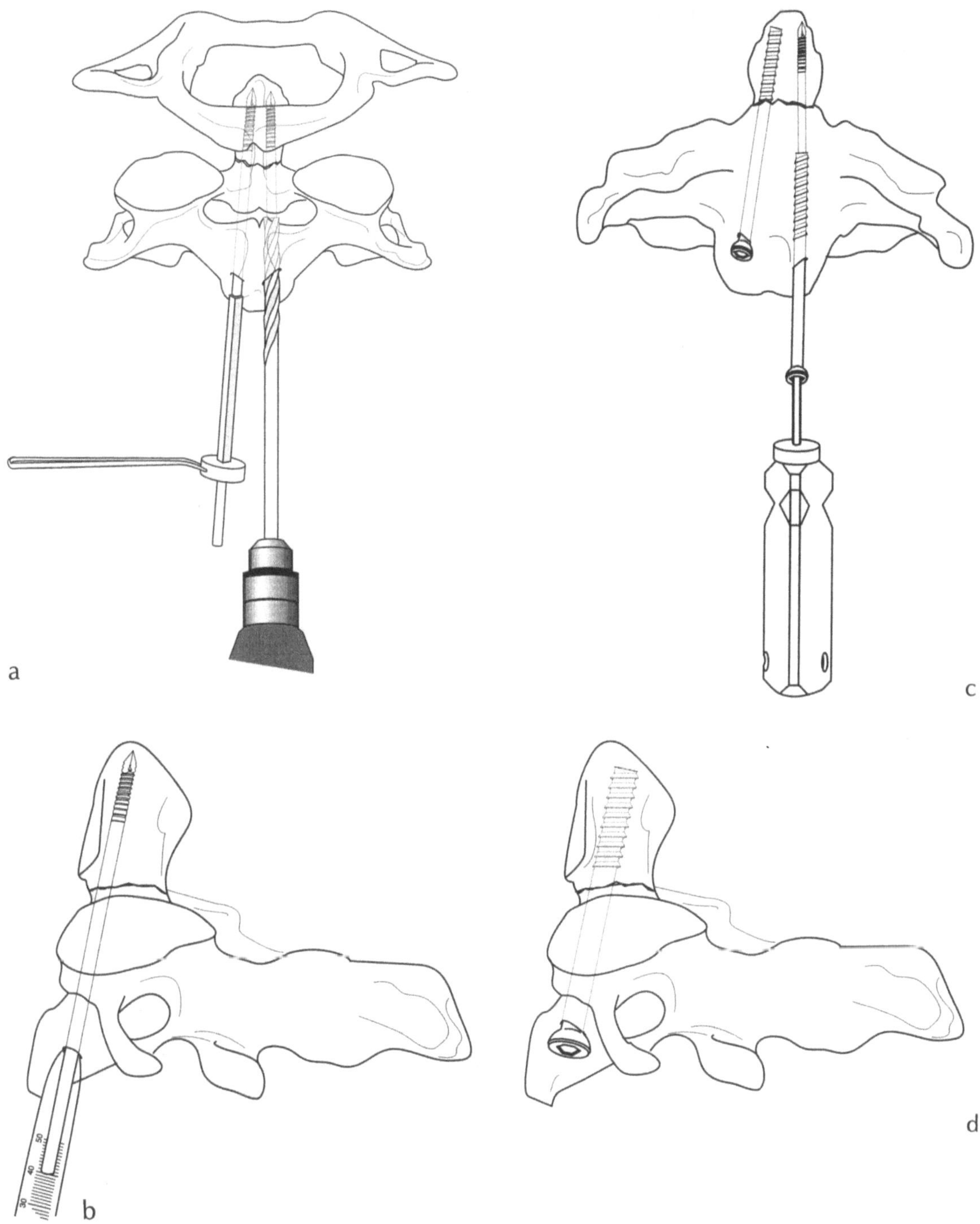


**FIGURE 17.2.** (a) The appropriate placement of the guide wires in the odontoid. A soft tissue protection sleeve is shown on the left and the cannulated overdrill on the right. (b) The screw length can be read directly from a depth gauge (as shown) or by measuring the length of guide wire not in the bone with an identical-length guide wire. The difference between the two measurements is the length of screw required. (c) After tapping the near cortex, screws are inserted taking care that guide pins do not advance with screw placement. (d) The threaded portion of the screw should not cross the fracture to minimize risk of nonunion.

## Posterior Stabilization of C-1–C-2

Magerl and Seemann[4] described the technique for stabilization of the C-1–C-2 articulation in which screws are placed from the posterior aspect of the lateral mass of C-2, crossing the C-1–C-2 joint, and then into the lateral mass of C-1, using a C-1 sublaminar wire to stabilize a posterior bone graft from C-1 to C-2. The original description recommended that the skin incision be extended to the upper thoracic level in order to facilitate correct drill placement to cross the C-1–C-2 articulation and gain sufficient purchase in the C-1 lateral mass to provide stability. The use of cannulated screws provides a method to attain bony stability with minimal soft tissue disruption.

Biomechanically, the transarticular C-1–C-2 technique imparts rigid stability to this segment and resists shearing moments to a greater extent than do other posterior methods of C-1–C-2 stabilization.[12,13]

Posterior C-1–C-2 transarticular stabilization is indicated in transverse ligament disruptions allowing atlantoaxial instability, odontoid nonunions, odontoid fractures with concomitant C-1 ring fractures that would prevent direct posterior wiring, and unstable Jefferson's fractures.[14]

### Anatomy

The C-1–C-2 bony articulation, designed for motion, offers little intrinsic stability due to the horizontal plane in which the facet joints lie. Disruption of the soft tissue structures, consisting of the alar ligaments, apical ligaments, accessory ligaments, and transverse ligament, can lead to a grossly unstable segment.

### Author's Preferred Equipment

*Guide pin:* 1.25 mm by 150 mm with a threaded tip. *Screw head:* Round head with an internal 3.5-mm hexagon. *Screw thread:* Cortical type; outer diameter—3.5 mm fully threaded. *Material:* 316 LVM stainless steel or titanium. *System accessory equipment:* soft tissue protection sleeve, cannulated tap, direct reading depth gauge. *Drill* (optional): 2.7-mm by 150-mm steel drill, which can be used with a direct reading depth gauge.

The patient is anesthetized and the radiolucent three-point head holder is placed. The patient is then carefully turned to the prone position and the head stabilized (Figure 17.3). Lateral plane fluoroscopy is used to check the position to assure correct reduction of the lateral masses. The image must not be oblique at the C-1–C-2, otherwise incorrect positioning of the guide pin may result. After the spinal position has been verified, the neck is then surgically prepped and draped.

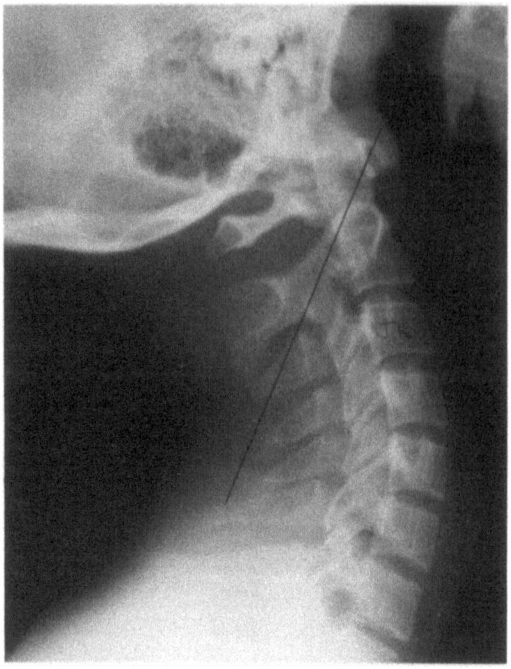

**FIGURE 17.3.** For correct screw placement, true lateral visualization must be obtained with the fracture reduced.

The incision is made in the midline, beginning at the skull base and extending caudally to the C-2-3 interspace. Lateral subperiosteal dissection exposes the C-1–C-2 and C-2–C-3 facets. The capsule of the C-2–C-3 joint must not be disturbed. The capsule of the C-1–C-2 facet is elevated from caudal to cephalad, taking care to avoid the vessels and nerve. Should the venous plexus be damaged at this level, brisk bleeding can occur.

Following exposure, subperiosteal elevation of the tissues around the posterior arch of C-1 is accomplished. A sublaminar wire or braided cable is then passed to secure the graft after screw placement. It is important to pass the C-1 sublaminar wire prior to lateral mass screw

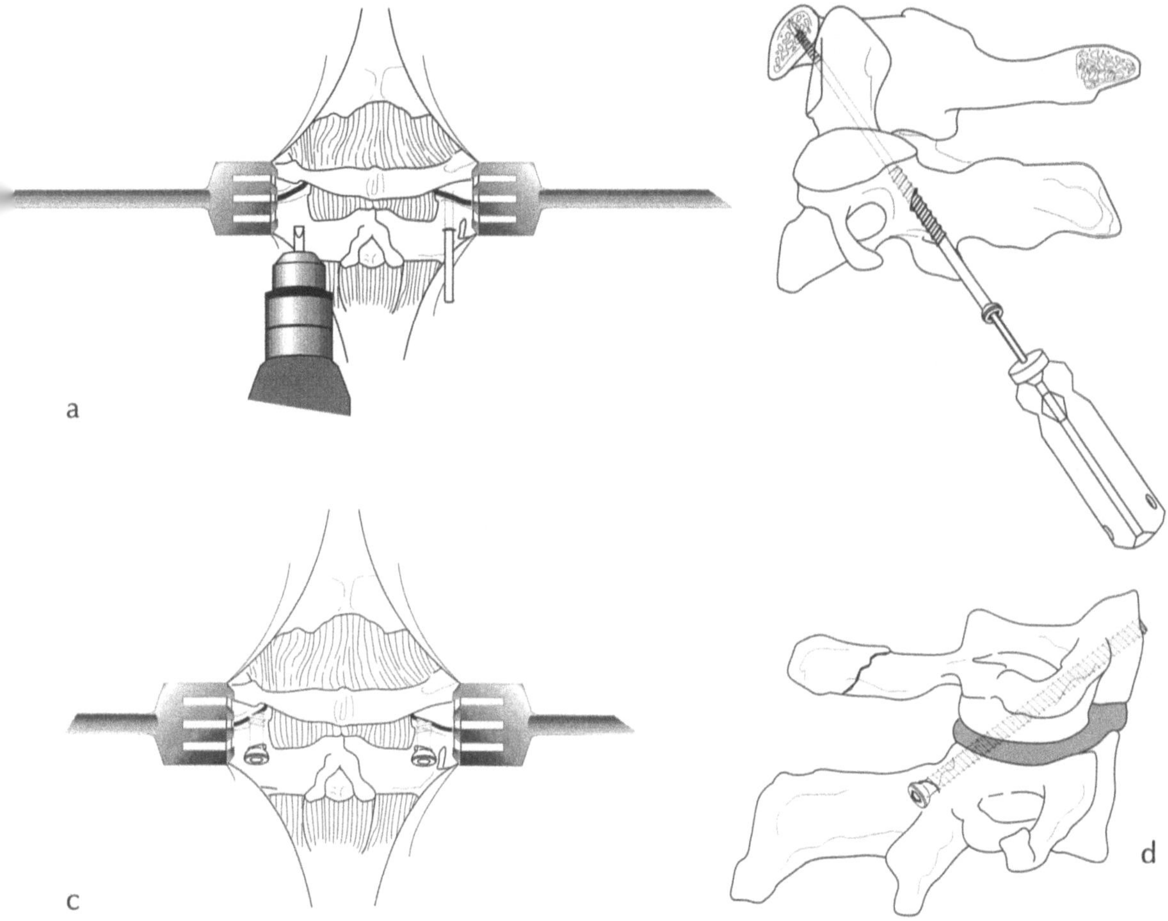


**FIGURE 17.4.** (a) The Kirschner wire is placed in the lateral mass of C-2 and directed cephalad toward the superior margin of the C-1 lateral mass. This position will allow optimal bone-screw interface for stabilization. (b) The near cortex is tapped and the appropriate length screw is inserted to assure purchase of the anterior cortex of the lateral mass of C-1. The author prefers the use of fully threaded cannulated screws for this application rather than the lag screws that are demonstrated here. (c and d) The correct final position of the lateral mass transarticular screws.

placement, which stabilizes the segment and renders wire passage more difficult and dangerous.

A 1.25-mm guide pin is then placed percutaneously in a cephalad direction. The insertion point on C-2 is in the fossa, slightly lateral to the junction of the lamina and lateral mass (Figure 17.4a). Using fluoroscopic guidance, the guide pin is then carefully directed toward the superior border of the lateral mass of C-1, just lateral to the C-2 pars intraarticularis. The guide pin must not be directed laterally as this puts the vertebral artery in jeopardy. It must be directed either straight ahead or slightly medial to avoid the vessel. A preoperative computed tomography (CT) or magnetic resonance imaging (MRI) scan can assist in attaining the correct orientation for guide pin direction. Great care must be taken at the point that the guide pin crosses the C-1–C-2 joint because the wire may bend slightly as it penetrates the cortical bone and produce impingement of the drill, with subsequent advancement of the guide pin into the posterior oropharyngeal fossa. The tip of the guide pin should engage the anterosuperior margin of the C-1 lateral mass. The near cortex is then tapped and a fully threaded 3.5-mm cortical screw of appropriate length (usually 40–45 mm) is placed (Figure 17.4b). The anterior cortex of the C-1 lateral mass should be purchased with the screw (Figure 17.4c,d). Autogenous iliac crest graft is obtained, contoured, and held in position with the C-1 sublaminar wire.

Postoperative management includes immobilization in a hard collar for 6 to 8 weeks and then weaning as pain diminishes and healing progresses.

A potential complication of this technique is that of penetration of the intervertebral foramen with subsequent vertebral artery injury. Should this problem occur with placement of the first screw, the procedure should be abandoned because of potential risk to the remaining vessel. Other complications include possible guide pin breakage during overdrilling with a cannulated bit or incarceration of guide pin and screw during insertion due to bending of the guide pin as it penetrated cortical bone at oblique angles (Figure 17.5). Inadvertent screw placement in the canal can be avoided by visualizing the medial border of the canal before the guide wire is placed.

### *Results*

Jeanneret and Magerl[14] reported a series of 13 patients in whom the transarticular technique was used. All patients achieved a solid arthrodesis. A comparable result was reported in another group of eight patients, all of whom achieved a solid fusion.[5]

### *Conclusion*

Posterior transarticular screw fixation provides an excellent biomechanical construct for stabilizing the C-1–C-2 articulation. Strict attention to detail is required throughout the procedure and clinical outcome and arthrodesis rate are excellent.

## Thoracic and Lumbar Spine

### *Author's Preferred Equipment*

*Guide pin:* 1.25 mm by 150 mm with a threaded tip. *Screw head:* Round head with an internal 3.5-mm hexagon. *Screw thread:* Cortical type; outer diameter—4.0 mm fully threaded. *Material:* 316 LVM stainless steel. *System accessory equipment:* Soft tissue protection sleeve, direct reading depth gauge. *Drill* (optional): 2.7 mm

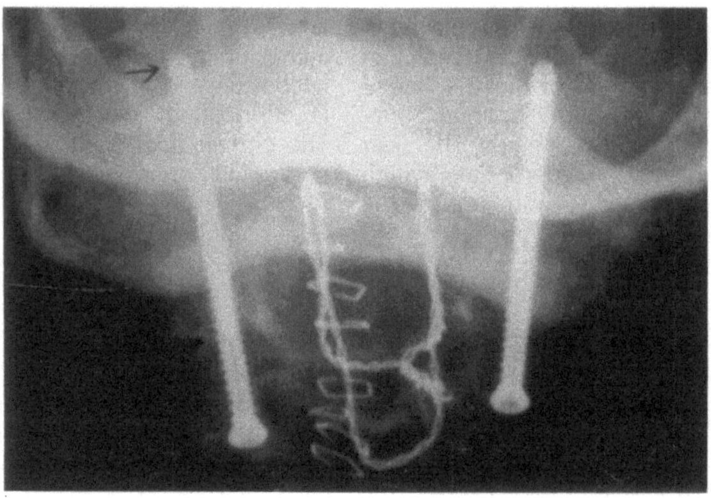

**FIGURE 17.5.** This AP radiograph reveals the remnant of a K-wire that was broken during the drilling of the lateral mass and was driven into the posterior pharynx with screw insertion. The transoral approach was utilized, but owing to the severe angle of the guide wire, it could not be removed. It was subsequently pushed back into the screw and the screw tip crushed. The patient ultimately achieved a solid fusion with no subsequent morbidity.

steel drill which can be used with a direct reading depth gauge.

## Alternate System

*Guide pin:* 2.0 mm with a threaded tip. *Screw head:* Round head with an internal hexagon. *Screw thread:* Cortical type; outer diameter—6.5 mm fully threaded, self-tapping. *Material:* 316 LVM stainless steel.

The most recent development in internal fixation of the spine has been the use of transpedicular screws to transfix a rod or plate to the vertebrae. This innovation provides a method to gain control of the vertebrae, even when the posterior elements are absent, thus facilitating reduction and stabilization of vertebral segments. The result has been an increased fusion rate in patients who are being treated for degenerative spinal conditions.[15] Placement of the screw through the pedicle into the vertebral body provides optimal holding power at the bone-screw interface, but potentially jeopardizes the neural elements in the event that the screw is placed out of the pedicle into the canal. Several methods have been developed to aid in identifying the pedicle and assist in screw placement, but a significant number of missed or penetrated pedicles have resulted.[16,17] Cannulated screw techniques are helpful in minimizing pedicle breakout using the "pedicle coaxial" technique.[18]

Using fluoroscopic assistance, an oblique image of the spine is obtained, which allows the pedicle to be viewed along its axis. This produces a "bull's-eye" effect for aiming the guide pin (Figure 17.6). The guide pin is then placed in the center of the pedicle and aligned parallel to the intensifier beam. The guide pin is then advanced to the anterior margin of the vertebral body, and the 6.5-mm cortical self-tapping cannulated screw is inserted over a 2.0-mm guide pin, or a 4.5-mm fully threaded cannulated screw is placed over a 1.25-mm guide pin. This maneuver is performed for as many segments as necessary, and the spine is then stabilized by connecting these screws to either a plate or rod.

Another method that can be utilized to enhance fusion of the lumbar spine is the translaminar facet joint technique described by Magerl.[19] This technique differs from previous descriptions by King[20] and Boucher[21] in that a much longer screw is placed through the entire lamina, exiting at the base of the transverse process (Figure 17.7).

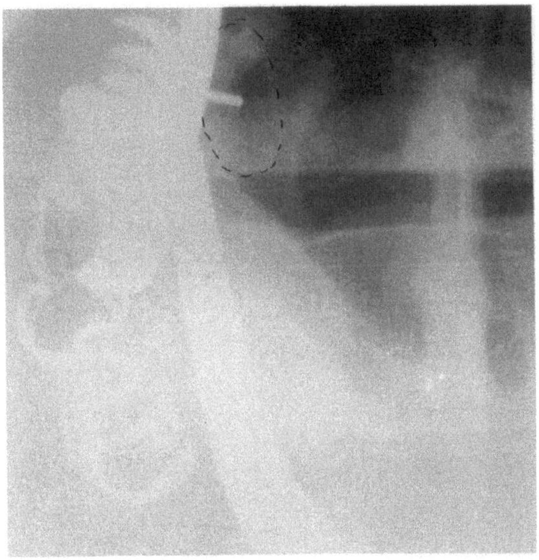

**FIGURE 17.6.** The "bull's-eye" is produced when the K-wire is viewed on end in the center of the pedicle. This minimizes the risk of thread cutout of the pedicle with screw insertion.

Following exposure of the lumbar spine segment to be fused, a guide pin is placed percutaneously and brought to rest on the side of the spinous process opposite the facet joint to be crossed. The angle is adjusted to permit the pin to pass between the two tables of the lamina, crossing the facet and exiting at the base of the transverse process. A self-tapping 4.0-mm cortical cannulated screw of appropriate length is then selected by direct measurement from the guide pin and placed. The opposite facet is then stabilized in the same manner and posterolateral bone grafting performed.

Jacobs et al.[22] reported on 43 patients who underwent lumbar fusion using the translaminar facet joint screw technique. Of the total, 91% of fusions were found to be solid. Clinical success was achieved in 93% of the patients, with a median time to fusion of 6 months.

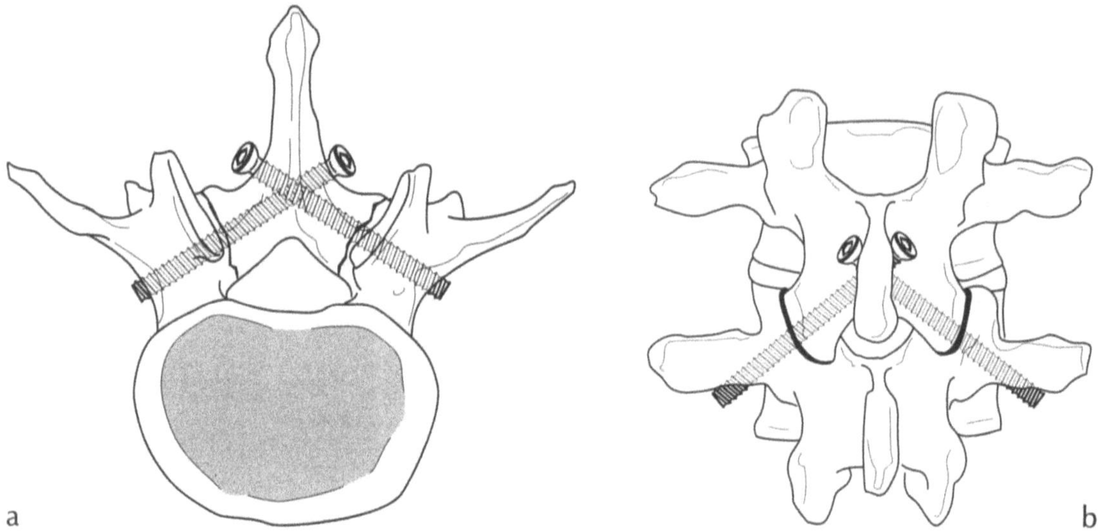


**FIGURE 17.7.** (a and b) Translaminar screws increase the screw working length biomechanically and have been shown to enhance the fusion rate when the anterior column is intact.

# Summary

Cannulated screws can reestablish spinal stability with minimal soft tissue damage in anatomical areas that are difficult to expose. Screw placement is possible without direct visualization of the fracture or surrounding area. Trial positioning is performed under fluoroscopic control with a small guide pin, which is relatively safe and if changed leaves very little loss of bone stock ultimately necessary for screw fixation. Accurate length estimates or measurements are possible, ensuring that the screw to be used will not be too long and impinge on more vital structures or too short and not give ideal fixation.

The use of cannulated screws can reestablish spinal stability in fractures of the cervical spine while soft tissue damage is minimized and motion maintained. The technique allows maximum bone-screw interface when the transpedicular approach is used, and the risk of pedicle breakout is reduced. In the lumbar spine, this technique provides a method by which the facet may be crossed safely, imparting stability and enhancing the rate of union.

# Acknowledgment

I would like to thank my son, Rob McGuire, for his assistance with the illustrations.

## References

1. Penning L. Normal movement of the cervical spine. *Am J Roentgenol* 1979;130:317–319.
2. Etter C, Coscia M, Jaberg H, Aebi M. Direct anterior fixation of dens fractures with a cannulated screw system. *Spine* 1991;16:S25–S32.
3. Bohler J. Anterior stabilization for acute fractures and nonunions of the dens. *J Bone Joint Surg* 1982;64A:18–27.
4. Magerl F, Seemann PS. Stable posterior fusion of the atlas and axis by transarticular screw fixation. In: Weidner PA, ed. *Cervical Spine*, vol 1. New York: Springer-Verlag, 1987;322–327.
5. McGuire R, Harkey HL. Modification of technique and results of transarticular C1 C2 stabilization. *Orthopedics* 1995;18:10, 1029–1032.
6. Anderson LD, D'Alonzo RT. Fractures of the odontoid process of the axis. *J Bone Joint Surg* 1974;56A:1663–1664.
7. Schatzker J, Rorabeek CH, Waddell JP. Fracture of the dens: an analysis of thirty-seven cases. *J Bone Joint Surg* 1971;53B:392–405.
8. Sasso RC, Heggeness MH, Dohrety BJ. Bio-

mechanics of odontoid fracture fixation: comparison of one and two screw techniques. *Spine* 1993;18:1950–1953.
9. Grazino G, Jaggers C, Lee M, Lynch W. A comparative study of fixation techniques for type II fractures of the odontoid process. *Spine* 1993; 18:2383–2387.
10. Heller JG, Also MD, Schaffler MB, Brahme SK, Miller CW, Garfin SR. Quantitive dens morphology. *Orthop Trans* 1990;14:693.
11. Montesano PX, Anderson PA, Schlehr F, Thalgott JS, Lowery G. Odontoid fractures treated by anterior odontoid screw fixation. *Spine* 1991;16: S33–37.
12. Grob D, Crisco JJ, Panjabi MM, Wang P, Devorak J. Biomechanical evaluation of four different posterior atlantoaxial fixation techniques. *Spine* 1992; 17:480–490.
13. Montesano P, Juach EC, Anderson PA, Benson DR, Hanson PB. Biomechanics of cervical fixation. *Spine* 1991;16:S10–S16.
14. Jeanneret B, Magerl F. Primary posterior fusion C1 C2 in odontoid fractures: indications, techniques, and results of transarticular screw fixation. *J Spinal Disorders* 1992;5:464–475.
15. Zdeblick TA. A prospective, randomized study of lumbar fusion. *Spine* 1993;18:983–991.
16. Saillant G. Etude anatomique des pedicules vertebraux: application chirurgicale. *Rev Chir Orthop* 1976;62:151–160.
17. Weinstein JN, Spratt KF, Spengler D, Brick C. Spinal pedicle fixation: reliability and validity of roentgenogram-based assessment and surgical factors on successful screw placement. *Spine* 1988; 13:1012–1018.
18. Krag MH, VanHal ME, Beynnon BD. Placement of transpedicular vertebral screws close to anterior vertebral cortex. *Spine* 1989;14:879–883.
19. Magerl F. Stabilization of the lower thoracic and lumbar spine with external skeletal fixation. *Clin Orthop* 1984;189:125–141.
20. King D. Internal fixation of lumbosacral fusion. *J Bone Joint Surg* 1959;41B:248–259.
21. Boucher HH. A method of spine fusion. *J Bone Joint Surg* 1959;41B:248–259.
22. Jacobs RR, Montesano PX, Jackson RP. Enhancement of lumbar spine fusion by use of translaminar facet joint screws. *Spine* 1989;14:12–15.

# 18
# The Shoulder

David M. Dines, Stanley E. Asnis, and Alexandra Page

Many fractures and fracture-dislocations about the shoulder girdle require open reduction and internal fixation. Numerous options exist for treating fractures of the proximal humerus and the scapula. In some cases, cannulated screws afford the optimal form of fracture treatment. Guide wires permit a provisional reduction of the fragments, followed by definitive fixation with cannulated screws. This chapter reviews salient anatomy, fracture mechanisms, and imaging studies, as well as the classification systems currently used for these fractures. Discussion of fracture repair will concentrate on the use of cannulated screw techniques.

The proximal humerus and the scapula constitute the bony architecture of the shoulder. Fractures of the proximal humerus are most significant, accounting for 4–5% of all fractures.[1] These fractures occur most frequently in the elderly population following low-energy trauma. The fracture pattern as well as the underlying bone quality contribute to determining the application of cannulated screws in fixation of these fractures. Fractures of the scapula occur less frequently, usually following high-energy trauma and therefore also have a high frequency of associated injuries. In the scapula, fractures of the glenoid rim and neck are most amenable to fixation with cannulated screw techniques.

## Anatomy

The anatomic features of the shoulder influence both the fracture patterns that occur as well as the options for successful surgical management (Figure 18.1). In the proximal humerus, the most common fractures occur along epiphyseal scars. Thus the anatomic development of the proximal humerus is fundamental to the understanding of fracture patterns that occur in adults. There are three ossification centers: (1) the humeral head, appearing at approximately 4 to 6 months; (2) the greater tuberosity, appearing at 3 years; and (3) the lesser tuberosity, appearing at 5 years. By age 6 the three centers have merged to form one epiphysis, although fusion does not occur until approximately 18 to 20 years in the female and 20 to 22 years in the male.

The adult proximal humerus can also be described using these same three segments, with the remaining humeral shaft providing a fourth segment. The articular surface is a large portion of a sphere, with the articular cartilage oriented posteriorly, superiorly, and medially. The anatomic neck separates the head from the greater and lesser tuberosities. The greater tuberosity is lateral, with three distinct facets for the attachment of the supraspinatus, infraspinatus, and teres minor tendons. Anteromedially is the lesser tuberosity, the insertion point of the subscapularis tendon. Between the tuberosities on the anterior aspect lies the bicipital groove. The surgical neck, just distal to the tuberosities, is the most common fracture site.

Prognosis for fracture healing in the proximal humerus is related to the preservation of the vascular supply to the fracture fragments. Blood supply to the humeral head originates primarily from the anterior and posterior circumflex arteries, which form an anastamosis around the neck. The arcuate artery, described by Liang,[2] ascends from the anterior circumflex. This anteromedial branch provides the greater portion of the vascular supply to both the tuberosities as well as the majority of the humeral head. A postero-

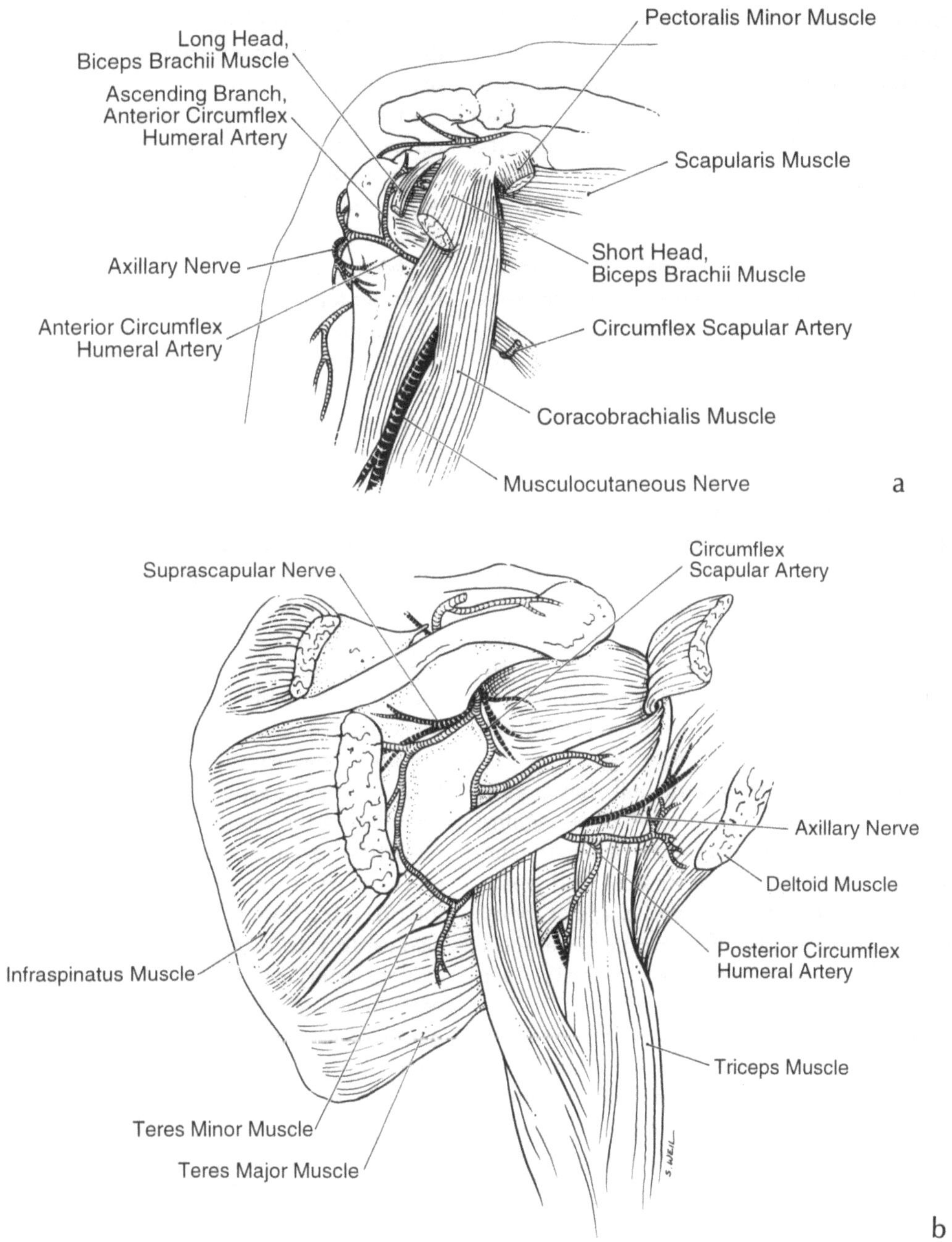


**FIGURE 18.1.** Anatomy of the shoulder. (a) Anterior aspect. (b) Posterior aspect.

medial arcuate artery also arises from the posterior circumflex, contributing blood supply to the greater tuberosity. Insertion of the tendons of the rotator cuff also provide a small portion of the blood supply to the humeral head via the suprascapular, subscapular, thoracoacromial, and suprahumeral arteries.[3] Because the blood supply to the humeral head enters proximal to the surgical neck, fractures at this level generally have a good prognosis for healing. Fractures of the anatomic neck, which are less common, usually result in disruption of the vascular supply with attendant high risk for avascular necrosis of the humeral head.

On the scapular side, the glenoid region of the scapula is the most common site of fractures.[3] The glenoid projects laterally from the body of the scapula via the sturdy glenoid neck. The small surface area is augmented by the glenoid labrum to enhance glenohumeral articulation. The labrum is occasionally traumatically detached, particularly in anterior dislocations. Blood supply to the glenoid region of the scapula is derived from the suprascapular and subscapular arteries. The subscapular artery runs along the inferior border of the scapula then divides into the circumflex scapular and thoracodorsal branches. The suprascapular artery descends down the posterior body. It forms an anastomosis with the circumflex scapular artery, a branch of the subscapular artery. Further blood supply to the shoulder comes from the acromial and deltoid branches of the thoracoacromial artery. In addition to supplying the scapula, the suprascapular and acromial arteries give a small contribution to humeral head vascularity via the rotator cuff insertions.[4,5]

The muscles of the rotator cuff, functioning to keep the humeral head positioned against the glenoid, originate from the anterior (subscapularis), superior (supraspinatus), and posterior (infraspinatus, teres minor) scapular body. Injuries to the rotator cuff can occur in association with fractures of either the proximal humerus or glenoid.

Several nerves and vessels in the shoulder area warrant specific attention due to their vulnerability either at the time of injury or during subsequent fracture management. The axillary nerve originates from the posterior cord of the brachial plexus, then passes along the upper edge of the teres major in the quadrangular space with the posterior humeral circumflex vessels. Next, it runs transversely through the body of the deltoid. Finally it passes anteriorly under the subscapularis tendon. Fracture fragments and stretching at the time of fracture can cause injury to the axillary nerve. To minimize risk to the axillary nerve during lateral, deltoid-splitting approaches, the muscle should never be split more than 5 cm distal to the acromion. Some authors recommend placing a suture across the deltoid at the inferior apex of the deltoid split to minimize risk of further deltoid dissection.[6]

In an anterior approach to the shoulder, the cephalic vein runs in the delto-pectoral groove. After incising the skin, dissection must proceed with care to preserve the vein. In the deeper dissection, the axillary nerve runs under the distal border of the subscapularis in the deepest layer. External rotation of the arm places the subscapularis muscle in tension. This both better defines the border of the subscapularis as well as pulls the incision through the tendon laterally, away from the axillary nerve. A triad of vessels (one artery with its two venae comitantes) are also present along the inferior border of the subscapularis. Known as the "three sisters," these vessels often require cauterization or ligation and can cause troublesome bleeding if inadvertently avulsed.

The *musculocutaneous* nerve lies medial to most anterior exposures for the shoulder, but the surgeon must remember its presence to avoid neuropraxia. Nerve supply to the coracobrachialis and short head of the biceps enters from the medial aspect, so all dissection must be done along the lateral border. Excessive medial retraction on the conjoint tendon can cause nerve injury. If the coracoid process is released, inferior retraction of the tendon and muscles can also cause a neuropraxia. The second part of the axillary artery passes deep to the coracoid process. Injury to both the axillary artery and the musculocutaneous nerve can be minimized by adducting the arm during exposure of the coracoid process.

During posterior approaches, both the axillary and suprascapular nerves are at risk. The axillary nerve, accompanied by the posterior humeral circumflex artery, passes beneath the teres minor. To avoid both structures, all posterior dissection should be done in the interval between the infraspinatus and the teres minor. The suprascapular nerve branches from the superior trunk, innervates the supraspinatus, then descends under the transverse scapular ligament at the scapular notch, giving fibers to the infraspinatus. The suprascapular nerve is located approximately 1 cm posterior to the lip of the glenoid. To minimize injury during a posterior approach to the shoulder, the suprascapular nerve should be identified and protected. Extensive medial retraction of the infraspinatus can also injure this nerve.

### Clinical Relevance: Safe Zones for Percutaneous Guide Pin Placement

1. Anterior: Pins should be proximal to the subscapularis tendon to avoid both the axillary nerve and the vessels on the inferior subscapularis border. Pins placed directly in the delto-pectoral groove can injure the cephalic vein.
2. Lateral: Pins should be placed either in the proximal 5 cm of the deltoid or more than 8 cm distally. The axillary nerve is at risk between 5 and 8 cm distal to the acromion.
3. Posterior: Do not insert pins posterior to the medial lip of the glenoid without dissection to identify and protect the suprascapular nerve. Avoid pins placed distal to the teres minor, which could injure the axillary nerve.

## Mechanisms of Injury

Fractures of the proximal humerus most frequently occur through low-energy trauma in patients with poor bone quality, most commonly following a fall on an outstretched arm from a standing height.[3] Impingement and pivoting of the greater tuberosity on the acromion can result in humeral head fracture, dislocation, or fracture-dislocation.[1] The greater tuberosity fragment usually displaces posteriorly and superiorly due to the pull of the attached rotator cuff; greater than 1 cm displacement of the fragment is considered pathognomonic for a rotator cuff tear.[7]

In uncontrolled muscle contraction such as seizures or electrical shock, the powerful internal rotators and adductors of the shoulder exert more force than the external rotators, thereby most often resulting in posterior dislocations and fracture-dislocations.[1]

Injury to the glenoid, in contrast, generally requires significant direct trauma.[8,9] The forces are usually applied via the humeral head. Forceful humeral head impingement on either the anterior or posterior glenoid rim can result in a rim fracture. Impaction of the humeral head directly into the glenoid fossa can create complex fracture patterns involving the fossa with subsequent fracture line propagation through the scapula.[10]

The less-common glenoid neck fractures also result from high-energy trauma, usually a direct anterior or posterior blow to the shoulder.[10] Additionally, impaction of the humeral head against the glenoid following a fall on an extended arm and, less commonly, a fall on the superior shoulder complex has been described.[3,11]

### Fracture Classifications

The two commonly used classifications for the proximal humerus are the Neer and the AO systems. The Neer classification[12] is based upon the four fragments described above in the development of the proximal humerus: the articular surface, the greater and lesser tuberosities, and the humeral shaft. The system was developed with consideration of the effects of each fracture on the humeral head vascular supply.

The minimally displaced fractures make up a group with any number of fracture lines at any position provided they are not displaced more than 1.0 cm or angulated more than 45°. Displacement greater than this poses a clinically significant threat to the blood supply of the fragment.

Two-part fractures occur when one fragment has displaced from the other three. This includes a surgical neck fracture with an intact humeral head, isolated fracture of one of the tuberosities, or an isolated anatomic neck fracture. Greater tuberosity fractures are commonly associated with rotator cuff tears. This fracture pattern not uncommonly occurs with anterior dislocation of the humeral head, which may have spontaneously reduced prior to the radiograph. Isolated lesser tuberosity fractures should raise the suspicion of an associated posterior dislocation. With the exception of the rare anatomic neck fracture, the blood supply to the articulating surface of the head is not compromised by a two-part fracture.

In three-part fractures, the greater or lesser tuberosity fragment has fractured, associated with a surgical neck fracture. This is more often associated with significant anatomic disruption, but vascular supply to the articular surface is usually maintained via the remaining tuberosity attachment.

Finally, the four-part fracture has separation of all four fragments. With both tuberosities detached, the articular surface is a free fragment without vascular supply. Additionally, Neer described the above fracture patterns associated with either an anterior or posterior dislocation of the humeral head.

The AO classification developed as a modification of the Neer system,[3] based on concern that vascular supply to the articular segment was not adequately addressed by the earlier classification. This system follows the AO system used for other joints, with each group subdivided numerically into more severe fractures. Type A fractures are extracapsular, with only two parts. There is usually no compromise of the blood supply in these fractures. Type B are partially intracapsular, with three segments involved, but either tuberosity still in contact with the humeral head, thus preserving some vascular supply. In type C, the fracture is intracapsular with four segments and complete disruption of the vascular supply to the humeral head.

There has been concern that both the Neer and the AO classifications have limitations. Even among shoulder and trauma specialists, intraobserver reproducibility in classifying fractures remains high. Despite this, the Neer and AO classification systems remain important tools for evaluating and planning treatment of proximal humerus fractures.

Fractures of the glenoid rim and fossa are most commonly classified by the system of Ideberg.[3,8,10] Type I represents a fracture of the glenoid rim: Ia, anterior rim; Ib, posterior rim. Small avulsion fractures that can occur with humeral head dislocation are not considered type I glenoid fractures.

Types II to VI in the Ideberg system involve the fossa of the glenoid. A transverse or oblique fracture through the fossa, extending through the lateral edge of the scapular body to create a free fragment of the inferior glenoid is a type II fracture. In type III fracture patterns, a transverse fracture through the fossa exits superiorly. This produces a fracture fragment containing the coracoid process and the superior portion of the glenoid. A type IV fracture also involves a transverse fossa fracture, but the fracture plane continues medially though the body of the scapula.

Higher energy injuries can result in the more comminuted type V fractures. Type V fractures are further divided into Va, Vb, and Vc.[8] These represent combinations of types II through IV. All involve a transverse fracture through the scapular body, as in type IV, and free fragments of the inferior glenoid (Va), superior glenoid and coracoid (Vb), or both (Vc). Finally, type VI fractures represent those with extensive comminution of the glenoid fossa.

The classification scheme of glenoid neck fractures is based on the evaluation of the glenoid fragment, lateral to the fracture line.[10] Those fractures with minimal or no displacement, leaving the glenoid in anatomic position, are type I fractures. Type II fractures have either translational or rotational displacement of the glenoid fragment. Translation of greater than 1 cm or rotation of greater than 40° has been determined as clinically significant.[10]

# Evaluation and Imaging

Following a careful physical examination to document the vascular and neurologic status of the upper extremity, adequate imaging studies are necessary for accurate diagnosis, particularly to evaluate for associated dislocation. The standard trauma shoulder series represents the minimum radiographs. The scapular anteroposterior (AP) view is taken with the posterior aspect of the affected shoulder against the plate and the contralateral shoulder rotated approximately 30° to 40° anteriorly to compensate for the anterior orientation of the glenoid. Similarly, the lateral—or scapular Y—view is taken perpendicular to the glenoid, with the anterior shoulder against the plate and the contralateral shoulder rotated 30° to 40° posteriorly. For the axillary view, the patient is supine with the arm abducted. If the patient is unable to comply with this positioning due to pain, alternatives have been described.[1,3] An axillary view should be considered mandatory to assess for an occult dislocation.

Additional views include the internal and external rotation AP views. The external rotation view places the greater tuberosity in profile. Absence of the greater tuberosity on this view indicates an avulsion that may not be recognized on other views due to overlap. For evaluating a Hills-Sachs lesion on the posterolateral humeral head, the internal rotation view should be obtained. A West Point axillary view can facilitate visualization of a Bankhart lesion on the glenoid.

Computed tomography (CT) scan provides the most accurate evaluation of complex proximal humeral fractures. This study is necessary in the setting of a pattern unclear on plain films. Castagno et al.[13] found CT altered the intended treatment plan in 15 of 17 patients. The most frequent finding was less displacement than suggested by plain films, necessitating less-aggressive intervention.

Evaluating fractures of the glenoid cavity and neck requires the same AP and lateral radiographs in the plane of the scapula described above. Additionally, an axillary view illustrates fractures of the glenoid rim.

Use of CT scanning can more clearly define glenoid fractures, with three dimensional reconstructions possibly assisting operative planning in complex fractures. Some authors feel that CT scanning is necessary to fully assess the complex scapular anatomy.[9] Additionally, three-dimensional reconstruction of CT scans may be helpful in assessing fracture anatomy and determining the appropriate fixation techniques.

## Fracture Treatment and Use of Cannulated Screws

Of the fracture patterns discussed, several of those occurring in the proximal humerus are amenable to open reduction and internal fixation (ORIF) with cannulated screws. The recurring theme of preservation of blood supply dictates that repair by ORIF is only acceptable in situations where the blood supply to the humeral head has not been compromised. Nondisplaced fractures heal well with closed treatment and four-part fractures usually require hemiarthroplasty. However, the displaced fractures with retained articular surface vascularity remain challenging surgical problems.

## Advantages of Cannulated Screws

The use of cannulated screws in the treatment of shoulder fractures can at times replace or frequently supplement the standard open reduction and internal fixation procedures. There are several advantages for using cannulated screws in fracture fixation.

1. The shoulder is very accessible to fluoroscopy and fluoroscopic placement of guide pins.
2. The incision and soft tissue dissection can often be minimized, being smaller than the wide exposures used with complete open reduction and fixation of the fracture. The guide pins can then be placed either through the primary wound or percutaneously through new puncture wounds to provide ideal pin orientation.
3. The guide pin can be used as a handle to reduce fracture fragment. It can also stabilize two fragments while a third fragment is manipulated for reduction. For example, in a three-part fracture, the head and greater tuberosity can be pinned while the shaft is reduced.
4. Guide pins provide preliminary fixation, and give greater flexibility to identify the ideal location for fixation with screw placement.
5. The guide pin can be used to establish the length of the ideal screw prior to placement of the screw. This is important in the shoulder where length is often critical. Too short a screw may result in threads across the fracture site, while too long a screw may penetrate the glenohumeral joint.

## Authors' Preferred Equipment

### System 1: Cannulated 6.5-mm Lag Screw

*Screw thread:* Outer diameter—6.5 mm; pitch—2.5 mm; reverse cutting flutes; self-cutting, self-tapping positive rake tip. *Drill:* A 3.2-mm steel drill, which can be used directly with a direct reading depth gauge. *Guide pin:* 3.2 mm with a threaded tip and tapered root diameter. *Screw head:* Round head with a 4.8-mm internal hexagon. *Material:* 22-13-5 stainless steel. *System accessory equipment:* Washers, depth gauge, pin guide, soft tissue protection sleeve, cannulated overdrill.

### System 2: Cannulated 5.0-mm Lag Screw

*Screw thread:* Outer diameter—5.0 mm; pitch 1.6 mm; reverse cutting flutes; self-cutting, self-tapping positive rake tip. *Screw shaft:* Smooth 3.5 mm. *Guide pin:* 2.0 mm with a threaded tip and tapered root diameter. *Screw head:* Round head with an internal 3.5-mm hexagon. *Material:* 316 LVM stainless steel. *System accessory equipment:* Washers, depth gauge, 2.0-mm pin guide, soft tissue protection sleeve, cannulated overdrill.

### System 3: Cannulated 4.5-mm Fully Threaded Screw (Occasional)

*Screw thread:* Outer diameter—4.5 mm; pitch—1.0 mm; self-cutting, self-tapping positive rake tip. *Screw shaft:* Fully threaded 4.5-mm root diameter. *Guide pin:* 2.0 mm with a threaded tip and tapered root diameter. *Screw head:* Round head with an internal 3.5-mm hexagon. *Material:* 316 LVM stainless steel. *System accessory equipment:* Washers, depth gauge, 2.0-mm pin guide, soft tissue protection sleeve, cannulated overdrill.

### System 4

*Screw thread:* Cancellous; outer diameter—3.5 mm; pitch—1.25 mm; not self-cutting. *Screw shaft:* 2.5 mm. *Guide pin:* 1.25 mm with a threaded tip. *Screw head:* Round head with an internal 2.5-mm hexagon. *Material:* 316 LVM stainless steel. *System accessory equipment:* Washers, depth gauge, pin guide, soft tissue protection sleeve, cannulated overdrill.

## Two-Part Proximal Humerus Fractures

### Greater Tuberosity

Fractures of the greater tuberosity are not common, and are usually associated with anterior shoulder dislocation. Open reduction and internal fixation are advised when the greater tuberosity is displaced following closed reduction. Depending upon the author, the critical displacement is either 5 mm or 1 cm.[14–16] Fractures with this amount of displacement not treated with internal fixation can result in impingement and limited range of motion.[16] Screw fixation is appropriate when the fragment is sufficiently large. For small avulsions, repair with suture through the rotator cuff and bony substance of the fragment has been advocated.[1,16,17] Alternatively, a small fragment may be discarded and a primary rotator cuff repair can be carried out. This fracture pattern is frequently associated with a rotator cuff tear,[12] which should be repaired at the time of surgery.

#### Authors' Technique

If the fragment is large enough to support screw fixation, then it should be appropriately reduced and fixed with a cannulated screw. This can occasionally be done almost percutaneously through a 1-cm incision or with a larger exposure through a deltoid-splitting approach, oriented anterolaterally. Either incision should not extend more than 5 cm distal to the acromium to avoid injury to the axillary nerve.

If displacement is small yet the surgeon has reasons to prefer internal fixation, the shoulder should be positioned under the fluoroscope. A 1-cm incision is then made after planning its position with a guide pin against the skin. The deltoid is split with a hemostat. The 2.0-mm guide pin is then placed through a soft tissue protector sleeve and positioned in the midportion of the fragment with the aid of fluoroscopy. The guide pin can often be used as a handle on the fragment to aid in reduction. The protector sleeve can be left on the guide pin to also aid in reduction and help to place pressure on the fragment. Once the reduction is satisfactory the guide pin is advanced across the fracture and into the proximal humerus. The fracture reduction and the position of the guide pin are confirmed by rotation of the shoulder under fluoroscopy. The direct reading depth gauge is used to determine the proper screw length. If the fragment is to be lagged into position by the screw, then a slightly shorter screw is used. A washer can optionally be placed around the 5.0-mm self-tapping cannulated lag screw in the more osteoporotic bone. If the bone fragment is small, the appropriate cannulated overdrill can be used to enlarge the hole in the fragment only and decrease the chance of weakening or breaking the fragment by the thread of the screw. In larger fragments in the younger patient, two 5.0-mm cannulated screws may be used or a 6.5-mm cannulated lag screw over a 3.2-mm guide pin.

If an open reduction is planned or necessary, the anterolateral deltoid splitting incision is used. The deltoid may be detached proximally to facilitate wider exposure. The fracture is reduced and guide pin(s) placed to provisionally fix the fragment. Fluoroscopic evaluation of the pin length and position is then performed. The application of the cannulated screw(s) is (are) performed as previously discussed.

Postoperative treatment includes sling and swathe with early passive range of motion. On postoperative day 2 or 3, passive range of motion should begin. Active assisted and strengthening exercises are deferred until there is evidence of clinical union. Abduction and external rotation against resistance are avoided until there is evidence of radiographic and clinical union.

## Lesser Tuberosity

Isolated lesser tuberosity fractures are extremely rare, most commonly seen with posterior dislocations. If there is more than 45° of angulation or 1 cm of displacement, open reduction and internal fixation is the treatment of choice. Repair of this fracture can be done with cannulated screw fixation.[1]

A delto-pectoral incision exposing the lesser tuberosity should be carried out. The tuberosity should be dissected free of its surrounding soft tissues and then reduced into its normal bed. Provisional cannulated 2.0-mm guide wires can be used to hold it in this position until intraoperative radiographic confirmation of reduction is obtained. Next, a cannulated 5.0-mm lag screw of the appropriate size should be placed. Postoperative care is similar to that for greater tuberosity fractures: sling and swathe with early passive motion, and avoidance of external rotation past 30°. Active and strengthening exercises are delayed until there is evidence of fracture healing.

## Anatomic Neck

The displaced anatomic neck fracture is rare, and carries a high risk of avascular necrosis. For this reason, a primary hemiarthroplasty is usually indicated in older patients. However, some authors feel internal fixation is warranted in young patients[1,17]; closed reduction alone is insufficient. Schlegel and Hawkins[16] suggest use of interfragmentary screws, although noting screw purchase can be difficult to obtain. There is currently no experience with cannulated screws in this fracture type, but the experience of Schlegel and Hawkins may indicate a possible role using the guide wires to improve initial fracture stabilization. In these fractures the femoral head fragment may be thin and screw positioning critical to give fixation and yet not penetrate the joint. Provisional guide pin positioning with the aid of fluoroscopy is very advantageous in facilitating ideal screw length and position.

## Surgical Neck

The most common two-part fracture occurs at the surgical neck. Closed reduction may result in a stable fracture. However, many such fractures also are unstable and readily displace with closed reduction and conservative management. Internal fixation is indicated if the fracture remains unstable or in polytrauma, where stability is necessary for patient management. There is no significant literature describing cannulated screw use for this fracture type. Other treatment techniques include percutaneous pinning,[7,17] but it can be a challenging procedure. Tension band wiring, with and without the use of intramedullary rods, has been described.[13,16] Using plate and screw technique in this area is not commonly accepted due to the increased tissue stripping required as well as the risks of screw loosening in poor-quality bone.[4,18] It could, however, be considered in a younger patient with better bone stock. Risks include impingement from prominent hardware and varus deformity. If open reduction is performed utilizing a buttress plate, cannulated screw techniques may add accuracy in determining screw length and position by placing cannulated screws through the proximal plate holes.

### Authors' Technique

The authors have found percutaneous cannulated screw fixation very effective in the treatment of the unstable two-part fracture, as shown in Figure 18.2a. The patient is placed in a supine position on the fluoroscopic operating table with the affected shoulder elevated with a roll of sheets under the scapula. A 1-cm incision is made over the area of the greater tuberosity. A 3.2-mm drill or guide wire is placed through a soft tissue protection sleeve and aimed with the aid of fluoroscopy. This drill is then driven into the proximal fragment and used as a handle to manipulate the fragment as the distal fragment fracture is reduced by moving the arm. When fracture alignment is obtained, the drill is driven across the fracture and into the medial cortex of the distal fragment (Figure 18.2b). A 1-cm incision is then made over the lateral arm in a position determined by fluoroscopy. A 3.2-mm drill is then driven through the lateral humeral cortex of the distal fragment, across the fracture, and into the superior portion of the humeral head. A parallel hole jig is placed over this distal drill and a second 3.2-mm drill is placed in a parallel hole at the desired distance distal to the first and driven through the lateral humeral cortex, across the fracture and into the middle to lower portion of the humeral head (Figure 18.2c). Position of all guide pins is confirmed by fluoroscopy while rotating the arm. The direct reading depth gauge is used to determine screw lengths. An appropriate 6.5-mm cannulated self tapping lag screw is then placed over each drill (Figure 18.2d). The 3.2-mm drills are used rather than the 3.2-mm guide pins for this procedure, particularly for the distal screws because they penetrate the hard bone of the cortex of the humeral shaft at an oblique angle more easily than the guide pins. They are the same length as the guide pins, thus can be used with the routine direct reading depth gauge. The decision of using drills or guide pins is left to the individual surgeon's discretion.

## Three-Part Proximal Humerus Fractures

Three-part fractures are common in the elderly population. They are often seen in patients with osteoporosis. Based upon the Neer classification system, this fracture pattern may include one of the tuberosities, the humeral shaft, and the humeral head and remaining tuberosity as a unit. This fracture is often associated with a dislocation.

In a younger patient with good bone stock, an attempt at reduction and internal fixation should be made. Closed reduction with percutaneous pinning has also been recommended for three-part fractures.[16] This technique involves minimal disruption of the surrounding tissues, therefore preserving blood supply.

### *Authors' Technique*

Closed reduction of the three-part fracture is obtained. To facilitate reduction, an image intensifier can be used. Additionally a guide pin can be used as a joystick to manipulate fracture fragments. The first guide pin secures the greater tuberosity fragment to the humeral shaft. This pin should be directed from posterosuperior to anteroinferior to maximize purchase in the greater tuberosity fragment. Next, two additional pins secure the shaft onto the humeral head. Two parallel pins are used to control rotation. Finally, the cannulated screws are placed over the guide pins.

Recently Cornell[19] described a technique for the open reduction and internal fixation of

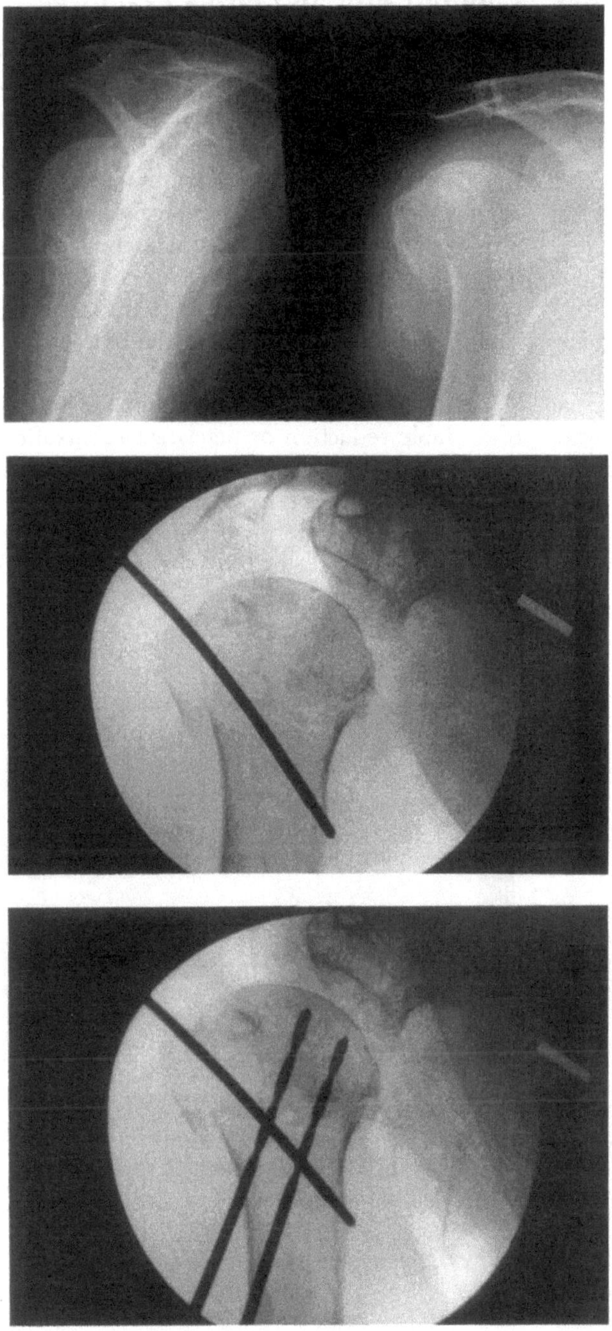

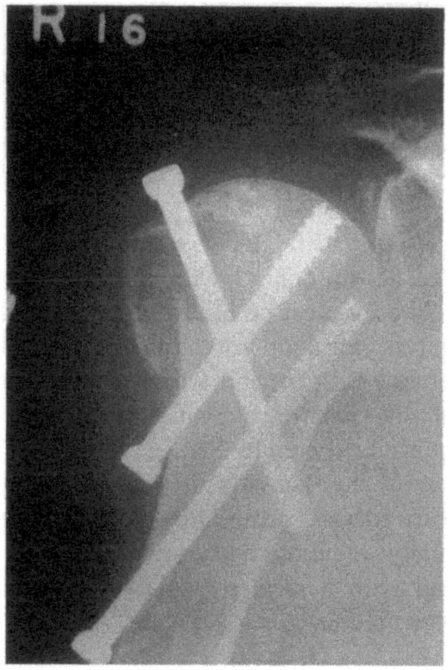

**FIGURE 18.2.** Technique for percutaneous pinning of a proximal humerous fracture. (a) Radiograph of a 76-year-old patient with a clinically unstable surgical neck fracture. (b) The first 3.2-mm (9-inch) guide pin secures the reduction of the proximal fragment to the humeral shaft. The percutaneous pin enters through the greater tuberosity. (c) Two additional 3.2-mm (9-inch) drill bits are used to secure the shaft to the humeral head. (d) Postoperative radiographs showing the three 6.5-mm cannulated screws used for final fixation.

three-part fractures. The combined head and tuberosity fragment is reduced to the humeral shaft using guide wires. The remaining tuberosity fragment is then attached using a figure-of-eight tension band wire. They report successful results in 15 patients. We have recently employed this method of fixation using cannulated screws. Preliminary results support excellent fixation. We suggest using a technique similar to that discussed above in the section Surgical Neck. One 5.0- or 6.5-mm screw is used to fix the free tuberosity to the humeral head. A tension band can be used of either wire or no. 5 surgical polyester suture.

## Four-Part Proximal Humerus Fractures

In a four-part fracture by definition the humeral head has no contact with either tuberosity and therefore almost no blood supply. There may be limited indication for attempting internal fixation in young patients with excellent bone stock, but the risk of avascular necrosis has been reported to be up to 90%.[7] Additionally, internal fixation that subsequently fails can complicate future surgical procedures. Successful treatment usually requires replacement of the humeral head with a hemiarthroplasty with tuberosity reconstruction.

## Glenoid Rim and Fossa Fractures

Fractures that involve the articular surface of the glenoid require open reduction and internal fixation when there is more than 5-mm displacement and 3-mm articular stepoff. In repairs of the glenoid fossa fractures, various authors have suggested using interfragmentary compression screws, 3.5-mm pelvic reconstruction plates, heavy sutures, Kirschner wires, or combinations of these.[9,15] Repair of any tears in the labrum or rotator cuff should be done at the time of fracture fixation.

Type I fractures are repaired in the setting of unstable reduction or persistent subluxation. Significant fractures usually involve greater than 25% of the fossa or have significant displacement.[3,8] A large anterior or posterior rim fragment can be reattached to the scapular neck

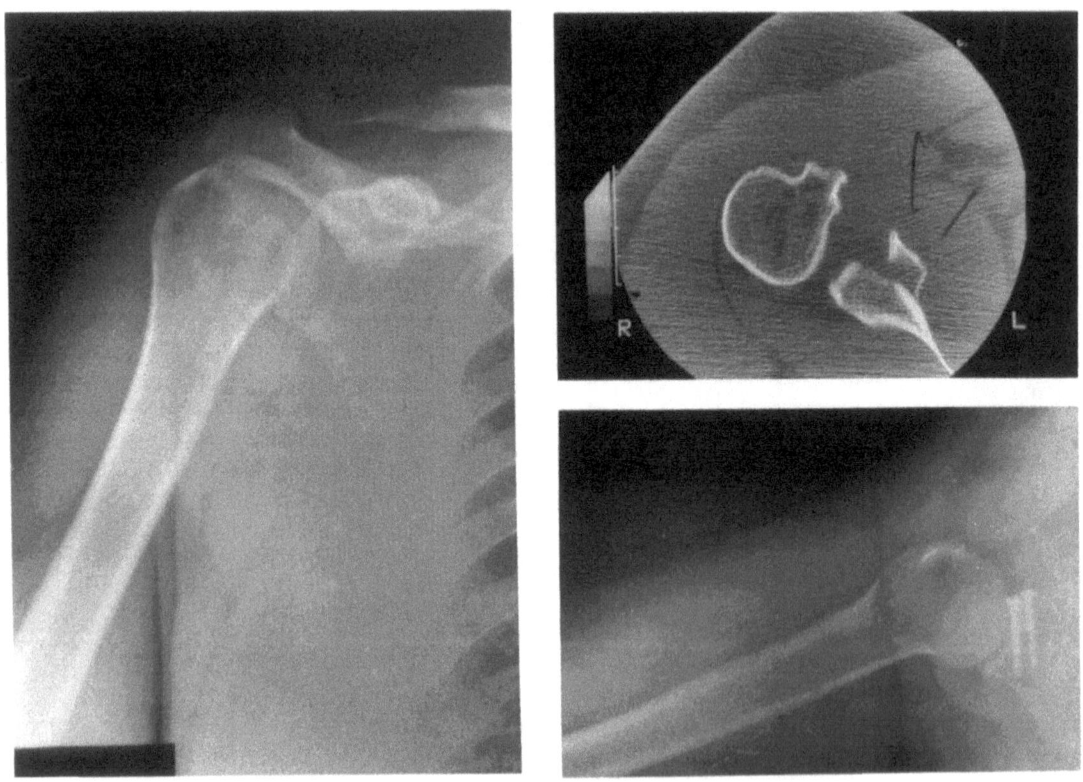

a b c

**FIGURE 18.3.** Fixation of an anterior glenoid rim fracture. (a) AP radiograph of anterior glenoid rim fracture. (b) The fracture is better visualized by CT. (c) Fixation with 3.5-mm cannulated screws.

with a compression screw. When extensive comminution of the rim exists, a technique using a tricortical iliac crest graft has been described.[8]

## Authors' Technique

### Anterior Rim Fracture

Figure 18.3 illustrates an anterior rim fracture and fixation. The authors' preferred method for an anterior rim fracture using cannulated screws entails an extended delto-pectoral incision. The subscapularis and capsule are detached to provide both an inside and outside view of the anterior glenoid rim. After retracting the subscapularis medially, the fracture fragments can be reduced and held in place with 2.0-mm and/or 1.25-mm guide pins from anterior to posterior. Next, cannulated screws are placed over the guide wires. The 5.0-mm screws can be used over the 2.0-mm guide pins, whereas 3.5-mm cannulated screws are placed over the 1.25-mm pins. Patients are treated in a sling and swathe for 3 weeks and then begun on passive range of motion. Active assisted range of motion is not begun until the fourth week.

### Posterior Rim Fracture

Posterior glenoid rim fractures are approached through a posterior deltoid-splitting incision for internal fixation. A posterior rim fracture with subsequent internal fixation is shown in Figure 18.4. The posterior third raphe of the deltoid is split from the posterior third of the acromion laterally approximately 5 cm. The incision may be enlarged by keying the deltoid proximally off the spine of the scapula. Next, the interval between the teres minor and the infraspinatus is identified. A longitudinal split is done, protecting the axillary nerve below the teres minor. The capsule is identified, and with appropriate retraction the fracture site can be seen. A longitudinal capsulotomy is necessary to assess the

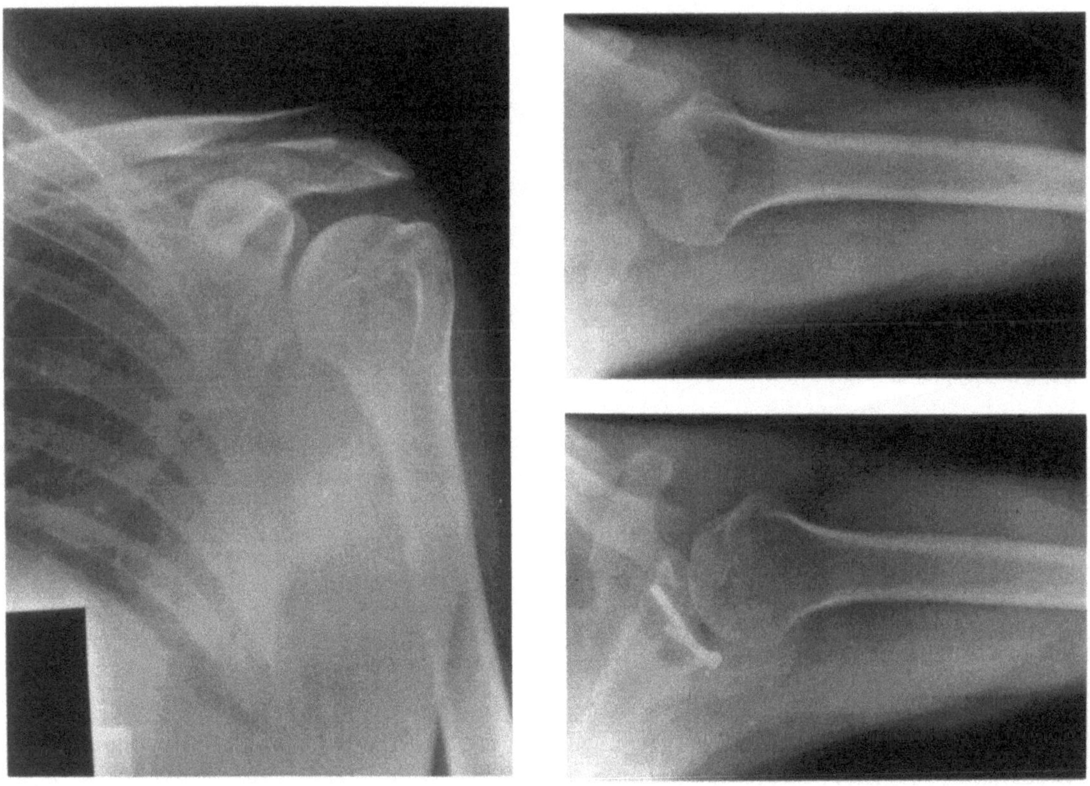

a b c

**FIGURE 18.4.** Fixation of posterior glenoid rim fracture. (a) AP radiograph of posterior glenoid rim fracture. (b) Axillary view of fracture. (c) Fixation with 3.5-mm cannulated screws.

reduction. Two 1.25-mm (or occasionally 2.0-mm) guide pins are placed from posterior to anterior through the fracture fragment. After radiographs to document the reduction, 3.5-mm cannulated lag screws (occasionally 5.0-mm cannulated screws) are passed over the wires in the routine fashion. The articular surface is assessed for congruity. The capsule is closed with 0 Tevdek suture. Care must be taken to avoid the suprascapular nerve, which runs 1 cm medial to the rim of the glenoid, coursing inferior to innervate the infraspinatus. The nerve can be palpated and in some cases should be identified.

The shoulder is placed in 10° of abduction and 30° of external rotation using an outrigger harness for 3 weeks. This position increases stability while the capsular repair heals. Passive motion is begun at 4 weeks. Active and active-assisted exercises are avoided until 6 to 8 weeks.

In a type II fracture, open reduction and internal fixation is advised for greater than 5-mm stepoff or glenohumeral instability. A lag screw can be passed from the inferior glenoid fragment into the glenoid neck. Similarly, for both type III and type IV fractures, a lag screw from the superior fragment into the glenoid neck secures fractures with more than 5 mm of articular displacement.[8] Because the type V fracture represents combinations of types II through IV, surgical repair is done using the technique for the corresponding two-part fracture. Type VI fractures are treated nonoperatively. Due to extensive comminution, these fractures are usually not amenable to internal fixation.[8]

## Glenoid Neck Fractures

Type II glenoid neck fractures are indicated for internal fixation. Depending upon the amount of comminution and the preference of the surgeon, cannulated lag screws, Kirschner wires, or 3.5-mm reconstruction plates can be used.

## References


1. Norris TR. Fractures of the proximal humerus and dislocations of the shoulder. In: Browner BD, Jupiter JB, Levine AM, Trafton PG, eds. *Skeletal Trauma*. Philadelphia: WB Saunders, 1992;1201–1290.
2. Liang PG. The arterial supply of the adult humerus. *J Bone Joint Surg* 1970;52A:1105–1116.
3. Bigliani LU, Craig EV, Butters KP. Fractures of the shoulder. In: Rockwood CA, Green DP, Bucholz RW, eds. *Fractures in Adults*. Philadelphia: JB Lippincott, 1991;871–1019.
4. Jobe CM. Gross anatomy of the shoulder. In: Rockwood CA, Matsen FA, eds. *The Shoulder*. Philadelphia: WB Saunders, 1990;34–97.
5. Netter FH. *Musculoskeletal System. Part I: Anatomy, Physiology, and Metabolic Disorders*. Summit, NJ: Ciba-Geigy, 1987;20–41.
6. Hoppenfeld S. *Surgical Exposures in Orthopaedics*, 2nd ed. Philadelphia: JB Lippincott, 1994.
7. Neer SC. Displaced proximal humeral fractures. Part II. *J Bone Joint Surg* 1970;52A:1090–1103.
8. Goss TP. Fractures of the glenoid cavity. *J Bone Joint Surg* 1992;74A:299–305.
9. Goss TP. Fractures of the glenoid cavity: operative principles and techniques. *Tech Orthop* 1994; 8:199–204.
10. Goss TP. Fractures of the glenoid neck. *J Shoul Elbow Surg* 1994;3:42–52.
11. Bigliani LU. Fractures of the proximal humerus. In: Rockwood CA, Matsen FA, eds. *The Shoulder*. Philadelphia: WB Saunders, 1990;278–334.
12. Neer SC. Displaced proximal humeral fractures. Part I. *J Bone Joint Surg* 1970;38A:1077–1089.
13. Castagno AA, Schuman WP, Kilcoyne RF, et al. Complex fractures of the proximal humerus: role of CT treatment. *Radiology* 1987;165(3):759–776.
14. Flatlow EL, Cuomo F, Maday MG, Miller SR, et al. Open reduction and internal fixation of two-part displaced fractures of the greater tuberosity of the proximal part of the humerus. *J Bone Joint Surg* 1991;73A:1213–1218.
15. Rockwood CA, Thomas SC, Matsen FA. Subluxations and dislocations about the glenohumeral joint. In: Rockwood CA, Green DP, Bucholz RW, eds. *Fractures in Adults*. Philadelphia: JB Lippincott, 1991;1021–1179.
16. Schlegel TF, Hawkins RJ. Displaced proximal humeral fractures: evaluation and treatment. *J AAOS* 1994;2:54–66.
17. Bigliani LU. Treatment of two- and three-part fractures of the proximal humerus. *Instr Course Lect* 1989;38:231–244.
18. Szyskowitz R, Seggl W, Schleifer P, Cundy PJ. Proximal humeral fractures. Management techniques and expected results. *Clin Orthop Rel Res* 1993;292:13–25.
19. Cornell CN. Tension-band wiring supplemented by lag-screw fixation of proximal humerus fractures: a modified technique. *Orthop Rev* 1994;May (suppl):19–23.

# 19
# Fractures About the Elbow

Jesse B. Jupiter

Injuries about the elbow represent a constellation of complex articular fractures. Recommendations for treatment have extended from essentially no treatment to operative reduction and stable internal fixation.[1–10] In the past decade there has been a worldwide acceptance of the operative approach to articular fractures of the distal end of the humerus, olecranon, and in some cases radial head. The publication of successful outcomes with operative treatment has led to the development of more precise methods of stable fixation of the small articular fragments supported by a rather limited amount of subchondral bone. Given the complex articular anatomy combined with the unique capsular and ligamentous architecture, operative treatment is not without potential and real problems, including soft tissue contracture, instability of fixation, malunion, nonunion, posttraumatic arthrosis, ulnar neuropathy, and an overall functional disability.[9,11–14] There is a well-defined role for the use of cannulated screws in some complex fracture patterns, and with the development of smaller cannulated screws the future holds even more promise for their usefulness.

## Anatomy

A number of difficulties exist in the surgical approach and operative management of fractures of the distal humerus, many of which are due to the intricate anatomy of this articulation (Figure 19.1). The elbow is in fact composed of three distinct articulations encased in one synovial-lined capsule. The proximity of the neurovascular structures, the meager skeletal support of the articular surfaces, and the lack of soft tissue attachments to the osseous structures all contribute to the unforgiving nature of these fractures and have led many to express concern as to the outcome of the operative treatment of these injuries.

The distal end of the humerus comprises two bony columns, one medial and one lateral, which flare out distally separated by the olecranon fossa and more distally the trochlea itself. The lateral humeral column diverges at approximately a 20° angle to the perpendicular of the humeral shaft, while the medial column diverges at a 40° to 45° angle from the longitudinal axis of the humerus. Many have viewed the distal end of the humerus as a triangle, with the spool-shaped trochlea interposed between the divergent medial and lateral columns.

The capitellum represents the anterior aspect of the most distal part of the lateral column with the most distal aspect of the medial column represented by the medial epicondyle, terminating just proximal to the trochlea. The articulation between the trochlear notch of the olecranon and the trochlea represents the fundamental element of the flexion-extension arc of elbow motion providing as much as 50% of the intrinsic stability of the elbow.[9,15] In addition, the medial and lateral ridges of the trochlea add to this intrinsic stability. It is not surprising, therefore, that the restoration of the anatomic dimensions of the trochlea is of paramount importance in the management of fractures of the distal end of the humerus and represents one of the major areas of application of cannulated screws.

Even in patients with osteopenia, the cortical bone at the margins of both medial and lateral columns are adequate for the purchase of bone screws. Thus, screws placed either independently

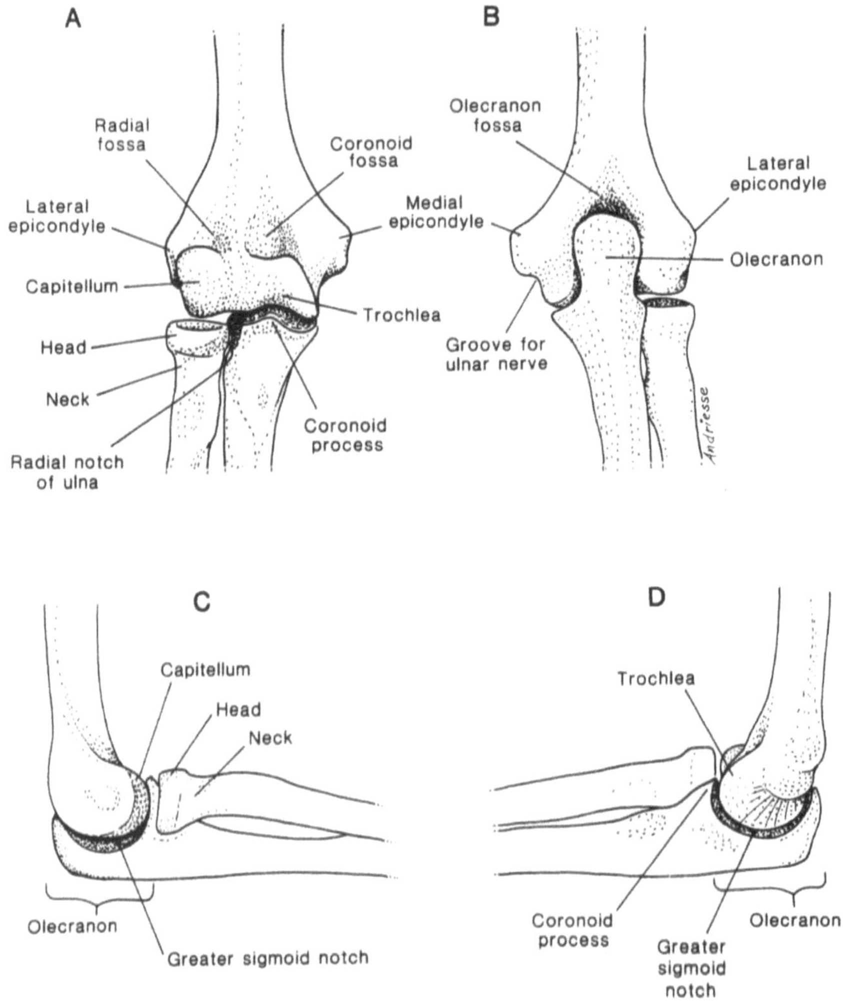


**FIGURE 19.1.** The skeletal and articular anatomy of the elbow. (A) Anterior view. (B) Posterior view. (C) Lateral view. (D) Medial view.

or through plates, whenever possible, should be directed toward the cortical margins of these bony columns in order to provide for acceptable screw purchase.

Articulating with the distal end of the humerus are the proximal end of the ulna, represented by the olecranon, and the radial head. The olecranon is a rather unique structure as it not only provides for the attachment of the powerful triceps as well as brachialis muscles but also plays a critical role in the intrinsic stability of the elbow. Developed on an evolutionary basis from a rather flat articulation with the end of the humerus to a rounded sulcus with a longitudinal groove congruent with the central groove of the trochlea, the vast majority of the articular cartilage of the olecranon is found at its proximal and distal regions rather than in the central zone of the olecranon. This is of fundamental importance when considering the location of olecranon osteotomies as well as the operative stabilization of olecranon fractures, many of which have a depressed segment in the central part of the olecranon sulcus. Also of critical importance, particularly when considering the placement of longitudinal screws, is the angulation of the proximal olecranon of about 7° from the perpendicular of the diaphysis of the midulna.

The olecranon also represents the insertion

sites of the stabilizing ligamentous structures of the elbow. These include the lateral ulnar collateral ligament, which inserts in the vicinity of the crista supinatorum on the radial side of the olecranon, and the coronoid region, to which insert the anterior oblique component of the medial collateral ligament as well as the capsule itself. Fractures of the coronoid are found not too infrequently in association with extensive soft tissue injuries and dislocations and represent an important fracture in the indications for cannulated screws about the elbow.

Lastly, the junction of the metaphyseal region of the proximal ulna and its diaphysis is of structural significance in the consideration of longitudinal screw placement. In addition to an angular alignment of approximately 7°, this region in some patients, particularly younger individuals, may have a very narrow medullary canal with substantial thickness of the surrounding cortex. This feature may impede the full placement of longer screws and should be borne in mind when the placement of screws is contemplated.

The final articulation to be considered is that of the radial head and its relationship with the capitellum. The radial head is not truly in the round but represents an articulation, not only with the capitellum but also with the proximal ulna. The rim of the radial head is composed of hyaline cartilage of a substantial thickness, which is supported by a rather limited amount of subchondral bone. At the juncture of the head and neck is found the annular ligament and oblique ligament, which are important in the stability of this articulation. The radiocapitellar articulation adds to the lateral stability of the elbow, and shearing fractures of the capitellum as well as some fractures of the radial head represent viable options for the use of cannulated screws for internal fixation (Figure 19.2).

# Classification

Along with the increased amount of operative intervention for fractures about the elbow has come a substantial increase in the understanding of the nature of the fracture patterns. Historically, when viewing distal humerus fractures, these were often described in a T or Y pattern, which did little to reflect the specificity of the intraarticular component.

A classification established by Mehne and Matta divided the distal humerus fractures into six major types (Figure 19.3)[9]:

1. High T fracture: This is represented by a fracture that divides both columns proximal or at the proximal limits of the olecranon fossa.
2. Low T fracture: This represents a fracture with a transverse fracture line crossing the olecranon fossa just proximal to the trochlea. This may be among the most common fracture patterns of the distal humerus in the elderly population and among the more difficult to effectively treat.
3. Y fracture: In this pattern oblique fracture lines cross each bony column at or about the olecranon to extend distally in a sagittal plane splitting the trochlea into two major fragments.
4. H fracture: The medial column has a fracture line proximal or distal to the medial epicondyle of the lateral column and fractured in a T or Y pattern. The trochlea is free-floating and may be further fragmented.
5. Medial lambda fracture: The most proximal fracture line exits medially and the lateral fracture line exits distal to the level of the lateral epicondyle.
6. Lateral lambda fracture: The pattern is similar to the H fracture but the lateral column is uninvolved.

Another type of fracture involving the distal part of the humerus is that of a shearing injury in which the anterior articular surface of the distal end is fractured in the coronal plane. This may occur in conjunction with sagittal transverse fracture lines extending into the distal humerus, or it may represent an isolated injury in which the capitellum and part of the trochlea are separated from the distal end of the humerus. In the latter case, it's recognition of the successful restoration of the articular surface (Figure 19.2). In some instances with the shearing fractures, cannulated screw fixation may be optimal.

A more universal classification that has been utilized now effectively throughout the world is the comprehensive classification of fractures. In

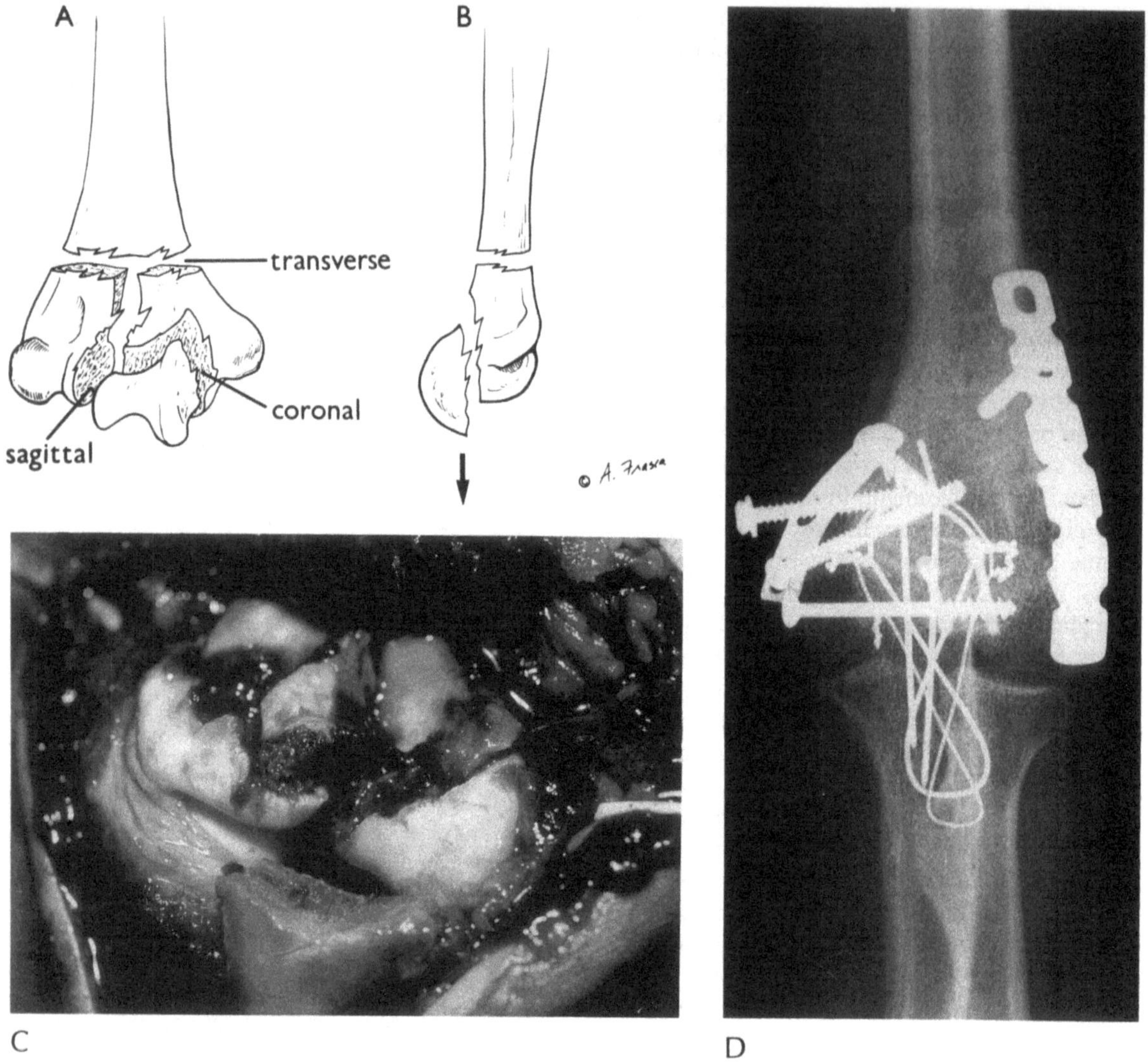


**FIGURE 19.2.** A complex distal humerus fracture may have fracture planes in multiple directions. (A and B) Anteroposterior and lateral view of a shearing articular fracture. (C) An intraoperative view of a complex articular fracture. (D) The anteroposterior x-ray of the fixation.

this classification all fractures involving the metaphysis and articular surfaces are divided into three main groups: group A, extraarticular fractures; group B, partial articular fractures in which a portion of the joint is disrupted, leaving intact a part of the joint attached to the more proximal osseous support; and group C, complete articular fractures in which there is complete disruption between the joint surface and the supporting bony structures. The three basic types are further divided on the basis of location and orientation of the major fracture lines and the amount of metaphyseal and articular comminution. As a result, there are 27 different categories in this classification for fractures at the distal end of the humerus[16] (Figure 19.4).

## Classification of Olecranon Fractures

Several classification systems have been effectively utilized in identifying various patterns of

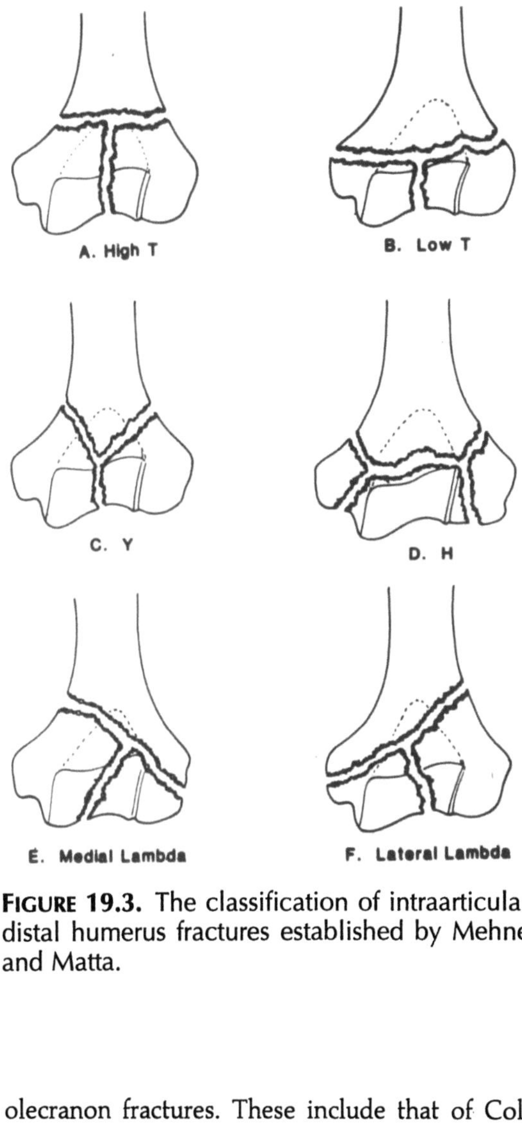


**FIGURE 19.3.** The classification of intraarticular distal humerus fractures established by Mehne and Matta.

olecranon fractures. These include that of Colton,[17] Schatzker and Tile[18] and the comprehensive classification of fractures.[16]

Colton classified olecranon fractures into two major groups: undisplaced (type I) and displaced (type II). A type I undisplaced fracture is defined as having less than 2 mm of separation and no increase in displacement with flexion to 90°, with the patient able to extend the elbow against gravity. Displaced fractures were subdivided into type IIA—avulsion, type IIB—oblique and transverse, type IIC—comminuted, and type IID—fracture-dislocations.[19]

Schatzker and Tile[18] addressed mechanical considerations of fractures with specific reference to the requirements placed on internal fixation. In this classification transverse fractures were defined as being either simple, i.e., two fragments, or complex, involving comminution or depression of the articular surface. An additional classification included oblique fractures extending distally from the midpoint of the trochlear notch. These particular fractures proved important as they are less stable with tension band wiring alone. The last group defined by Schatzker and Tile is that of comminuted fractures. These can include fractures of the coronoid process, those extending distally beyond the midpoint of the trochlear notch, and those fractures involving fractures or dislocations of the radial head.

The comprehensive classification of fractures also divides the olecranon fractures into group A—extraarticular, group B—single fragment, and group C—multiple fragments of both the radial head and olecranon (Figure 19.5).

## Radial Head Classification

The radial head fracture has had a number of classifications. The early classification of radial head fractures by Carstam,[20] Bakalim,[21] and Mason[22] were based solely on radiographs and failed to take into account associated injuries. Bakalim's classification is type I—nondisplaced, type II—split fracture, type III—comminuted fracture, type IV—impacted neck fracture, and type V—displaced neck fracture. The Mason classification is type I—nondisplaced fractures of the head or neck; type II—displaced, two-part fractures involving the head or neck; and type III—comminuted fractures of the head and neck or displaced fractures of the neck alone. Johnston[23] added a fourth category to Mason's classification, identifying those fractures associated with an elbow dislocation.

Schatzker and Tile[18] devised a classification system for radial head fractures: type I—a wedge fracture of the head that may or may not be displaced, type II—an impaction where part of the head and neck remain intact with the fracture tilted and/or impacted, and type III—a severely comminuted fracture where no portion of the head or neck remains in continuity.[24]

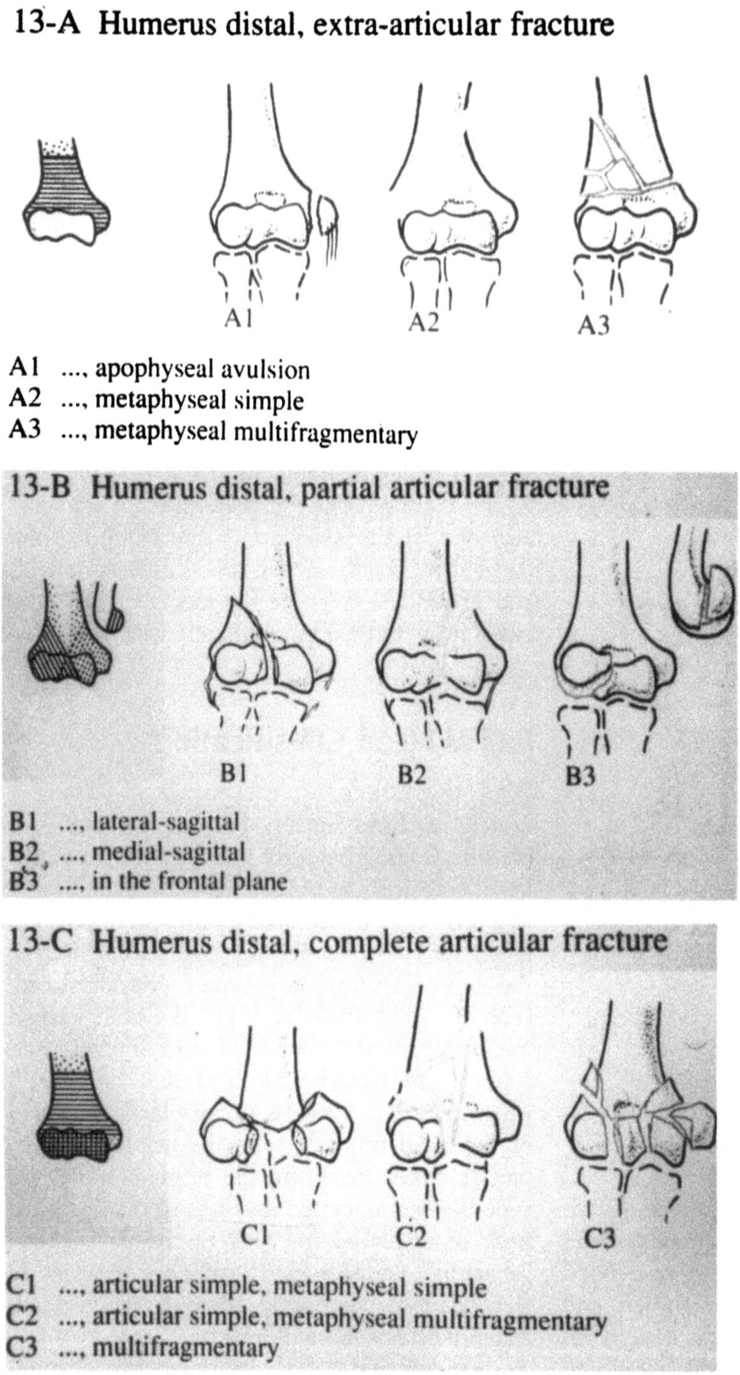


**FIGURE 19.4.** The comprehensive classification of fractures of the distal end of the humerus. (A) Extra-articular fracture. (B) Partial articular fracture. (C) Complete articular fracture.

# Treatment

## Distal Humerus Fractures

The operative treatment of intraarticular fractures of the distal humerus can be lengthy and complex. For this reason, general endotracheal anesthesia is preferred, with the patient positioned either on his or her side with the arm supported on soft bolsters or prone with the arm on a small extension off the operative table. It is my personal preference for the patient to be positioned on his or her side to avoid the potential for the involved arm being hyper-

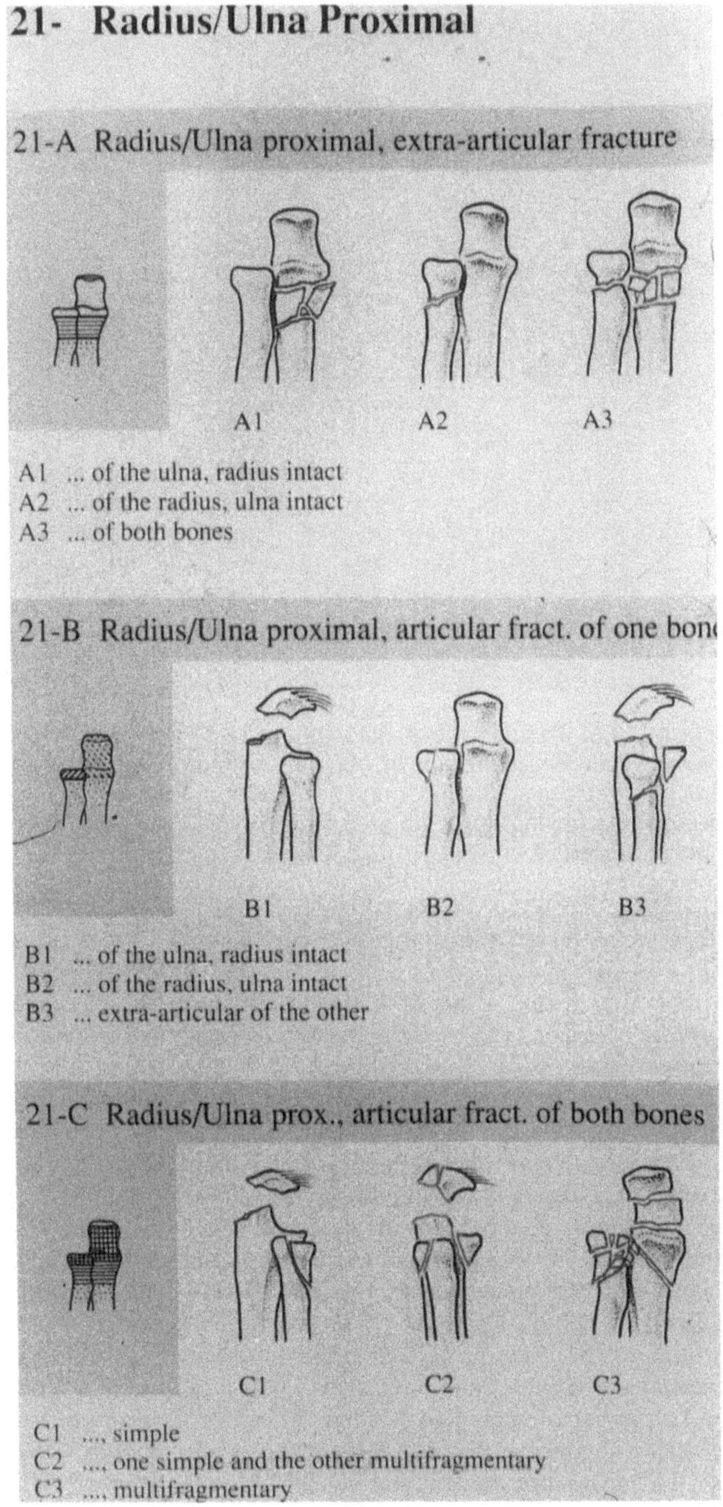


**FIGURE 19.5.** The comprehensive classification of fractures of the radial head and olecranon.

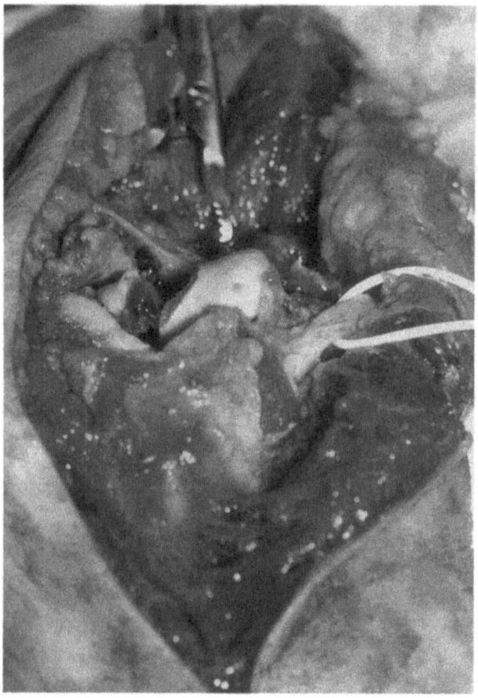

**FIGURE 19.6.** Through a transolecranon osteotomy, excellent visualization is obtained of the articular fragments. The ulnar nerve is held in a vessel loop having been mobilized out of the cubital tunnel.

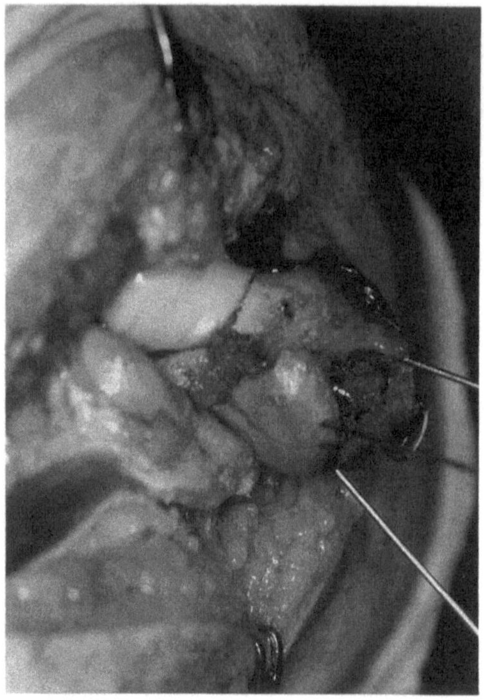

**FIGURE 19.7.** The articular fragments are secured provisionally with smooth Kirschner wires. A cannulated screw can be placed directly over these wires.

abducted at the shoulder during a lengthy operative procedure.

The skin incision is that of a straight midline posterior incision. This incision is extensile and rarely results in any sensitivity at the scar despite its being located over the posterior part of the elbow.

The ulnar nerve should be identified and protected. Neuritis involving the ulnar nerve is regrettably all too common after operative manipulation. It should be not only elevated from the cubital tunnel but also dissected proximally and distally for at least 6 to 8 cm. This will allow the nerve to lie free in the subcutaneous tissue (Figure 19.6).

To approach the fracture one has the option of either a transolecranon approach or elevation of the triceps from the medial or lateral side of the olecranon. In most situations the transolecranon approach has proven to be preferable in both the degree of exposure of the articular surfaces as well as the postoperative healing. When faced with a complex fracture in the elderly, however, one might find that an alternative to stable internal fixation is that of total elbow arthroplasty. In these instances we have preferred to elevate the triceps off the olecranon from the medial side, thereby preserving the option of a total elbow arthroplasty.

A lateral approach elevating the triceps off the olecranon from the lateral side may be preferential for fractures involving the lateral column, capitellum, and or radial head.

Once the fracture anatomy has been confirmed under direct vision, the fracture fragments are optimally reduced and provisionally held to their origins on the bony columns using smooth 0.045- or 0.062-inch Kirschner wires. Attempts should be made to reposition the trochlea at its anatomic width. On occasion there may be fragmentation and loss of substance in the middle of the trochlea. Rather than

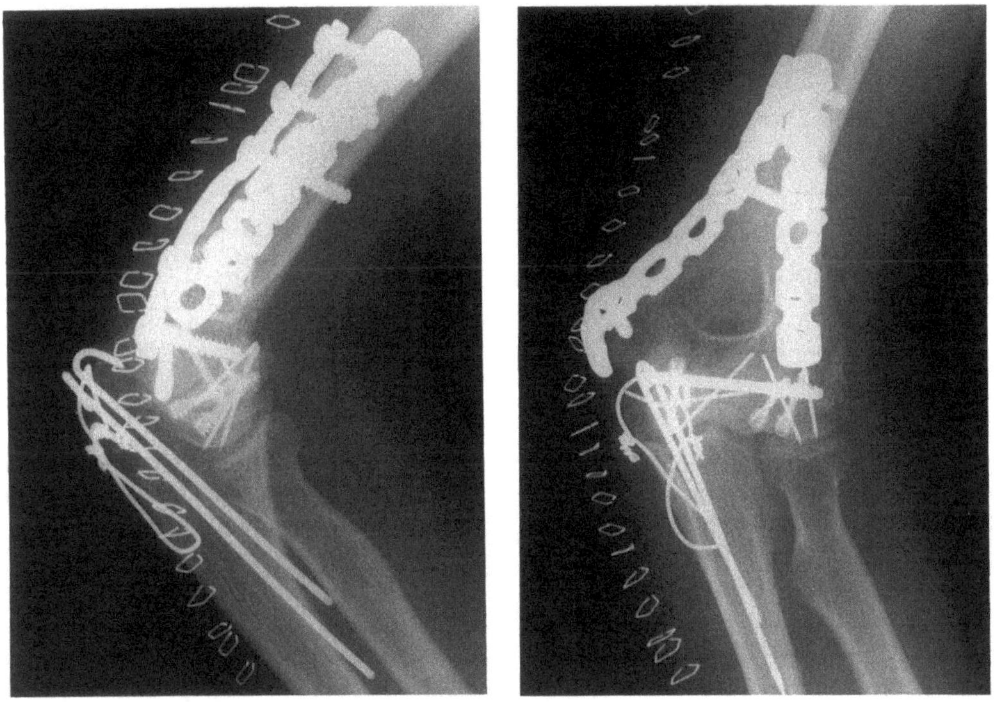

A B

**FIGURE 19.8.** This complex intraarticular fracture was secured with plates and screws. A cannulated screw was placed across the trochlear fracture (A,B).

excise these fragments, bringing the intact pieces together at a narrowed width, it is preferable to provide a cancellous bone graft to maintain the width. In conjunction with this would be the need to avoid using compression of one major trochlear fragment onto the other when fixing the fragments together with a screw (Figure 19.7).

The restoration of the trochlear fragments may represent the optimal indication for cannulated screw fixation. The advantage of the cannulated screw in this setting is that the provisional fixation of a Kirschner wire can be placed in an optimal position for both provisional fixation as well as screw placement. Given the fragile nature of these fragments and the limited amount of subchondral bone, there may be few options for placement of both Kirschner wires as well as screws. Therefore, the opportunity to limit the amount of surgical manipulation of these fragments is enhanced by the use of cannulated screws. As a general rule, a 3.5-mm screw is preferable in this anatomic region.

In the setting of articular disruption, in not only the sagittal plane but also the coronal plane, interfragmentary screw fixation is also useful. There have been occasions in which the use of self-compressing threaded Herbert screws or interfragmentary lag screws placed from posterior to anterior have been effective. At times in these cases, the concept of a cannulated screw can minimize the surgical manipulation of the fragments, offsetting the potential for fragmentation (Figure 19.8).

The articular reconstructions are then brought back to a secure fixation of the bony columns, ordinarily using contoured plates and screws. These plates can be strategically placed to achieve definitive fixation that is tailored to the specific fracture patterns of both the articular as well as bony columns (Figure 19.9). By having plates placed at different directions, the mechanical strength is enhanced.

Once the fractures appear stably secured, the elbow should be put through full range of motion to visually assess the stability of the internal fixation. In the event that motion is observed at the fracture line, additional fixa-

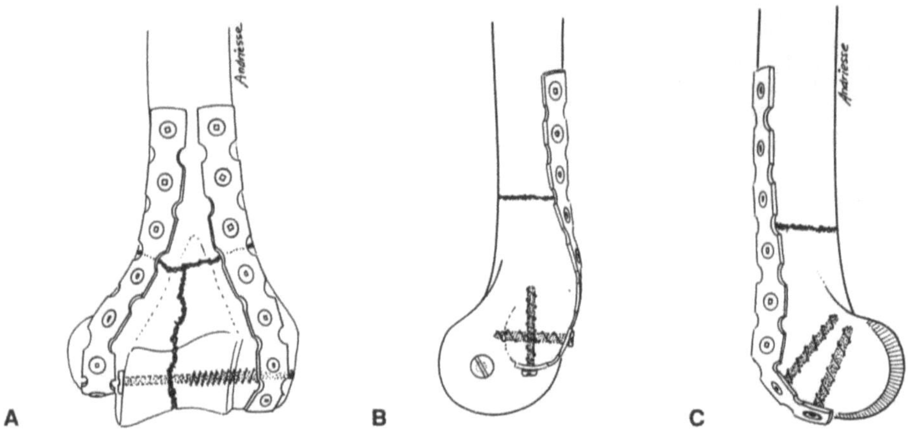


FIGURE 19.9. The articular reconstruction is placed back onto the bony columns with strategically placed and contoured 3.5-mm reconstruction plates. (A) dorsal view. (B) contoured plate around medial epicondyle. (C) posterior plate along lateral columns.

tion should be provided. Tenuous fixation can be supplemented by cancellous bone graft to enhance and speed healing. In the event that one or two carefully placed screws do not provide sufficient purchase, the screw purchase can be enhanced by the use of polymethyl methacrylate. The methyl methacrylate is mixed and, while still in the liquid phase, poured into a 12-cm syringe with a straight tip. The tip is then placed into the screw hole and enough cement placed to just fill the hole. Extravasation of cement, particularly near the fracture lines, should be carefully avoided. The screws are then reinserted and allowed to remain in place until the cement begins to become firm, at which point the screw should be advanced a final one or two turns. Excess cement is removed only after it is completely hard.

When an olecranon osteotomy has been performed, fixation can be either with the tension band technique or with a longitudinal screw placed preferably along with a tension band wire. In these instances, the use of a 4.5- or 6.5-mm cannulated screw is an effective means of providing stable fixation. If longitudinal screw fixation is chosen, the surgeon should be mindful of the modest angular relationship of the proximal ulna to its shaft. Failure to keep this in mind will potentially inhibit the screw from passage into the medullary space.

Postoperative management is contingent upon stability achieved at surgery. If this is present, it is useful to begin active mobilization once soft tissue swelling has diminished. This can ordinarily be begun either on the first or second postoperative day. Splints and braces are preferred by some but these may tend to limit patient activity and lead to surrounding soft tissue and capsular fibrosis.

There are specific fractures of the distal humerus that may be amenable to percutaneous screw fixation. These include the low transverse supracondylar fracture in the elderly individual or complex fractures associated with soft tissue injury. In these instances the cannulated screw offers the enhanced stability of a compression screw but can be applied percutaneously (Figure 19.10). In some instances the fragile nature of the bone will require a placement of a washer to prevent the screw head from impacting and fragmenting the underlying cortical bone.

## Radial Head Fractures

Fractures of the radial head with minimal or no displacement are felt to be stable and can be treated nonoperatively. In most cases there is no urgency to have a rapid mobilization but rather aspiration of the hematoma and instillation of Marcaine may provide transient pain relief, and

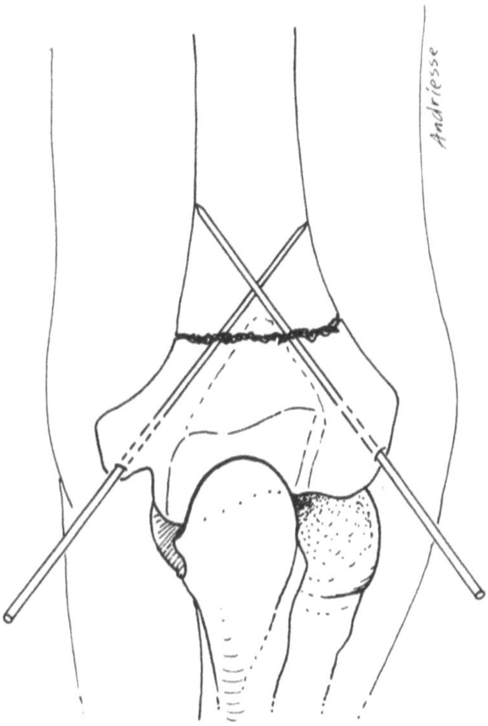


**FIGURE 19.10.** A low transverse supracondylar fracture can be percutaneously fixed with smooth Kirschner wires over which cannulated screws can be placed under control of an image intensifier.

then splint or sling immobilization for 7 to 10 days will prevent a fracture from displacing.

Two-part displaced radial head fractures represent an optimal indication for internal fixation. If aspiration of a fracture hematoma and instillation of analgesic is accomplished, the surgeon can examine forearm rotation effectively. If there is a mechanical block or a palpable incongruence, operative fixation is indicated.

Improvement in small implant design and application has made internal fixation more reliable. The surgical approach is that of standard lateral incision identifying an interval between the anconeus and extensor carpi ulnaris muscles; 2.0-mm screws, screws and plates, or self-compressing Herbert screws are the usual implants applied for these fractures. Some have recommended bioabsorbable pins. While the author has no experience with cannulated screws in this area, the potential for smaller cannulated screws would offer a decided advantage to the treatment of these fractures given that there is little room for both provisional Kirschner wire and screw fixation. Additionally, the opportunity should exist for manipulation of two-part fractures under arthroscopic guidance and internal fixation through a percutaneous approach (Figure 19.11).

Displaced fractures, particularly those associated with soft tissue injury, are important indications for internal fixation. Often the soft tissue injury is a combination of capsule and ligament—both lateral as well as medial. The operative approach to the radial head should include a more proximal extension to explore the origin of the lateral capsular ligament complex. Quite often these will be avulsed from their origin and failure to repair them in conjunction with excision of the radial head can result in chronic instability and ultimate disability and posttraumatic arthrosis. Even the comminuted fractures of the radial head and neck can be repaired, in many cases using multiple small screws, threaded wires, and even small implant plates (Figure 19.12).

In the expectation of a complex reconstruction, additional exposure can be achieved by performing an osteotomy of the lateral epicondyle and elevating this with its attached ligament and muscles distally to permit excellent exposure. Should this be considered, recommendations are to explore the path of the posterior interosseous nerve to prevent injury to this structure, which runs quite close to the surgical site. By doing this the surgeon can be more comfortable and confident in the manipulation of the fragments, knowing exactly the location of the nerve.

Although radial head resection still represents the most commonly performed procedure for comminuted fractures, it has been observed to be associated with problems such as instability, late posttraumatic arthrosis, and proximal migration of the radius when associated with disruption of the interosseous membrane.[13,25] In fact, complications associated with radial head fractures can be looked at in two particular groups—those associated with a fracture and those following a radial head excision.[9]

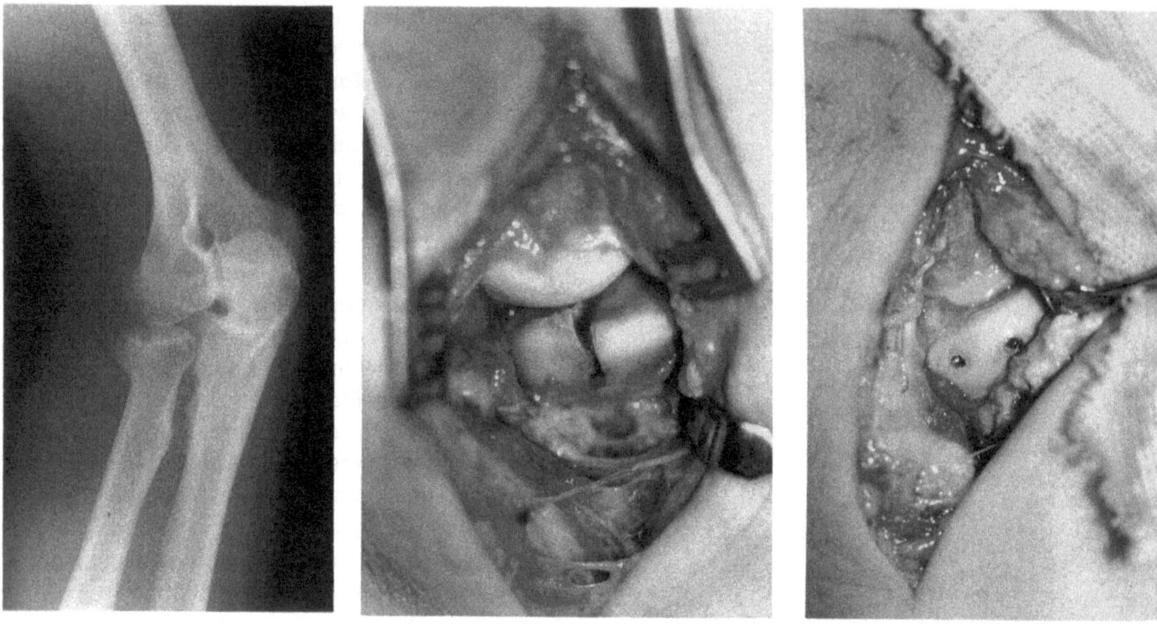

A B C

**FIGURE 19.11.** A displaced two-part fracture of the radial head is amenable to screw fixation. (A) The oblique radiograph reveals the displaced fracture. (B) At surgery, the fracture is seen displaced with a mechanical block to rotation. (C) Two buried screws provide stable fixation.

A

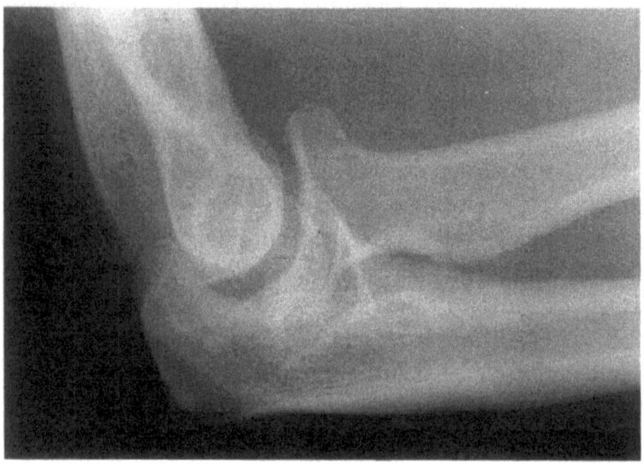

B

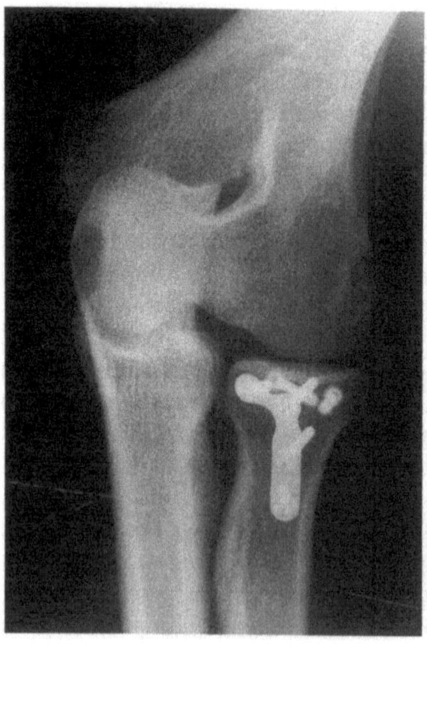

**FIGURE 19.12.** A complex radial head fracture with a distal radioulnar joint injury. (A) The lateral x-ray of the impacted fracture. (B) Stable fixation was achieved with a small plate and screws.

## Olecranon Fractures

Given that the olecranon provides the distal unit of the elbow flexion-extension joint, articular realignment as well as stable fixation to permit mobilization represents the fundamental approaches to treatment. The subcutaneous position of the olecranon renders it vulnerable to direct trauma. By the same token, in some instances fractures occur as part of an axial-directed force due to the patient falling on an outstretched arm with the elbow held in some degree of flexion and the forearm experiencing a torque injury.

Nondisplaced fractures, although uncommon, can be successfully treated by immobilization of the limb in a long arm splint or cast with the elbow flexed at 90° for approximately 3 to 4 weeks. The surgeon is obligated to obtain an x-ray within a week to 10 days following the beginning of this treatment to make certain that displacement of the fracture has not occurred.

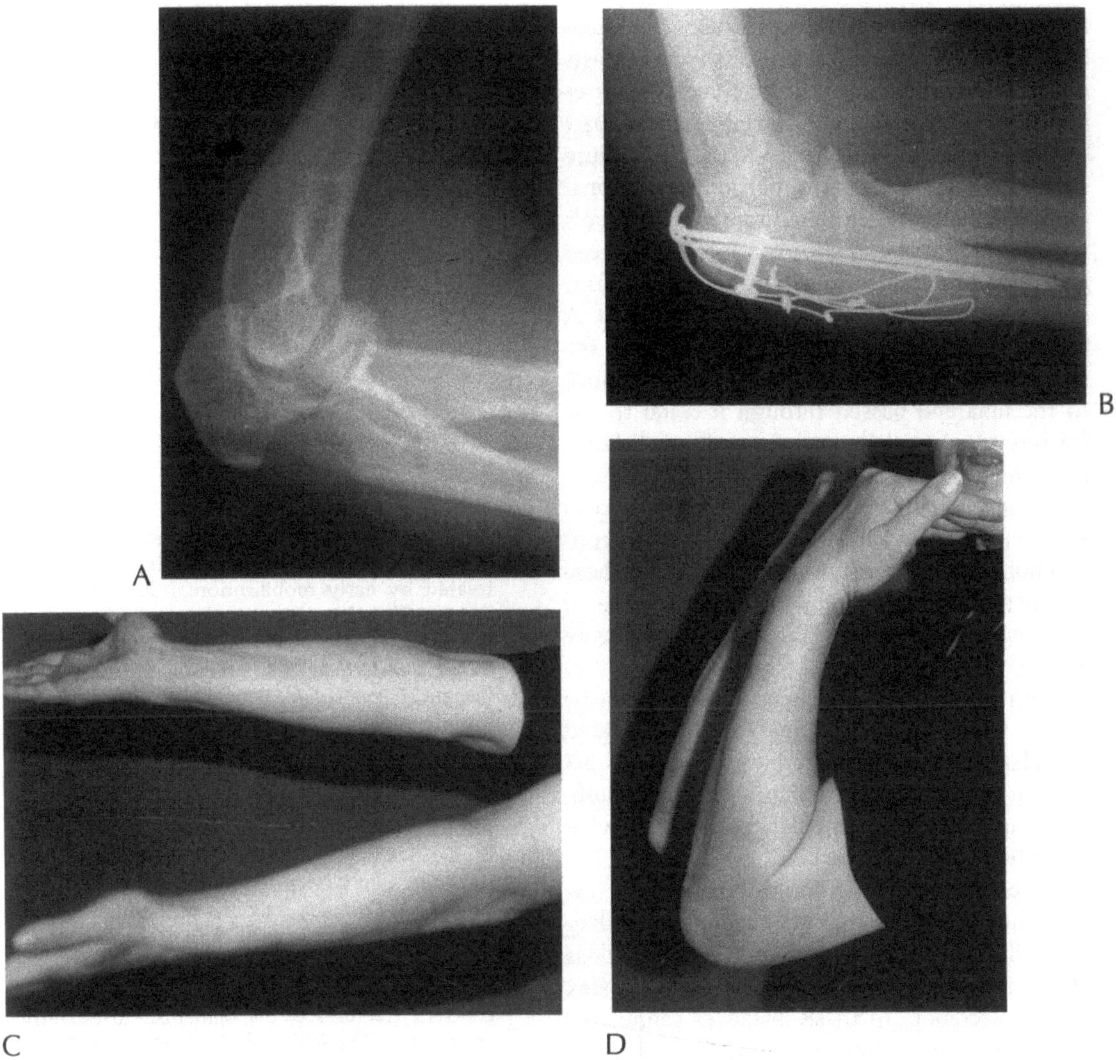


**FIGURE 19.13.** A complex displaced olecranon fracture is secured with a tension band and interfragmentary screw. (A) The lateral radiograph of the displaced articular fracture of the olecranon. (B) The stable fixation of a tension band and cannulated screw. (C and D) Excellent functional recovery.

Displaced fractures require operative treatment. While the surgeon should strive for reposition and internal fixation of the fracture fragments, in some instances enthusiasm has been voiced for fragment excision and triceps reconstruction.[26,27]

The transverse fracture, either by itself or when associated with a comminuted or depressed fracture of the articular surface, is amenable to tension band fixation. This is a mechanically sound approach with the wire loop placed dorsal to the mid-axis of the ulna, transforming tensile or distraction forces at the fracture site into compressive forces. The standard approach for tension band fixation consists of two longitudinally placed Kirschner wires obliquely placed from the dorsal proximal part of the olecranon tip passing across the fracture site to purchase the anterior part of the proximal ulna. These Kirschner wires represent controls against rotational and shearing forces. If placed in this manner with a purchase on the anterior cortex, proximal migration will be minimized. A loop of wire is then placed underneath the triceps through Sharpey's fibers extending dorsal to the ulna and passed through it distal to the fracture by at least the same margin of distance from the tip of the olecranon to the fracture line. Some surgeons have utilized a screw placed in the same position as the Kirschner wires in conjunction with a tension band loop. In these instances there is the possibility of the use of a cannulated screw for this approach (Figure 19.13).

With elevation of fragments, a screw can be placed to serve as a buttress for the elevated articular fragments. The screws are usually 3.5 mm in size and placed obliquely to have sufficient purchase on the opposite cortex somewhat distal to the fracture line.

An optimal use of an interfragmentary screw is in those fractures that are oblique, extending from the distal part of the olecranon sulcus at the joint line distally into the dorsal cortex of the olecranon. In these instances cannulated screws offer an option to control accurately the placement of these interfragmentary screws. Screws alone will not be sufficient to withstand the tensile forces occurring at this fracture, and therefore neutralization of these forces will be required by either the use of tension band wire techniques or by a dorsally applied plate.

As the fractures extend distally, particularly those involving the coronoid process, plate fixation is necessary. The coronoid can be secured in some instances with screws alone, either placed through the plate or independent of the plate. These fractures may be the result of high-energy trauma and can be associated with instability of the elbow. They may represent among the more difficult fractures about the elbow. Cancellous bone graft may be required to help the support the articular reconstructions and fill in any defects in the cortex opposite the plate.[18]

# Complications

Complications specific to fracture of the olecranon include loss of elbow flexion-extension, malposition with posterior displacement of the radial head, failure to unite, and posttraumatic arthrosis.

## References

1. Brown RF, Morgan RG. Intercondylar T-shaped fractures of the humerus. Results in ten cases treated by early mobilization. *J Bone Joint Surg* 1971;53B(3):425–428.
2. Evans EB. Heterotopic bone formation in thermal burns. *Clin Orthop* 1991;263:94–101.
3. Gabel GT, Hanson G, Bennett JB, Noble PC, Tullos HS. Intraarticular fractures of the distal humerus in the adult. *Clin Orthop* 1987;216:99–108.
4. Horne G. Supracondylar fractures of the humerus in adults. *J Trauma* 1980;20:71–74.
5. Josefsson PO, Gentz CF, Johnell O, Wendeberg B. Dislocation of the elbow and intraarticular fractures. *Clin Orthop* 1988;246:126–130.
6. Jupiter JB. Complex fractures of the distal part of the humerus. *J Bone Joint Surg* 1994;76A:1252–1263.
7. Jupiter JB, Neff U, Holzach P, Allgöwer M. Intercondylar fractures of the humerus. An operative approach. *J Bone Joint Surg* 1985;67A:226–239.
8. Keon-Cohen BT. Fractures of the elbow. *J Bone Joint Surg* 1966;48A:1623–1639.
9. Mehne DK, Jupiter JB. Fractures of the distal humerus. In: Browner BD, Jupiter JB, Levine AM,

Trafton PG, eds. *Skeletal Trauma, Fractures, Dislocations, Ligamentous Injuries.* Philadelphia: WB Saunders, 1992;1146–1176.
10. Waddell JP, Hatch J, Richards R. Supracondylar fractures of the humerus—results of surgical treatment. *J Trauma* 1988;28:1615–1621.
11. Ackerman G, Jupiter JB. Nonunion of fractures of the distal end of the humerus. *J Bone Joint Surg* 1988;70A:75–83.
12. Dellon AL. Review of treatment results for ulnar nerve entrapment at the elbow. *J Hand Surg* 1989; 14A:688–700.
13. Essex-Lopresti P. Fractures of the radial head with distal radioulnar dislocation. *J Bone Joint Surg* 1951;33B:244–247.
14. McKee M, Jupiter J, Toh CL, Wilson L, Colton C, Karras KK. Reconstruction after malunion and nonunion of intraarticular fractures of the distal humerus. Methods and results in 13 adults. *J Bone Joint Surg* 1994;76B(4):614–621.
15. Morrey BF. Post-traumatic contracture of the elbow. Operative treatment, including distraction arthroplasty. *J Bone Joint Surg* 1990;72A:601–618.
16. Müller ME, Nazarian S, Koch P. *AO Classification of Fractures.* Berlin: Springer-Verlag, 1987.
17. Colton CL. Fractures of the olecranon in adults. Classification and management. *Injury* 1973–74;5: 121–129.
18. Schatzker J. Olecranon fractures. In: Schatzker J, Tile M, eds. *The Rational Basis of Operative Fracture Care.* New York: Springer-Verlag, 1987;89–96.
19. Broberg MA, Morrey BF. Results of treatment of fracture-dislocation of the elbow. *Clin Orthop* 1987;216:109–119.
20. Carstam N. Operative treatment of fractures of the upper end of the radius. *Acta Orthop Scand* 1950;19:502–526.
21. Bakalim C. Fractures of the radial head and their treatment. *Acta Orthop Scand* 1970;41:320.
22. Mason M. Some observations on fractures of the head of the radius with a review of one hundred cases. *Br J Surg* 1954;42:123–132.
23. Johnston GW. Follow-up of one hundred cases of fracture of the head of the radius with a review of the literature. *Ulster Med J* 1962;31:51–56.
24. Schatzker J. Fractures of the radial head. In: Schatzker J, Tile M, eds. *The Rational Basis of Operative Fracture Care.* New York: Springer-Verlag, 1987;97–102.
25. Curr J, Coe W. Dislocation of the inferior radio-ulnar joint. *Br J Surg* 1946;34:74–77.
26. Gartsman GM, Sculco TP, Otis JC. Operative treatment of olecranon fractures—excision or open reduction with internal fixation. *J Bone Joint Surg* 1981;63A:718–721.
27. McAusland WR. The treatment of fractures of the olecranon by longitudinal screw or nail fixation. *Ann Surg* 1942;116:293–296.

# Index

T

MIX
Papier aus verantwortungsvollen Quellen
Paper from responsible sources
FSC® C105338

If you have any concerns about our products,
you can contact us on
**ProductSafety@springernature.com**

In case Publisher is established outside the EU,
the EU authorized representative is:
**Springer Nature Customer Service Center GmbH**
**Europaplatz 3, 69115 Heidelberg, Germany**

Printed by Libri Plureos GmbH
in Hamburg, Germany